Current Progress in Prostate Cancer Research

Current Progress in Prostate Cancer Research

Editor: Peter Hayes

FOSTER ACADEMICS

www.fosteracademics.com

www.fosteracademics.com

FOSTER ACADEMICS

Cataloging-in-Publication Data

Current progress in prostate cancer research / edited by Peter Hayes.
p. cm.
Includes bibliographical references and index.
ISBN 978-1-63242-750-2
1. Prostate--Cancer. 2. Prostate--Cancer--Research. I. Hayes, Peter.
RC280.P7 C87 2019
616.994 63--dc23

Foster Academics,
118-35 Queens Blvd., Suite 400,
Forest Hills, NY 11375, USA

ISBN 978-1-63242-750-2 (Hardback)

Printed and bound in China.

Contents

Preface

This book has been an outcome of determined endeavour from a group of educationists in the field. The primary objective was to involve a broad spectrum of professionals from diverse cultural background involved in the field for developing new researches. The book not only targets students but also scholars pursuing higher research for further enhancement of the theoretical and practical applications of the subject.

The prostate is an endocrine gland of the male reproductive system, which secretes the alkaline fluid component of semen. The cancer which develops in the prostate is known as prostate cancer. In the initial stage, it may not cause any symptom, but it can cause several complications in the later stage. Some of the common symptoms include problems associated with urination, like frequent urination, nocturia, hematuria and dysuria. It may also cause problems associated with sexual organs, such as painful ejaculation and difficulty in achieving erection. Ultrasound, digital rectal examination (DRE), cystoscopy, transrectal ultrasonography and magnetic resonance imaging (MRI) are some of the common diagnostic methods useful in the diagnosis of prostate cancer. Treatment methods include radiation therapy and radical prostatectomy. Prostate cancer research is an upcoming field of medical research that has undergone rapid development over the past few decades. It presents researches and studies performed by experts across the globe. The book is appropriate for students seeking detailed information in this area as well as for experts.

It was an honour to edit such a profound book and also a challenging task to compile and examine all the relevant data for accuracy and originality. I wish to acknowledge the efforts of the contributors for submitting such brilliant and diverse chapters in the field and for endlessly working for the completion of the book. Last, but not the least; I thank my family for being a constant source of support in all my research endeavours.

Editor

1

Pharmacokinetic and Biodistribution Assessment of a Near Infrared-Labeled PSMA-Specific Small Molecule in Tumor-Bearing Mice

Joy L. Kovar,[1] Lael L. Cheung,[1] Melanie A. Simpson,[2] and D. Michael Olive[3]

[1] *Translational Research, LI-COR Biosciences, 4647 Superior Street, Lincoln, NE 68504, USA*
[2] *Department of Biochemistry, University of Nebraska, Lincoln, NE 68588-0664, USA*
[3] *SVS Consulting, Lincoln, NE 68516, USA*

Correspondence should be addressed to Joy L. Kovar; joy.kovar@licor.com

Academic Editor: William L. Dahut

Prostate cancer is the most frequently diagnosed cancer in men and often requires surgery. Use of near infrared (NIR) technologies to perform image-guided surgery may improve accurate delineation of tumor margins. To facilitate preclinical testing of such outcomes, here we developed and characterized a PSMA-targeted small molecule, YC-27. IRDye 800CW was conjugated to YC-27 or an anti-PSMA antibody used for reference. Human 22Rv1, PC3M-LN4, and/or LNCaP prostate tumor cells were exposed to the labeled compounds. *In vivo* targeting and clearance properties were determined in tumor-bearing mice. Organs and tumors were excised and imaged to assess probe localization. YC-27 exhibited a dose dependent increase in signal upon binding. Binding specificity and internalization were visualized by microscopy. *In vitro* and *in vivo* blocking studies confirmed YC-27 specificity. *In vivo*, YC-27 showed good tumor delineation and tissue contrast at doses as low as 0.25 nmole. YC-27 was cleared via the kidneys but bound the proximal tubules of the renal cortex and epididymis. Since PSMA is also broadly expressed on the neovasculature of most tumors, we expect YC-27 will have clinical utility for image-guided surgery and tumor resections.

1. Introduction

Prostate cancer is the most frequently diagnosed cancer in men, affecting one in six, and is a leading cause of cancer mortality [1–4]. Current methods for prostate cancer detection include imaging by ultrasound and multiparametric MRI for guidance in biopsy procedures and single-photon emission computed tomography (SPECT) with ^{111}In-capromab pendetide (Prostascint) for evaluation and management of the disease [5–7]. Dual modality imaging agents are being developed to take advantage of radionuclide sensitivity and the resolution of near infrared (NIR) fluorescence [8] for possible use in pre- and intraoperative applications. Clinically available NIR dyes (indocyanine green and methylene blue) are contrast agents with no tumor specificity [9, 10]. However, imaging resolution is increased using agents that couple strong tumor-targeting properties with sensitive detection and relatively rapid clearance [11]. Recent reports have described the successful intraoperative use of small molecule targeting agents in several types of cancer for evaluation of tumor margins, image-assisted resection, and laparoscopic removal of lymph nodes [12–18].

Effective targeting of tumor cells has been achieved by use of a variety of agents that are designed to recognize aspects of the tumor cell surface in a specific manner [11, 13, 19, 20]. Particularly promising results have been obtained by targeting prostate-specific membrane antigen (PSMA), a type II transmembrane glycoprotein also known as glutamate carboxypeptidase II, and folate hydrolase I, which is basally expressed by prostate epithelial cells and overexpressed in primary and metastatic prostate cancer [3, 4, 15]. Moreover, PSMA expression has been detected in a variety of other solid tumors, specifically and strongly associated with endothelial cells of the peritumoral and intratumoral neovasculature [3, 4, 21, 22]. Thus, PSMA is an attractive molecular target, both for advancing basic mechanistic studies of prostate cancer progression in preclinical models and for surgical applications [15, 21–23].

Available tools for PSMA targeting include monoclonal antibodies and a variety of small molecule or peptide ligands, each of which has advantages and limitations associated with its use [24]. Antibody-based probes are attractive because of the high level of specificity for the target and the picomolar-range affinities that can often be achieved. These properties, coupled with a longer circulating half-life than that of many small molecules, significantly lower the required dose for optimal detection [25]. Slower clearance (2-3 days) of monoclonal antibody probes may be favorable for presurgical routines, but this extended waiting period is then necessary before sufficiently high tumor-to-background signal is realized and surgery can be performed with confidence [11, 13, 20]. These probes are also potentially immunogenic. In contrast, small molecule probes can often be generated with nanomolar affinity ranges and rapid clearance rates that not only facilitate tissue penetration but also minimize potential toxicity resulting from exposure times [26–28]. Several groups have developed PSMA-specific small molecule urea-based compounds that have been successfully applied to optical imaging of tumor tissue [27–31].

In this report, we evaluate near infrared (NIR) fluorescence-based imaging of prostate tumor cells that were targeted by a small molecule PSMA targeting agent, YC-27. Comparisons to a commercially available anti-PSMA antibody were made to illustrate biodistribution and clearance issues. Both molecules were labeled with IRDye 800CW and characterized for specific binding to PSMA-positive cells in culture, followed by an evaluation of clearance and tumor-targeting efficacy in mice. Our results support the specificity of PSMA targeting for tumor detection, provide optimized conditions for its use in mice, and suggest benefits to the use of YC-27 as a targeting agent based on its pharmacokinetic properties.

2. Materials and Methods

2.1. Cell Culture, Materials, and Reagents. LNCaP and 22Rv1 human prostate carcinoma cells purchased from American Type Culture Collection (Rockville, MD) were maintained in RPMI 1640 medium containing 10% fetal bovine serum. PC3 M-LN4 cells, derived from PC3 human prostate adenocarcinoma cells, were kindly provided by Dr. Isaiah J. Fidler (MD Anderson Cancer Center, Houston, TX) and maintained in minimal essential medium containing 10% fetal bovine serum, sodium pyruvate, and nonessential amino acids. Human PSMA/FOLH1/NAALADase I antibody was purchased from R & D Systems (Minneapolis, MN). DAPI and TO-PRO-3 were purchased from Life Technologies Corporation (Carlsbad, CA). Rabbit polyclonal β-tubulin antibody was purchased from Santa Cruz Biotechnology (Santa Cruz, CA). Fluoromount Reagent and poly-D-lysine hydrobromide were obtained from Sigma-Aldrich Chemicals (St. Louis, MO) and Zeba Spin Desalting Column was from Thermo Fisher Scientific (Waltham, MA). Poly-D-lysine coated 96-well plates were purchased from BD Biosciences (Bedford, MA). Amino acid synthons, synthetic resin supports, and peptide coupling reagents (NovaBioChem) were purchased from EMD Millipore (Billerica, MA). IRDye 800CW NHS ester was provided by LI-COR Biosciences (Lincoln, NE). All other reagents for chemical synthesis, purification, and analysis were purchased from Sigma-Aldrich (Milwaukee, WI), VWR (Radnor, PA), Glen Research (Sterling, VA), and Thermo Fisher Scientific (Waltham, MA). High-performance liquid chromatography (HPLC) analysis and purification were performed on an Agilent 1100 Series HPLC with appropriate reverse-phase columns, Ultraviolet and Visible (UV/Vis) spectral analysis was performed on an Agilent 8453 Series Spectrophotometer, and low-resolution mass spectrometry (LRMS) was performed using electrospray (ES) techniques on an Agilent 1100 Series LC/MSD Trap (Agilent Technologies, Santa Clara, CA). The Odyssey Classic Infrared Imaging System, Aerius Automated Infrared Imaging System, and Pearl Impulse Small Animal Imager were provided by LI-COR Biosciences (Lincoln, NE).

2.2. Synthesis and Labeling of YC-27 and Anti-PSMA Antibody. The bioactive moiety of YC-27 was synthesized as previously reported [28] and labeled with IRDye 800CW NHS ester (YC-27 800CW) [28]. The analytical data for YC-27 from *de novo* synthesis were consistent with earlier reported results [28, 29] and the dye-to-protein ratio was 1 : 1. IRDye 800CW anti-PSMA antibody (PSMA 800CW) was prepared by the addition of IRDye 800CW NHS ester at 3 : 1 dye-to-antibody molar ratio. The solution was incubated for 3 h at room temperature followed by spin column purification to remove any remaining unconjugated dye. The final product dye-to-protein ratio was 1.9.

2.3. Microscopy. Three human prostate cancer cell lines with different levels of PSMA expression were used to evaluate localization and internalization of probes: PC3 M-LN4 (negative), 22Rv1 (low), and LNCaP (high) [32, 33]. PC3 M-LN4 and 22Rv1 cells were incubated at 37°C for 1 h with 300 nM YC-27 800CW or 1 μg PSMA 800CW. Cells were rinsed and fixed with 4% formaldehyde for 20 min and nuclei stained with DAPI. Images were obtained by fluorescence microscopy using an Olympus IX81 Inverted Microscope equipped with a halogen bulb and NIR filters (EX:HQ760/40x, 790DCXR, EM:HQ830/50 m; Chroma Technology Corp., Rockingham, VT).

2.4. In Vitro Examination of YC-27 800CW in Cell Culture. Human A431, MCF7, U87 GM, PC3 M-LN4, and 22Rv1 cells were rinsed with PBS and lysed with Laemmli Sample buffer. After electrophoresis, proteins were transferred to a nitrocellulose membrane, blocked for 1 h with Odyssey Blocking Buffer, and incubated with primary antibodies at 1 : 2000 dilution (PSMA 800CW and rabbit polyclonal β tubulin) for 1 h at room temperature with shaking. Proteins were detected with IRDye 680RD-conjugated goat anti-rabbit IgG secondary antibody (LICOR Biosciences) visualized on an Odyssey Infrared Imaging System (LI-COR Biosciences).

Binding and specificity of YC-27 800CW and PSMA 800CW were further evaluated by fluorescent cell-based assays. 22Rv1, PC3 M-LN4, and LNCaP cells were grown to approximately 80% confluency in a 96-well microtiter plate. Poly-D-lysine coated plates were required for LNCaP assays. Growth media were replaced with media containing increasing concentrations of PSMA 800CW only (0.01 to 5 μg/mL), YC-27 800CW (0.1 nM to 1 μM), unlabeled YC-27 (0.026 nM to 50 μM, 1:5 dilution series) plus 28 nM YC-27 800CW, and YC-27 800CW (28 nM) plus 2-PMPA, a competitive inhibitor of the NAALADase activity of PSMA (0.5 nM to 50 μM, 1:10 dilution series). All treatments were done in triplicate and incubated at 37°C in 5% CO_2 for approximately 15 min. Wells were rinsed in 1x PBS and stopped by fixing with 4% formaldehyde solution for 20 min followed by four washes in 1x PBS + 0.02% Triton X-100 to remove unbound dye and permeabilize the cells. The plates were blocked in Odyssey Blocking Buffer (LI-COR Biosciences, Lincoln, NE) for 1 hour and incubated for an additional hour with TO-PRO-3 DNA stain (diluted 1:5000) for normalization of cell number. Washing steps were repeated with Odyssey Buffer + 0.02% Tween-20 and the plate was scanned with an Odyssey SA Automated Infrared Imaging System. Quantification was achieved by ratiometric analysis of the fluorescent intensities obtained from 700 nm (representing cell number) and 800 nm (representing labeled probe) channels. Binding (apparent K_d) and competition (IC_{50}) parameters were calculated by nonlinear curve fit analysis using GraphPad Prism 5 (GraphPad Software, San Diego, CA).

2.5. In Vivo Animal Imaging. Male SCID Hairless Outbred mice (SHO, Crl:SHO-*Prkdc*^{SCID}*Hr*^{hr}) were purchased from Charles River (Willington, MA) and maintained on a purified irradiated maintenance diet (AIN-93 M) from Harlan Teklad (Madison, WI). All experimental procedures for animal use were previously reviewed and approved by the Institutional Animal Care and Use Committee at the University of Nebraska-Lincoln and conducted in accordance with the Guide for the Care and Use of Laboratory Animals published by the US National Institutes of Health.

Six-week-old mice were implanted subcutaneously with 22Rv1 (PSMA positive, right flank) and PC3 M-LN4 (PSMA negative, left flank) cells (1×10^6 cells/100 μL saline) and maintained until tumor size reached approximately 3 mm in diameter. At this time, tumor-bearing animals received either 1x PBS (100 μL), IRDye 800CW carboxylate (1 nmol), IgG 800CW (IgG 800CW, 75 μg), YC-27 800CW (1 nmol), or PSMA 800CW (75 μg) injected via the tail vein. Three doses, 0.25, 0.5, and 1.0 nmol, were evaluated in mice with 22Rv1 tumors ($n = 3$ per dose). Specificity was further confirmed by inhibition with 2-PMPA. For this experiment, preinjection of 2-PMPA (2 μg, intravenous administration) was followed by YC-27 800CW dose (0.5 nmole). Images were captured 24 h after injection of all compounds using the Pearl Impulse Small Animal imaging system.

2.6. Organ and Tissue Analysis. After final imaging, animals were sacrificed and tumors and organs were removed for imaging to confirm signal content and assess agent targeting. Tumors and organs were snap-frozen in OCT compound for cryosectioning. Sections (8 μm thickness) were scanned using the Odyssey CLx imaging system to measure 800 nm fluorescence signal. The 800 nm fluorescence signal per pixel was used to compare targeting agent specificity and retention in tissues.

3. Results

3.1. Western Blot Analysis and Microscopic Examination. We first confirmed the selectivity of the PSMA-specific antibody chosen for our study reference using western analysis (Figure 1(a)). PSMA protein (85 kDa) was specifically detected in the PSMA-expressing cell line, 22Rv1. No significant nonspecific binding was noted for the nonexpressing cell lysates. Prostate tumor cell lines that were positive or negative for PSMA expression (22Rv1 and PC3 M-LN4, resp.) were incubated with PSMA 800CW (1 μg, Figures 1(b) and 1(c)) or YC-27 800CW (300 ng, Figures 1(d) and 1(e)) and counterstained with DAPI to visualize nuclei. Both probes bound the PSMA-expressing cell lines and showed negligible binding to the nonexpressing cell line.

3.2. Cellular Specificity of YC-27 800CW. To evaluate the affinity and targeting specificity of YC-27 800CW, we performed cell-based dose response assays. Three human prostate tumor cell lines were chosen based on differing expression of PSMA. YC-27 800CW showed dose dependent increases in fluorescence, indicating high affinity binding to 22Rv1 cells (apparent $K_d = 8$ nM, Figure 2(a)). No significant signal increase was obtained upon addition of YC-27 800CW to the PSMA-negative cell line, PC3 M-LN4 (Figure 2(a)). Importantly, LNCaP cells, which express levels of PSMA that are higher than those of other commercially available lines, exhibited comparable affinity for YC-27 800CW (apparent $K_d = 36$ nM, Figure 2(b)) with a significantly higher (~200-fold) fluorescence intensity at saturation, reflecting a higher number of binding sites for the probe on these cells.

Specificity was further confirmed by competition studies. LNCaP cells were treated with YC-27 800CW in combination with either unlabeled YC-27 (Figure 2(c)) or with 2-PMPA, a potent competitive inhibitor of PSMA enzymatic activity (Figure 2(d)). Both compounds inhibited effectively as seen by dose response decreases in signal intensity. The IC_{50} for unlabeled YC-27 and 2-PMPA were 1.7 μM and 0.1 μM, respectively, confirming PSMA as the target for the small molecule.

3.3. In Vivo Probe Performance. Male mice were injected subcutaneously with 22Rv1 cells in the right flank and PC3 M-LN4 cells in the left for direct comparison of PSMA targeting probes. As expected, animals receiving any of the three control compounds 1x PBS, 800CW carboxylate, or IgG 800CW showed minimal retention in either tumor (white arrows, Figures 3(a)–3(c)). Both YC-27 800CW and PSMA

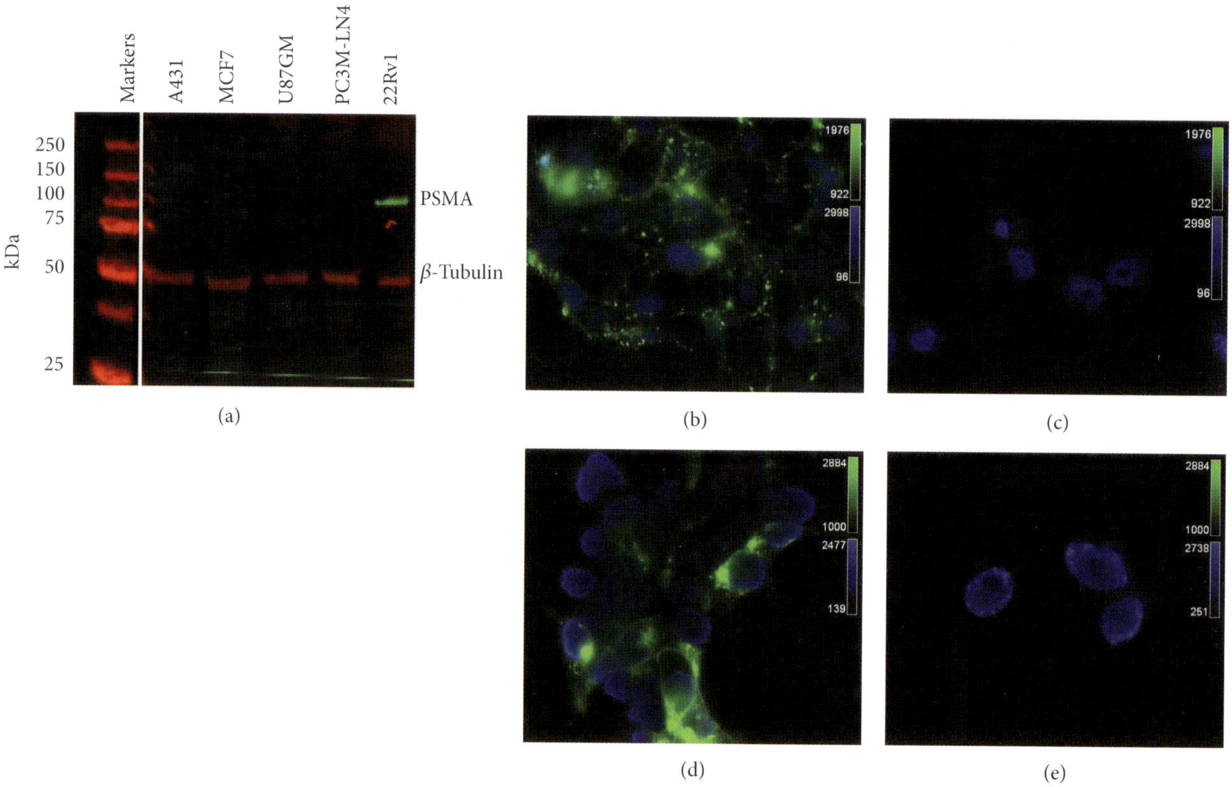

FIGURE 1: Western blot and probe localization. Human A431, MCF7, U87 GM, PC3 M-LN4, and 22Rv1 cell lysates were prepared for western blot analysis (a) to confirm PSMA reactivity of anti-PSMA antibody candidate. PSMA 800CW distinguished between 22Rv1 (PSMA positive) and PC3 M-LN4 (PSMA negative) prostate tumor cell lysates, with no signal detected for cell lysates of nonprostate origin (A431, MCF-7, and U-87 MG). Microscopy images captured cell binding for PSMA 800CW ((b) and (c)) and YC-27 800CW ((d) and (e)) to 22Rv1 (PSMA positive, (b) and (d)) and PC3 M-LN4 (PSMA negative, (c) and (d)). Images were obtained by fluorescence microscopy using an Olympus IX81 Inverted Microscope.

800CW bound the 22Rv1 tumor (white arrows, Figures 3(d) and 3(e), resp.), while little or no signal was visible in the PC3 M-LN4 tumors. As anticipated, animals injected with PSMA 800CW showed incomplete clearance of the probe at the 24 h time point (Figure 3(e)).

Examination of excised liver, kidney, and tumors from animals given YC-27 800CW and PSMA 800CW is presented in Figures 4(a) and 4(b), respectively. As expected, YC-27 800CW showed negligible signal in the liver and high signal in the kidneys, indicating no significant liver retention. PSMA 800CW on the other hand showed the opposite with high fluorescent signal in the liver and low signal in the kidneys indicating a higher liver retention. Both probes were specific for the PSMA-expressing tumor, 22Rv1, with negligible signal in the PC3 M-LN4 tumor. Signals quantified in sections from multiple organs further supported these results (Figure 4(c)). In general, all tissues retained higher levels of PSMA 800CW, including the PC3 M-LN4 tumor, which is consistent with incomplete clearance of the free probe. Both probes accumulated in the epididymis. In considering the higher signal of PSMA 800CW in 22Rv1 tumors, liver, and epididymis, it is important to recognize that the optimal clearance and imaging time point for an antibody-based probe is closer to 72 h rather than the 24 h time point that was optimal for YC-27 800CW [2].

Sections of liver, kidney, testes, and epididymis, which had higher signal retention, were examined in greater detail (Figure 5). Fluorescence intensity of both control IgG 800CW and specific PSMA 800CW was high in liver sections (Figure 5(a)), consistent with the reported clearance of antibody-based reagents [2]. Low signal was noted in the kidney. YC-27 800CW exhibited significant signal in the kidney, with little or no signal retention in the liver. As noted previously, the epididymis showed residual signal for both PSMA-specific probes and, to a lesser extent, the labeled controls. Interestingly, YC-27 800CW showed strong localized signal in the kidney renal cortex, which houses the proximal tubules. A representative microscopic image of the renal cortex region (40X; Figure 5(b)) showed specific signal in the brush border housing the proximal tubules.

3.4. Minimal Effective Dose Determination for YC-27 800CW. SCID Hairless mice bearing 22Rv1 (right flank, white arrows) and PC3 M-LN4 (left flank) xenografts received intravenous injections of 0.25, 0.5, or 1.0 nmol YC-27 800CW or YC-27 800CW (0.5 nmol) plus 2-PMPA (2 μg). Animals were

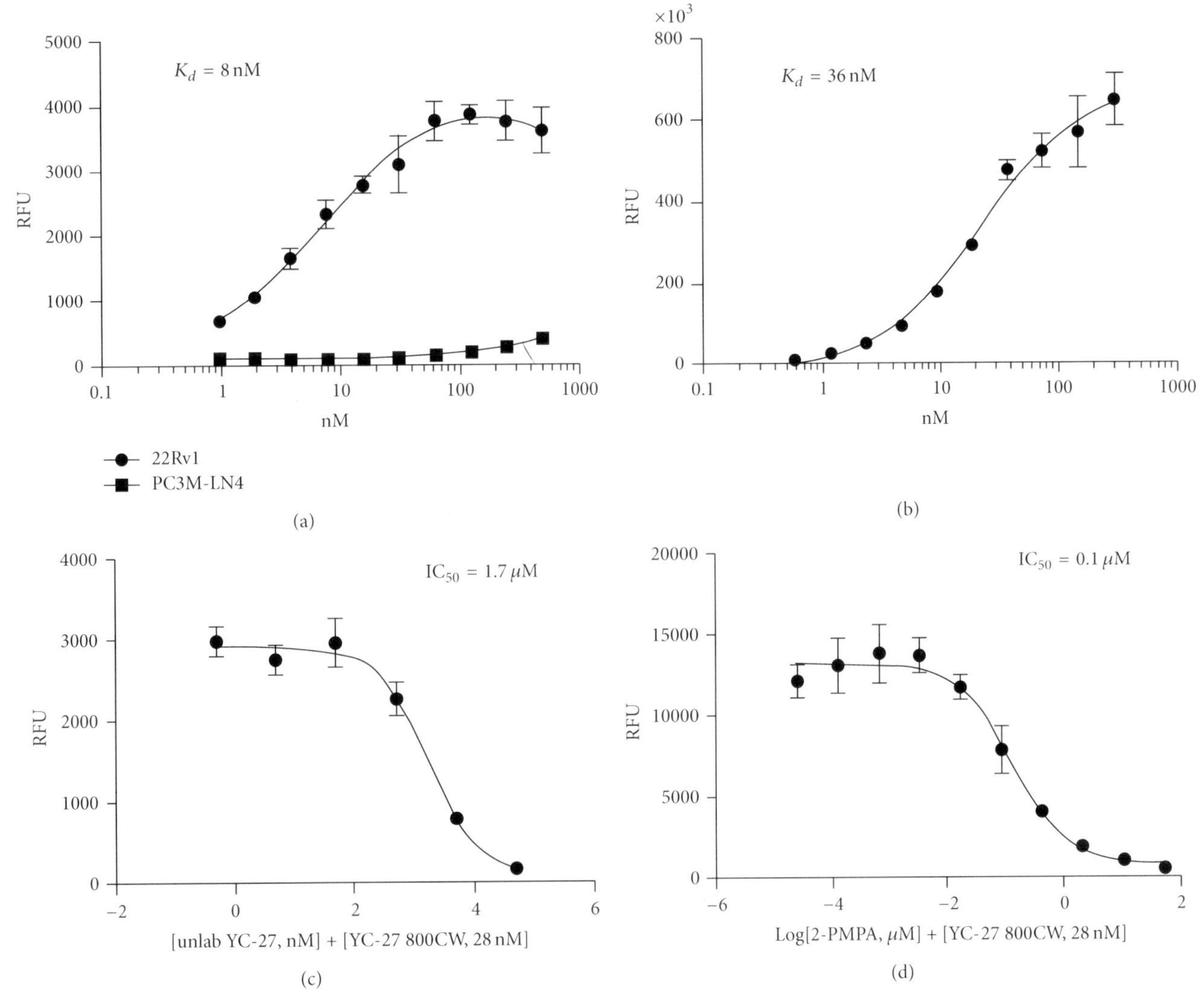

Figure 2: Immunofluorescent cell-based comparison of binding and inhibition. (a) 22Rv1 and PC3 M-LN4 cells were incubated with YC-27 800CW (1 nM to 0.5 μM). Apparent K_d = 8 nM. K_d for PC3 M-LN4 could not be determined. (b) LNCaP cells were incubated with YC-27 800CW (0.5 nM to 0.5 μM, apparent K_d = 36 nM). Competition of YC-27 800CW binding to LNCaP cells by unlabeled YC-27 ((c), IC_{50} = 1.7 μM) or inhibition by 2-PMPA preincubation ((d), IC_{50} = 0.1 μM).

imaged 24 h after injection and tumors excised for further analysis. As shown in Figures 6(a) and 6(b), reasonable tumor-to-background was achieved at the lowest dose of 0.25 nmol. To demonstrate that the observed signals were due to specific binding of the YC-27 800CW probe to PSMA, animals receiving 0.5 nmol of the probe were challenged with 2-PMPA prior to probe injection. The resulting ~50% decrease in signal confirmed the probe bound to its intended target *in vivo*.

4. Discussion

YC-27 is chemically optimized from a lead compound that exploited the inhibitory properties of a PSMA-binding urea scaffold [27, 28], which improved pharmacokinetics for detection of prostate and nonprostate tumors [29]. In the current report, we characterized a YC-27 based NIR conjugate and compared its properties to an antibody-based PSMA targeting agent. Our cell-based and *in vivo* data confirmed that the attachment of IRDye 800CW to YC-27 did not alter its target binding characteristics and showed the conjugate bound PSMA-positive cells and tumors with high affinity and specificity. YC-27 800CW produced a strong, specific fluorescent signal in PSMA-positive tumors of intact animals within 24 h, leaving minimal nonspecific background signal.

At the cellular level, PSMA is known to be internalized from its residence at the cell surface via clathrin-coated pits, which are subsequently recycled to the surface to reexpose PSMA [23, 34]. Our cell-based analysis confirmed that YC-27 800CW successfully bound extracellular PSMA, and fluorescence microscopy revealed that significant quantities were specifically internalized by the PSMA-positive cells. The endocytic internalization and recycling of the PSMA target

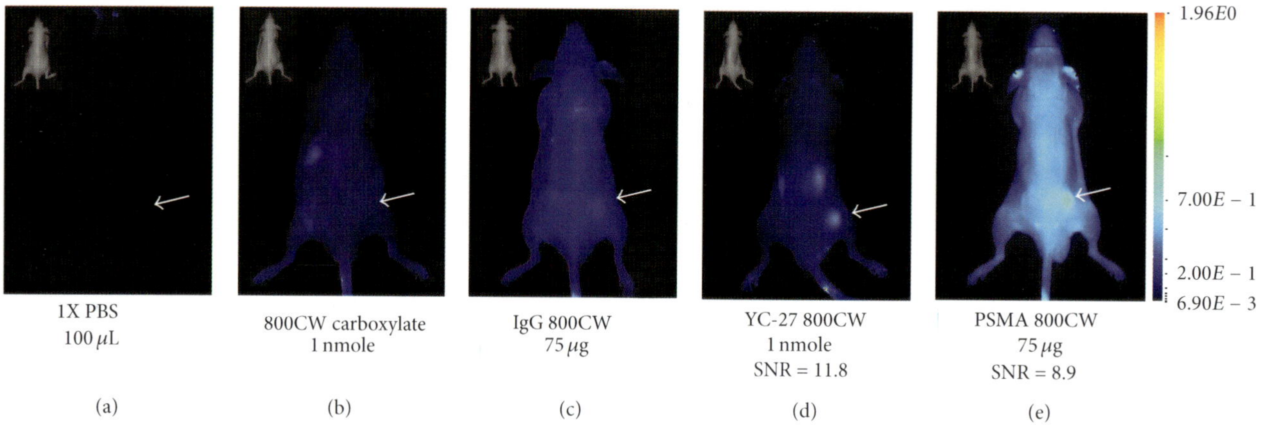

FIGURE 3: Tumor imaging with YC-27 800CW. SCID Hairless mice implanted with 22Rv1 (right flank) and PC3 M-LN4 (left flank) cells received (a) 1X PBS, 100 μL; (b) 800CW carboxylate, 1 nmol; (c) IgG 800CW, 75 μg; (d) YC-27 800CW, 1 nmol (D/P = 1; SNR = 11.8); or (e) PSMA 800CW, 75 μg (D/P = 1; SNR = 8.9), which was allowed to clear for 24 h prior to imaging on Pearl Impulse Imaging System. Signal is presented in pseudocolor. All images were normalized to the same LUT. White arrows indicate the location of the 22Rv1 tumor. Inset panels show the white light image of the mouse.

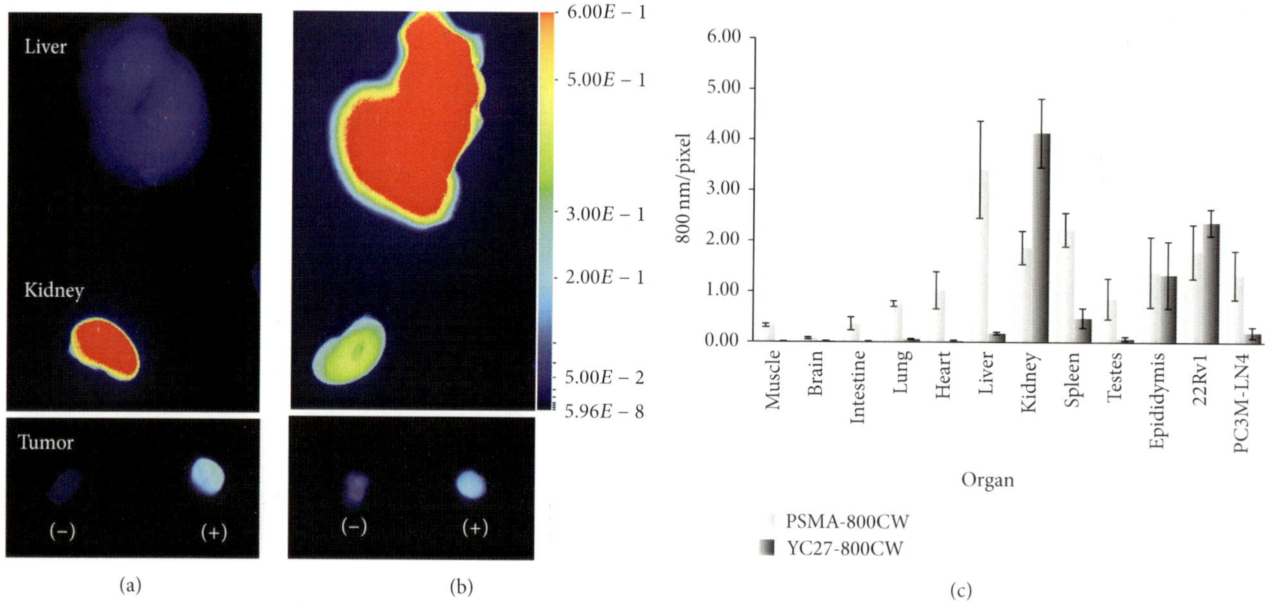

FIGURE 4: Tissue distribution of fluorescence signal. Tissues were excised at endpoint from animals given YC-27 800CW (column (a)) or PSMA 800CW (column (b)). Representative whole organs (liver, kidney, and tumors) were imaged on the Pearl Impulse and reviewed for residual fluorescence of each probe 24 h after intravenous administration. (c) Tissue sections (8 μm; frozen) were prepared from muscle, brain, intestine, lung, heart, liver, kidney, spleen, testes, epididymis, and tumors, 22Rv1 and PC3 M-LN4. Sections were imaged on Odyssey CLx (21 μm) and 800 nm signal intensity per pixel was plotted for both probes.

is a mechanism that has afforded significant tumor-targeting sensitivity by other receptor-targeted NIR fluorescent probes, such as IRDye 800CW EGF [35], because the fluorophore label accumulates within the cell while the receptor is returned to the surface for additional probe binding.

YC-27 800CW cleared quickly in intact animals, yielding high tumor-to-background signal within 24 h. In contrast, antibodies are known to have prolonged circulating half-lives [11, 20, 36, 37], so it was not surprising that the antibody-based agent PSMA 800CW did not achieve optimal clearance in this period. The clearance profiles were reflected in the quantitative analysis of fluorescence accumulation in excised organs and tissues, which demonstrated greater signal in all tissues of animals receiving PSMA 800CW. YC-27 800CW fluorescence was most prominent in the renal cortex, particularly in the brush border housing the proximal tubules. Several reports have found PSMA expressed in mouse kidneys [38, 39], but the implications for clinical use are unknown. Basal PSMA expression is also reported in salivary gland, brain, and small intestine [40]. No significant

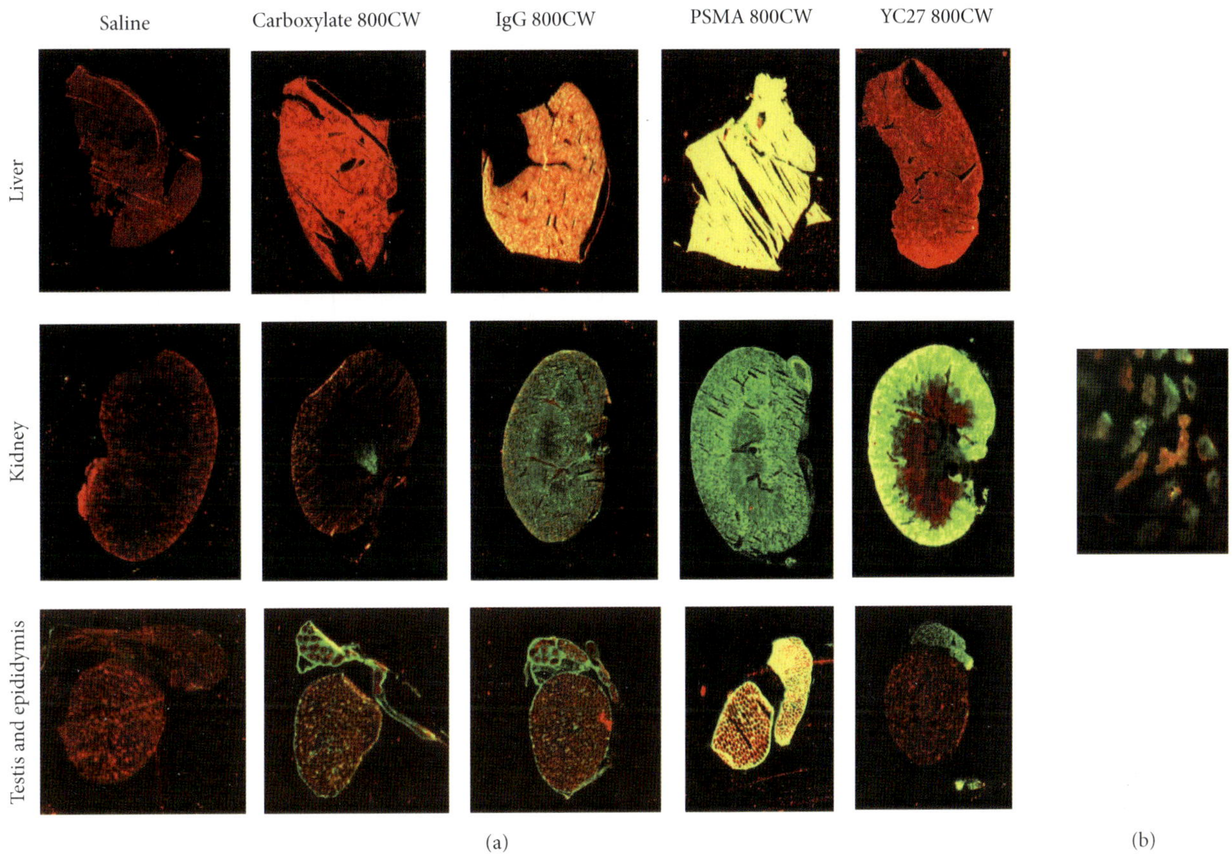

FIGURE 5: Fluorescence signal retention in specific clearance organs. (a) Tissue sections from mice receiving 1X PBS, carboxylate 800CW, IgG 800CW, PSMA 800CW, and YC-27 800CW were scanned on Odyssey CLx (21 micron). In all images, green indicates signals captured at 800 nm and red represents autofluorescence at 700 nm. Colocalization of the signals is yellow. (b) Higher magnification image (40x) of kidney renal cortex from YC-27 800CW treated mouse.

signal was detected 24 h after injection in the prostatic region including the bladder. These distribution patterns support future testing of YC-27 800CW for sensitive and specific distinction between normal, benign, and malignant tissue. The binding of YC-27 800CW noted in the epididymis may be attributable to recognition of the probe by glutamate receptors (GluR). Previously, it was suggested that GluR may be involved in spermatogenesis, spermatozoa motility, and testicular development [41, 42]. In addition, glutamate binding could be partially displaced by *N*-methyl-D-aspartate in the seminal vesicles [42]. The small molecule, YC-27, has a glutamate component that may be exposed and available for receptor binding. Another potential explanation is that epididymal signals for all labeled agents, probes, and controls may result from a bottleneck in clearance through this highly vascular region coinciding with the imaging time point. Nonetheless, binding to the epididymis is not expected to be problematic in prostate surgery since this tissue is usually removed during prostatectomy.

It has been suggested that the long circulating time exhibited by antibody-based fluorescent contrast agents could be advantageous, because lower doses of the agent would be needed [2, 11, 20, 43]. However, the dose dependence of the small molecule, YC-27 800CW, showed that 22Rv1 tumors were detectable with good tumor-to-background using 0.25 nmol. Thus, rapid clearance of a targeting agent does not compromise its efficacy when the agent has high affinity for the target, and the rapid clearance would be entirely compatible with clinical workflow. This has important implications for translation, since visualization of tumor margins at the primary site, unambiguous identification of tumor-involved secondary sites [12, 13, 20, 44–46], and image-guided real time localization of tumor-involved nodes or residual tissue following resection [14, 47] could potentially benefit long-term patient outcomes.

Currently, ^{111}In-capromab pendetide (Prostascint), an antibody that recognizes an intracellular epitope of PSMA, is used as an imaging agent in SPECT. These scans are useful in early phases of diagnosis or postsurgery but may be a disadvantage in the operating suite where exposure to ionizing radiation to patient and surgeon could occur. NIR-labeled optical imaging agents are also gaining attention for tumor resection of a variety of cancers [11, 13, 20, 48, 49]. Due to the cost of clinical trials, single agents with broad

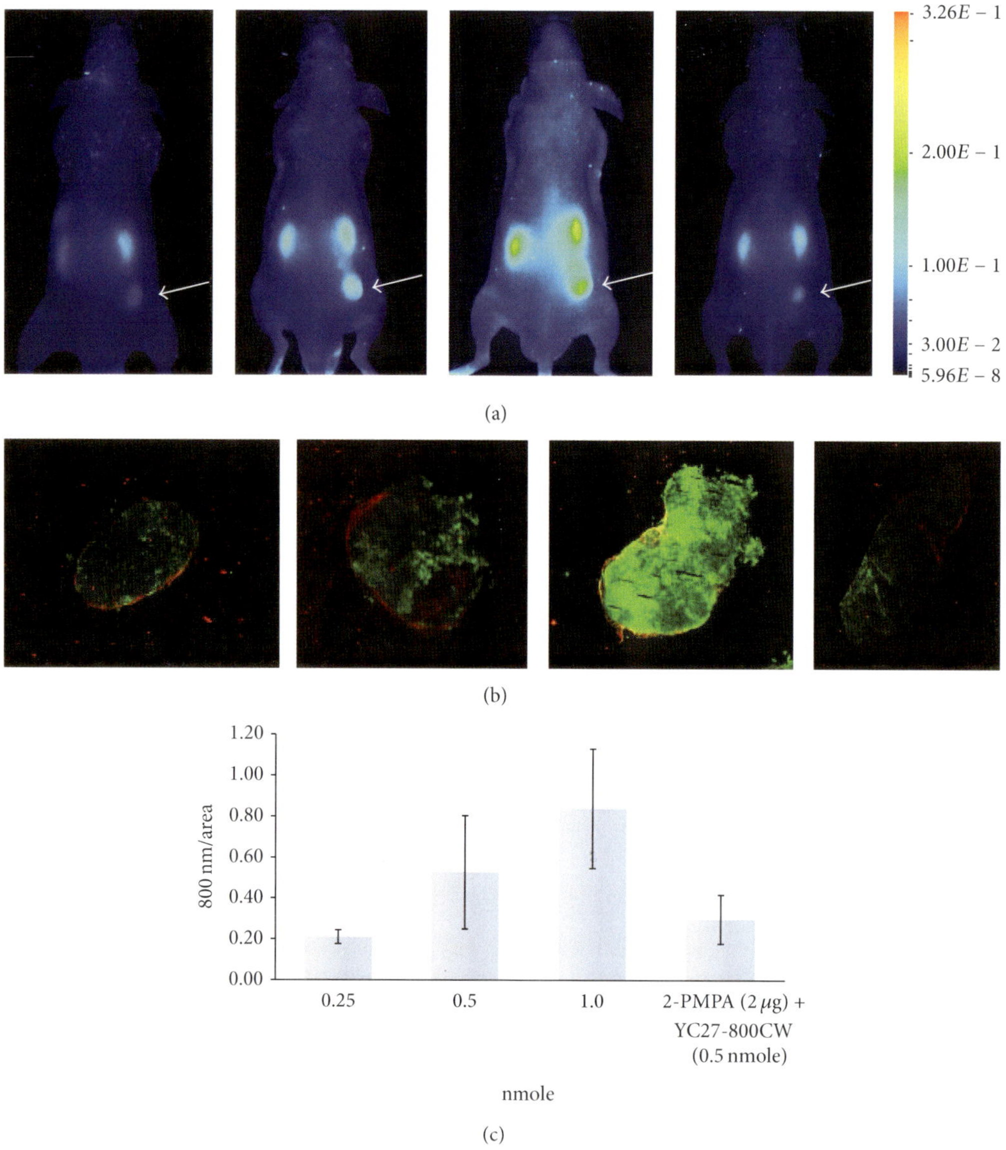

FIGURE 6: Specificity of YC-27 800CW for tumor imaging *in vivo*. SCID Hairless mice implanted with 22Rv1 (right flank, white arrows) and PC3 M-LN4 (left flank) cells received intravenous injections of 0.25, 0.5, or 1.0 nmol YC27-800CW or 2-PMPA (2 μg) plus YC-27 800CW (0.5 nmol). (a) Animals were imaged intact after 24 hours, using Pearl Impulse; (b) 22Rv1 tumor sections from each animal at endpoint were imaged on Odyssey CLx; (c) signal intensity of each tumor was quantified and normalized to unit area. Intact animal images are presented in pseudocolor. All images are normalized to the same LUT. Odyssey CLx images for tumor sections are shown in green (800 nm) and red (700 nm) and standardized to the same LUT.

reactivity against a number of cancers are desirable because this approach reduces preclinical toxicity work and development of new GMP manufacturing and formulation processes for individual agents [50]. PSMA is broadly expressed on the neovasculature of many solid tumors [3, 4, 21, 51], so agents targeting this protein are good candidates for clinical translation [21, 22], and it may prove valuable to add YC-27 800CW to the toolkit. Use of NIR fluorophore-labeled PSMA targeting agents produced 100% resection with no residual positive margins in PSMA-positive tumor-bearing animals, supporting the use of this approach for prostate tumor resections [15]. Future studies will be needed to define the broad tumor-targeting efficacy of YC-27-based agents for solid tumors.

References

[1] R. Siegel, D. Naishadham, and A. Jemal, “Cancer statistics, 2012,” *CA Cancer Journal for Clinicians*, vol. 62, no. 1, pp. 10–29, 2012.

[2] K. Imai and A. Takaoka, "Comparing antibody and small-molecule therapies for cancer," *Nature Reviews Cancer*, vol. 6, no. 9, pp. 714–727, 2006.

[3] R. S. Israeli, C. T. Powell, J. G. Corr, W. R. Fair, and W. D. W. Heston, "Expression of the prostate-specific membrane antigen," *Cancer Research*, vol. 54, no. 7, pp. 1807–1811, 1994.

[4] D. A. Silver, I. Pellicer, W. R. Fair, W. D. W. Heston, and C. Cordon-Cardo, "Prostate-specific membrane antigen expression in normal and malignant human tissues," *Clinical Cancer Research*, vol. 3, no. 1, pp. 81–85, 1997.

[5] J. J. Futterer and J. O. Barentsz, "MRI-guided and robotic-assisted prostate biopsy," *Current Opinion in Urology*, vol. 22, pp. 316–319, 2012.

[6] M. J. Manyak, "Indium-111 capromab pendetide in the management of recurrent prostate cancer," *Expert Review of Anticancer Therapy*, vol. 8, no. 2, pp. 175–181, 2008.

[7] A. K. Gregorakis, E. H. Holmes, and G. P. Murphy, "Prostate-specific membrane antigen: current and future utility," *Seminars in Urologic Oncology*, vol. 16, no. 1, pp. 2–12, 1998.

[8] S. R. Banerjee, M. Pullambhatla, Y. Byun et al., "Sequential SPECT and optical imaging of experimental models of prostate cancer with a dual modality inhibitor of the prostate-specific membrane antigen," *Angewandte Chemie—International Edition*, vol. 50, no. 39, pp. 9167–9170, 2011.

[9] T. Kitai, T. Inomoto, M. Miwa, and T. Shikayama, "Fluorescence navigation with indocyanine green for detecting sentinel lymph nodes in breast cancer," *Breast Cancer*, vol. 12, no. 3, pp. 211–215, 2005.

[10] N. Tagaya, R. Yamazaki, A. Nakagawa et al., "Intraoperative identification of sentinel lymph nodes by near-infrared fluorescence imaging in patients with breast cancer," *The American Journal of Surgery*, vol. 195, no. 6, pp. 850–853, 2008.

[11] A. G. T. Terwisscha van Scheltinga, G. M. van Dam, W. B. Nagengast et al., "Intraoperative near-infrared fluorescence tumor imaging with vascular endothelial growth factor and human epidermal growth factor receptor 2 targeting antibodies," *Journal of Nuclear Medicine*, vol. 52, no. 11, pp. 1778–1785, 2011.

[12] L. Jacobs, "Positive margins: the challenge continues for breast surgeons," *Annals of Surgical Oncology*, vol. 15, no. 5, pp. 1271–1272, 2008.

[13] G. M. van Dam, G. Themelis, L. M. A. Crane et al., "Intraoperative tumor-specific fluorescence imaging in ovarian cancer by folate receptor-α targeting: first in-human results," *Nature Medicine*, vol. 17, no. 10, pp. 1315–1319, 2011.

[14] L. M. A. Crane, G. Themelis, R. G. Pleijhuis et al., "Intraoperative multispectral fluorescence imaging for the detection of the sentinel lymph node in cervical cancer: a novel concept," *Molecular Imaging and Biology*, vol. 13, no. 5, pp. 1043–1049, 2011.

[15] H. Laydner, S. S. Huang, W. D. Heston et al., "Robotic real-time near infrared targeted fluorescence imaging in a murine model of prostate cancer: a feasibility study," *Urology*, vol. 81, pp. 451–456, 2013.

[16] N. S. van den Berg, O. R. Brouwer, W. M. C. Klop et al., "Concomitant radio- and fluorescence-guided sentinel lymph node biopsy in squamous cell carcinoma of the oral cavity using ICG-(99m)Tc-nanocolloid," *European Journal of Nuclear Medicine and Molecular Imaging*, vol. 39, pp. 1128–1136, 2012.

[17] A. C. van Leeuwen, T. Buckle, G. Bendle et al., "Tracer-cocktail injections for combined pre- and intraoperative multimodal imaging of lymph nodes in a spontaneous mouse prostate tumor model," *Journal of Biomedical Optics*, vol. 16, no. 1, Article ID 016004, 2011.

[18] S. Tobis, J. Knopf, C. Silvers et al., "Near infrared fluorescence imaging with robotic assisted laparoscopic partial nephrectomy: initial clinical experience for renal cortical tumors," *The Journal of Urology*, vol. 186, no. 1, pp. 47–52, 2011.

[19] S. Achilefu, S. Bloch, M. A. Markiewicz et al., "Synergistic effects of light-emitting probes and peptides for targeting and monitoring integrin expression," *Proceedings of the National Academy of Sciences of the United States of America*, vol. 102, no. 22, pp. 7976–7981, 2005.

[20] C. H. Heath, N. L. Deep, L. Sweeny, K. R. Zinn, and E. L. Rosenthal, "Use of panitumumab-IRDye800 to image microscopic head and neck cancer in an orthotopic surgical model," *Annals of Surgical Oncology*, vol. 19, pp. 3879–3887, 2012.

[21] S. S. Chang, V. E. Reuter, W. D. W. Heston, N. H. Bander, L. S. Grauer, and P. B. Gaudin, "Five different anti-prostate-specific membrane antigen (PSMA) antibodies confirm PSMA expression in tumor-associated neovasculature," *Cancer Research*, vol. 59, no. 13, pp. 3192–3198, 1999.

[22] U. Elsässer-Beile, P. Bühler, and P. Wolf, "Targeted therapies for Prostate cancer against the prostate specific membrane antigen," *Current Drug Targets*, vol. 10, no. 2, pp. 118–125, 2009.

[23] H. Liu, A. K. Rajasekaran, P. Moy et al., "Constitutive and antibody-induced internalization of prostate-specific membrane antigen," *Cancer Research*, vol. 58, no. 18, pp. 4055–4060, 1998.

[24] J. R. Osborne, N. H. Akhtar, S. Vallabhajosula, A. Anand, K. Deh, and S. T. Tagawa, "Prostate-specific membrane antigen-based imaging," *Urologic Oncology*, vol. 31, pp. 144–154, 2013.

[25] M. Longmire, P. L. Choyke, and H. Kobayashi, "Clearance properties of nano-sized particles and molecules as imaging agents: considerations and caveats," *Nanomedicine*, vol. 3, no. 5, pp. 703–717, 2008.

[26] R. S. Agnes, A. M. Broome, J. Wang, A. Verma, K. Lavik, and J. P. Basilion, "An optical probe for noninvasive molecular imaging of orthotopic brain tumors overexpressing epidermal growth factor receptor," *Molecular Cancer Therapeutics*, vol. 11, pp. 2202–2211, 2012.

[27] S. R. Banerjee, C. A. Foss, M. Castanares et al., "Synthesis and evaluation of technetium-99m- and rhenium-labeled inhibitors of the prostate-specific membrane antigen (PSMA)," *Journal of Medicinal Chemistry*, vol. 51, no. 15, pp. 4504–4517, 2008.

[28] Y. Chen, S. Dhara, S. R. Banerjee et al., "A low molecular weight PSMA-based fluorescent imaging agent for cancer," *Biochemical and Biophysical Research Communications*, vol. 390, no. 3, pp. 624–629, 2009.

[29] Y. Chen, M. Pullambhatla, S. R. Banerjee et al., "Synthesis and biological evaluation of low molecular weight fluorescent imaging agents for the prostate-specific membrane antigen," *Bioconjugate Chemistry*, vol. 23, pp. 2377–2385, 2012.

[30] S. A. Kularatne, K. Wang, H.-K. R. Santhapuram, and P. S. Low, "Prostate-specific membrane antigen targeted imaging and therapy of prostate cancer using a PSMA inhibitor as a homing ligand," *Molecular Pharmaceutics*, vol. 6, no. 3, pp. 780–789, 2009.

[31] T. Liu, L. Y. Wu, M. R. Hopkins, J. K. Choi, and C. E. Berkman, "A targeted low molecular weight near-infrared fluorescent probe for prostate cancer," *Bioorganic and Medicinal Chemistry Letters*, vol. 20, no. 23, pp. 7124–7126, 2010.

[32] M. J. Evans, P. M. Smith-Jones, J. Wongvipat et al., "Noninvasive measurement of androgen receptor signaling with a positron-emitting radiopharmaceutical that targets prostate-specific membrane antigen," *Proceedings of the National Academy of Sciences of the United States of America*, vol. 108, no. 23, pp. 9578–9582, 2011.

[33] X. Wang, D. Ma, W. C. Olson, and W. D. W. Heston, "In vitro and in vivo responses of advanced prostate tumors to PSMA ADC, an auristatin-conjugated antibody to prostate-specific membrane antigen," *Molecular Cancer Therapeutics*, vol. 10, no. 9, pp. 1728–1739, 2011.

[34] K. Bouchelouche, P. L. Choyke, and J. Capala, "Prostate specific membrane antigen- a target for imaging and therapy with radionuclides," *Discovery Medicine*, vol. 9, no. 44, pp. 55–61, 2010.

[35] J. L. Kovar, M. A. Johnson, W. M. Volcheck, J. Chen, and M. A. Simpson, "Hyaluronidase expression induces prostate tumor metastasis in an orthotopic mouse model," *The American Journal of Pathology*, vol. 169, no. 4, pp. 1415–1426, 2006.

[36] V. Kenanova, T. Olafsen, D. M. Crow et al., "Tailoring the pharmacokinetics and positron emission tomography imaging properties of anti-carcinoembryonic antigen single-chain Fv-Fc antibody fragments," *Cancer Research*, vol. 65, no. 2, pp. 622–631, 2005.

[37] M. Tabrizi, G. G. Bornstein, and H. Suria, "Biodistribution mechanisms of therapeutic monoclonal antibodies in health and disease," *AAPS Journal*, vol. 12, no. 1, pp. 33–43, 2010.

[38] D. J. Bacich, J. T. Pinto, W. P. Tong, and W. D. W. Heston, "Cloning, expression, genomic localization, and enzymatic activities of the mouse homolog of prostate-specific membrane antigen/NAALADase/folate hydrolase," *Mammalian Genome*, vol. 12, no. 2, pp. 117–123, 2001.

[39] P. D. Gregor, J. D. Wolchok, V. Turaga et al., "Induction of autoantibodies to syngeneic prostate-specific membrane antigen by xenogeneic vaccination," *International Journal of Cancer*, vol. 116, no. 3, pp. 415–421, 2005.

[40] J. K. Troyer, M. L. Beckett, and G. L. Wright Jr., "Detection and characterization of the prostate-specific membrane antigen (PSMA) in tissue extracts and body fluids," *International Journal of Cancer*, vol. 62, no. 5, pp. 552–558, 1995.

[41] R. Dingledine, K. Borges, D. Bowie, and S. F. Traynelis, "The glutamate receptor ion channels," *Pharmacological Reviews*, vol. 51, no. 1, pp. 7–61, 1999.

[42] S. S. Gill and O. M. Pulido, "Glutamate receptors in peripheral tissues: current knowledge, future research, and implications for toxicology," *Toxicologic Pathology*, vol. 29, no. 2, pp. 208–223, 2001.

[43] W. Scheuer, G. M. van Dam, M. Dobosz, M. Schwaiger, and V. Ntziachristos, "Drug-based optical agents: infiltrating clinics at lower risk," *Science Translational Medicine*, vol. 4, article 134ps11, 2012.

[44] M. Deeter, R. Dorer, M. K. Kuppusamy, R. P. Koehler, and D. E. Low, "Assessment of criteria and clinical significance of circumferential resection margins in esophageal cancer," *Archives of Surgery*, vol. 144, no. 7, pp. 618–624, 2009.

[45] R. E. Emerson, M. O. Koch, T. D. Jones, J. K. Daggy, B. E. Juliar, and L. Cheng, "The influence of extent of surgical margin positivity on prostate specific antigen recurrence," *Journal of Clinical Pathology*, vol. 58, no. 10, pp. 1028–1032, 2005.

[46] N. V. Zhukov and S. A. Tjulandin, "Targeted therapy in the treatment of solid tumors: practice contradicts theory," *Biochemistry (Moscow)*, vol. 73, no. 5, pp. 605–618, 2008.

[47] N. Wada, N. Sakemura, S. Imoto, T. Hasebe, A. Ochiai, and N. Moriyama, "Sentinel node biopsy in primary breast cancer: radioactive detection and metastatic disease," *European Journal of Surgical Oncology*, vol. 33, no. 6, pp. 691–695, 2007.

[48] L. M. A. Crane, M. van Oosten, R. G. Pleijhuis et al., "Intra-operative imaging in ovarian cancer: fact or fiction?" *Molecular Imaging*, vol. 10, no. 4, pp. 248–257, 2011.

[49] M. van Oosten, L. M. A. Crane, J. Bart, F. W. van Leeuwen, and G. M. van Dam, "Selecting potential targetable biomarkers for imaging purposes in colorectal cancer using target selection criteria (TASC): a novel target identification tool," *Translational Oncology*, vol. 4, no. 2, pp. 71–82, 2011.

[50] A. D. Nunn, "The cost of developing imaging agents for routine clinical use," *Investigative Radiology*, vol. 41, no. 3, pp. 206–212, 2006.

[51] M. J. Morris, N. Pandit-Taskar, C. R. Divgi et al., "Phase I evaluation of J591 as a vascular targeting agent in progressive solid tumors," *Clinical Cancer Research*, vol. 13, no. 9, pp. 2707–2713, 2007.

2

Galectins as New Prognostic Markers and Potential Therapeutic Targets for Advanced Prostate Cancers

Diego J. Laderach, Lucas Gentilini, Felipe M. Jaworski, and Daniel Compagno

Laboratorio de Glicómica Funcional, IQUIBICEN-CONICET, Departamento de Química Biológica, Facultad de Ciencias Exactas y Naturales, Universidad de Buenos Aires, C1428, Buenos Aires, Argentina

Correspondence should be addressed to Diego J. Laderach; diegoladerach@qb.fcen.uba.ar and Daniel Compagno; danielcompagno@qb.fcen.uba.ar

Academic Editor: James L. Gulley

A better understanding of multimolecular interactions involved in tumor dissemination is required to identify new effective therapies for advanced prostate cancer (PCa). Several groups investigated protein-glycan interactions as critical factors for crosstalk between prostate tumors and their microenvironment. This review both discusses whether the "galectin-signature" might serve as a reliable biomarker for the identification of patients with high risk of metastasis and assesses the galectin-glycan lattices as potential novel targets for anticancer therapies. The ultimate goal of this review is to convey how basic findings related to galectins could be in turn translated into clinical settings for patients with advanced PCa.

1. Introduction

Prostate cancer (PCa) is the second most common cancer in men and represents a significant cause of mortality worldwide [1]. About 15%–20% of men with PCa will certainly develop metastatic disease and die. Early diagnosis and rapid treatment play a critical role in the final outcome of the disease. At present, surgical and radiation treatments are efficient against clinically localized PCa, whereas androgen ablation is mainly recommended for advanced PCa [2]. However, metastatic cancer is essentially fatal due to disease evolution towards a castration-resistant PCa (CRPC). Novel alternative approaches are therefore essential to prevent tumor dissemination and progression to this incurable stage.

Effective cancer therapies for PCa typically capitalize on molecular differences between healthy and neoplastic tissues that can be targeted with drugs [3]. In the past years, delineating gene and protein expression profiles has been critical in dissecting the molecular underpinnings of cellular function; the arising information has been exploited for the design of rational therapeutic strategies. In the postgenomic era, the study of the "glycome" has enabled the association of specific glycan structures with the transition from normal to neoplastic tissue [4]. Glycans abundantly decorate the surface of all mammalian cells and the extracellular matrix with which they interact [5]. In general, mammalian glycans are the product of a repertoire of glycosyltransferases and glycosidases acting sequentially and dictating the glycosylation signature of each cell type [6]. It has been recognized that the structure of cell surface glycans can change under different physiological and pathological conditions. In fact, malignant transformation is associated with abnormal glycosylation resulting in the synthesis of altered glycan determinants in the tumor microenvironment [7]. The responsibility of decoding the information displayed by cell surface glycan structures is attributed in part to endogenous glycan-binding proteins or lectins, whose expression and function are also regulated during oncogenesis and metastasis [8].

Galectins (Gals) are a family of evolutionarily conserved glycan-binding proteins characterized by their affinity for N-acetyllactosamine sequences which can be displayed on cell surface glycoconjugates [9, 10]. Through this type of interactions, Gals promote lattice formation, strengthening the avidity and half-life of ligand/receptor interactions, and organize centers for molecular signaling [11]. Therefore, these particular lectins are the molecular links between changes in glycophenotype and signaling processes that underlie cellular responses to exogenous stimuli. In addition, Gals are also involved in endogenous regulation of different intracellular pathways with high impact on controlling cellular behavior [12–14].

Interestingly, alterations in Gal expression are observed in pathologic processes such as inflammation, cancer, and autoimmunity [9, 15–17]. A series of studies in experimental models and cancer patients have reported significant associations among the expression of Gals and tumorigenesis, metastatic potential, and tumor-immune escape. This review focuses on the role of Gals in PCa progression and how could they be used as diagnostic markers of PCa evolution as well as new therapeutic targets for metastatic and castration-resistant PCa (mCRPC) patients.

2. Basic Biochemistry and Molecular Biology of Galectins

Galectins are a family of fifteen described lectins that bind to the carbohydrate portion of cell surface glycoproteins or glycolipids and are defined by at least one carbohydrate recognition domain (CRD) with affinity for beta-galactosides through a conserved sequence motif [18]. However, each of the members of this family has subtle differences in their glycan-binding specificity and tissue distribution (for detailed information see The Center of Functional Glycomics (CFG) database http://www.functionalglycomics.org/CFGparadigms/index.php/Main_Page). Members of the Gal family are found in vertebrates, invertebrates, and protists; Gal-related sequences have also been found in plants and viruses. The high degree of conservation of Gal sequences suggests that they have an important role in basic cellular mechanisms [19, 20]. However, from the fifteen defined members only 11 are expressed in humans (see Table 1, [18]).

Galectins have been subdivided into three groups (Figure 1(a)) based on their structure and the number of CRD: (a) prototype Gals are constituted by a single CRD (Gals-1, -2, -5, -7, -10, -11, -13, and -14); (b) tandem-repeat Gals, by 2 different but homologous CRDs, connected by a linker region (Gals-4, -6, -8, -9, and -12); (c) chimera-Gals, represented by a unique member: Gal-3, consisted by a single CRD fused to a tail of short tandem repeats. These different structures allow oligomerization of Gals required for effective signaling through binding to cell surface glycoconjugates containing N-acetyllactosamine moieties (Figures 1(b) and 2) [11]. As an example, Gal-3 is a chimera-type Gal containing a single carbohydrate recognition domain (CRD) with an extended proline and glycine rich-N-terminus that promotes oligomerization towards highly structured forms. As other Gals, extracellular and membrane triggered functions of Gal-3 strongly depend on CDR-mediated recognition of glycan chains on glycoproteins, inducing the assembly of lattices in membrane through direct engagement of specific cell surface glycoconjugates by traditional ligand-receptor binding [10].

Galectins are synthesized in the cytoplasm and secreted using a nonclassical pathway [44]; thus, these lectines are found in a variety of intracellular compartments, as well as in the extracellular milieu of almost all cell types and tissues. Membrane-bound or soluble forms of Gals have been described with some different functions: it is well established that glycoconjugate recognition by Gals plays key roles during anoikis resistance, metastatic dissemination, and escape of tumor cells from the immune response (see for review [9, 45]).

Galectins could be affected by posttranscriptional modifications such as cleavage or phosphorylation. In fact, phosphorylation or proteolysis affects Gal-3 structure and localization altering important biologic functions of this lectin in human carcinomas [46–48]. Gal-3 cleavage by matrix metalloprotease (MMP)-2/-9 is observed in breast and prostate cancers and is responsible for tumor growth, angiogenesis, and apoptosis resistance in mouse models and influence cell migration, angiogenesis, and tumor progression [48, 49].

The expression pattern of different Gals changes during tissue development and is altered at sites of inflammation and tumor. Different reports in colon, breast, prostate, thyroid, and laryngeal cancers have demonstrated an important role of Gals in tumor emergence and progression (see for review [15]). At this respect, the expression level of some Gals by tumor cells has been shown to be correlated with metastatic potential. Gals can contribute to tumor progression through many different mechanisms [50, 51]. Most studies have evaluated defined Gals, particularly Gals-1 and -3. However, existing data indicate that other Gals, especially those whose expression is altered in cancer, probably contribute to various steps in tumor progression. Mechanisms by which those Gals are involved in such effects remain poorly understood especially in the PCa field.

3. Expression of Galectins in Normal and Cancerous Human Prostate Tissues

Few studies investigated the expression of Gals in normal prostate [52, 53] and Gals-1; -3, and -8 are the most studied proteins in prostate carcinoma [23, 29, 52–55]. Pioneer studies by Lotan's group found that Gal-1 and Gal-3 are expressed in the cytoplasm of the majority of prostate cancer cell lines, except LNCaP which is the most studied human androgen-sensitive cell line. In fact, LNCaP does not express both Gals [25]. It is important to note that although LNCaP cells were clearly negative for Gal-1 expression in this first published work, we and others have demonstrated that LNCaP cell line does express low levels of Gal-1 mRNA and these transcripts are upregulated when cells underwent castration resistance (CR) [56]. In our study, we were able to detect the expression of Gal-1 at transcriptional levels with a 20-fold lower level when compared with androgen unresponsive 22Rv1 and PC-3 cells (Figure 3(a)). Additionally, we have been able to detect low protein levels by immunocytochemistry and western blot (see Figure 3(a)). Even more, LNCaP cells that have been rendered androgen unresponsive (by culturing them for several weeks in the absence of hormones) expressed higher levels of Gal-1 as detected by RT-qPCR (see Figure 3(b), left panel). Our studies have been performed on cells in the log phase of growth, as we used to observe variation of Gal expression

Table 1: Summary of reported galectin functions in prostate cancers.

Galectin	Tumor cell growth/survival/apoptosis		Metastasis		Immune response	
	In vitro	*In vivo*	*In vitro*	*In vivo*	*In vitro*	*In vivo*
Gal-1	Promotes apoptosis in LNCaP [21] O-glycosylation protects PCa cell from Gal-1-induced apoptosis [22] Promotes tubulogenesis [23]	Gal-1 principal inducer of neovascularization [23]	Promotes cell adhesion to ECM, EC [24, 25] Osteoblasts proliferation and differentiation, effects inhibited by IGF [26]	?	Invasion of T cell in matrigel assays and adhesion of T cell to Gal-1-expressing EC [27]	?
Gal-3	Promotes apoptosis or survival depending of cell subcellular localization or cell type [28–30] Drug resistance [31, 32]	Gal-3 as inducer of angiogenesis [33]	Interaction with blood vessel allowing metastasis process such as arrest in certain organs [34, 35] PCa cell with preferential binding to HBME through collagen XXIII and Gal-3 could explain bone metastasis [36, 37]	Anti-Gal-3 Abs or MCP inhibits spontaneous metastasis in Copenhagen rat-injected Dunning rat PCa cells [38], influences bone metastasis as indirect inhibition of Gal-3, and inhibits skeleton metastasis after Luc-PC-3 intracardiac injection [39] Using Gal-3 inhibitors inhibits tumor growth or lung metastasis [33, 40, 41]	?	?
Gal-8	Exclusive expression at the neoplasic stage in prostate tissue (PCTA-1); links to integrin to inhibit cell adhesion [42]	?	Links to integrin to inhibit cell adhesion and promote metastasis and cell spreading. In contrary, in soluble form Gal-8 promotes cell-adhesion to ECM [43]	?	?	?
Gal-4	Gal-4 as inducer of tubulogenesis [33]	?	?	?	?	?
Gal-9	Gal-9 as inducer of tubulogenesis [33]	?	?	?	?	?
Gal-12	?	?	?	?	?	?
Others Gals	?	?	?	?	?	?

depending on cell culture conditions such as confluency (data not shown), situation that is not referred to in previous cited references. Moreover, two different sources of androgen-responsive and PSA/Gal-1-producing LNCaP cells were evaluated as we do infer that some phenotypic differences may appear in such largely used PCa cell line (Figure 3(b), right panel). Results clearly demonstrate that the LNCaP cell line (either castration-sensitive or a clone that undergoes castration-resistant) as well as a PSA-negative LNCaP clone (selected *in vitro* by Vaarala and colleagues [56]) is able to produce Gal-1, at least under some culture conditions. However, when expressed, Gal-1 plays an important function in cell-extracellular matrix (ECM) interactions, conferring adhesion properties to some PCa cell lines. Gals-1 and -3 have been thus suggested to play a role in the development and progression of cancer [25].

Studying the role of Gals in PCa cell lines is certainly not enough to validate relevance in the human pathology. For clinical relevance, Lotan's group has studied by immunohistochemistry (IHC) the expression of Gals in normal human prostate tissue and prostate adenocarcinoma, containing formalin-fixed, paraffin-embedded sections of 7 normal human prostates, 8 cases of prostatic intraepithelial neoplasia (PIN), 20 primary adenocarcinomas of the prostate, and 12 PCa metastases. Gal-1 was expressed in most cases, irrespective of the histology stages. In contrast, Gal-3 expression

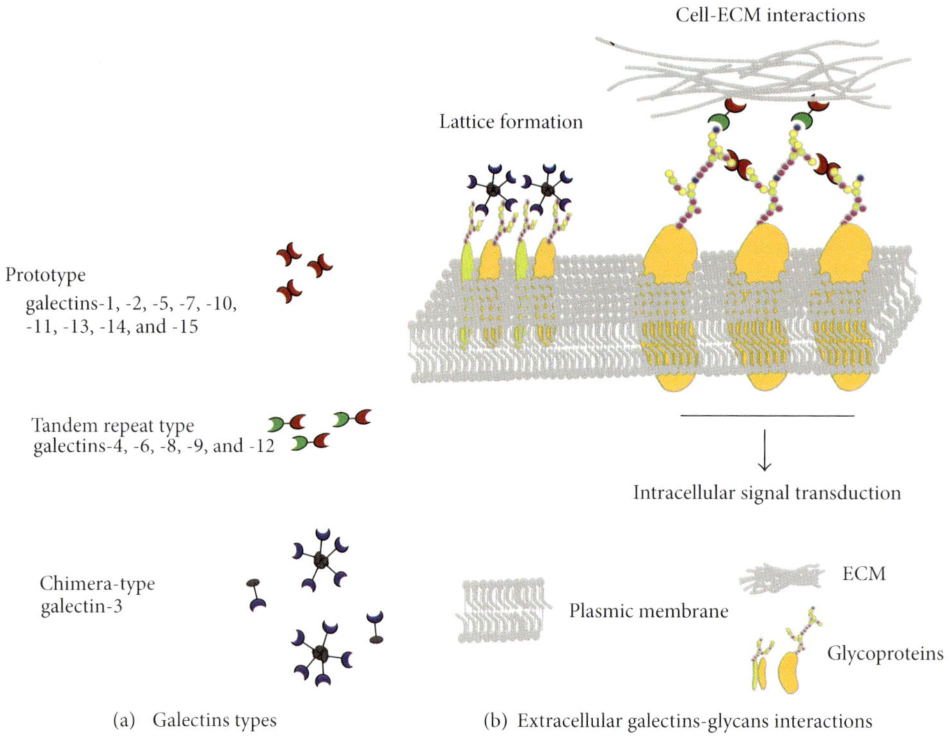

Figure 1: Interactions of galectins with extracellular glycoconjugates.

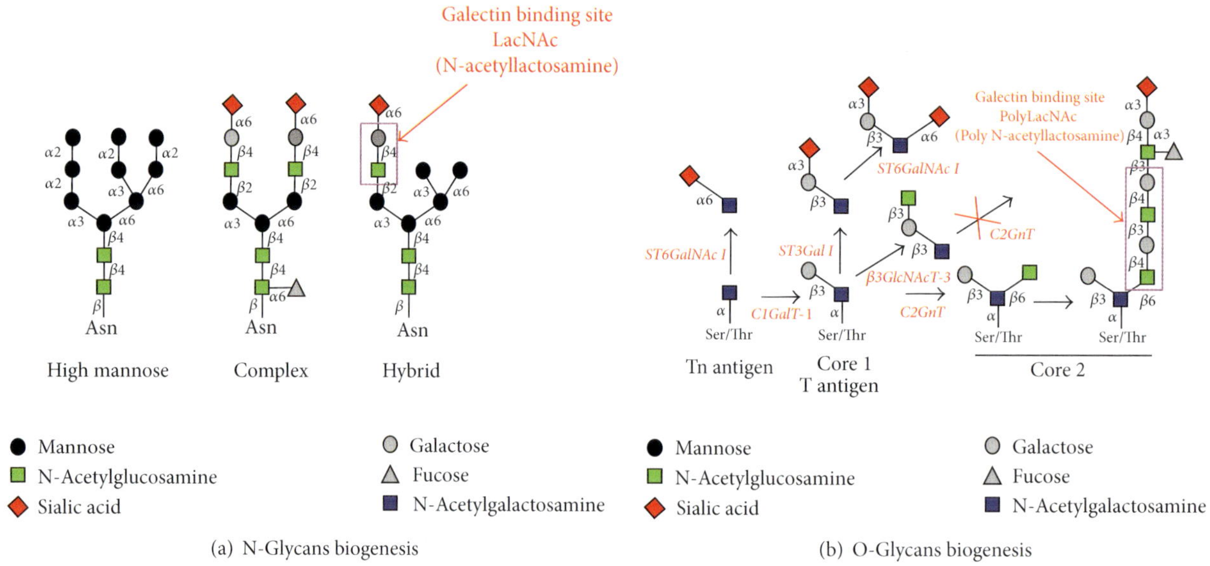

Figure 2: Glycans biogenesis and galectins recognition. (a) N-Glycans and (b) O-Glycans.

significantly decreased in primary carcinoma and metastatic disease compared with normal and premalignant tissue, suggesting that loss of Gal-3 expression may be associated with the evolution of the disease [52]. Additionally, analyses of the Gal-1 expression in 148 human primary PCa samples by IHC revealed that this Gal was not detected in normal, PIN, or carcinoma cells but accumulated in the stroma, including associated fibroblasts. Gal-1 was significantly increased in the tumor-associated stroma compared with the nonneoplastic gland-associated stroma in more than 21% of the cases. The authors hypothesized that the accumulation of Gal-1 in the stroma of malignant tissue may indicate both a possible role for this Gal in the acquisition of an invasive phenotype and poor prognosis [53].

Furthermore, alteration in the nuclear/cytoplasmic expression ratio of Gal-3 correlates with PCa progression [54], and decreasing expression of Gal-3 in benign, adjacent-benign, and tumor tissues suggests that Gal-3 expression

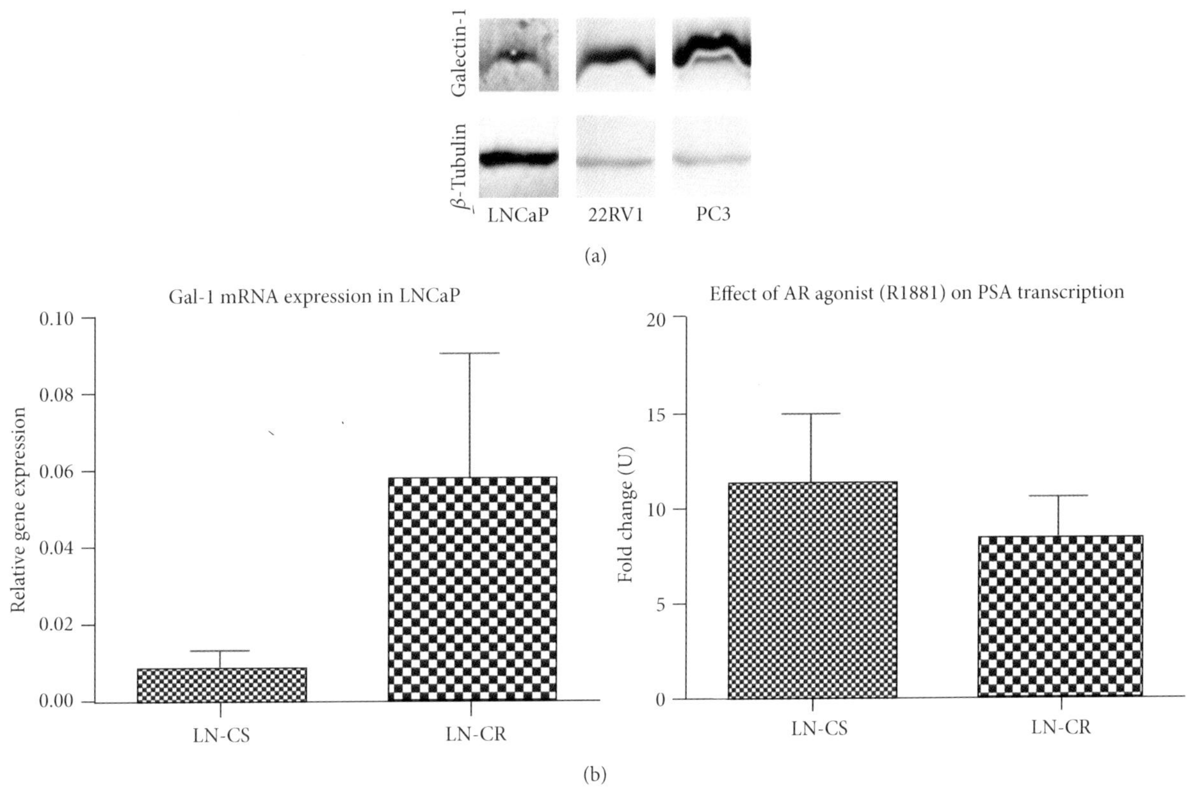

Figure 3: Galectin-1 expression in LNCaP cells. (a) Protein levels of Gal-1 in castration sensitive LNCaP and castration resistant 22Rv1 and PC-3 PCa cell lines. (b) Transcriptional levels of Gal-1 in castration sensitive (CS) or resistant (CR) LNCaP cells. Induction of prostate specific antigen (PSA) in response to androgen receptor agonist (R18.81; 3 days, 10^{-10} M) is shown in both cases as fold change between cultures in absence of hormones and in presence of R18.81. Cells were cultured in absence of hormones (medium complemented with 10% stripped charcoal-treated serum) for 48 h and then cultured for 3 days in absence or presence of R18.81 (10^{-10} M) before mRNA extraction and RT-qPCR for Gal-1 and PSA expression analyses.

could be useful for predicting biochemical recurrence [55]. Moreover, Raz's group was the first to show Gal-3 as a cell adhesion molecule involved in tumor progression [29]. In this study, IHC analysis revealed that Gal-3 is cleaved during the progression of PCa, implicating this Gal both as a diagnostic marker and therapeutic target for future disease treatments [29]. Not only Gal-3 expression levels but also its cleavage by matrix metalloprotease (MMP)-2/-9 are related to both breast and prostate cancers and are responsible for tumor growth, angiogenesis, and apoptosis resistance in mouse models [48]. Increased chemotaxis, invasion, and interactions with endothelial cells resulting in angiogenesis and morphologic changes are induced by transfecting BT-459, a Gal-3 negative breast cancer cell line, with either cleavable full-length Gal-3 or its fragmented peptides [48]. Additionally, amino acids 1–62 and 33–250 from cleaved Gal-3 were identified to stimulate migration and morphogenesis of endothelial cells. Thus, cleavage of the aminoterminus of Gal-3 followed by its release in the tumor microenvironment leads in part to breast cancer angiogenesis and progression [48]. In PCa, Gal-3 functions are dependent on both its localization [30] and posttranslational modifications such as cleavage and phosphorylation. Gal-3 can be phosphorylated at Tyr-107 by c-Abl and then cleaved between Tyr107 and Gly108 by prostate-specific antigen (PSA) [49]. Similarities in the role of cleaved Gal-3 with breast cancer could be postulated: Gal-3 cleavage results in loss of lectin multivalency while preserving its carbohydrate binding activity. The authors also showed that Tyr-107 phosphorylation by c-Abl affects Gal-3 cleavage by PSA and influences the localization and role of this lectin in PCa [49].

An evaluation of Gal-3 expression in tissue microarrays prepared from 83 tumor, 78 adjacent-benign, and 75 benign tissues obtained from 83 patients who had undergone prostatectomy for clinically localized PCa suggests that the expression of this lectin could be used as predictor of biochemical recurrence [55]. In this study, multivariate analysis (including age, Gleason score, T stage, seminal vesicle invasion, or pre-operative PSA and Gal-3 staining) demonstrated nuclear and cytoplasmic localization of Gal-3 in benign, adjacent-benign and tumor tissues with a significant decrease of its expression from benign to adjacent-benign, and to tumor tissues. These results convincingly demonstrate that Gal-3 staining intensity correlates with biochemical recurrence.

As Gal-1 and Gal-3 are the two best studied Gal members in cancer and particularly in PCa, we wondered if other Gals could show a particular profile of expression. As Gals play fundamental, although divergent, roles in diverse tumor

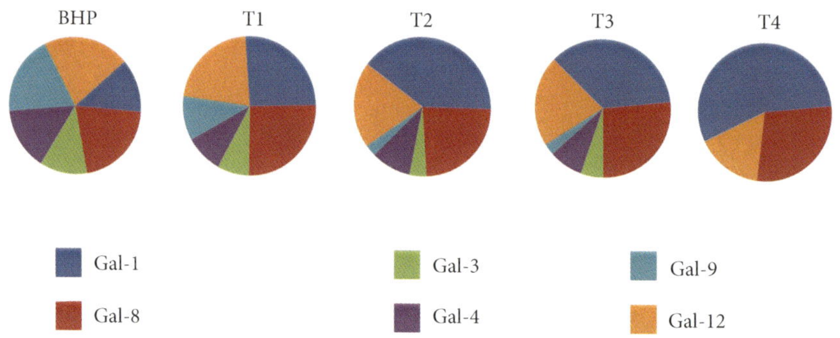

FIGURE 4: Profile of expression of galectins through PCa evolution. Radical prostatectomies were classified according to TNM scale. Specimens ($n = 61$) covered all stages of prostate cancer evolution, including T1 (tumor detected in less or 5% of the tissue), T2 (tumor confined to the prostate), T3 (tumor that extends beyond the prostatic capsule), and T4 (tumor that invades structures other than seminal vesicles), in addition to BHP. Immunohistochemistry was conducted on paraffin-embedded tissue samples as previously described [23]. The figure shows proportional expression of each Gal at different stages of PCa.

microenvironments [57], identification of the "galectin-specific signature" of PCa is critical for diagnostic, prognostic, and therapeutic purposes. For this, we decided to study the expression of almost all Gals in human prostate cancer cells. Firstly, in order to delineate the Gal expression profile of PCa progression, we examined the Gal transcriptional pattern of several human PCa cell lines, which are representative of different stages of the disease. These include LNCaP and castration-resistant cell lines 22Rvl or PC-3, which either express or do not express the androgen receptor (AR), respectively, and display a more aggressive behavior *in vivo* [58–60]. Total RNA was extracted in the log phase of growth in culture and analyzed by quantitative RT-PCR. Remarkably, Gal-1 was found to be the most abundantly expressed Gal in all cells analyzed and its expression was higher in those PCa cells exhibiting a more aggressive behavior *in vivo*. Gal-8 mRNA, which has been postulated as a PCa marker [42, 61], was found to be ubiquitously expressed, although being at modest levels in all cell lines tested. Gal-3 mRNA was only detected in androgen-independent, AR negative PC-3 cells. Transcripts for all other Gal family members (Gal-2, -4, -7, -9, -10, and 13), however, were found to be expressed at very low levels. To further delineate "the galectin-specific PCa signature," we profiled expression of Gals at the protein level (mainly focusing on those members of the family showing higher transcriptional levels). Immunocytochemical analysis of PCa cells confirmed that Gal-1 is the most abundantly expressed Gal in all PCa cells analyzed showing a pronounced upregulation in stages of more aggressive behavior. On the other hand, Gal-3 was predominantly expressed in the PC-3 cell line, and Gals-8 and -9 showed the modest expression in all cell lines analyzed. In agreement with transcriptional profiles, other Gal family members showed lower levels of protein expression. Altogether, these results indicate a fine regulation of Gal expression, mostly at the transcriptional level, in PCa cells characterized by distinct phenotypes, hormone-dependence, and aggressive behavior [23].

The differential expression of Gals in PCa cell lines prompted us to investigate the profile of these lectins in biopsies obtained from 60 patients naive of any therapeutic treatment. Samples were classified according to TNM classification (UICC, 2002). A large spectrum of PCa phases, T1, T2, T3, and T4 in addition to a benign stage (BHP), were represented. Gal expression was analyzed by IHC in paraffin embedded tissue samples. These results are summarized in Figure 4 and show the evolution of the expression of Gals, essentially Gals-1, -3, -4, -8, -9, and -12 during the progression of PCa. Similar to tumor cell lines, Gal-1 exhibited the highest expression levels which increased progressively during tumor evolution towards more aggressive stages. Further analysis revealed that, in addition to its expression in tumor cells, Gal-1 is also expressed, although at a lower levels, in tumor-associated stroma and normal adjacent tissue. These findings broaden the results reported previously by Ellerhorst et al. [52] and Clausse et al. [24], who showed selective Gal-1 expression in endothelial cells (EC) in PCa. On the other hand, although typically expressed at lower levels, Gals-3, -4, -9, and -12 gradually decrease as the disease advances. Conversely, Gal-8 was highly expressed, but no apparent regulation could be observed during disease progression. Thus, a "galectin-specific signature" characterized by up-, down-, or nonregulated family members delineates PCa progression in patients biopsies, suggesting novel biomarkers of disease evolution. Particularly, we show for the first time Gal-1 expression as a hallmark of PCa aggressiveness, suggesting a major target for anticancer therapies [23]. These changes on Gal profiles may have important impacts on tumor biology as they are reported to affect several cellular processes, developed in the following chapters.

4. Effects of Galectins on Apoptosis

Galectins have contrasting effects on apoptosis. While Gal-1 is an apoptosis promoter, Gal-3 shows both pro- or anti-apoptotic effects depending on its subcellular localization in PCa. For instance, induction of differentiation and apoptosis by butyrate was investigated in four human PCa cell lines including LNCaP [21]. Treatment of PCa cells with butyrate resulted in increased Gal-1 expression in a time- and dose-dependent manner followed by induction of apoptosis. As

LNCaP cells do not express (or express low levels of) Gal-1, transfection with a Gal-1 expression vector inhibits LNCaP cell growth and increases the apoptosis rate. Therefore, Gal-1 may function downstream in the pathway of butyrate-induced differentiation and apoptosis [21].

It is well demonstrated that Gal-1 could act extracellularly to induce apoptosis in glycopermissive cells [62]. In PCa, Gal-1-induced apoptosis is highly dependent on the O-glycosylation of cells. Expression of alpha-2,3-sialyltransferase-1 blocks O-glycans elongation and protects LNCaP subclone from Gal-1-induced apoptosis [22]. This original work shows that the expression of Gal *per se* is not the final determinant of cell apoptosis; instead, regulation of lectin expression and the glycan repertoire determines the final phenotype, sensitivity, or resistance to apoptosis induction.

In an opposite way, Gal-3 has a dual role in controlling cell apoptosis depending on the PCa cell model. To study whether Gal-3 regulates drug-induced apoptosis, Raz's group either transfected LNCaP cells with Gal-3 or silenced Gal-3 expression in PC-3 cells. They tested sensitivity to cis-diamminedichloroplatinum and showed apoptosis induction in Gal-3 expressing LNCaP, more precisely through inhibition of cytochrome c release and caspase-3 activation [28]. On the contrary, Gal-3 knockdown in PC-3 cells leads to cell-cycle arrest at G(1) phase, upregulation of nuclear p21, and hypophosphorylation of the retinoblastoma tumor suppressor protein (pRb), with no effect on cyclin D1, cyclin E, cyclin-dependent kinases (CDK2 and CDK4), and p27 protein expression levels [29].

More interestingly, Gal-3 also shows a dual role upon its subcellular localization promoting or alternatively inhibiting apoptosis in Gal-3 transfected LNCaP cells. While nuclear Gal-3 targeting allowed by fusion with nuclear localization sequences was found to have proapoptotic properties, the cytoplasmic form is antiapoptotic and promotes tumor progression [30]. These results clearly demonstrate a fine participation of Gals in the control of survival and proliferation processes in tumor cells.

5. Galectins in Cancer Cell Adhesion and Metastasis

During tumor progression, malignant cells acquire the ability to overcome cell-cell adhesion and invade surrounding tissues, a state known as metastatic disease. It is important to understand this process and identify inducers of tumor metastasis in order to develop treatments that target metastatic cells for long-term tumor regression.

Galectin-1 is involved in numerous biological functions including capillaries formation. Gal-1 is expressed by endothelial cells (EC) from capillaries infiltrating the tumor tissue in 64% of the cases of 100 human prostate carcinoma samples, but in only few cases (7%) in endothelial cells in the adjacent nontumoral stroma. These results strongly suggest that tumor cells induce Gal-1-expressing EC allowing tumor adhesion to vessel endothelium. To verify this hypothesis, Clausse and colleagues incubated HUVECs cells with conditioned media from PC-3 or DU145 prostate carcinoma cells and they observed a significant increase of Gal-1 protein expression. Additionally, both PC-3 conditioned medium and recombinant Gal-1 induced increased PC-3 cells adhesion to EC, while conditioned media complemented by an anti-Gal-1 antiserum abolished this modulation [24]. It is important to note that no cell adhesion to EC was observed when normal lymphocytes were used instead of PC-3 cells under the same conditions. This places Gal-1 as a molecular link of the specific EC/tumor interaction and suggests an additional tumor-based immune escape mechanism. In the same way, expression of Gal-1 in the cell surface of LNCaP also showed the lectin ability to modulate adhesion to the ECM [25] revealing a general function of Gal-1 in PCa cell-matrix interactions.

Capillary formation is essential for tumors to obtain nutriments as well as for migration and the metastasis process. Interactions of metastatic cancer cells with blood vessels are critical during early stages of cancer metastasis but also in the lodge of tumor cells in specific organs and tissues. In 2005, Glinskii and colleagues demonstrated that mechanical entrapment alone, in the absence of tumor cell adhesion to blood vessel walls, is not sufficient for metastatic cell arrest in the microvasculature of the target organ. The analysis of the frequency and location of fluorescent tumor cells in different organs and tissues following intravenous inoculation revealed that PCa cells go into a wide variety of tissues and organs but not to the lung capillary bed. Results showed that arrest of metastatic cells in target organ microvessels is not a consequence of mechanical trapping, but is supported predominantly by intercellular adhesive interactions mediated by cancer-associated Thomsen-Friedenreich (TF) antigen and Gal-3 [35]. Additionally, carbohydrate moieties of the TF antigen (Galβ1,3GalNAc) on the surface of endothelial cells could be efficiently recognized by Gal-3, thus priming them for harboring metastatic cancer cells [34].

In mCRPC, bones are a privilege site for the metastatic disease that causes osteoblastic growth. However, the mechanisms that contribute to bone metastasis are poorly understood. It was suggested that the bone provides a favorable environment for PCa cells growth and that tumor cells preferentially bind to bone marrow EC. To verify this hypothesis, cancer cell adhesion to a human bone marrow endothelial (HBME-1) cell and EC lines from other organs was assessed. *In vitro*, PCa cells adhered preferentially to HBME-1 when compared with endothelium derived from other sources, and this adhesion was inhibited by anti-Gal-3 and anti-LFA-1 sera [36]. These data showed that bone metastasis of PCa cells is essentially caused by their preferential binding to bone marrow endothelial cell and in part mediated by cell-cell adhesion via Gal-3 [36]. As in non-small-cell lung cancer, collagen XXIII is a transmembrane protein previously shown to be upregulated, at least in part, through Gal-3, and whose expression facilitates metastases formation in PCa model [37]. This suggests a potential role for collagen XXIII in combination with Gal-3 in mediating metastasis by facilitating cell-cell and cell-matrix adhesion as well as anchorage-independent cell growth.

Being currently incurable, PCa metastasis has a remarkable ability to spread to the skeleton. Advanced PCa cells are essentially characterized by bone metastasis that predominantly causes an osteolytic phenotype. In a PC-3 cellular model, it has been shown that both the conditioned media from these PCa cells containing Gal-1 and recombinant Gal-1 inhibited the osteoblastic proliferation and differentiation of human bone marrow stromal (hBMS) cells. Thus, the authors hypothesized that Gal-1 could be involved in the osteoblastic response caused by PCa cells metastasizing to the bone, by affecting the matrix mineralization [26]. To date, studies in animal models still fail to demonstrate the role of Gal-1 in PCa metastasis process.

Gal-3 is the only member of this family of lectins that was studied *in vivo*: Gal-3 expression drives spontaneous metastasis using rat PCa models such as Dunning or Copenhagen rat [38]. The oral administration of modified citrus pectin (MCP, pH-modified), a soluble component of plant fiber derived from citrus fruit, revealed inhibition of cell-cell interactions mediated by cell surface carbohydrate-binding Gal-3 molecules. In fact, the presence of Gal-3 in Dunning PCa cell lines (MAT-LyLu cells) and primary human prostate carcinoma was demonstrated by immunoblotting and IHC. Lung metastatic colonies were observed after subcutaneous injections of MAT-LyLu cells in posterior legs of male Copenhagen rats, while continuous administration of MCP in drinking water reduced the number of lung metastases. MCP had no effect on the growth of the primary tumors suggesting that the reduction of lung metastases was caused by both interference with migration or tumor adhesion such as cell adhesion to EC, and the spreading of tumor cells. As MCP is not an exclusive inhibitor of Gal-3, further studies are still required to specifically target this galectin and determine its role in normal and cancerous prostate tissues and the ability of Gal-3 targeting to inhibit prostate metastasis in animal models. As we previously described, interactions mediated by the cancer-associated TF glycoantigen and Gal-3 play an important role in several rate-limiting steps of cancer metastasis such as cell adhesion to bone marrow endothelium, homotypic tumor cell aggregation, and clonogenic survival and growth [34, 35], and it was only recently shown that Gal-3 influences bone metastasis in a mouse model after intracardiac injection of luciferase-expressing PC-3 cells in nude mice [39]. Indirect targeting of Gal-3 by using daily intraperitoneal administration of Lac-l-Leu, which binds and inhibits Gals by mimicking essential structural features of the TF-Ag, affects PCa cell adhesion to bone marrow endothelium, homotypic aggregation, transendothelial migration, clonogenic growth, and final spreading of tumor cells to the skeleton [39]. These results were recently confirmed by others demonstrating inhibition of tumor-endothelial cell interactions and lung metastasis using TFD100 (a purified glycopeptide acting as competitor in Gal-3 binding to TF-Ag on the surface of most cancer cells [33]), or using MCP in combination with other drugs such as ProstaCaid [41]. Altogether, they highlight the impact of Gal-3 on invasive behavior in human PCa cells *in vitro*. As Gal-3 is not expressed in advanced stages of the disease, other factors act to promote spreading of tumor cells and have to be identified to attempt to cure mCRPC patients.

Galectin-8 was initially called Prostate Cancer Tumor Antigen-1 (PCTA-1) because of its exclusive expression in neoplastic prostate cells and its absence in normal prostate tissue. In fact, Gal-8 levels of expression positively correlate with certain human neoplasms [42]. Gal-8, like other galectins, is a regulator of cell adhesion depending on its formulation. Thus, immobilized protein acts as a potent matrix protein in promoting cell adhesion by ligation and clustering of a selective subset of cell surface integrin receptors and triggering signaling cascades including Tyr phosphorylation of focal adhesion kinase and paxillin [63]. In contrast, when present in excess as a soluble ligand, Gal-8 forms complexes with integrin that negatively regulates cell adhesion and tumor properties such as growth and metastasis [43]. No current evidence exists about these potential roles of Gal-8 in animal models to understand why Gal-8 is only expressed in prostate tissue at neoplastic stages.

Interestingly, glycosyltransferase-mediated regulation of carbohydrate expression on cell membrane-glycoconjugates has been recently shown to be involved in migration and invasion properties of the PC-3 cell line. It is well known that Gals link to tri- and tetrabranched N-glycans forming multivalent lattices that enhance cell surface residency of growth factor receptors and focal adhesion turnover. Silencing N-acetylglucosaminyltransferase I (MGAT1, the first enzyme of N-glycans biogenesis) by RNA interference in PC-3 was enough to inhibit cell invasion by affection of focal adhesion and microfilament organization, thus generating a less motile phenotype. More importantly, orthotopic injection of MGAT1-silenced PC-3 in nude mice revealed a decrease in primary tumor growth and poor incidence of lung metastases as well [64]. Not only N-glycans should be considered as potential regulators of Gal functions in PCa but also O-glycosylation confers LNCaP cells susceptibility to Gal-1-induced apoptosis [22].

6. Galectins as Inducers of Tumor Angiogenesis

Cancer metastasis involves a series of steps including angiogenesis, detachment of tumor cells from the primary tumor, intravasation, evasion of host defense, arrest and attachment at a distant site, extravasation, dormant survival, and establishment of new growth. During extravasation, tumor cells bind to endothelial cells through protein, carbohydrate interactions and penetrate through the endothelium and basement membrane. Besides providing tumors with nutrients, newly formed capillaries constitute a potential escape route for tumor cells, thus favoring metastatic dissemination, and also provide an access to host immune cells.

Analysis of Gal-1 expression in EC from 100 PCa patients who had undergone a radical prostatectomy for localized prostate cancer (Gleason score from 2 to 10) revealed increased frequency of Gal-1 expression in capillaries infiltrating the tumor compared to those present in the non tumoral adjacent tissue [24]. Although EC do express Gal-1, *in vitro* culture of HUVEC cells in normal medium complemented by conditional media from PC-3 or DU145 led to enhanced Gal-1 expression in EC [24]. These results demonstrate that secreted factors from tumor cells influence

Gal-1 expression in capillaries cells and promote specific attachment of tumor cells to EC. This heterotypic cell interaction is essentially due to Gal-1 produced by tumor cells as Gal-1 blocking antibodies inhibited this effect [24]. However, further experiments are required to unveil the role of this interaction in the evolution of the disease.

Because Gal-1 expression is associated with PCa aggressiveness and has emerged as a novel proangiogenic factor in other tumor types [65, 66], we decided to further examine whether expression of this lectin correlates with the frequency of blood vessels in low grade or high grade human PCa [23]. For this purpose, we evaluated coexpression of Gal-1 and CD34 by IHC analysis of a human PCa tissue array comprised of 29 paired cores of invasive PCa. A positive correlation between Gal-1 and CD34 was selectively detected in arrays of human PCa, but not in arrays of human breast cancer which served as control, suggesting a tissue-specific proangiogenic effect of this lectin in cancer. This selectivity is consistent with the ability of Gal-1 to induce angiogenesis of oligodendroglioma [65], B16 melanoma [67], and Kaposi's sarcoma [68], but not Lewis lung carcinoma [69]. This correlation between Gal-1 expression and the number of blood vessels was also verified when the tumor compartment was compared to nonmalignant areas and was even more pronounced in high grade compared to low grade tumors [23]. Complementary to what was previously reported by Clausse and colleagues [24], we demonstrated that tumor cells are the major source of Gal-1. While some inconsistencies are observed between studies addressing the relative expression of Gal-1 by stroma versus tumor cells probably by differences in methodological approaches, its functional impact on other cancers such as melanoma or lung carcinoma was elegantly assessed in mice by comparing the functionality of these cellular compartments under Gal-1 deficiency or wildtype conditions. Those results clearly demonstrated tumor as the main Gal-1 source in controlling tumor growth [69]. Another possibility that must be taken into consideration is the hypothesis that EC are able to capt tumor derived-Gal-1 through mechanisms that must be fully understood [67].

Given the promising therapeutic value of anti-angiogenic strategies in advanced androgen-refractory PCa [70], we were prompted to examine the role of Gal-1 in PCa angiogenesis. We first evaluated the effect of conditioned medium obtained from 22Rv1 (PCa CM), a Gal-1-positive PCa cell line, on *in vitro* tubulogenesis. PCa CM induced the formation of tubular-like structures when added to EC. The involvement of Gal-1 in this process was assessed by using an anti-Gal-1 neutralizing mAb, which considerably reduced the formation of these structures [23]. These *in vitro* effects of Gal-1-expressing PCa cells on endothelial cell morphogenesis prompted us to investigate the role of this lectin in angiogenesis *in vivo*. Our experimental approach consisted in the s.c. injection of 22Rv1 PCa cells in Matrigel plugs. Importantly, we were able to differentiate the source of Gal-1 (tumor and microenvironment versus tumor alone): firstly, a blocking anti-Gal-1 mAb was added to the mix (total Gal-1 inhibition independently of its source is to be expected); alternatively, we used 22Rv1 tumor cells transduced with a human specific Gal-1 shRNA-coding lentivirus (thus inhibiting tumoral Gal-1 expression alone). A marked reduction of microvessel density was observed using both experimental approaches, indicating that tumor cells are the main source of Gal-1, at least at early time points of tumor implantation and neovascularization. Confirming this reasoning, intermediate effects were observed when Gal-1 was partially downregulated in PCa cells. Altogether, these *in vitro* and *in vivo* results reveal a key role of Gal-1 in PCa-induced angiogenesis. More importantly, we showed that *in vivo* silencing of Gal-1 expression by tumor cells does not interfere with other pro- or anti-angiogenic factors such as VEGF or thrombospondin and bFGF, revealing the preponderant role of Gal-1 in promoting PCa neovascularization and suggesting Gal-1 as a new potent target for clinic therapeutic approaches in advanced PCa patients [23].

Gal-3 could also act as an angiogenic inducer by recognizing the TF disaccharide antigen present on the surface of most cancer cells. Using a purified glycopeptide TFD100 that binds Gal-3 with picomolar affinity, the authors blocked Gal-3-mediated interactions and inhibited angiogenesis of PC-3 tumors in mice [33]. In this PC-3 model, Gal-4 and Gal-9 also efficiently bind to TFD100 and thus are implicated in PCa. Consequently, silencing of these molecules causes strong reduction of *in vitro* tubulogenesis and VEGF-induced blood vessels formation in Matrigel plug assays [33]. Altogether, these results highlight a major role of the interactions between Gals and their corresponding glycoligands in determining tumor-associated angiogenesis.

7. Galectins as Immune Tolerance Inducers in Prostate Cancer

An efficient immune response against pathogens or tumors needs effective egress of lymphocytes from the blood into the target tissue. This process is allowed in part by specific EC proteins promoting lymphocyte adhesion to and migration across endothelium. Other molecules negatively regulate transendothelial migration of lymphocytes. Gal-1 is one of the best studied members that acts as inducer of immune tolerance in cancer [10]. As it was previously showed, Gal-1 expression could be induced in EC by neighbor tumor cells [24], but it is well known that this lectin could regulate the inflammatory setting, modulating T cell cytokine production and triggering T-cell death [17, 27]. Migration of T-cell lines through Matrigel is inhibited by EC treated with either PCa conditioned media containing Gal-1 or with Matrigel coated with recombinant Gal-1. This inhibition is reverted by using an anti-Gal-1 serum, demonstrating that transendothelial migration of T cells is negatively regulated by Gal-1-producing EC. More importantly, the inhibition is due to decreased adhesion of T-cells to Gal-1 expressing EC rather than T cell death. In fact, T-cell treatment with benzyl-a-GalNAc, which reduces core 2 O-glycan expression thus blocking Gal-1 recognition, inhibits Gal-1-induced T cell death. Polarization of CD43 molecule on T cells is essential for T cell migration. Interestingly, Gal-1-coated ECM enhanced clustering of CD43, which contributes to the inhibitory effect on T-cell migration [27]. The role of Gals as active controllers of immunological tolerance in PCa is a field that is still open to new discoveries.

8. Galectins as Molecules with Prognosis and Therapeutic Value in Prostate Cancer: From Animal Models to Clinical Settings

PCa is curable only when detected in its early stages as a result of both prostate-specific antigen (PSA) blood test screening and digital rectal exam. When patients suffer from metastatic disease and undergo mCRPC, docetaxel-based combination chemotherapy is the only available therapy that has demonstrated a survival benefit in 50% of these advanced stages of PCa. Moreover, FDA approved new therapies, most are being evaluated on clinical trials and are based on targeting the angiogenesis, the tumor microenvironment, or immunotherapy [71]. All these drugs showed improved overall survival (OS) of the mCRPC patients for 3–5 months. One of these drugs is PROVENGE (sipuleucel-T), a dendritic cell-based immunotherapy targeting the prostatic acid phosphate (PAP), an antigen expressed in more than 95% of PCa [72]. The treatment consists in *ex-vivo* loading of autologous dendritic cells with the recombinant antigen which is PAP-GM-CSF: chimera of PAP and the granulocyte-macrophage colony-stimulating factor (GM-CSF), an immune adjuvant. This new treatment is only intended for men with asymptomatic or minimally symptomatic and metastasized PCa that are resistant to standard hormone treatment. In controlled and multicenter clinical trials, several adverse events have been reported in the PROVENGE group, which include acute infusion reactions (occurring within 1 day of infusion) and cerebrovascular events. The most common adverse events (incidence $\geq$ 15%) reported were chills, fatigue, fever, back pain, nausea, joint ache, and headache [73].

Xtandi (enzalutamide), an androgen receptor antagonist, is a new PCa treatment approved by FDA in August 2012 to treat mCRPC patients, with spreading or recurred cancer even with medical or surgical therapy and resistant to docetaxel-based chemotherapy.

Finally, Xofigo was approved by FDA in mid-2013 for patients with CRPC, symptomatic metastases that spread to bones but not to other organs as in visceral metastatic disease. Xofigo binds with minerals in the bone to deliver radiation directly to bone tumors, limiting the damage to the surrounding normal tissues. Xofigo is an alpha particle-emitting radioactive therapeutic agent (radium-223 dichloride). The most common side effects were nausea, diarrhea, vomiting, swelling of the leg, ankle, or foot, and blood cells abnormalities with less than 5 months of improved OS.

Therefore, it is critical to identify new molecular targets to efficiently cure advanced cancers. A limited number of studies consider potential implications of individual Gals in the modulation of the metastatic process, yet the role of these essential proteins *in vivo* is still unclear. Under this scenario, a more deeply comprehension of the influence of Gals in evolution of PCa could help to define new drugs that treat advanced and mCRPC patients. For instance, the ratio of phosphorylated/dephosphorylated Gal-3 might be used as a complementary value to that of PSA for prognosis of PCa [49].

From a therapeutic point of view, Gal-3 has been conjugated to the chemotherapy drug 5-Fluoracil and delivered to PC-3 tumors by using a copolymer system named Gal-3-targeted HPMA copolymer-(G3-C12-)5-Fluorouracil conjugates. This drug showed *in vitro* inhibition of PC-3 cell migration after wounding and displayed a potent antitumor activity against PC-3 tumor xenografts in *nude* mice [40].

Drug resistance is a major obstacle for PCa therapy, but its underlying mechanisms are not clear, especially in patients with advanced stages of the disease. A comparative proteomic profiling of camptothecin- (CPT-) resistant PC-3 and CPT-sensitive LNCaP human PCa cell lines identified a signature of 144 proteins with different expression levels between the two cell lines that are suggested to contribute to the development of drug resistance [74]. In this respect, Gal-3 is highly expressed in PC-3 cells, whereas it is not detectable in LNCaP. The expression level of these proteins and/or mRNAs could be a useful parameter to evaluate chemotherapy resistance in clinical specimens of PCa [74]. The same conclusion was drawn when Gal-3 silencing induced increased cisplatin-induced apoptosis of PC-3 cells [31]. Resistance to apoptosis is a critical feature of neoplastic cells; Gal-3 either inhibits anticancer drug-induced apoptosis or promotes cell death depending on its subcellular localization. These findings suggest that Gal-3 targeting could improve the efficacy of anticancer drug chemotherapy in PCa [28]. In fact, Gal-3 presents a domain like NWGR anti-death motif of Bcl-2 family which confers antiapoptotic properties through regulation of Bad protein and suppression of the mitochondrial apoptosis pathway [75]. Thus, Gal-3 shows multifunctional oncogenic functions such as the regulation of tumor proliferation, angiogenesis and apoptosis. In this sense, sensibility to proapoptotic agents like cis-platin and etoposide is higher in Gal-3 negative PCa cell lines than in Gal-3 expressing cells [28, 32]. These observations imply that Gal-3 inhibits anticancer drug-induced apoptosis and, consequently, Gal-3 targeting could improve the efficacy of anticancer drug chemotherapy in PCa. However, as Gal-3 is only expressed in early but not in late stages, it is unlikely that this kind of treatment could serve as new curative options for mCRPC patients.

Recently, we confirmed pioneer studies of Gal-1 as a tumoral marker of poor prognosis for PCa patients [53], and we showed a regulated expression of several Gals with diagnostic value. In fact, strong increase of Gal-1, decrease of Gals-4, -9, and -12, and gradual decrease to complete extinction of Gal-3 expressions could define the stage of PCa progression using IHC as a simple method to analyse Gal expression in available patients samples (Figure 4 and [23]). As shown in Figure 4, comparison of Gal expression could define PCa patient stage: T1, T2-T3, and T4; however, while T1 and T4 could be easily identified, it appears difficult to differentiate T2 to T3 stages since Gal profile is similar between these two intermediate stages.

Galectins are not only shown to be involved in anti-apoptotic functions and edition of immune tolerance; several studies clearly revealed their proangiogenic functions in cancers [68, 76–78]. Interactions of metastatic cancer cells with vascular endothelium are critical during early stages of cancer metastasis. Various investigations, not developed in this review due to space limitations, showed Gals as angiogenic-regulatory proteins. For instance, Gal-3 was suggested as a new target to treat breast cancer patients [34], and Gal-8 as a new modulator of EC migration and angiogenesis [79]. In the case of PCa, we recently demonstrated that Gal-1 is the principal inducer of neoangiogenesis [23] and could be used as a novel target for anti-angiogenic therapies in human advanced PCa.

9. Conclusion

While localized PCa can be cured, metastatic and advanced prostate cancers pose a significant therapeutic challenge. We and others identified a "galectin-regulated signature" as new prognostic markers and molecular targets of novel therapeutic avenues for preventing metastasis. Tumor metastasis is a multistep process involving several cellular and molecular interactions. Recognition of glycoconjugates by galectins regulates tumor behavior through both intrinsic as well as extrinsic signals involving modulation of homotypic cell aggregation, tumor cell apoptosis, angiogenesis, and tumor immune escape [9]. In fact, Gal-1 expression regulates prostate tumor cell resistance to apoptosis before becoming castration resistant [22]. As shown in breast cancer, Gal-3 containing NWGR amino acid domain sequence as bcl-2 gene family also could act as antiapoptotic protein independently of Bcl-2, Bcl-X_L, or Bax proteins [80]. Thus, both Gals may contribute to tumor survival and to the selection process that is characteristic of the evolution of this type of cancer. However, not only the tumor itself but also the surrounding tissues and the complex network of stromal, endothelial, and immune cells that interact within the tumor microenvironment should be considered. In this respect, cancer cells not only control the expression of their own Gals but also modulate Gal expression in environmental tissues [24]. Gals regulate cell-cell and cell-ECM interactions. Surprisingly, different members of the family elicit particular and sometimes antagonic effects. In fact, anti-Gal-3 monoclonal antibodies (mAbs) prevent the adhesion of prostate tumor cells to bone marrow endothelial cells [36]. In addition, Gal-1 increases, while Gal-8 reduces tumor cell-ECM interactions [52, 63, 81]. Altogether, these effects may contribute to shaping a favorable tumor microenvironment that allows distant dissemination of transformed cells.

Despite these observations, there are relatively few *in vivo* studies addressing the source and function of Gals and exploring these phenotypes in PCa [35, 38, 82, 83]. In fact, expression levels of Gals-1 and -3 were reported to be associated with the growth and metastatic properties of prostate tumors and may correlate with a poor prognosis [24, 35, 38, 52, 82, 84]. During the last two decades, Gal-3 was the only member of the family whose role has been addressed using *in vivo* experimental models. A key role of this glycan-binding protein in the formation of spontaneous metastasis was demonstrated using peptide inhibitors in experimental animal models of PCa [38, 39]. Moreover, tumor cell expression of Gal-3 has been shown to delineate the transition from benign prostate glands to hormone-resistant malignant disease [84], and its regulated expression is associated with promoter methylation [85]. Silencing Gal-3 results in decreased migration, invasion, and proliferation of PCa cells [29]. Taking into consideration these results, Gal-3 emerges as a key lectin that plays an essential role in the formation of metastases but not in the progression of advanced disease. Moreover, Gals-1 and -3 were both found in the nucleus of cells [86, 87]. The importance of both Gals in presplicing RNA activity has been demonstrated by depleting these lectins from nuclear extracts, which causes inhibition of the splicing activity [88, 89]. These properties and the relation with other nuclear factors such as splicing or transcriptional factors should be explored in PCa to identify new intracellular partners that could represent new therapeutic targets and signaling pathways as well.

Galectin profile in cancer may be intrinsically determined and consequently considered as biomarkers of cell transformation. In this respect, we can assume that each type of tumor can be associated with characteristic profiles of Gals. Our study on PCa cell lines and patient samples proposes a particular profile of Gals through disease progression [23, 76]. However, tumor cell must be considered in association with its microenvironment. In this respect, most of the cancers are characterized by particular inflammatory processes where bidirectional dialogues between tumor, resident, and infiltrating cells result in changes on cell surface expression of glycans and lectins. It is possible that Gals may be an acute phase reactants produced in response to tumor-associated stress. Under this view, changes in Gal profiles could represent an epiphenomenon due to associations with inflammation. Whatever the real cause/effect, changes in Gal expression may be exploited as accurate tools for diagnosis, prognosis, and probably therapeutic purposes in cancer.

In spite of considerable progress in dissecting the functions of individual Gals, an integrated portrait of the "galectin signature" of the human PCa microenvironment is still missing. In addition, it is not clear which cellular compartment expresses a given Gal and when this expression is required for cancer progression. While only Gals-1 and -3 were extensively studied in PCa, these Gals have been already shown to be potential new factors that participate directly in PCa progression and cancer drug resistance. In fact, Raz's group showed that phosphorylated Gal-3 is responsible for drug resistance in PCa and should be considered as new target to improve efficiency of chemotherapeutic agents such as cisplatin and etoposide [32]. We demonstrated that Gal-1 expressed by the tumor is essential and sufficient to promote neovascularization independently of classical angiogenic pathways. This strongly supports the idea of Gal-1 targeting as a new anti-angiogenic therapy for advanced PCa. Additionally, we showed that Gals-4 and -12 suffered decreased expression through PCa evolution, but the role of these Gals in PCa is a field that lacks a more deeply understanding.

Finally, Gal-8 is another tandem-repeat Gal of importance in PCa. This Gal has been defined first in 1996 [42] and 2000 [61] as PCa biomarkers and six years after as a potential responsible for hereditary PCa [90]. To date, no study has been performed to understand why this particular

Gal is generally expressed in all tissues but it only turned on in neoplasic prostatic tissues and is absent in normal prostate. Despite these important characteristics, studies about the role of Gal-8 in PCa are still missing. Thus, its use as a therapeutic target in this disease should be further explored.

Acknowledgments

The authors apologize to the many authors whose papers could not be cited owing to space limitations. This study is supported by Agencia Nacional de Promoción Científica y Técnica (PICT2008-0134), Association pour la Recherche sur les Tumeurs de la Prostate (ARTP), Fundación Florencio Fiorini, and Consejo Nacional de Investigaciones Científicas y Técnicas (CONICET).

References

[1] A. Jemal, F. Bray, M. M. Center, J. Ferlay, E. Ward, and D. Forman, "Global cancer statistics," *CA Cancer Journal for Clinicians*, vol. 61, no. 2, pp. 69–90, 2011.

[2] S. R. Denmeade and J. T. Isaacs, "A history of prostate cancer treatment," *Nature Reviews Cancer*, vol. 2, no. 5, pp. 389–396, 2002.

[3] N. Taniguchi, K. Nakamura, H. Narimatsu, C.-W. Von Der Lieth, and J. Paulson, "Human disease glycomics/proteome initiative workshop and the 4th HUPO annual congress," *Proteomics*, vol. 6, no. 1, pp. 12–13, 2006.

[4] N. H. Packer, C.-W. Von Der Lieth, K. F. Aoki-Kinoshita et al., "Frontiers in glycomics: bioinformatics and biomarkers in disease: an NIH white paper prepared from discussions by the focus groups at a workshop on the NIH campus, bethesda MD (September 11-13, 2006)," *Proteomics*, vol. 8, no. 1, pp. 8–20, 2008.

[5] J. B. Lowe, "Glycosylation, immunity, and autoimmunity," *Cell*, vol. 104, no. 6, pp. 809–812, 2001.

[6] M. A. Daniels, K. A. Hogquist, and S. C. Jameson, "Sweet 'n' sour: the impact of differential glycosylation on T cell responses," *Nature Immunology*, vol. 3, no. 10, pp. 903–910, 2002.

[7] D. H. Dube and C. R. Bertozzi, "Glycans in cancer and inflammation—potential for therapeutics and diagnostics," *Nature Reviews Drug Discovery*, vol. 4, no. 6, pp. 477–488, 2005.

[8] C. D. Rillahan and J. C. Paulson, "Glycan microarrays for decoding the glycome," *Annual Review of Biochemistry*, vol. 80, pp. 797–823, 2011.

[9] F.-T. Liu and G. A. Rabinovich, "Galectins as modulators of tumour progression," *Nature Reviews Cancer*, vol. 5, no. 1, pp. 29–41, 2005.

[10] G. A. Rabinovich and D. O. Croci, "Regulatory circuits mediated by lectin-glycan interactions in autoimmunity and cancer," *Immunity*, vol. 36, no. 3, pp. 322–335, 2012.

[11] O. B. Garner and L. G. Baum, "Galectin-glycan lattices regulate cell-surface glycoprotein organization and signalling," *Biochemical Society Transactions*, vol. 36, no. 6, pp. 1472–1477, 2008.

[12] D. Compagno, F. Jaworski, L. Gentilini et al., *Galectins: Major Signaling Modulators Inside and Outside the Cell*, 2013.

[13] F. Yu, R. L. Finley Jr., A. Raz, and H.-R. C. Kim, "Galectin-3 translocates to the perinuclear membranes and inhibits cytochrome c release from the mitochondria. A role for synexin in galectin-3 translocation," *The Journal of Biological Chemistry*, vol. 277, no. 18, pp. 15819–15827, 2002.

[14] A. Paz, R. Haklai, G. Elad-Sfadia, E. Ballan, and Y. Kloog, "Galectin-1 binds oncogenic H-ras to mediate ras membrane anchorage and cell transformation," *Oncogene*, vol. 20, no. 51, pp. 7486–7493, 2001.

[15] I. Camby, M. Le Mercier, F. Lefranc, and R. Kiss, "Galectin-1: a small protein with major functions," *Glycobiology*, vol. 16, no. 11, 2006.

[16] M. T. Elola, C. Wolfenstein-Todel, M. F. Troncoso, G. R. Vasta, and G. A. Rabinovich, "Galectins: matricellular glycan-binding proteins linking cell adhesion, migration, and survival," *Cellular and Molecular Life Sciences*, vol. 64, no. 13, pp. 1679–1700, 2007.

[17] G. A. Rabinovich and M. A. Toscano, "Turning 'sweet' on immunity: galectin-glycan interactions in immune tolerance and inflammation," *Nature Reviews Immunology*, vol. 9, no. 5, pp. 338–352, 2009.

[18] R. Y. Yang, G. A. Rabinovich, and F. T. Liu, "Galectins: structure, function and therapeutic potential," *Expert Reviews in Molecular Medicine*, vol. 10, p. e17, 2008.

[19] D. N. W. Cooper, "Galectinomics: finding themes in complexity," *Biochimica et Biophysica Acta*, vol. 1572, no. 2-3, pp. 209–231, 2002.

[20] G. A. Rabinovich, M. A. Toscano, S. S. Jackson, and G. R. Vasta, "Functions of cell surface galectin-glycoprotein lattices," *Current Opinion in Structural Biology*, vol. 17, no. 5, pp. 513–520, 2007.

[21] J. Ellerhorst, "Induction of differentiation and apoptosis in the prostate cancer cell line LNCaP by sodium butyrate and galectin-1," *International Journal of Oncology*, vol. 14, no. 2, pp. 225–232, 1999.

[22] H. F. Valenzuela, K. E. Pace, P. V. Cabrera et al., "O-glycosylation regulates LNCaP prostate cancer cell susceptibility to apoptosis induced by galectin-1," *Cancer Research*, vol. 67, no. 13, pp. 6155–6162, 2007.

[23] D. J. Laderach, L. Gentilini, L. Giribaldi et al., "A unique galectin signature in human prostate cancer progression suggests galectin-1 as a key target for treatment of advanced disease," *Cancer Research*, vol. 73, pp. 86–96, 2013.

[24] N. Clausse, F. Van Den Brûle, D. Waltregny, F. Garnier, and V. Castronovo, "Galectin-1 expression in prostate tumor-associated capillary endothelial cells is increased by prostate carcinoma cells and modulates heterotypic cell-cell adhesion," *Angiogenesis*, vol. 3, no. 4, pp. 317–325, 1999.

[25] J. Ellerhorst, "Differential expression of endogenous galectin-1 and galectin-3 in human prostate cancer cell lines and effects of overexpressing galectin-1 on cell phenotype," *International Journal of Oncology*, vol. 14, no. 2, pp. 217–224, 1999.

[26] H. Andersen, O. N. Jensen, E. P. Moiseeva, and E. Eriksen, "A proteome study of secreted prostatic factors affecting osteoblastic activity: galectin-1 is involved in differentiation of human bone marrow stromal cells," *Journal of Bone and Mineral Research*, vol. 18, no. 2, pp. 195–203, 2003.

[27] J. He and L. G. Baum, "Endothelial cell expression of galectin-1 induced by prostate cancer cells inhibits T-cell transendothelial migration," *Laboratory Investigation*, vol. 86, no. 6, pp. 578–590, 2006.

[28] T. Fukumori, N. Oka, Y. Takenaka et al., "Galectin-3 regulates mitochondrial stability and antiapoptotic function in response to anticancer drug in prostate cancer," *Cancer Research*, vol. 66, no. 6, pp. 3114–3119, 2006.

[29] Y. Wang, P. Nangia-Makker, L. Tait et al., "Regulation of prostate cancer progression by galectin-3," *American Journal of Pathology*, vol. 174, no. 4, pp. 1515–1523, 2009.

[30] S. Califice, V. Castronovo, M. Bracke, and F. Van Den Brûle, "Dual activities of galectin-3 in human prostate cancer: tumor supp-res-sion of nuclear galectin-3 vs tumor promotion of cytoplasmic galectin-3," *Oncogene*, vol. 23, no. 45, pp. 7527–7536, 2004.

[31] Y. Wang, P. Nangia-Makker, V. Balan, V. Hogan, and A. Raz, "Calpain activation through galectin-3 inhibition sensitizes prostate cancer cells to cisplatin treatment," *Cell Death and Disease*, vol. 1, no. 11, article e101, 2010.

[32] T. Fukumori, H.-O. Kanayama, and A. Raz, "The role of galectin-3 in cancer drug resistance," *Drug Resistance Updates*, vol. 10, no. 3, pp. 101–108, 2007.

[33] P. Guha, E. Kaptan, G. Bandyopadhyaya et al., "Cod glycopeptide with picomolar affinity to galectin-3 suppresses T-cell apoptosis and prostate cancer metastasis," *Proceedings of the National Academy of Sciences of the United States of America*, vol. 110, no. 13, pp. 5052–5057, 2013.

[34] V. V. Glinsky, G. V. Glinsky, K. Rittenhouse-Olson et al., "The role of thomsen-friedenreich antigen in adhesion of human breast and prostate cancer cells to the endothelium," *Cancer Research*, vol. 61, no. 12, pp. 4851–4857, 2001.

[35] O. V. Glinskii, V. H. Huxley, G. V. Glinsky, K. J. Pienta, A. Raz, and V. V. Glinsky, "Mechanical entrapment is insufficient and intercellular adhesion is essential for metastatic cell arrest in distant organs," *Neoplasia*, vol. 7, no. 5, pp. 522–527, 2005.

[36] J. E. Lehr and K. J. Pienta, "Preferential adhesion of prostate cancer cells to a human bone marrow endothelial cell line," *Journal of the National Cancer Institute*, vol. 90, no. 2, pp. 118–123, 1998.

[37] K. A. Spivey, I. Chung, J. Banyard, I. Adini, H. A. Feldman, and B. R. Zetter, "A role for collagen XXIII in cancer cell adhesion, anchorage-independence and metastasis," *Oncogene*, vol. 31, no. 18, pp. 2362–2372, 2012.

[38] K. J. Pienta, H. Naik, A. Akhtar et al., "Inhibition of spontaneous metastasis in a rat prostate cancer model by oral administration of modified citrus pectin," *Journal of the National Cancer Institute*, vol. 87, no. 5, pp. 348–353, 1995.

[39] O. V. Glinskii, S. Sud, V. V. Mossine et al., "Inhibition of prostate cancer bone metastasis by synthetic TF antigen mimic/galectin-3 inhibitor lactulose-L-leucine," *Neoplasia*, vol. 14, no. 1, pp. 65–73, 2012.

[40] Y. Yang, Z. Zhou, S. He et al., "Treatment of prostate carcinoma with (Galectin-3)-targeted HPMA copolymer-(G3-C12)-5-Fluorouracil conjugates," *Biomaterials*, vol. 33, no. 7, pp. 2260–2271, 2012.

[41] J. Jiang, I. Eliaz, and D. Sliva, "Synergistic and additive effects of modified citrus pectin with two polybotanical compounds, in the suppression of invasive behavior of human breast and prostate cancer cells," *Integrative Cancer Therapies*, vol. 12, no. 2, pp. 145–152, 2013.

[42] Z.-Z. Su, J. Lin, R. Shen, P. E. Fisher, N. I. Goldstein, and P. B. Fisher, "Surface-epitope masking and expression cloning identifies the human prostate carcinoma tumor antigen gene PCTA-1 a member of the galectin gene family," *Proceedings of the National Academy of Sciences of the United States of America*, vol. 93, no. 14, pp. 7252–7257, 1996.

[43] Y. Zick, M. Eisenstein, R. A. Goren, Y. R. Hadari, Y. Levy, and D. Ronen, "Role of galectin-8 as a modulator of cell adhesion and cell growth," *Glycoconjugate Journal*, vol. 19, no. 7–9, pp. 517–526, 2002.

[44] C. Seelenmeyer, C. Stegmayer, and W. Nickel, "Unconventional secretion of fibroblast growth factor 2 and galectin-1 does not require shedding of plasma membrane-derived vesicles," *FEBS Letters*, vol. 582, no. 9, pp. 1362–1368, 2008.

[45] E. Gorelik, U. Galili, and A. Raz, "On the role of cell surface carbohydrates and their binding proteins (lectins) in tumor metastasis," *Cancer and Metastasis Reviews*, vol. 20, no. 3-4, pp. 245–277, 2001.

[46] N. Mazurek, J. S. Yun, K.-F. Liu et al., "Phosphorylated galectin-3 mediates tumor necrosis factor-related apoptosis-inducing ligand signaling by regulating phosphatase and tensin homologue deleted on chromosome 10 in human breast carcinoma cells," *The Journal of Biological Chemistry*, vol. 282, no. 29, pp. 21337–21348, 2007.

[47] N. Mazurek, Y. J. Sun, J. E. Price et al., "Phosphorylation of galectin-3 contributes to malignant transformation of human epithelial cells via modulation of unique sets of genes," *Cancer Research*, vol. 65, no. 23, pp. 10767–10775, 2005.

[48] P. Nangia-Makker, Y. Wang, T. Raz et al., "Cleavage of galectin-3 by matrix metalloproteases induces angiogenesis in breast cancer," *International Journal of Cancer*, vol. 127, no. 11, pp. 2530–2541, 2010.

[49] V. Balan, P. Nangia-Makker, D. H. Kho, Y. Wang, and A. Raz, "Tyrosine-phosphorylated galectin-3 protein is resistant to prostate-specific antigen (PSA) cleavage," *The Journal of Biological Chemistry*, vol. 287, no. 8, pp. 5192–5198, 2012.

[50] M. Salatino and G. A. Rabinovich, "Fine-tuning antitumor responses through the control of galectin-glycan interactions: an overview," *Methods in Molecular Biology*, vol. 677, pp. 355–374, 2011.

[51] V. Balan, P. Nangia-Makker, and A. Raz, "Galectins as cancer biomarkers," *Cancers*, vol. 2, no. 2, pp. 592–610, 2010.

[52] J. Ellerhorst, P. Troncoso, X.-C. Xu, J. Lee, and R. Lotan, "Galectin-1 and galectin-3 expression in human prostate tissue and prostate cancer," *Urological Research*, vol. 27, no. 5, pp. 362–367, 1999.

[53] F. A. van den Brule, D. Waltregny, and V. Castronovo, "Increased expression of galectin-1 in carcinoma-associated stroma predicts poor outcome in prostate carcinoma patients," *The Journal of Pathology*, vol. 193, no. 1, pp. 80–87, 2001.

[54] F. A. Van Den Brûle, D. Waltregny, F.-T. Liu, and V. Castronovo, "Alteration of the cytoplasmic/nuclear expression pattern of galectin-3 correlates with prostate carcinoma progression," *International Journal of Cancer*, vol. 89, no. 4, pp. 361–367, 2000.

[55] J. S. Knapp, S. D. Lokeshwar, U. Vogel et al., "Galectin-3 expression in prostate cancer and benign prostate tissues: correlation with biochemical recurrence," *World Journal of Urology*, vol. 31, no. 2, pp. 351–358, 2013.

[56] M. H. Vaarala, K. Porvari, A. Kyllönen, and P. Vihko, "Differentially expressed genes in two LNCaP prostate cancer cell lines reflecting changes during prostate cancer progression," *Laboratory Investigation*, vol. 80, no. 8, pp. 1259–1268, 2000.

[57] L. Ingrassia, I. Camby, F. Lefranc et al., "Anti-galectin compounds as potential anti-cancer drugs," *Current Medicinal Chemistry*, vol. 13, no. 29, pp. 3513–3527, 2006.

[58] D. Compagno, C. Merle, A. Morin et al., "SIRNA-directed in vivo silencing of androgen receptor inhibits the growth of castration-resistant prostate carcinomas," *PLoS ONE*, vol. 2, no. 10, Article ID e1006, 2007.

[59] M. E. Kaighn, K. Shankar Narayan, and Y. Ohnuki, "Establishment and characterization of a human prostatic carcinoma cell line (PC-3)," *Investigative Urology*, vol. 17, no. 1, pp. 16–23, 1979.

[60] R. M. Sramkoski, T. G. Pretlow II, J. M. Giaconia et al., "A new human prostate carcinoma cell line, 22Rv1," *In Vitro Cellular and Developmental Biology*, vol. 35, no. 7, pp. 403–409, 1999.

[61] R. V. Gopalkrishnan, T. Roberts, S. Tuli, D.-C. Kang, K. A. Christiansen, and P. B. Fisher, "Molecular characterization of prostate carcinoma tumor antigen-1, PCTA-1, a human galectin-8 related gene," *Oncogene*, vol. 19, no. 38, pp. 4405–4416, 2000.

[62] M. A. Toscano, G. A. Bianco, J. M. Ilarregui et al., "Differential glycosylation of TH1, TH2 and TH-17 effector cells selectively regulates susceptibility to cell death," *Nature Immunology*, vol. 8, no. 8, pp. 825–834, 2007.

[63] Y. Levy, R. Arbel-Goren, Y. R. Hadari et al., "Galectin-8 functions as a matricellular modulator of cell adhesion," *The Journal of Biological Chemistry*, vol. 276, no. 33, pp. 31285–31295, 2001.

[64] R. B. Zavareh, M. A. Sukhai, R. Hurren et al., "Suppression of cancer progression by MGAT1 shRNA knockdown," *PLoS ONE*, vol. 7, no. 9, Article ID e43721, 2013.

[65] M. Le Mercier, S. Fortin, V. Mathieu et al., "Galectin 1 proangiogenic and promigratory effects in the Hs683 oligodendroglioma model are partly mediated through the control of BEX2 expression1," *Neoplasia*, vol. 11, no. 5, pp. 485–496, 2009.

[66] V. L. Thijssen, S. Hulsmans, and A. W. Griffioen, "The galectin profile of the endothelium: altered expression and localization in activated and tumor endothelial cells," *American Journal of Pathology*, vol. 172, no. 2, pp. 545–553, 2008.

[67] V. L. Thijssen, B. Barkan, H. Shoji et al., "Tumor cells secrete galectin-1 to enhance endothelial cell activity," *Cancer Research*, vol. 70, no. 15, pp. 6216–6224, 2010.

[68] D. O. Croci, M. Salatino, N. Rubinstein et al., "Disrupting galectin-1 interactions with N-glycans suppresses hypoxia-driven angiogenesis and tumorigenesis in Kaposi's sarcoma," *The Journal of Experimental Medicine*, vol. 209, no. 11, pp. 1985–2000, 2012.

[69] A. Banh, J. Zhang, H. Cao et al., "Tumor galectin-1 mediates tumor growth and metastasis through regulation of T-cell apoptosis," *Cancer Research*, vol. 71, no. 13, pp. 4423–4431, 2011.

[70] M. Karlou, V. Tzelepi, and E. Efstathiou, "Therapeutic targeting of the prostate cancer microenvironment," *Nature Reviews Urology*, vol. 7, no. 9, pp. 494–509, 2010.

[71] J. Semenas, C. Allegrucci, S. A. Boorjian, N. P. Mongan, and J. L. Persson, "Overcoming drug resistance and treating advanced prostate cancer," *Current Drug Targets*, vol. 13, no. 10, pp. 1308–1323, 2012.

[72] P. W. Kantoff, C. S. Higano, N. D. Shore et al., "Sipuleucel-T immunotherapy for castration-resistant prostate cancer," *The New England Journal of Medicine*, vol. 363, no. 5, pp. 411–422, 2010.

[73] X. Huang, C. H. Chau, and W. D. Figg, "Challenges to improved therapeutics for metastatic castrate resistant prostate cancer: from recent successes and failures," *Journal of Hematology & Oncology*, vol. 5, p. 35, 2012.

[74] N. Hasegawa, K. Mizutani, T. Suzuki, T. Deguchi, and Y. Nozawa, "A comparative study of protein profiling by proteomic analysis in camptothecin-resistant PC3 and camptothecin-sensitive LNCaP human prostate cancer cells," *Urologia Internationalis*, vol. 77, no. 4, pp. 347–354, 2006.

[75] R.-Y. Yang, D. K. Hsu, and F.-T. Liu, "Expression of galectin-3 modulates T-cell growth and apoptosis," *Proceedings of the National Academy of Sciences of the United States of America*, vol. 93, no. 13, pp. 6737–6742, 1996.

[76] D. Compagno, D. J. Laderach, L. Gentilini, F. M. Jaworski, and G. A. Rabinovich, "Delineating the "galectin signature" of tumor microenvironment," *Oncoimmunology*, vol. 2, no. 4, Article ID e23565, 2013.

[77] P. Nangia-Makker, Y. Honjo, R. Sarvis et al., "Galectin-3 induces endothelial cell morphogenesis and angiogenesis," *American Journal of Pathology*, vol. 156, no. 3, pp. 899–909, 2000.

[78] V. L. J. L. Thijssen, R. Postel, R. J. M. G. E. Brandwijk et al., "Galectin-1 is essential in tumor angiogenesis and is a target for antiangiogenesis therapy," *Proceedings of the National Academy of Sciences of the United States of America*, vol. 103, no. 43, pp. 15975–15980, 2006.

[79] V. M. C. Delgado, L. G. Nugnes, L. L. Colombo et al., "Modulation of endothelial cell migration and angiogenesis: a novel function for the "tandem-repeat" lectin galectin-8," *FASEB Journal*, vol. 25, no. 1, pp. 242–254, 2011.

[80] S. Akahani, P. Nangia-Makker, H. Inohara, H.-R. C. Kim, and A. Raz, "Galectin-3: a novel antiapoptotic molecule with a functional BH1 (NWGR) domain of Bcl-2 family," *Cancer Research*, vol. 57, no. 23, pp. 5272–5276, 1997.

[81] F. Van den Brûle, S. Califice, F. Garnier, P. L. Fernandez, A. Berchuck, and V. Castronovo, "Galectin-1 accumulation in the ovary carcinoma peritumoral stroma is induced by ovary carcinoma cells and affects both cancer cell proliferation and adhesion to laminin-1 and fibronectin," *Laboratory Investigation*, vol. 83, no. 3, pp. 377–386, 2003.

[82] S. Califice, V. Castronovo, and F. Van Den Brûle, "Galectin-3 and cancer," *International Journal of Oncology*, vol. 25, no. 4, pp. 983–992, 2004.

[83] J. Heimburg, J. Yan, S. Morey et al., "Inhibition of spontaneous breast cancer metastasis by anti-Thomsen-friedenreich antigen monoclonal antibody JAA-F11," *Neoplasia*, vol. 8, no. 11, pp. 939–948, 2006.

[84] A. S. Merseburger, M. W. Kramer, J. Hennenlotter et al., "Involvement of decreased galectin-3 expression in the pathogenesis and progression of prostate cancer," *Prostate*, vol. 68, no. 1, pp. 72–77, 2008.

[85] H. Ahmed, P. P. Banerjee, and G. R. Vasta, "Differential expression of galectins in normal, benign and malignant prostate epithelial cells: silencing of galectin-3 expression in prostate cancer by its promoter methylation," *Biochemical and Biophysical Research Communications*, vol. 358, no. 1, pp. 241–246, 2007.

[86] A. Vyakarnam, A. J. Lenneman, K. M. Lakkides, R. J. Patterson, and J. L. Wang, "A comparative nuclear localization study of galectin-1 with other splicing components," *Experimental Cell Research*, vol. 242, no. 2, pp. 419–428, 1998.

[87] I. Paron, A. Scaloni, A. Pines et al., "Nuclear localization of Galectin-3 in transformed thyroid cells: a role in transcriptional regulation," *Biochemical and Biophysical Research Communications*, vol. 302, no. 3, pp. 545–553, 2003.

[88] A. Vyakarnam, S. F. Dagher, J. L. Wang, and R. J. Patterson, "Evidence for a role for galectin-1 in pre-mRNA splicing," *Molecular and Cellular Biology*, vol. 17, no. 8, pp. 4730–4737, 1997.

[89] S. F. Dagher, J. L. Wang, and R. J. Patterson, "Identification of galectin-3 as a factor in pre-mRNA splicing," *Proceedings of the National Academy of Sciences of the United States of America*, vol. 92, no. 4, pp. 1213–1217, 1995.

[90] C. Maier, K. Rösch, K. Herkommer et al., "A candidate gene approach within the susceptibility region PCaP on 1q42.2-43 excludes deleterious mutations of the PCTA-1 gene to be responsible for hereditary prostate cancer," *European Urology*, vol. 42, no. 3, pp. 301–307, 2002.

3

CHEK2* 1100delC Mutation and Risk of Prostate Cancer

Victoria Hale,[1] Maren Weischer,[2] and Jong Y. Park[1]

[1] *Department of Cancer Epidemiology, Moffitt Cancer Center, 12902 Magnolia Drive, Tampa, FL 33612, USA*
[2] *Department of Clinical Biochemistry, Herlev Hospital, 2730 Herlev, Denmark*

Correspondence should be addressed to Jong Y. Park; jong.park@moffitt.org

Academic Editor: Alexandre R. Zlotta

Although the causes of prostate cancer are largely unknown, previous studies support the role of genetic factors in the development of prostate cancer. *CHEK2* plays a critical role in DNA replication by responding to double-stranded breaks. In this review, we provide an overview of the current knowledge of the role of a genetic variant, 1100delC, of *CHEK2* on prostate cancer risk and discuss the implication for potential translation of this knowledge into clinical practice. Currently, twelve articles that discussed *CHEK2**1100delC and its association with prostate cancer were identified. Of the twelve prostate cancer studies, five studies had independent data to draw conclusive evidence from. The pooled results of OR and 95% CI were 1.98 (1.23–3.18) for unselected cases and 3.39 (1.78–6.47) for familial cases, indicating that *CHEK2**1100delC mutation is associated with increased risk of prostate cancer. Screening for CHEK2*1100delC should be considered in men with a familial history of prostate cancer.

1. Introduction

Prostate cancer is the most common nonskin malignancy among men worldwide. In the US, an estimated 233,000 new cases and 29,480 deaths are expected in 2014 [1]. Prostate cancer is nevertheless a little understood disease. Unlike other common cancers, environmental risk factors appear to be of minor consequence. The strongest risk factor is for the individual man with a family history of the disease. Indeed, twin studies have suggested that about 42% of the individual's risk of prostate cancer may be attributed to heritable factors [2]. Further, recent genome wide association studies (GWAS) have identified susceptibility variants [3–5], providing evidence in support of the role of genetic susceptibility in the development of prostate cancer.

The cell cycle checkpoint kinase 2 (*CHEK2*) encodes the CHEK2 enzyme, which plays a critical role in ensuring accurate DNA repair in response to double-stranded breaks. Located on chromosome 22q12.1 [6], *CHEK2* spans 50 kb [7] and contains 14 exons [6]. CHEK2 kinase is activated by ataxia telangiectasia mutated (ATM) and phosphorylates TP53 and BRCA1, which activates the homologous recombination repair pathway [8, 9]. Because of the role of CHEK2 kinase in activating the repair mechanism of double-stranded DNA breaks, CHEK2 kinase acts as a tumor suppressor promoting genomic stability and thereby preventing tumorigenesis [10, 11]. Therefore, any mutation causing a malfunction of the CHEK2 protein decreases cellular ability to protect the integrity of DNA. Among numerous mutations identified in *CHEK2*, the best studied mutations in prostate cancer are 1100delC, IVS2+1G>A, I157T, and del5395 [12–17]. Three mutations (1100delC, IVS2+1G>A, and del5395) cause *CHEK2* protein-truncation. A missense variant I157T affects the forkhead-associated (FHA) domain, where it mediates ATM-dependent CHEK2 phosphorylation and targeting of CHEK2 to bind partners such as BRCA1 [18] and is associated with reduced DNA repair ability and increased risk for various cancers [19].

We decided to focus on the 1100delC mutation as it is a frame-shift mutation that abrogates kinase activity and renders the protein ineffective. In the following, we provide an overview of the current knowledge of the role of a genetic variant, 1100delC, of *CHEK2* in prostate cancer risk along with a meta-analysis and discuss the implication for potential translation of this knowledge into clinical practice.

2. Methods

An online search in PubMed was performed in December 2013 using the following keywords: (CHEK2*1100delC prostate), (CHEK2*1100delC), (CHEK2 prostate), (CHEK2 cancer), or (susceptibility gene prostate). Respectively, the PubMed provided 9, 36, 98, 326, and 1,590 results. References of the identified studies were scrutinized in order to make sure all possible studies could be included in this review. The titles and abstracts of articles identified by PubMed were reviewed and unmatched articles which did not meet with selection criteria were excluded. We included articles that examined *CHEK2**1100delC heterozygosity and risk of prostate cancer. Overall, we found 12 articles that met this criterion [20–31].

In case results from the same individuals were reported in more than one publication, the newest or most informative article was selected [25–31]. Among the seven articles published by Cybulski et al. [20, 25, 26, 30, 31, 69, 70], we considered the most recent case/control study [20] as the most informative study. Additionally, three studies from Wu et al. [27], Dong et al. [23], and Zheng et al. [28] seem to contain data from the same cohorts. Therefore, Dong et al. study [23] was taken into consideration for analysis. Thompson et al. reported nonsignificant ($P = 0.26$) risk increase among *CHEK2* mutation carriers [29]. However, the population of this study was based on families with breast cancer history and incidence rates of prostate cancer were based on questionnaire. In addition, genotyping analysis was done with only a fraction of study participants (1,324/11,116). Thus, out of 12 articles, five articles contained independent results applicable to be analyzed (Table 1) [20–24]. The seven excluded articles for conclusion were listed in Table 2 [25–28, 30, 31, 70]. There are a few studies that investigated associations between *CHEK2**del1100C and prostate cancer risk. However, the investigators combined multiple mutations into a group. Therefore, we could not evaluate a role of *CHEK2**1100delC mutation in these articles [56, 69, 70].

3. Results

The five included studies examined CHEK2*1100delC heterozygosity and risk of cancer in 6,228 prostate cancer cases including 830 familial cases and 9,258 male controls. Selected characteristics of studies are shown in Table 1 [20–24]. Overall, *CHEK2**1100delC was identified in 0.7% (36/5,124) of sporadic prostate cancer cases, 1.2% (13/1084) of familial prostate cancer cases, and 0.36% (33/9,258) of male controls. The pooled results of OR and 95% CI were 1.98 (1.23–3.18) for unselected cases and 3.39 (1.78–6.47) for familial cases, showing that *CHEK2**1100delC heterozygosity is associated with increased risk of prostate cancer.

Cybulski et al. sequenced the coding region of *CHEK2* using genomic DNA from 140 Polish prostate patients and investigated a role of three variants, including *CHEK2**1100delC in prostate cancer risk. The numbers of *CHEK2**1100delC carriers were 4, 3, and 1 in 1,921 controls, 690 unselected cases, and 98 familial cases, respectively. The publication concluded that prostate cancer risk was nonsignificantly increased 2.0- and 4.9-fold for unselected and familial cases [30]. This however may have been a question of insufficient statistical power. Gene variants of *CHEK2* have been associated with predisposition of multiple cancers. Therefore, Cybulski et al. [31] tested whether *CHEK2* is a multisite cancer susceptibility gene using 4,000 controls and 4,008 various cancer cases. For prostate cancer, the *CHEK2**1100delC mutation increased a nonsignificant risk (OR = 1.74, 95% CI = 0.48–6.35) based on 690 prostate cases and 4,000 controls. Later, Cybulski et al. [25, 26] reported a significant risk increase for *CHEK2**1100delC mutation in unselected (OR = 3.5, 95% CI = 1.6–7.5) and familial cases (OR = 5.6, 95% CI = 1.6–19.9) as compared with controls. Recently, Cybulski et al. (2013) further investigated that four variants of *CHEK2*, including 1100delC mutation on risk and progression using expanded 3,750 Polish unselected prostate cancer patients, 412 familial cases, and 3,956 controls. Strong associations were observed for both unselected (OR = 3.2, 95% CI = 1.4–7.5) and familial cases (OR = 5.5, 95% CI = 1.6–19.0) [20].

Mayo investigators [23, 27, 28] analyzed gene mutations of *CHEK2*. Thirty-three different mutations were identified in *CHEK2* from 876 DNA samples from various prostate cancer patients. Most *CHEK2* mutations identified in prostate cancer patients were not detected in 423 control men. Frequencies of *CHEK2**1100delC mutation were 0.022 (4/178 prostate tissues), 0.0025 (1/400 cases without familial history), 0.003 (1/298 cases with family history), and 0.0 (0/423 control men). The authors also investigated the functional importance of *CHEK2**1100delC mutation [23]. Western blot analysis of *CHEK2**1100delC mutation in the EBV-transformed cell lines showed a significant reduction of CHEK2 protein, which is involved in the DNA damage pathway. Based on these results, the authors concluded that CHEK2 may contribute to prostate cancer risk because the DNA-damage-signaling pathway probably plays a significant role in prostate cancer development [23].

Seppälä et al. reported that the frequency of *CHEK2** 1100delC was elevated in sporadic cases (OR = 3.14; 95% CI = 0.65–15.16) and in 120 prostate cancer patients with family history (OR = 8.24; 95% CI = 1.49–45.5) compared to 480 controls. These data suggest strong association between the 1100delC mutation and prostate cancer risk, especially in individuals with family history. Based on these data, the authors concluded that the *CHEK2**1100delC mutation is a low-penetrance prostate cancer predisposition allele that contributes significantly to familial clustering of prostate cancer at the population level [22].

Weischer et al. reported whether *CHEK2**1100delC mutation affected prostate cancer risk in the Danish general population with a prospective study design. They reported that multifactorially adjusted hazard ratio by *CHEK2**1100delC heterozygosity versus noncarriers was 2.3 (95% CI = 0.6–9.5) for prostate cancer [24].

However, Wagenius et al. could not confirm results from Cybulski study. They assessed the significance of the *CHEK2**1100delC mutation for prostate cancer in the population of Southern Sweden. Frequency of the *CHEK2**1100delC mutation was not different in sporadic cases (1/145, 0.007) and

TABLE 1: Characteristics and results of 5 prostate cancer studies.

Carrier/Total	Population	Country	OR/HR (95% CI)	*P* value	Ref.
21/3,750	Unselected cases	PL	3.2 (1.4–7.5)	0.009	[20]
4/412	Familial cases		5.5 (1.6–19.0)	0.01	
7/3,956	Controls		Reference		
1/145	Without family history	SW	0.70 (0.07–6.78)	0.76	[21]
4/254	Familial cases		1.61 (0.36–7.27)	0.53	
3/305	Controls		Reference		
7/537	Unselected cases	FI	3.14 (0.65–15.16)	0.15	[22]
4/120	Familial cases		8.24 (1.49–45.54)	0.02	
2/480	Controls		Reference		
4/178	Cases	US	NA	NA	[23]
1/400	Without family history		NA	NA	
1/298	Familial cases		NA	NA	
0/423	Controls		NA	NA	
2/114	Cases	DE	2.3 (0.6–9.5)	NA	[24]
21/4,094	Controls		Reference		
36/5,124	**Unselected cases**	**Pooled**	**1.98 (1.23–3.18)**	**0.004**	**Combined**
13/1,084	**Familial cases**		**3.39 (1.78–6.47)**	**0.0001**	
33/9,258	**Controls**		**Reference**		

PL: Poland, SW: Sweden, FI: Finland, US: United States, DE: Denmark, NA: not available.

TABLE 2: Characteristics and results of 7 excluded prostate cancer studies.

Carrier/Total	Population	Country	OR/HR (95% CI)	*P* value	Ref.
14/1,864	Unselected cases	PL	3.5 (1.6–7.5)	0.002	[25, 26]
3/249	Familial cases		5.6 (1.6–19.9)	0.02	
12/5,496	Controls		Reference		
3/84	Cases	US	NA	NA	[27, 28]
	Families with breast cancer history	UK, NE, DE, US	2.68 (ratio of carrier RR versus noncarrier RR)	0.26	[29]
3/690	Unselected cases	PL	2.1 (0.5–9.4)	0.32	[30]
1/98	Familial cases		4.9 (0.5–44.6)	0.11	
4/1,921	Controls		Reference		
3/690	Unselected cases	PL	1.74 (0.48–6.35)	0.39	[31]
10/4,000	Controls		Reference		

PL: Poland, UK: United Kingdom, NE: Netherlands, DE: Denmark, US: United States, NA: not available.

in prostate cancer patients with family history (4/254, 0.016) compared to controls (3/305, 0.01) [21].

Thompson et al. assessed the risk of various cancers in association with *CHEK2**1100delC mutation by using incidence data from 11,116 individuals from 734 non-BRCA1/2 families with breast cancer history. These data were from the United Kingdom (236 families), the Netherlands (233 families), Germany (17 families), and the United States (248 families) [29]. Thompson et al. tested 1,324 individuals from 734 families for *CHEK2**1100delC mutation and identified 115 carriers from 67 families. Based on these data, the authors estimated relative risk to carriers and noncarriers by maximum likelihood via the expectation-maximization algorithm. Seventy-five prostate cancers were observed. Among these patients, six patients were in *CHEK2*1100*delC-positive families. The ration of carrier RR (1.42) to the noncarrier RR (0.53) was 2.68 ($P = 0.26$). This study has a limitation because of the heavy reliance on family members' reports of cancer in their relatives. Therefore, the extent of the underreporting for male relatives was hindered to obtain meaningful estimates of the risk to male carriers because families were collected for breast cancer research projects.

4. Discussion

We reviewed the current knowledge of the role of a genetic variant, 1100delC, of *CHEK2* in prostate cancer risk and found pooled odds ratios of prostate cancer for *CHEK2**1100delC heterozygote of 1.98 (95% CI: 1.23–3.18) for unselected cases and 3.39 (95% CI: 1.78–6.47) for familial cases versus noncarriers, suggesting that screening for CHEK2*1100delC should be considered in men with a familial history of prostate cancer.

The *CHEK2**1100delC mutation was first identified in patients with Li-Fraumeni syndrome in 1999 [71]. This mutation was presented as a cause of breast cancer by Meijers-Heijboer et al. [42] and has emerged as a potential risk factor of prostate cancer by Dong et al. [23]. This association was supported by other studies [20–22, 24, 25]. The prevalence rate of *CHEK2**1100delC mutation is about 0.5–1% in Northern and Eastern European population [72]. However, this rate is much less frequent in other European countries. Furthermore, the *CHEK2**1100delC mutation is very rare or absent in Hispanics, Blacks, and Asian populations [35, 39, 45, 52, 73, 74]. Although the prevalence of the *CHEK2**1100delC mutation varies, risk of prostate cancer was found to be doubled for White men of Northern or Eastern European descent with heterozygous genotype for the *CHEK2**1100delC mutation.

Bahassi et al. demonstrated the biological role of *CHEK2**1100delC *in vivo*. They showed an increased tumor formation in multiple cancer sites, including lung and breast in homozygous *CHEK2**1100delC mutant ($P = 0.025$) and heterozygous mice ($P = 0.13$) as compared with wild-type [75].

4.1. Role of CHEK2 Mutation in Other Cancers. A role of *CHEK2**1100delC was also evaluated in various cancers, including breast [32, 76], colorectal, glioma, melanoma [24, 59, 77], esophageal, ovarian, pancreatic, leukemia, and lung cancers (Table 3). Generally, *CHEK2**1100delC heterozygosity increases the risk for breast, colon, melanoma, and prostate cancers. However, larger studies are needed to evaluate a potential association with *CHEK2**1100delC mutation in other cancers, such as glioma, and pancreas.

The *CHEK2**1100delC has been most studied in breast cancer. Weischer et al. investigated the association of the *CHEK2**1100delC mutant with risk for breast cancer (OR = 3.01, 95% CI = 2.53–3.58) using a meta-analysis with 22 independent studies containing 25,571 cases and 30,056 controls [32]. Based on these data, they suggested that this mutation should be screened for when testing for BRCA1/2 mutations. Overall, the majority of the studies found some degree of association between breast cancer and the *CHEK2**1100delC mutant.

Xiang et al. [62] reported a significant association between *CHEK2**1100delC and risk for colorectal cancer (CRC) in a meta-analysis with 6 studies [60]. The *CHEK2**1100delC mutant was associated with sporadic CRC (OR = 2.80, 95% CI = 0.49–4.30), unselected CRC (OR 2.11, 95% CI = 1.41–3.16), and familial CRC (OR 2.80, 95% CI = 1.74–4.51).

Weischer et al. performed an association study on the Danish and German population while also conducting a meta-analysis with four different studies [24, 77]. The odds ratio for malignant melanoma for *CHEK2**1100delC heterozygotes compared with noncarriers was 2.01 (95% CI = 1.03–3.91) in Danes, 1.41 (95% CI = 0.46–4.31) in Germans, and 1.71 (95% CI = 1.02–3.17) in both Danes and Germans. In the meta-analysis with 2,619 cases and the 17,481 controls, the authors found that there was an odds ratio of 1.81 (95% CI = 1.07–3.05) of malignant melanoma for *CHEK2**1100delC heterozygotes in comparison to the noncarriers. The author concluded that *CHEK2**1100delC heterozygotes have a twofold risk of malignant melanoma compared with noncarriers [59].

However, several studies reported inconsistent results. Three small studies were performed to see whether there was an association between *CHEK2**1100delC and risk for glioma [68, 78, 79]. However, independent and combined data suggest that the *CHEK2* variant is not associated with glioma risk.

In an esophageal cancer study, Koppert et al. found 1.5% of 551 cases and 1.4% of 644 controls carry the *CHEK2**1100delC mutation [63]. Similarly, there is no patient with *CHEK2**1100delC mutation among 91 German head and neck cancer patients [64]. Therefore, the authors concluded that the *CHEK2**1100delC mutation has no major contribution in carcinogenesis in the esophagus [63] and head and neck [64].

Only one study described *CHEK2**1100delC and its association with ovarian cancer risk. Among 268 randomly recruited Russian ovarian cancer patients, two patients had the *CHEK2**1100delC mutation, while one carrier was found in 821 controls. Thus, the author concluded that there is no significant association between *CHEK2**1100delC and risk for ovarian cancer [65].

Sellick et al. found that there may be a low penetrance effect on risk of chronic lymphocytic leukemia (CLL) based on 973 cases and 1,620 UK controls. But there was no significant association found between *CHEK2**1100delC and familial or sporadic leukemia (OR = 0.74, 95% CI = 0.32–1.7) [67].

In the lung cancer study, Huijts et al. could not confirm an association between *CHEK2**1100delC mutation and lung cancer risk in 457 unrelated lung cancer patients [58].

Results from multiorgan cancer study by Cybulski et al. suggested an increased risk in thyroid and renal cancers although they were not in the significant level [31].

The studies performed in Malaysia [39], France [68], USA [54], Chile [53], Spain [52], Turkey [16], Malaysia [39], Czech [66], and Korea [45] did not find any individual with the *CHEK2**1100delC allele. In many cases, sample sizes were often not large enough to detect a case with *CHEK2**1100delC mutation. Further, as described, there are significant differences of prevalence of the *CHEK2**1100delC mutation among different populations.

We are aware of some limitations of this meta-analysis. First, because of the lack of the individual level data of the reviewed studies, our reports were based on unadjusted published estimates; therefore, we were unable to adjust them by possible confounders such as age and other environmental risk factors. Second, the prevalence of *CHEK2**1100delC was only sufficient in the European population but not in other ethnic groups. Therefore, the role of this mutation in other ethnic groups could not be assessed.

Table 3: Characteristics and results of various cancer studies.

Cancer Site	Case/control	Population	Country	OR/HR (95% CI)	*P* value	Ref.
Breast	(459) 25,571/(179) 30,056	(Meta-analysis)		3.01 (2.53–3.58)		[32]
Breast	1,828/7,030	(Cases/controls)	UK, FI, NE, GE, RU	6.43 (4.33–9.56)	<0.0001	[33]
Breast	(120) 2,554/(37) 3,267	(Familial cases)	NE	4.30 (2.97–6.25)	<0.0001	[34]
Breast	3,882/8,609	(Cases/controls)	CA	2.6 (1.1–5.8)	0.05	[35]
Breast	75/300	(Cases/controls)	SW	2.5	0.26	[36]
Breast	708 bilateral + 1,395 unilateral	(Cases only)	US, DE	1.8 (0.6–5.4)		[37]
Breast	71/1,692	(Cases/controls)	NE	4.1 (1.2–14.3)	0.05	[38]
Breast	(0) 668	(Cases only)	MAL			[39]
Breast	1,101/4,665	(Cases/controls)	DE	1.2 (0.7–2.1)		[24]
		(Breast)		3.2 (1.0–9.9)		
		(Colorectal)		1.6 (0.4–6.5)		
Breast	161/153		US	NS		[40]
Breast	2,311/496	(Female cases/controls)	CA	6.65 (2.37–18.68)		[41]
			US	0.12 (0.02–0.89)		
Breast	1,071/1,620		UK, NE, CA, US, GE	1.1% of controls versus 5.1% of cases	0.00000003	[42]
Breast	300/1,665		US	1% among cases versus 0.3% of controls	0.1	[43]
Breast	10,860/9,065	(Aggregate)	UK, NE, FI, GE, AU	2.34 (1.72–3.20)	0.0000001	[44]
Breast	(0) 493	(Cases only)	KO			[45]
Breast	903/1,016		IR	0.5% of cases versus 0.1% of controls; 5.65 (0.66–48.46)	0.09	[46]
Breast	1,479	(Cases only)	US	2.1 (1.0–4.3)	0.049	[47]
Breast	1,035/1,885	(Positive family history)	FI	2.27 (1.11–4.63)	0.021	[48]
		(Bilateral)		6 (1.87–20.32)	0.007	
Breast	300	(Cases only)	AU	0.6% of cases		[49]
Breast	237/331	(Cases/controls)	NE	11.4% of cases versus 2.8% of controls	0.001	[50]
Breast	302	(Cases only)	RU	3% of cases.		[51]
Breast	(0) 400/(0) 400		SP			[52]
Breast	(0) 196/(0) 1,024		CHL			[53]
Breast	(0) 102	(Familial cases)	US			[54]
Breast	507/513	(Cases/controls)	FR	1.14% in cases versus 0.29% in controls; 5.18	0.004	[55]
Breast	5,953	(Cases only)	PL	3.6 (2.1–6.2)	0.0001	[56]
		(Prostate)		4.4 (2.2–8.7)	0.0001	
		(Colon)		4.2 (2.4–7.8)	0.0001	
Breast	8,612	(Cases only)	UK			[57]
Breast, Colorectal	75	(Cases only)	SW	2.5%	0.26	[36]
Breast	(3) 1,434	(Cases only)	NE	3.4 (0.4–32.6)	0.3	[58]
Melanoma	(15) 1,889/(59) 12,801	(Combined)		1.79 (1.02–3.17)		[59]
			DE	2.01 (1.03–3.91)		
			GE	1.42 (0.46–4.31)		
Melanoma	(18) 2,619/(67) 17,481	(Meta-analysis)		1.81 (1.07–3.05)		[59]

Table 3: Continued.

Cancer Site	Case/control	Population	Country	OR/HR (95% CI)	*P* value	Ref.
Colorectal	(8) 818/(5) 760	(Unselected)	SW	1.49 (0.49–4.58)	0.48	[60]
	(2) 174/(5) 760	(Familial)		1.76 (0.34–9.13)	0.50	
Colorectal	369	(Cases only)	NE	4.2% HNPCC cases		[61]
Colorectal	4,194/10,010	(Meta-analysis)		2.11 (1.41–3.16)	0.0003	[62]
	1,050/3,784	(Familial)		2.80 (1.74–4.51)	<0.0001	
	652/2,115	(Sporadic)		1.45 (0.49–4.30)	0.50	
Colorectal	(0) 210/(0) 446	(Cases/controls)	TUK			[16]
Esophagus	(8) 551/(9) 644	(Cases/controls)	NE	1.04 (0.35–3.06)	0.94	[63]
Head & Neck	(0) 91	(Case only)	GE			[64]
Ovary	(2) 268/(1) 821	(Cases/controls)	RU	6.17 (0.56–68.3)	0.09	[65]
Pancreas	(0) 270/(0) 683	(Cases/controls)	CZ			[66]
Leukemia	(8) 973/(18) 1,620	(Cases/controls)	UK	0.74 (0.32–1.7)		[67]
Lung	(0) 457	(Cases only)	NE			[58]
Brain	(0) 79	(Familial cases)	FR			[68]

UK: United Kingdom, FI: Finland, NE: Netherlands, GE: Germany, RU: Russia, CA: Canada, SW: Sweden, US: United States, DE: Denmark, GE: Germany, MAL: Malaysia, AU: Australia, KO: Korea, IR: Ireland, SP: Spain, CHL: Chile, FR: France, PL: Poland, TUK: Turkey, and CZ: Czech.

4.2. Future Perspective. The screening for the *CHEK2** 1100delC mutation was suggested for cancer pre-vention, especially for breast cancer [32, 80]. The rationale is that (1) *CHEK2** 1100delC was demonstrated numerously as a risk factor for various cancers, (2) the lifetime prostate cancer risk for men with *CHEK2** 1100delCmutation is 25–45%, and (3) *CHEK2** 1100delC analysis would be a single genotyping test with a low cost.

Because odds ratios were reported for prostate cancer with this mutation range between 2.0 and 3.0, it is reasonable to suggest screening for *CHEK2* mutations in men. Men with *CHEK2* mutations and family history of prostate cancer show a higher risk of prostate cancer. Therefore, *CHEK2* screening would be a useful strategy for prostate cancer among individuals with familial history. Unfortunately, the role of this mutation in survival or response to treatment in prostate cancer is not established yet. However, a recent study reported that breast cancer with *CHEK2** 1100delC is associated with a worse survival [81]. Thus, *CHEK2* could be a future target of cancer genetic test that could help in the detection and prevention of various cancers [82]. Genotyping for *CHEK2** 1100delC should be considered in men of Northern or Eastern European descent with a familial history of prostate cancer.

Acknowledgment

The development of this paper was supported in part by R01CA128813 (PI: Park).

References

[1] R. Siegel, J. Ma, Z. Zou, and A. Jemal, "Cancer statistics, 2014," *CA Cancer Journal for Clinicians*, vol. 64, no. 1, pp. 9–29, 2014.

[2] P. Lichtenstein, N. V. Holm, P. K. Verkasalo et al., "Environmental and heritable factors in the causation of cancer—analyses of cohorts of twins from Sweden, Denmark, and Finland," *The New England Journal of Medicine*, vol. 343, no. 2, pp. 78–85, 2000.

[3] L. A. Hindorff, E. M. Gillanders, and T. A. Manolio, "Genetic architecture of cancer and other complex diseases: lessons learned and future directions," *Carcinogenesis*, vol. 32, no. 7, pp. 945–954, 2011.

[4] F. Wiklund, "Prostate cancer genomics: can we distinguish between indolent and fatal disease using genetic markers?" *Genome Medicine*, vol. 2, no. 7, article 45, 2010.

[5] J. S. Varghese and D. F. Easton, "Genome-wide association studies in common cancers—what have we learnt?" *Current Opinion in Genetics & Development*, vol. 20, no. 3, pp. 201–209, 2010.

[6] Y. Pommier, O. Sordet, V. A. Rao, H. Zhang, and K. W. Kohn, "Targeting Chk2 kinase: molecular interaction maps and therapeutic rationale," *Current Pharmaceutical Design*, vol. 11, no. 22, pp. 2855–2872, 2005.

[7] J. Bartek, J. Falck, and J. Lukas, "Chk2 kinase—a busy messenger," *Nature Reviews Molecular Cell Biology*, vol. 2, no. 12, pp. 877–886, 2001.

[8] W. Roeb, J. Higgins, and M.-C. King, "Response to DNA damage of CHEK2 missense mutations in familial breast cancer," *Human Molecular Genetics*, vol. 21, no. 12, pp. 2738–2744, 2012.

[9] N. Tung and D. P. Silver, "Chek2 DNA damage response pathway and inherited breast cancer risk," *Journal of Clinical Oncology*, vol. 29, no. 28, pp. 3813–3815, 2011.

[10] J. Bartek and J. Lukas, "Chk1 and Chk2 kinases in checkpoint control and cancer," *Cancer Cell*, vol. 3, no. 5, pp. 421–429, 2003.

[11] G. Zoppoli, S. Solier, W. C. Reinhold et al., "CHEK2 genomic and proteomic analyses reveal genetic inactivation or endogenous activation across the 60 cell lines of the US National Cancer Institute," *Oncogene*, vol. 31, no. 4, pp. 403–418, 2012.

[12] U. Teodorczyk, C. Cybulski, D. Wokołorczyk et al., "The risk of gastric cancer in carriers of CHEK2 mutations," *Familial Cancer*, vol. 12, no. 3, pp. 473–478, 2013.

[13] P. Pohlreich, Z. Kleibl, P. Kleiblová et al., "The clinical importance of a genetic analysis of moderate-risk cancer susceptibility genes in breast and other cancer patients from the Czech Republic," *Klinicka Onkologie*, vol. 25, pp. S59–S66, 2012.

[14] C. Liu, Q.-S. Wang, and Y.-J. Wang, "The CHEK2 I157T variant and colorectal cancer susceptibility: a systematic review and meta-analysis," *Asian Pacific Journal of Cancer Prevention*, vol. 13, no. 5, pp. 2051–2055, 2012.

[15] S. G. Angelova, M. E. Krasteva, Z. I. Gospodinova, and E. I. Georgieva, "CHEK2 gene alterations independently increase the risk of death from breast cancer in Bulgarian patients," *Neoplasma*, vol. 59, no. 6, pp. 622–630, 2012.

[16] S. Bayram, M. Topaktaş, H. Akkiz, A. Bekar, and E. Akgöllü, "CHEK2 1100delC, IVS2+1G>A and I157T mutations are not present in colorectal cancer cases from Turkish population," *Cancer Epidemiology*, vol. 36, no. 5, pp. 453–457, 2012.

[17] D. J. Novak, L. Q. Chen, P. Ghadirian et al., "Identification of a novel CHEK2 variant and assessment of its contribution to the risk of breast cancer in French Canadian women," *BMC Cancer*, vol. 8, article 239, 2008.

[18] J. Li, B. L. Williams, L. F. Haire et al., "Structural and functional versatility of the FHA domain in DNA-damage signaling by the tumor suppressor kinase Chk2," *Molecular Cell*, vol. 9, no. 5, pp. 1045–1054, 2002.

[19] F.-F. Han, C.-L. Guo, and L.-H. Liu, "The effect of CHEK2 variant I157T on cancer susceptibility: evidence from a meta-analysis," *DNA and Cell Biology*, vol. 32, no. 6, pp. 329–335, 2013.

[20] C. Cybulski, D. Wokołorczyk, W. Kluźniak et al., "An inherited NBN mutation is associated with poor prognosis prostate cancer," *British Journal of Cancer*, vol. 108, no. 2, pp. 461–468, 2013.

[21] M. Wagenius, A. Borg, L. Johansson, A. Giwercman, and O. Bratt, "CHEK2* 1100delC is not an important high-risk gene in families with hereditary prostate cancer in southern Sweden," *Scandinavian Journal of Urology and Nephrology*, vol. 40, no. 1, pp. 23–25, 2006.

[22] E. H. Seppälä, T. Ikonen, N. Mononen et al., "CHEK2 variants associate with hereditary prostate cancer," *British Journal of Cancer*, vol. 89, no. 10, pp. 1966–1970, 2003.

[23] X. Dong, L. Wang, K. Taniguchi et al., "Mutations in CHEK2 associated with prostate cancer risk," *The American Journal of Human Genetics*, vol. 72, no. 2, pp. 270–280, 2003.

[24] M. Weischer, S. E. Bojesen, A. Tybjærg-Hansen, C. K. Axelsson, and B. G. Nordestgaard, "Increased risk of breast cancer associated with *CHEK2∗1100delC*," *Journal of Clinical Oncology*, vol. 25, no. 1, pp. 57–63, 2007.

[25] C. Cybulski, D. Wokołorczyrk, T. Huzarski et al., "A large germline deletion in the Chek2 kinase gene is associated with an increased risk of prostate cancer," *Journal of Medical Genetics*, vol. 43, no. 11, pp. 863–866, 2006.

[26] C. Cybulski, "Selected aspects of inherited susceptibility to prostate cancer and tumours of different site of origin," *Hereditary Cancer in Clinical Practice*, vol. 5, no. 3, pp. 164–179, 2007.

[27] X. Wu, X. Dong, W. Liu, and J. Chen, "Characterization of CHEK2 mutations in prostate cancer," *Human Mutation*, vol. 27, no. 8, pp. 742–747, 2006.

[28] L. Zheng, F. Wang, C. Qian et al., "Unique substitution of CHEK2 and TP53 mutations implicated in primary prostate tumors and cancer cell lines," *Human Mutation*, vol. 27, no. 10, pp. 1062–1063, 2006.

[29] D. Thompson, S. Seal, M. Schutte et al., "A multicenter study of cancer incidence in CHEK2 1100delC mutation carriers," *Cancer Epidemiology, Biomarkers & Prevention*, vol. 15, no. 12, pp. 2542–2545, 2006.

[30] C. Cybulski, T. Huzarski, B. Górski et al., "A novel founder CHEK2 mutation is associated with increased prostate cancer risk," *Cancer Research*, vol. 64, no. 8, pp. 2677–2679, 2004.

[31] C. Cybulski, B. Górski, T. Huzarski et al., "CHEK2 is a multiorgan cancer susceptibility gene," *The American Journal of Human Genetics*, vol. 75, no. 6, pp. 1131–1135, 2004.

[32] M. Weischer, S. E. Bojesen, C. Ellervik, A. Tybjærg-Hansen, and B. G. Nordestgaard, "*CHEK2∗*1100delC genotyping for clinical assessment of breast cancer risk: meta-analyses of 26,000 patient cases and 27,000 controls," *Journal of Clinical Oncology*, vol. 26, no. 4, pp. 542–548, 2008.

[33] O. Fletcher, N. Johnson, I. D. S. Silva et al., "Family history, genetic testing, and clinical risk prediction: pooled analysis of CHEK2∗1100delC in 1,828 bilateral breast cancers and 7,030 controls," *Cancer Epidemiology Biomarkers and Prevention*, vol. 18, no. 1, pp. 230–234, 2009.

[34] M. A. Dank, M. A. Jonker, I. Kluijt et al., "CHEK2∗1100delC homozygosity is associated with a high breast cancer risk in women," *Journal of Medical Genetics*, vol. 48, no. 12, pp. 860–863, 2011.

[35] S. Zhang, C. M. Phelan, P. Zhang et al., "Frequency of the CHEK2 1100delC mutation among women with breast cancer: an international study," *Cancer Research*, vol. 68, no. 7, pp. 2154–2157, 2008.

[36] A. Isinger, M. Bhat, A. Borg, and M. Nilbert, "*CHEK2* 1100delC in patients with metachronous cancers of the breast and the colorectum," *BMC Cancer*, vol. 6, article 64, 2006.

[37] L. Mellemkjær, C. Dahl, J. H. Olsen et al., "Risk for contralateral breast cancer among carriers of the CHEK2∗1100delC mutation in the WECARE Study," *British Journal of Cancer*, vol. 98, no. 4, pp. 728–733, 2008.

[38] M. Wasielewski, M. A. Den Bakker, A. van Den Ouweland et al., "CHEK2 1100delC and male breast cancer in the Netherlands," *Breast Cancer Research and Treatment*, vol. 116, no. 2, pp. 397–400, 2009.

[39] E. Thirthagiri, L. S. Cheong, C. H. Yip, and S.-H. Teo, "CHEK2*1100delC does not contribute to risk to breast cancer among Malay, Chinese and Indians in Malaysia," *Familial Cancer*, vol. 8, no. 4, pp. 355–358, 2009.

[40] J. Huang, S. M. Domchek, M. S. Brose, T. R. Rebbeck, K. L. Nathanson, and B. L. Weber, "Germline *CHEK2∗*1100delC mutations in breast cancer patients with multiple primary cancers," *Journal of Medical Genetics*, vol. 41, no. 11, article e120, 2004.

[41] J. L. Bernstein, S. N. Teraoka, E. M. John et al., "The CHEK2∗1100delC allelic variant and risk of breast cancer: screening results from the breast cancer family registry," *Cancer Epidemiology Biomarkers and Prevention*, vol. 15, no. 2, pp. 348–352, 2006.

[42] H. Meijers-Heijboer, A. van den Ouweland, J. Klijn et al., "Low-penetrance susceptibility to breast cancer due to CHEK2∗1100delC in noncarriers of BRCA1 or BRCA2 mutations: The CHEK2-breast cancer consortium," *Nature Genetics*, vol. 31, no. 1, pp. 55–59, 2002.

[43] K. Offit, H. Pierce, T. Kirchhoff et al., "Frequency of *CHEK2∗1100delC* in New York breast cancer cases and controls," *BMC Medical Genetics*, vol. 4, article 1, 2003.

[44] D. Easton, "CHEK2∗1100delC and susceptibility to breast cancer: a collaborative analysis involving 10,860 breast cancer cases and 9,065 controls from 10 studies," *The American Journal of Human Genetics*, vol. 74, no. 6, pp. 1175–1182, 2004.

[45] D. H. Choi, D. Y. Cho, M. H. Lee et al., "The CHEK2 1100delC mutation is not present in Korean patients with breast cancer cases tested for BRCA1 and BRCA2 mutation," *Breast Cancer Research and Treatment*, vol. 112, no. 3, pp. 569–573, 2008.

[46] N. M. McInerney, N. Miller, A. Rowan et al., "Evaluation of variants in the CHEK2, BRIP1 and PALB2 genes in an Irish breast cancer cohort," *Breast Cancer Research and Treatment*, vol. 121, no. 1, pp. 203–210, 2010.

[47] M. K. Schmidt, R. A. E. M. Tollenaar, S. R. De Kemp et al., "Breast cancer survival and tumor characteristics in premenopausal women carrying the CHEK2*1100delC germline mutation," *Journal of Clinical Oncology*, vol. 25, no. 1, pp. 64–69, 2007.

[48] P. Vahteristo, J. Bartkova, H. Eerola et al., "A CHEK2 genetic variant contributing to a substantial fraction of familial breast cancer," *The American Journal of Human Genetics*, vol. 71, no. 2, pp. 432–438, 2002.

[49] C. R. Jekimovs, X. Chen, J. Arnold et al., "Low frequency of *CHEK2* 1100delC allele in Australian multiple-case breast cancer families: functional analysis in heterozygous individuals," *British Journal of Cancer*, vol. 92, no. 4, pp. 784–790, 2005.

[50] R. A. Oldenburg, K. Kroeze-Jansema, J. Kraan et al., "The CHEK2∗1100delC variant acts as a breast cancer risk modifier in non-BRCA1/BRCA2 multiple-case families," *Cancer Research*, vol. 63, no. 23, pp. 8153–8157, 2003.

[51] A. P. Sokolenko, M. E. Rozanov, N. V. Mitiushkina et al., "Founder mutations in early-onset, familial and bilateral breast cancer patients from Russia," *Familial Cancer*, vol. 6, no. 3, pp. 281–286, 2007.

[52] A. Osorio, R. Rodríguez-López, O. Díez et al., "The breast cancer low-penetrance allele 1100delC in the CHEK2 gene is not present in Spanish familial breast cancer population," *International Journal of Cancer*, vol. 108, no. 1, pp. 54–56, 2004.

[53] P. González-Hormazábal, V. G. Castro, R. Blanco et al., "Absence of CHEK2 1100delC mutation in familial breast cancer cases from a South American population," *Breast Cancer Research and Treatment*, vol. 110, no. 3, pp. 543–545, 2008.

[54] M. D. Iniesta, M. A. Gorin, L.-C. Chien et al., "Absence of *CHEK2∗*1100delC mutation in families with hereditary breast

cancer in North America," *Cancer Genetics*, vol. 202, no. 2, pp. 136–140, 2010.

[55] A. Desrichard, Y. Bidet, N. Uhrhammer, and Y.-J. Bignon, "CHEK2 contribution to hereditary breast cancer in non-BRCA families," *Breast Cancer Research*, vol. 13, no. 6, article R119, 2011.

[56] J. Gronwald, C. Cybulski, W. Piesiak et al., "Cancer risks in first-degree relatives of CHEK2 mutation carriers: effects of mutation type and cancer site in proband," *British Journal of Cancer*, vol. 100, no. 9, pp. 1508–1512, 2009.

[57] H. Naseem, J. Boylan, D. Speake et al., "Inherited association of breast and colorectal cancer: limited role of *CHEK2* compared with high-penetrance genes," *Clinical Genetics*, vol. 70, no. 5, pp. 388–395, 2006.

[58] P. E. Huijts, A. Hollestelle, B. Balliu et al., "CHEK2∗1100delC homozygosity in the Netherlands—prevalence and risk of breast and lung cancer," *European Journal of Human Genetics*, vol. 22, no. 1, pp. 46–51, 2014.

[59] M. Weischer, I. M. Heerfordt, S. E. Bojesen et al., "CHEK2∗1100delC and risk of malignant melanoma: Danish and German studies and meta-analysis," *Journal of Investigative Dermatology*, vol. 132, no. 2, pp. 299–303, 2012.

[60] T. Djureinovic, A. Lindblom, J. Dalén et al., "The CHEK2 1100delC variant in Swedish colorectal cancer," *Anticancer Research*, vol. 26, no. 6C, pp. 4885–4888, 2006.

[61] M. Wasielewski, H. Vasen, J. Wijnen et al., "CHEK2 1100delC is a susceptibility allele for HNPCC-related colorectal cancer," *Clinical Cancer Research*, vol. 14, no. 15, pp. 4989–4994, 2008.

[62] H.-P. Xiang, X.-P. Geng, W.-W. Ge, and H. Li, "Meta-analysis of CHEK2 1100delC variant and colorectal cancer susceptibility," *European Journal of Cancer*, vol. 47, no. 17, pp. 2546–2551, 2011.

[63] L. B. Koppert, M. Schutte, M. Abbou, H. W. Tilanus, and W. N. M. Dinjens, "The *CHEK2*∗1100delC mutation has no major contribution in oesophageal carcinogenesis," *British Journal of Cancer*, vol. 90, no. 4, pp. 888–891, 2004.

[64] K. Scheckenbach, G. Papadopoulou, T. K. Hoffmann et al., "The checkpointkinase 2 (CHK2) 1100delC germ line mutation is not associated with the development of squamous cell carcinoma of the head and neck (SCCHN)," *Journal of Negative Results in BioMedicine*, vol. 9, no. 1, article 10, 2010.

[65] N. Y. Krylova, D. N. Ponomariova, N. Y. Sherina et al., "CHEK2 1100delC mutation in Russian ovarian cancer patients," *Hereditary Cancer in Clinical Practice*, vol. 5, no. 3, pp. 153–156, 2007.

[66] B. Mohelnikova-Duchonova, O. Havranek, I. Hlavata et al., "*CHEK2* gene alterations in the forkhead-associated domain, 1100delC and del5395 do not modify the risk of sporadic pancreatic cancer," *Cancer Epidemiology*, vol. 34, no. 5, pp. 656–658, 2010.

[67] G. S. Sellick, K. Sullivan, D. Catovsky, and R. S. Houlston, "CHEK2∗1100delC and risk of chronic lymphocytic leukemia," *Leukemia and Lymphoma*, vol. 47, no. 12, pp. 2659–2660, 2006.

[68] S. E. Hallani, B. Boisselier, Y. Marie et al., "*TP53* mutations but no *CHEK2∗1100DelC* variant in familial gliomas," *Cancer Genetics and Cytogenetics*, vol. 188, no. 2, pp. 126–128, 2009.

[69] C. Cybulski, B. Gliniewicz, A. Sikorski et al., "Epistatic relationship between the cancer susceptibility genes CHEK2 and p27," *Cancer Epidemiology Biomarkers and Prevention*, vol. 16, no. 3, pp. 572–576, 2007.

[70] C. Cybulski, D. Wokołorczyk, W. Kluźniak et al., "A personalised approach to prostate cancer screening based on genotyping of risk founder alleles," *British Journal of Cancer*, vol. 108, no. 12, pp. 2601–2609, 2013.

[71] D. W. Bell, J. M. Varley, T. E. Szydlo et al., "Heterozygous germ line hCHK2 mutations in Li-Fraumeni syndrome," *Science*, vol. 286, no. 5449, pp. 2528–2531, 1999.

[72] C. Cybulski, D. Wokołorczyk, T. Huzarski et al., "A deletion in CHEK2 of 5,395 bp predisposes to breast cancer in Poland," *Breast Cancer Research and Treatment*, vol. 102, no. 1, pp. 119–122, 2007.

[73] M. A. Caligo, S. Agata, G. Aceto et al., "The CHEK2 c.1100delC mutation plays an irrelevant role in breast cancer predisposition in Italy," *Human Mutation*, vol. 24, no. 1, pp. 100–101, 2004.

[74] A. S. G. Lee and P. Ang, "CHEK2∗1100delC screening of asian women with a family history of breast cancer is unwarranted," *Journal of Clinical Oncology*, vol. 26, no. 14, pp. 2419–2420, 2008.

[75] E. M. Bahassi, S. B. Robbins, Y. Moying et al., "Mice with the *CHEK2*∗1100delC SNP are predisposed to cancer with a strong gender bias," *Proceedings of the National Academy of Sciences of the United States of America*, vol. 106, no. 40, pp. 17111–17116, 2009.

[76] M. Weischer, B. G. Nordestgaard, P. Pharoah et al., "*CHEK2* *1100delC heterozygosity in women with breast cancer associated with early death, breast cancer-specific death, and increased risk of a second breast cancer," *Journal of Clinical Oncology*, vol. 30, no. 35, pp. 4308–4316, 2012.

[77] T. Dębniak, B. Górski, C. Cybulski et al., "Rarity of germline 1100delC mutation in CHK2 in patients with malignant melanoma of the skin," *Melanoma Research*, vol. 14, no. 2, pp. 121–124, 2004.

[78] Y. Ino, D. C. Wahrer, D. W. Bell, D. A. Haber, and D. N. Louis, "Mutation analysis of the hCHK2 gene in primary human malignant gliomas," *Neurogenetics*, vol. 3, no. 1, pp. 45–46, 2000.

[79] S.-L. Sallinen, T. Ikonen, H. Haapasalo, and J. Schleutker, "CHEK2 mutations in primary glioblastomas," *Journal of Neuro-Oncology*, vol. 74, no. 1, pp. 93–95, 2005.

[80] S. Gutiérrez-Enríquez, J. Balmaña, M. Baiget, and O. Díez, "Detection of the *CHEK2* 1100delC mutation by MLPA *BRCA1/2* analysis: a worthwhile strategy for its clinical applicability in 1100delC low-frequency populations?" *Breast Cancer Research and Treatment*, vol. 107, no. 3, pp. 455–457, 2008.

[81] M. Kriege, A. Hollestelle, A. Jager et al., "Survival and contralateral breast cancer in CHEK2 1100delC breast cancer patients: impact of adjuvant chemotherapy," *British Journal of Cancer*, vol. 111, no. 5, pp. 1004–1013, 2014.

[82] S. A. Narod, "Testing for CHEK2 in the cancer genetics clinic: ready for prime time?" *Clinical Genetics*, vol. 78, no. 1, pp. 1–7, 2010.

4

Evaluating the Impact of PSA as a Selection Criteria for Nerve Sparing Radical Prostatectomy in a Screened Cohort

Shyam K. Tanguturi,[1,2] Ming-Hui Chen,[3] Marian Loffredo,[4,5] Jerome P. Richie,[4] and Anthony V. D'Amico[4,5]

[1] *Harvard Radiation Oncology Program, Harvard Medical School, Boston, MA 02115, USA*
[2] *Brigham and Women's Hospital, 75 Francis Street, ASB1 L2, Boston, MA 02115, USA*
[3] *Department of Statistics, University of Connecticut, Storrs, CT 06269, USA*
[4] *Lank Center for Genitourinary Oncology, Dana Farber Cancer Institute, Boston, MA 02115, USA*
[5] *Department of Radiation Oncology, Dana Farber Cancer Institute and Brigham and Women's Hospital, Boston, MA 02115, USA*

Correspondence should be addressed to Shyam K. Tanguturi; stanguturi@partners.org

Academic Editor: Cristina Magi-Galluzzi

Purpose. We investigated whether NS-RP increased risk of PSA failure and whether PSA should be included as a selection criterion for NS. *Methods.* We evaluated 357 consecutive men with screen-detected PC who underwent open RP without adjuvant radiotherapy between 9/11/2001 and 12/30/2008. Criteria for NS included Gleason score $\leq 3 + 4$, percentage of positive biopsies (PPB) $\leq 50\%$, percentage of core involvement $\leq 50\%$, nonapical location, no perineural invasion, and no palpable disease on pre- or intraoperative exam but did not include a PSA threshold. Cox multivariable regression assessed whether increasing PSA or unilateral- or bilateral-NS versus non-NS-RP was associated with PSA failure adjusting for prognostic factors. *Results.* After a median follow-up of 3.96 years, 34 men sustained PSA failure (9.5%). Increasing PSA was significantly associated with increased risk of PSA failure in the interaction model (adjusted hazard ratio (AHR): 1.09 [95% CI: 1.03–1.16]; $P = 0.005$), whereas unilateral (AHR: 1.24 [95% CI: 0.36–4.34]; $P = 0.73$) or bilateral NS (AHR: 0.41 [95% CI: 0.06–2.59]; $P = 0.34$) versus non-NS RP was not. *Conclusion.* NS-RP in a screened cohort did not increase risk of PSA failure using NS criteria not including PSA.

1. Introduction

Nerve-sparing (NS) radical prostatectomy (RP) was introduced in 1984 by Dr. Patrick Walsh as a means of preserving potency and maintaining patient reported health related quality of life following NS RP [1, 2]. This procedure involves preservation of the neurovascular bundles (NVB), which travel dorsolateral to the prostate and are believed to supply neurophysiologic control of erectile tissue [3]. NS RP has been found to correlate with early return of urinary continence when applied in a risk-stratified approach [4], which is another potential benefit of this approach.

Since that time, the procedure has been widely used, with rates of patient reported postoperative potency ranging from 21 to 89.7% after RP [5–11]. Despite the wide adoption of NS RP, prospective randomized assessment of prostate cancer control outcomes with or without NS is lacking. Some have raised the concern that this procedure may place select patients with large tumor burden at increased risk of post-RP prostate-specific antigen (PSA) failure by increasing the risk of positive surgical margins due to the close proximity of the NVBs to the posterolateral aspect of the prostatic fascia [12–14]. However, this concern has been debated [12, 15, 16].

Different investigators have attempted to define tumor factors believed to optimize selection for NS to thereby reduce the risk of a positive margin [12, 17, 18]. Earlier series from the Washington University Medical Center describe ideal candidates for NS RP as young patients with clinical stage not exceeding T2 and well-differentiated tumors [18]. An algorithm from New York University (NYU) reserves NS RP for patients with Gleason 6 or less tumors with percentage of positive biopsies (PPB) less than 50% or no perineural invasion (PNI), Gleason 7 tumors with PPB less than 30% and no PNI, and Gleason 8 to 10 tumors with PPB less than 10% and no PNI [17]. At the University of Miami, Florida, similar criteria include preoperative potency, desire to maintain potency, biopsies with tumor on one side only, T2b disease or less, intraoperative absence of palpable induration or periprostatic fibrosis, Gleason score of 7 or less, PSA of 10 ng/mL or less, and nonapical location of tumor [12, 16].

At the Brigham and Women's Hospital, criteria for NS by side included Gleason score 3 + 4 or less, PPB and percentage of core involvement 50% or less, nonapical location, and no perineural invasion or palpable disease on pre- or intraoperative exam but did not include a maximum PSA value. Therefore using these criteria as the basis for NS or not, the current study was designed to investigate whether an increasing PSA level and whether unilateral (UNS) or bilateral (BNS) versus non-NS RP were associated with an increased risk of PSA failure adjusting for known predictors for PSA recurrence in men who did not undergo adjuvant radiation therapy.

2. Patients and Methods

2.1. Patient Population and Treatment. We identified 357 consecutively treated men with screen-detected biopsy proven prostate cancer (PC) who underwent an open radical prostatectomy by a single urologic oncologist between 9/11/2001 and 12/30/2008 at a single academic center. Determination of the use of bilateral and unilateral NS was judged on each side separately and was based on the presence of Gleason score 3 + 4 or less, PPB and percentage of core involvement 50% or less, nonapical location, and no perineural invasion or palpable disease on pre- or intraoperative exam but did not include a maximum PSA value.

2.2. Pathologic Processing of the RP Specimen. RP pathologic specimens were step-sectioned and reviewed by an expert genitourinary pathologist as previously described [19]. The apical and basal margins were amputated to a thickness of 5 mm and sectioned at 3 mm intervals parasagittally or perpendicular to the initial transverse incision. The base of the seminal vesicles was amputated and the basal cross-section submitted. The prostate was sectioned as thinly as possible perpendicularly to the long axis (apical to basal) of the gland, typically at 3 mm intervals, with most specimens requiring four to seven cross-sections. For each cross-section, a single section each of the right and left posterior region was submitted, with most cases entirely submitting the posterior zone. Finally, at least one section of the mid-anterior prostate was also submitted, although frequently more than one section was submitted for histology analysis.

Evidence of extraprostatic disease including seminal vesicle invasion (SVI), extracapsular extension (ECE), nodal involvement (pN1), and/or positive surgical margins was recorded, and tumor staging was defined using the 2010 American Joint Committee on Cancer (AJCC) categorization. All biopsy and prostatectomy Gleason scores were centrally reviewed and determined using a primary and secondary Gleason grade +/− a tertiary pattern in a manner similar to that outlined in the 2005 International Society of Urological Pathology (ISUP) consensus recommendations [20]. This study was approved by the institutional review board at the Brigham and Women's Hospital.

2.3. Follow-Up and Determination of PSA Failure. Adjuvant radiation therapy was not used. Patient follow-up consisted of a serum PSA measurement and digital rectal examination every 3 months for the first 2 years, every 6 months for the next 3 years, and annually thereafter. PSA failure was defined in accordance with American Urological Association (AUA) guidelines as a postoperative serum PSA level greater than 0.2 ng/mL, confirmed on a second measurement at least one month later [21].

2.4. Statistical Methods

2.4.1. Comparison of the Distribution of Clinical and Pathologic Factors in Men Selected for Bilateral or Unilateral versus Non-Nerve Sparing Radical Prostatectomy. The distribution of PSA, PPB, age, clinical tumor category, biopsy and prostatectomy Gleason score, and prostatectomy tumor category and margin status was compared across men who had bilateral, unilateral, or non-NS RP. The distributions of these characteristics were compared using a Mantel-Haenszel Chi Squared metric for categorical factors and [22] a nonparametric Wilcoxon statistic for continuous covariates [23] (Table 1). In the case of small sample size, a Fisher's exact test was employed [22].

2.4.2. Time to PSA Failure Analyses. A Cox Proportional Hazards multivariable regression model was used to evaluate whether increasing PSA or use of UNS or BNS versus non-NS RP was associated with the risk of PSA failure after adjusting for known predictors of PSA failure, including an interaction term between PPB and PSA in the absence of adjuvant radiation therapy use [24]. Because PPB was used whereas PSA level was not used as a selection criterion for NS RP and because both PSA and PPB are associated with tumor volume, which may in turn increase the risk of positive surgical margins and subsequent PSA failure following NS RP, we included an interaction term in the model between PSA and PPB. Other variables included in the multivariable model included age, PSA and PPB (both continuous) at diagnosis, Gleason Score (8–10 versus 7 versus 6 or less as baseline), tumor category (cT2-3 versus T1c as baseline), and type of NS RP (UNS or BNS versus non-NS as baseline). Unadjusted and adjusted hazard ratios with 95% confidence intervals and associated P values were calculated for each covariate. A 2-sided P value < 0.05 was considered statistically significant. SAS version 9.3 was used for all statistical analyses (SAS Institute, Inc. Cary, NC).

2.4.3. Estimates of PSA Failure. The Kaplan-Meier method was used to estimate PSA failure-free survival for men following RP stratified by whether bilateral, unilateral, or non- NS was employed [7]. Comparison of these Kaplan-Meier estimates was performed using a log rank test [25]. A Bonferroni

Table 1: Comparison of the distribution of clinical and pathologic factors in men selected for bilateral or unilateral versus non-nerve sparing radical prostatectomy.

Clinical factor	Non-nerve sparing (non-NS) $N = 19$	Unilateral nerve sparing (UNS) $N = 151$	Bilateral nerve sparing (BNS) $N = 187$	*P* value comparing non-NS, UNS, and BNS
Median PSA (IQR) (ng/mL)	4.6 [4.0, 10.0]	5.0 [4.0, 6.2]	4.6 [3.5, 6.0]	0.137
Median PPB (IQR) (%)	50.0 [18.2, 70.0]	33.3 [25.0, 50.0]	16.7 [10.0, 25.0]	<0.0001
PSA and PPB category*				
Both > median	8 (10.39%)	50 (64.94%)	19 (24.68%)	<0.0001**
PSA > median PPB ≤ Median	1 (1.04%)	30 (31.25%)	65 (67.71%)	<0.0001**
PSA ≤ median PPB > median	5 (6.25%)	49 (61.25%)	26 (32.50%)	<0.0001**
Both ≤ median	5 (4.81%)	22 (21.15%)	77 (74.04%)	<0.0001**
Median age (IQR) (yrs)	60.2 [52.0, 67.2]	61.4 [57.4, 64.9]	57.8 [52.9, 61.9]	<0.0001
AJCC clinical tumor category				<0.0001**
1c	16 (84%)	109 (72%)	170 (91%)	
2-3	3 (16%)	42 (28%)	17 (9%)	
Biopsy Gleason score				<0.0001**
7 or less	11 (58%)	131 (87%)	187 (100%)	
8 to 10	8 (42%)	20 (13%)	0 (0%)	
AJCC prostatectomy tumor category				<0.0001**
2	12 (63%)	119 (79%)	174 (93%)	
3-4	7 (37%)	32 (21%)	13 (7%)	
Prostatectomy Gleason score				<0.0001**
7 or less	13 (68%)	129 (85%)	187 (100%)	
8–10	6 (32%)	22 (15%)	0 (0%)	
Margin status				<0.0001**
Positive	8 (42%)	18 (12%)	10 (5%)	
Negative	11 (58%)	133 (88%)	177 (95%)	

PSA: prostate-specific antigen; PPB: percentage of positive prostate biopsies; IQR: interquartile range; AJCC: American Joint Commission on Cancer. *Overall, median PPB = 25%; overall, median PSA = 4.8 ng/mL; overall, 7% had PSA ≥ 10 ng/mL. **Fisher exact test *P* value.

correction was applied to adjust for multiple comparisons ($n = 3$), such that a significant *P* value was <0.05/3 or 0.0167 [26]. Point estimates of PSA failure-free survival with associated 95% confidence intervals were calculated and reported.

3. Results

3.1. Comparison of the Distribution of Clinical and Pathologic Factors in Men Selected for Bilateral or Unilateral versus Non-Nerve Sparing Radical Prostatectomy. As shown in Table 1, men undergoing BNS compared to UNS and non-NS were significantly younger and had more favorable disease characteristics including median PPB, clinical tumor category, biopsy Gleason score, as well as prostatectomy findings of tumor category, Gleason score, and margin status (all *P* values for trend < 0.0001). However, median PSA was not significantly different between men undergoing BNS, UNS, or non-NS, respectively, 4.6 ng/mL, 5.0 ng/mL, and 4.6 ng/mL (*P* value for trend = 0.137). Overall, 7% of men in this study had a PSA of 10 ng/mL or more.

As indicated by the distribution of BNS, UNS, non-NS across PPB and PSA categories, Table 1 also illustrates that PPB was used as a selection criteria for NS whereas PSA level was not. Specifically, high PPB (>median of 25%) led to lower rates of BNS between 25 and 33%, whereas high PSA (>median of 4.8 ng/mL) did not correlate to increased or decreased use of BNS ranging from a high of 68% when the PPB was ≤median to a low of 25% when the PPB was greater than the median. Among men with low PPB (<median), rates of BNS remained high at 68% and 74% irrespective of whether the PSA level was greater than median or less than median, respectively.

3.2. Time to PSA Failure Analysis. After a median follow-up of 3.96 years (interquartile range 1.92–5.00), 34 out of 357 men sustained PSA failure (9.5%). While increasing PSA was significantly associated with an increased risk of PSA failure in the interaction model (adjusted hazard ratio (AHR): 1.09 [95% Confidence Interval (CI): 1.03 to 1.16]; $P = 0.005$) the use of UNS (AHR: 1.24 [95% CI: 0.36 to 4.34]; $P = 0.73$) or BNS (AHR: 0.41 [95% CI: 0.06–2.59]; $P = 0.34$) versus non-NS RP was not.

TABLE 2: Univariable and Multivariable hazard ratios for clinical factors from the Cox regression analysis for the risk of PSA-failure.

Clinical factor	Number of men	Number of events	Univariable analysis		Multivariable analysis	
			HR (95% CI)	P value	AHR (95% CI)	P value
Age at diagnosis (years)	357	34	0.99 (0.95, 1.04)	0.814	0.98 (0.92, 1.05)	0.542
PSA (ng/mL)	357	34	1.09 (1.04, 1.15)	0.001	1.09 (1.03, 1.16)	0.005
PPB (%)	357	34	1.04 (1.02, 1.06)	<0.001	1.03 (1.01, 1.05)	0.009
PSA & PPB interaction	357	34	0.999 (0.998, 1.000)	0.177	0.999 (0.998, 1.000)	0.054
Highest Gleason score						
6	208	2	1 (Ref)	—	1 (Ref)	—
7	121	17	15.24 (3.52, 65.99)	<0.001	9.70 (2.17, 43.37)	0.003
8–10	28	15	67.60 (15.45, 295.75)	<0.001	25.01 (5.08, 123.14)	<0.001
AJCC clinical tumor category						
T1c	295	19	1 (Ref)	—	1 (Ref)	—
T2-3	62	15	3.77 (1.91, 7.42)	<0.001	1.49 (0.72, 3.08)	0.283
Type of nerve sparing RP						
BNS	187	3	0.043 (0.011, 0.173)	<0.001	0.407 (0.064, 2.589)	0.341
UNS	151	25	0.473 (0.193, 1.156)	0.101	1.242 (0.355, 4.342)	0.734
Non-NS	19	6	1 (Ref)	—	1 (Ref)	—

HR: hazard ratio; AHR: adjusted hazard ratio; PSA: prostate-specific antigen; PPB: percentage of positive prostate biopsies; AJCC: American Joint Commission on Cancer; RP: radical prostatectomy; BNS: bilateral nerve sparing; UNS: unilateral nerve sparing; Non-NS: non-nerve sparing.

Other factors significantly associated with an increased risk of PSA failure included increasing PPB (AHR: 1.03 [95% CI: 1.01 to 1.05]; $P = 0.009$), biopsy Gleason score 7 (AHR: 9.70 [95% CI: 2.17 to 43.37]; $P = 0.003$), and biopsy Gleason score 8–10 (AHR: 25.01 [95% CI: 5.08 to 123.14]; $P < 0.001$) compared to 6 or less.

3.3. Estimates of PSA Failure. As shown in Figure 1, the univariable estimates of PSA failure-free survival decreased significantly in men undergoing non-NS as compared to UNS as compared to BNS (overall log-rank test P value < 0.0001). Specifically, 4-year point estimates of PSA failure-free survival for men undergoing BNS, UNS, and non-NS were 98.7% (95% CI: 94.9 to 99.7%), 84.4% (95% CI: 75.9 to 90.0%), and 58.0% (95% CI: 27.7 to 79.4%), respectively.

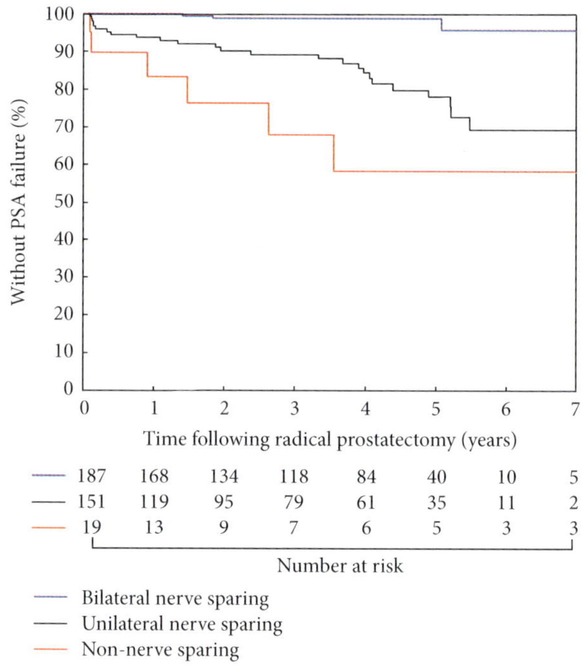

FIGURE 1: PSA failure-free survival following radical prostatectomy, stratified by whether one, both, or neither nerve was spared.

4. Discussion

In this study, we found that men undergoing UNS or BNS versus non-NS had more favorable prognostic factor distributions (Table 1) with respect to PPB, Gleason score, and T category but not PSA level, which is consistent with the selection criteria used for NS. This is in turn was reflected in more favorable PSA outcomes among men undergoing UNS or BNS versus non-NS RP, as illustrated in Figure 1. However, after adjusting for prognostic factors in the multivariable model, the use of UNS or BNS as compared to non-NS no longer predicted for a lower risk of PSA failure (Table 2), despite the lack of use of adjuvant radiation therapy. Together, these data support that the selection criteria used for NS in this study are effective and do not place men at increased risk of PSA failure.

Nevertheless, some investigators have published that a PSA < 10 ng/mL and no more than one high-grade core biopsy predicts for ipsilateral organ confined disease at a rate of 88.5% [27]. Therefore some have advocated for use of PSA < 15 ng/mL in addition to diffusion weighted MRI, PPB, and T category to select patients for NS RP [28]. Results in the current study cannot be used to design the optimal cut-point (i.e., <10 or <15 ng/mL), given that 93% of men in this cohort had a PSA < 10 ng/mL. While the results of this study support the hypothesis that the use of UNS or BNS did not impact the increased risk of PSA failure conferred by increasing preoperative PSA level, a prospective assessment in which men are randomly assigned to BNS versus non-NS if their PSA level exceeds a predetermined cut-point and if all other criteria for NS RP used in this study are met could be considered to determine the impact of preoperative PSA level on future risk of PSA failure. Such a study could ascertain whether the increased risk of PSA failure observed with increasing pre-RP PSA level is due to local persistence of disease that NS may have contributed to or micrometastatic disease, which NS would have no impact on.

Several points require further discussion. First, the decision to perform BNS in our study depended only on the PPB value being low and not on the value of the PSA, as shown in Table 1. Therefore we included an interaction term between PPB and PSA in our multivariable model, given that it is known that increasing PPB and PSA are both associated with increased tumor volume, risk of positive margins, and subsequent PSA failure following NS RP [29–31]. We found that in the multivariable model, the interaction term between PPB and PSA approached significance ($P = 0.054$) and had HR < 1, suggesting that these two factors contribute information regarding the risk of PSA failure interactively. Specifically, this near-significant interaction in our model between PPB and PSA lent support to the hypothesis that an increasing PSA level led to a higher risk of PSA failure, when PPB was less than 2/3. The value of 2/3 was determined by using a mathematical formulation involving taking the logarithms of the AHRs corresponding to PPB, PSA, and PPB*PSA from the Cox interaction model. Second, we know that not all PSA failures lead to clinically significant outcomes such as distant metastasis (DM) or death from prostate cancer. Specifically, as the PSA DT decreases, the risk of observing these clinically significant endpoints increases [32, 33]. Therefore, further follow-up of the data in this study is needed to ascertain if the association between increasing pre-RP PSA level and an increased risk of PSA failure translates to increased risks of DM and death from prostate cancer. Third, studies have not found inferior PSA outcomes when minimally invasive techniques such as robotic or laparoscopic RP as compared to open RP are performed. [34–36]. Therefore, these data using open RP should apply to patients undergoing robotic or laparoscopic RP. Fourth, the median PSA in this study was 4.8 ng/mL, with only 7% of men having a PSA ≥ 10 ng/mL. Therefore, prospective studies in which men who meet all requirements for NS as described in this study but have a PSA in excess of 10 ng/mL should be performed in order to rigorously assess the impact of PSA level as a NS criterion or not on future risk of PSA failure.

Despite these considerations, using criteria for NS that did not include PSA, the use of NS did not increase the risk of PSA failure in a cohort screened with PSA. Therefore it appears that while increasing PSA level was associated with an increased risk of PSA failure, the use of UNS or BNS as compared to non-NS RP was not suggesting that factors other than NS were responsible for the increased risk of PSA failure in men with high pre-RP PSA levels. Whether the increased risk of PSA failure observed with increasing pre-RP PSA level can be reduced by including a predetermined PSA cut-point to select for non-NS requires additional study.

References

[1] P. C. Walsh and P. J. Donker, "Impotence following radical prostatectomy: insight into etiology and prevention," *Journal of Urology*, vol. 128, no. 3, pp. 492–497, 1982.

[2] P. C. Walsh and J. L. Mostwin, "Radical prostatectomy and cystoprostatectomy with preservation of potency. Results using a new nerve-sparing technique," *British Journal of Urology*, vol. 56, no. 6, pp. 694–697, 1984.

[3] A. Takenaka, G. Murakami, H. Soga, S.-H. Han, Y. Arai, and M. Fujisawa, "Anatomical analysis of the neurovascular bundle supplying penile cavernous tissue to ensure a reliable nerve graft after radical prostatectomy," *Journal of Urology*, vol. 172, no. 3, pp. 1032–1035, 2004.

[4] A. Srivastava, S. Chopra, A. Pham et al., "Effect of a risk-stratified grade of nerve-sparing technique on early return of continence after robot-assisted laparoscopic radical prostatectomy," *European Urology*, vol. 63, no. 3, pp. 438–444, 2013.

[5] J. A. Talcott, P. Rieker, K. J. Propert et al., "Patient-reported impotence and incontinence after nerve-sparing radical prostatectomy," *Journal of the National Cancer Institute*, vol. 89, no. 15, pp. 1117–1123, 1997.

[6] J. Noldus, U. Michl, M. Graefen, A. Haese, P. Hammerer, and H. Huland, "Patient-reported sexual function after nerve-sparing radical retropubic prostatectomy," *European Urology*, vol. 42, no. 2, pp. 118–124, 2002.

[7] H. R. Kübler, T. Y. Tseng, L. Sun, J. Vieweg, M. J. Harris, and P. Dahm, "Impact of Nerve Sparing Technique on Patient Self-Assessed Outcomes After Radical Perineal Prostatectomy," *Journal of Urology*, vol. 178, no. 2, pp. 488–492, 2007.

[8] R. Katz, L. Salomon, A. Hoznek et al., "Patient reported sexual function following laparoscopic radical prostatectomy," *Journal of Urology*, vol. 168, no. 5, pp. 2078–2082, 2002.

[9] Y.-H. Lee, J.-K. Huang, and C.-M. Lu, "The impact on sexual function after nerve sparing and non-nerve sparing radical retropubic prostatectomy," *Journal of the Chinese Medical Association*, vol. 66, no. 1, pp. 13–18, 2003.

[10] E. Rodriguez Jr., D. S. Finley, D. Skarecky, and T. E. Ahlering, "Single institution 2-year patient reported validated sexual function outcomes after nerve sparing robot assisted radical prostatectomy," *Journal of Urology*, vol. 181, no. 1, pp. 259–263, 2009.

[11] Y. D. Dubbelman, G. R. Dohle, and F. H. Schröder, "Sexual function before and after radical retropubic prostatectomy: a systematic review of prognostic indicators for a successful outcome," *European Urology*, vol. 50, no. 4, pp. 711–720, 2006.

[12] J. A. Wieder and M. S. Soloway, "Incidence, etiology, location, prevention and treatment of positive surgical margins after radical prostatectomy for prostate cancer," *Journal of Urology*, vol. 160, no. 2, pp. 299–315, 1998.

[13] W. J. Catalona and S. W. Bigg, "Nerve-sparing radical prostatectomy: evaluation of results after 250 patients," *Journal of Urology*, vol. 143, no. 3, pp. 538–543, 1990.

[14] R. C. Smith, A. W. Partin, J. I. Epstein, and C. B. Brendler, "Extended followup of the influence of wide excision of the neurovascular bundle(s) on prognosis in men with clinically localized prostate cancer and extensive capsular perforation," *Journal of Urology*, vol. 156, no. 2, pp. 454–458, 1996.

[15] B. M. Moore, R. Savdie, R. A. Pebenito et al., "The impact of nerve sparing on incidence and location of positive surgical margins in radical prostatectomy," *BJU International*, vol. 109, no. 4, pp. 533–538, 2012.

[16] M. Sofer, K. L. Hamilton-Nelson, J. J. Schlesselman, and M. S. Soloway, "Risk of positive margins and biochemical recurrence in relation to nerve-sparing radical prostatectomy," *Journal of Clinical Oncology*, vol. 20, no. 7, pp. 1853–1858, 2002.

[17] O. Shah, D. A. Robbins, J. Melamed, and H. Lepor, "The New York University nerve sparing algorithm decreases the rate of positive surgical margins following radical retropubic prostatectomy," *Journal of Urology*, vol. 169, no. 6, pp. 2147–2152, 2003.

[18] W. J. Catalona, "Patient selection for, results of, and impact on tumor resection of potency-sparing radical prostatectomy," *Urologic Clinics of North America*, vol. 17, no. 4, pp. 819–826, 1990.

[19] A. A. Renshaw, "Correlation of gross morphologic features with histologic features in radical prostatectomy specimens," *American Journal of Clinical Pathology*, vol. 110, no. 1, pp. 38–42, 1998.

[20] J. I. Epstein, W. C. Allsbrook Jr., M. B. Amin et al., "The 2005 International Society of Urological Pathology (ISUP) consensus conference on Gleason grading of prostatic carcinoma," *American Journal of Surgical Pathology*, vol. 29, no. 9, pp. 1228–1242, 2005.

[21] M. S. Cookson, G. Aus, A. L. Burnett et al., "Variation in the definition of biochemical recurrence in patients treated for localized prostate cancer: the American Urological Association Prostate Guidelines for Localized Prostate Cancer Update Panel report and recommendations for a standard in the reporting of surgical outcomes," *Journal of Urology*, vol. 177, no. 2, pp. 540–545, 2007.

[22] A. Agresti, *Categorical Data Analysis*, Wiley Series in Probability and Statistics, Wiley, Hoboken, NJ, USA, 3rd edition, 2013.

[23] M. Hollander and D. A. Wolfe, *Nonparametric Statistical Methods*, Wiley Series in Probability and Statistics Texts and References Section, Wiley, New York, NY, USA, 2nd edition, 1999.

[24] D. R. Cox, "Regression models and life-tables," *Journal of the Royal Statistical Society. Series B*, vol. 34, no. 2, pp. 187–220, 1972.

[25] N. Mantel, "Evaluation of survival data and two new rank order statistics arising in its consideration," *Cancer Chemotherapy Reports*, vol. 50, no. 3, pp. 163–170, 1966.

[26] J. P. Shaffer, "Multiple hypothesis testing," *Annual Review of Psychology*, vol. 46, no. 1, pp. 561–584, 1995.

[27] M. Graefen, A. Haese, U. Pichlmeier et al., "A validated strategy for side specific prediction of organ confined prostate cancer: a tool to select for nerve sparing radical prostatectomy," *Journal of Urology*, vol. 165, no. 3, pp. 857–863, 2001.

[28] T. Naiki, T. Okamura, D. Nagata et al., "Preoperative prediction of neurovascular bundle involvement of localized prostate cancer by combined T2 and diffusionweighted imaging of magnetic resonance imaging, number of positive biopsy cores, and Gleason score," *Asian Pacific Journal of Cancer Prevention*, vol. 12, no. 4, pp. 909–913, 2011.

[29] T. J. Sebo, J. C. Cheville, D. L. Riehle et al., "Predicting prostate carcinoma volume and stage at radical prostatectomy by assessing needle biopsy specimens for percent surface area and cores positive for carcinoma, perineural invasion, Gleason score, DNA ploidy and proliferation, and preoperative serum prostate specific antigen: a report of 454 cases," *Cancer*, vol. 91, no. 11, pp. 2196–2204, 2001.

[30] L. Egevad, M. Norberg, S. Mattson, B. J. Norlén, and C. Busch, "Estimation of prostate cancer volume by multiple core biopsies before radical prostatectomy," *Urology*, vol. 52, no. 4, pp. 653–658, 1998.

[31] F. Dong, J. S. Jones, A. J. Stephenson, C. Magi-Galluzzi, A. M. Reuther, and E. A. Klein, "Prostate cancer volume at biopsy predicts clinically significant upgrading," *Journal of Urology*, vol. 179, no. 3, pp. 896–900, 2008.

[32] C. R. Pound, A. W. Partin, M. A. Eisenberger, D. W. Chan, J. D. Pearson, and P. C. Walsh, "Natural history of progression after PSA elevation following radical prostatectomy," *Journal of the American Medical Association*, vol. 281, no. 17, pp. 1591–1597, 1999.

[33] P. Zhou, M.-H. Chen, D. McLeod, P. R. Carroll, J. W. Moul, and A. V. D'Amico, "Predictors of prostate cancer-specific mortality after radical prostatectomy or radiation therapy," *Journal of Clinical Oncology*, vol. 23, no. 28, pp. 6992–6998, 2005.

[34] J. C. Hu, X. Gu, S. R. Lipsitz et al., "Comparative effectiveness of minimally invasive vs open radical prostatectomy," *Journal of the American Medical Association*, vol. 302, no. 14, pp. 1557–1564, 2009.

[35] J. C. Hu, Q. Wang, C. L. Pashos, S. R. Lipsitz, and N. L. Keating, "Utilization and outcomes of minimally invasive radical prostatectomy," *Journal of Clinical Oncology*, vol. 26, no. 14, pp. 2278–2284, 2008.

[36] W. T. Lowrance, E. B. Elkin, L. M. Jacks et al., "Comparative effectiveness of prostate cancer surgical treatments: a population based analysis of postoperative outcomes," *Journal of Urology*, vol. 183, no. 4, pp. 1366–1372, 2010.

5

Analysis of Prostate Cancer Susceptibility Variants in South African Men: Replicating Associations on Chromosomes 8q24 and 10q11

Pedro Fernandez,[1] Muneeb Salie,[2] Danielle du Toit,[3] and Andre van der Merwe[1]

[1] *Division of Urology and Tygerberg Hospital, Stellenbosch University, P.O. Box 241, Cape Town 8000, South Africa*
[2] *SA MRC Centre for TB Research and DST/NRF Centre of Excellence for Biomedical Tuberculosis Research, Division of Molecular Biology and Human Genetics, Stellenbosch University, P.O. Box 241, Cape Town 8000, South Africa*
[3] *Unistel Medical Laboratories, P.O. Box 241, Cape Town 8000, South Africa*

Correspondence should be addressed to Pedro Fernandez; pf3@sun.ac.za

Academic Editor: Manfred Wirth

Genome-wide association studies (GWAS) have implicated single nucleotide polymorphisms (SNPs) on chromosomes 2p15, 6q25, 7p15.2, 7q21, 8q24, 10q11, 10q26, 11q13, 17q12, 17q24, 19q13, and Xp11, with prostate cancer (PCa) susceptibility and/or tumour aggressiveness, in populations of African, European, and Asian ancestry. The objective of this study was to confirm these associations in South African Mixed Ancestry and White men. We evaluated 17 prioritised GWAS SNPs in South African cases (331 Mixed Ancestry and 155 White) and controls (178 Mixed Ancestry and 145 White). The replicated SNP associations for the different South African ethnic groups were rs7008482 (8q24) ($p = 2.45 \times 10^{-5}$), rs6983267 (8q24) ($p = 4.48 \times 10^{-7}$), and rs10993994 (10q11) ($p = 1.40 \times 10^{-3}$) in Mixed Ancestry men and rs10993994 ($p = 1.56 \times 10^{-9}$) in White men. No significant associations were observed for the analyses stratified by disease aggressiveness in the individual and the combined population group analysis. The present study demonstrates that a number of known PCa susceptibility variants may contribute to disease susceptibility in South African men. Larger genetic investigations extended to other South African population groups are warranted to confirm the role of these and other SNPs in disease susceptibility.

1. Introduction

Prostate cancer (PCa) is the most frequently diagnosed cancer in men in developed countries, with higher incidence rates in the United States of America (USA) in individuals of African ancestry [1]. African American (AA) men have a PCa incidence rate that is 1.6 times that in European American (EA) men and the mortality rate is 2.5 times greater than EA men [2]. In developing countries, recent estimates suggest that PCa is also the leading cancer in terms of incidence and mortality in men from Sub-Saharan Africa (SSA) and the Caribbean [3]. Moreover, underdiagnoses and underreporting have been shown to be widespread in men from SSA and the Caribbean [4], further indicating that incidence and mortality rates may be substantially underestimated in developing countries.

Numerous genome-wide association studies (GWAS) have identified close to 100 PCa susceptibility variants, primarily in populations of European ancestry [5–12], to a lesser extent in AA men [8, 12, 13], and, recently, in African men [14, 15]. Even though many of these associations exceeded or were close to genome-wide significance levels, it remains necessary to confirm these findings in multiple independent populations to rule out false positive results, thereby improving the likelihood that they represent true associations. To this end, several studies have replicated GWAS associations in AA, EA, and Asian men [16–29]. Although GWAS have generally been undertaken to a lesser extent in African descent populations, a recent meta-analysis of 82 PCa susceptibility variants identified primarily in GWAS in European and Asian descent populations generally demonstrated consistent replication of the direction of effects in men with African ancestry [30].

In the present study, we investigated PCa susceptibility single nucleotide polymorphisms (SNPs) in men from two separate South African population groups, one group of mixed Khoisan (San), African, European, and Asian descent and the other of European descent. We report replicating associations with PCa susceptibility for three of the 17 investigated SNPs among Mixed Ancestry (also termed South African Coloured) and White men.

2. Materials and Methods

2.1. Study Population. The study population comprised 331 Mixed Ancestry and 155 White cases (ethnicity was self-reported for all participants, as previously described) [31]. All cases had no prior cancer at any other site and were recruited from the Division of Urology, Tygerberg Hospital (Cape Town, South Africa). Clinical characteristics including prostate specific antigen (PSA), Gleason score, tumour node metastasis (TNM) stage, age at diagnosis, and other cancer diagnoses were obtained from medical records. All cases underwent radical prostatectomy, transurethral resection of the prostate, or prostatic biopsy and had histologically confirmed PCa. Cases were additionally stratified by risk of developing aggressive PCa using the D'Amico Cancer Risk Group Classification system. Probability of developing aggressive PCa in cases was categorized as "low" (tumour category < T1-2a or PSA ≤ 10 ng/mL or Gleason score < 7) or "high" (tumour category ≥ T2b or PSA > 10 or Gleason score ≥ 7) ("high" was defined here as the combination of intermediate + high risk).

Controls were selected among subjects admitted to Tygerberg Hospital for routine PSA examinations or benign prostatic hyperplasia (BPH) and comprised of 178 Mixed Ancestry men and 145 White men, matched for age and ethnicity (self-reported), and were from the same geographical region. Inclusion criteria for controls were PSA levels of ≤4.0 ng/mL and a normal digital rectal examination (DRE) or negative biopsy on histology.

All participants were informed and gave written consent to participate in the study and allow their biological samples to be genetically analysed, conducted in accordance with the Declaration of Helsinki. The study was approved by the Stellenbosch University Faculty of Medicine and Health Sciences Human Research Ethics Committee.

2.2. SNP Selection and Genotyping. Based on previously reported PCa GWAS and replication studies, we selected 17 SNPs on chromosomes 2p15, 6q25, 7p15.2, 7q21, 8q24, 10q11, 10q26, 11q13, 17q12, 17q24, 19q13, and Xp11. Given the diverse ancestral lineages of the South African population, the SNPs were prioritised for analyses primarily if they had been implicated in PCa susceptibility in GWAS and/or replication studies in European, African, and Asian descent populations. At the time of initial SNP selection, the novel PCa susceptibility variants identified in African men [14, 15] had not yet been reported and were thus not investigated in this study.

Genotyping was performed at the Stellenbosch University Central Analytical Facility (CAF) (Cape Town, South Africa) on the 17 selected SNPs using commercially available Taqman SNP Genotyping Assays (Life Technologies, USA). Quality control (QC) for exclusion from the study for individual samples was a genotype call rate <90%. For all SNPs, genotyping QC was assessed by including DNA duplicates (to an equivalent of 5% duplicates per 384-well plate), and the concordance genotype call rate between samples and duplicates was set at ≥95%. We excluded all SNPs whose genotype frequency departed from Hardy-Weinberg equilibrium (HWE) at $p < 0.01$ in the controls and SNPs that were monomorphic (had a frequency <1%) in our study populations.

2.3. Statistical Analyses. Descriptive analyses for discrete traits were carried out using contingency table methods and Fisher's exact tests (FET) or chi-square statistics. Medians were used to summarize continuously distributed traits. We tested the SNPs in the controls for departures of HWE and determined allele and genotype frequencies in cases and controls. For each SNP in each population group, logistic regression models were used to estimate PCa genotype and allelic odds ratios (OR), 95% confidence intervals (CI), and corresponding p values adjusted for age (i.e., age at diagnosis for cases and age at ascertainment for controls). We adjusted for age and ethnicity in the combined population logistic regression analysis. Logistic regression was similarly used to estimate OR, 95% CI, and p values for cases stratified by disease aggressiveness ("low" versus "high"). All analyses were performed in R, freely available from http://www.R-project.org/. In the present study, we adopted a conservative approach by only considering a Bonferroni corrected p value threshold of $p < 1.47 \times 10^{-3}$ statistically significant ($\alpha = 0.05/17$ SNPs × two population groups). This correction may be considered to be overly conservative [32]; however, because the number of multiple comparisons we performed was relatively small, we opted to use a family-wise error rate approach instead of a less stringent approach [33].

3. Results

The median age at diagnoses of PCa cases and the median age of controls were significantly different among the groups; PSA levels were significantly different between the groups, with Mixed Ancestry controls and cases showing higher median levels (Table 1). No significant differences were noted for Gleason score and tumour stage between the two groups, although Mixed Ancestry men showed significantly higher frequency of distant metastasis at the time of diagnosis (Table 1).

For the genotype QC analysis, two cases and one control Mixed Ancestry sample achieved a genotype call rate <90% and were thus excluded, leaving the analysed total of cases at 329 Mixed Ancestry and 155 White and a total number of controls at 177 Mixed Ancestry and 145 White. Additionally, four of the 17 selected SNPs were excluded from further study: rs721048 (2p15) and rs5945619 (Xp11) failed to meet the QC

TABLE 1: Clinical characteristics among South African cases and controls.

Variables of interest	Mixed Ancestry		White		p value
	Controls ($n = 178$)	Cases ($n = 331$)	Controls ($n = 145$)	Cases ($n = 155$)	
Median age (years)[a]	60	67	64	70	**<0.001**
Median PSA (ng/mL)[b]	0.89	18.4	0.86	11.7	**<0.001**
Gleason ≥ 7[‡]		84/177 (41.7%)		42/96 (43.8%)	0.557
Stage ≥ 2b[‡]		118/283 (41.7%)		39/123 (31.7%)	0.058
Metastasis[‡]		30/252 (11.9%)		4/116 (3.4%)	**0.009**

[a]For each of the respective population groups, $p < 0.05$ when comparing the median age between cases and controls.

[b]For each of the respective population groups, $p < 0.05$ when comparing the median PSA between cases and controls.

[‡]Gleason score, tumour stage, and/or metastases information were missing from the medical records of some of the clinically confirmed prostate cancer cases. Therefore, the numbers and percentages shown are for the available information and not that of the total number of cases included in the study for each population group.

concordance genotype call rate of ≥95%, and Bd11934905 (8q24) and rs7210100 (17q21) were monomorphic in both population groups.

Of the 13 remaining prioritised SNPs, three were significantly associated with PCa after correction for multiple testing in Mixed Ancestry men: rs7008482 (8q24) (OR = 0.41, 95% CI: 0.26–0.62; $p = 2.45 \times 10^{-5}$), rs6983267 (8q24) (OR = 0.35, 95% CI: 0.23–0.53; $p = 4.48 \times 10^{-7}$), and rs10993994 (10q11) (OR = 1.56, 95% CI: 1.56–6.08; $p = 1.40 \times 10^{-3}$) (Table 2). In White men, only rs10993994 (OR = 3.49, 95% CI: 2.28–5.54; $p = 1.56 \times 10^{-9}$) was significantly associated with PCa after correction for multiple testing (Table 2). In the combined population analysis, the associations for rs7008482, rs6983267, and rs10993994 and PCa susceptibility were statistically significant (Table 2). No significant associations were observed for the case-only analyses stratified by disease aggressiveness ("low" versus "high" risk) in the individual and the combined population group analysis (data not shown).

4. Discussion

The present study replicates previously reported associations for rs7008482, rs6983267, and rs10993994, in two different South African population groups. Men from the two population groups reported here have PCa age-standardized incidence rates that are between 1.4 and 2.4 times higher than men from other South African population groups (Mixed Ancestry: 39.1 per 100,000 and White: 52.0 per 100,000 compared to Asian: 28.6 per 100,000 and Black: 21.6 per 100,000) (National Cancer Registry, 2009) [44]. When we compared the age at diagnosis between the two groups, Mixed Ancestry men were shown generally to be diagnosed with PCa at an earlier age than White men (67 versus 70 years). Additionally, Mixed Ancestry men, who have substantial proportions of African ancestry (combination of San, European, Black, and Asian ancestry [45]), showed significantly higher frequency of distant metastasis at the time of diagnosis. A few studies have suggested that men with African ancestry more often present with aggressive disease compared to men of European ancestry [29, 46]. Though highly speculative, our observations may support this view, although our genetic analysis stratified by disease aggressiveness failed to provide supporting evidence.

Most GWAS and replication studies have consistently identified genetic associations with SNPs on chromosome 8q24 [5–8, 10, 11, 16, 19, 20, 22, 23, 25, 26]; two 8q24 SNPs were associated in our study, whereas in another study South African Black men showed associations with the rs6983561 [29]. It has been suggested that multiple, independent polymorphic variants on chromosome 8q24 may produce a common biological mechanism that contributes to disease, or, alternatively, the 8q24 regions may cumulatively influence the regulation of adjacent genes (cis-regulation) or genes on other chromosomes (trans-regulation) [47]. Additionally, it has been suggested that the 8q24 regions harbor previously unannotated microRNAs (miRNAs) and that the miRNA elements in these regions are involved in cis-regulation of distal genes, thereby affecting RNA expression [48]. However, it remains inconclusive why so many studies have shown PCa susceptibility associations to 8q24 given that it is a gene-poor region.

We showed that the SNP rs10993994 was associated with PCa susceptibility across both population groups, as well as in the combined populations. Pomerantz et al. [39] demonstrated that the T-allele of rs10993994 decreased expression in normal tissue of both isoforms of the beta-microseminoprotein gene (*MSMB*), as well as increasing the expression of the five isoforms of the nuclear receptor coactivator 4 gene (*NCOA4*). Furthermore, it was speculated that because rs10993994 is not a susceptibility allele for other cancers, such as colon or breast cancer, the associations observed with this SNP may thus be specific to prostate cancer [39].

In the present study, we opted to use a very conservative approach to reduce the chance of identifying false positive associations. However, we noted SNPs that would conventionally be considered associated with the disease if a less stringent statistical approach was employed. In the White group, rs1048657 (7p15), rs4430796 (17q12), and rs1859962 (17q24) were significant at $p < 0.05$ but not after correction for multiple testing (Table 2). For the Mixed Ancestry, because of the effect of population stratification, we only consider a $p < 4.1 \times 10^{-3}$ statistically significant (also applied

TABLE 2: Summary results for SNP genotyping analysis in South African men.

rs number	Cytoband	In/nearest gene[‡]	Effect allele; frequency (control | case); per effect allele OR (95% CI)[a]; p value (adjusted for age)		
			Mixed Ancestry	White	Combined[b]
rs9364554	6q25	*SLC22A3*	T; (0.13 | 0.11); 0.236	T; (0.20 | 0.21); 0.493	T; (0.17 | 0.15); 0.737
rs10486567	7p15	*JAZF1*	G; (0.17 | 0.22); 0.098	G; (0.15 | 0.19); 1.89 (1.11–3.28); 0.019	G; (0.16 | 0.21); 1.42 (1.08–1.85); 0.011
rs6465657	7q21	*LMTK2*	T; (0.18 | 0.14); 0.56 (0.36–0.87); 0.010	T; (0.18 | 0.23); 0.226	T; (0.18 | 0.17); 0.455
rs7008482	8q24	*NSMCE2*	T; (0.44 | 0.31); **0.41 (0.26–0.62); 2.45×10^{-5}**	G; (0.42 | 0.42); 0.877	T; (0.51 | 0.60); **0.48 (0.34–0.68); 3.87×10^{-5}**
rs6983561	8q24	*PRNCR1*	C; (0.16 | 0.18); 0.335	C; (0.06 | 0.10); 0.067	C; (0.11 | 0.15); 0.078
rs6983267	8q24	*POU5F1P1*	T; (0.41 | 0.26); **0.35 (0.23–0.53); 4.48×10^{-7}**	T; (0.39 | 0.37); 0.774	T; (0.40 | 0.30); **0.53 (0.39–0.73); 8.05×10^{-5}**
rs4242382	8q24	*POU5F1P1*	A; (0.24 | 0.19); 0.59 (0.39–0.89); 0.013	A; (0.20 | 0.19); 0.768	A; (0.22 | 0.19); 0.11
rs10993994	10q11	*MSMB*	T; (0.27 | 0.37); **1.56 (1.56–6.08); 1.40×10^{-3}**	T; (0.12 | 0.33); **3.49 (2.28–5.54); 1.56×10^{-9}**	T; (0.20 | 0.35); **2.09 (1.64–2.68); 3.03×10^{-9}**
rs4962416	10q26	*CTBP2*	C; (0.49 | 0.46); 0.61 (0.36–0.97); 0.035	T; (0.43 | 0.47); 0.305	T; (0.48 | 0.46); 0.338
rs7931342	11q13	*MYEOV*	T; (0.44 | 0.38); 0.064	T; (0.48 | 0.48); 0.664	T; (0.46 | 0.41); 0.091
rs4430796	17q12	*HNF1B*	A; (0.44 | 0.39); 0.433	A; (0.48 | 0.44); 0.48 (0.26–0.84); 0.010	A; (0.46 | 0.45); 0.424
rs1859962	17q24	*CASC17*	G; (0.28 | 0.28); 0.757	G; (0.29 | 0.36); 1.42 (1.01–2.01); 0.044	G; (0.28 | 0.30); 0.302
rs2735839	19q13	*KLK3*	A; (0.31 | 0.36); 0.149	A; (0.36 | 0.34); 0.734	A; (0.33 | 0.35); 0.377

Only $p < 1.47 \times 10^{-3}$ (Bonferroni correction) indicated in bold text was considered statistically significant.

[a]OR (95% CI) only shown for SNPs where $p < 0.05$.

[b]Adjusted for age and ethnicity.

[‡]Genes indicated have been shown to be involved in prostate tumour onset or progression or to have altered expression in prostate tumours [34–41], except *NSMCE2*, shown to alter growth rates of breast cancer cells [42], *MYEOV*, shown to be overamplified in breast and oesophageal carcinomas [43], and *CASC17*, a long nonprotein coding RNA gene.

when combining the Mixed Ancestry with other groups) [31]. For the Mixed Ancestry and the combined group, only rs7008482, rs6983267, and rs10993994 were significantly associated after correction for population stratification as well as for multiple testing (Table 2). The individual samples sizes in our study were small; therefore, larger genetic investigations in the population groups investigated here are required to conclusively establish whether or not the selected SNPs play a role in PCa susceptibility.

Our study findings should be interpreted in light of some limitations. We acknowledge that our investigations were only performed on men from the two South African population groups with the highest incidence of PCa and recognize that significant underreporting and underdiagnosis of PCa have been documented in other groups, particularly in South African Black men [49]; thus, future studies would need to be extended to other population groups. Our study sample was relatively small and this may have disadvantaged our power to detect statistical significance. We excluded two SNPs (Bd11934905 and rs7210100) with minor allele frequencies (MAFs) < 1%, because there may not be sufficient power to detect the effect of rare variants due to our sample size; however, larger studies should be undertaken as we cannot disregard them as potential disease-causative SNPs. Population stratification is an additional confounder in case-control association analyses. Daya and colleagues [45] have shown using ancestry informative markers (AIMs) specific for the South African Mixed Ancestry population that genetic associations may change after adjustment for ancestry (previous associations may be abolished or associations may only become apparent after adjustment for ancestry). However, the authors also noted that association results are more likely to be unaffected by adjustment for ancestry if the allele frequencies in the stratified population do not differ markedly from the source populations [45]. When we compared the allele frequencies of the selected SNPs in the Mixed Ancestry to likely source populations in the 1000 Genomes database (African, European, South, and East Asian), the allele frequencies we observed often differed by <5%.

5. Conclusions

We demonstrate that a number of reported susceptibility SNP variants may contribute to PCa susceptibility in South African Mixed Ancestry and White men. However, this was a relatively small study and only men from two population groups were investigated. Consequently, larger genetic investigations extended to different South African population groups are warranted to confirm the role of these and other SNPs in PCa susceptibility.

Acknowledgments

The authors would like to thank all the participants of the study and the urologists who facilitated the collection of samples. The study was supported by grants from the AORTIC/NCI BIG_CAT Programme and Cancer Association of South Africa (CANSA) (424366) (Pedro Fernandez).

References

[1] A. Jemal, F. Bray, M. M. Center, J. Ferlay, E. Ward, and D. Forman, "Global cancer statistics," *CA: A Cancer Journal for Clinicians*, vol. 61, no. 2, pp. 69–90, 2011.

[2] O. W. Brawley, "Trends in prostate cancer in the United States," *Journal of the National Cancer Institute—Monographs*, vol. 2012, no. 45, pp. 152–156, 2012.

[3] J. Ferlay, H.-R. Shin, F. Bray, D. Forman, C. Mathers, and D. M. Parkin, "Estimates of worldwide burden of cancer in 2008: GLOBOCAN 2008," *International Journal of Cancer*, vol. 127, no. 12, pp. 2893–2917, 2010.

[4] T. R. Rebbeck, S. S. Devesa, B. L. Chang et al., "Global patterns of prostate cancer incidence, aggressiveness, and mortality in men of African descent," *Prostate Cancer*, vol. 2013, Article ID 560857, 12 pages, 2013.

[5] J. Gudmundsson, P. Sulem, A. Manolescu et al., "Genome-wide association study identifies a second prostate cancer susceptibility variant at 8q24," *Nature Genetics*, vol. 39, no. 5, pp. 631–637, 2007.

[6] R. A. Eeles, Z. Kote-Jarai, G. G. Giles et al., "Multiple newly identified loci associated with prostate cancer susceptibility," *Nature Genetics*, vol. 40, no. 3, pp. 316–321, 2008.

[7] R. A. Eeles, Z. Kote-Jarai, A. A. Al Olama et al., "Identification of seven new prostate cancer susceptibility loci through a genome-wide association study," *Nature Genetics*, vol. 41, no. 10, pp. 1116–1121, 2009.

[8] F. R. Schumacher, S. I. Berndt, A. Siddiq et al., "Genome-wide association study identifies new prostate cancer susceptibility loci," *Human Molecular Genetics*, vol. 20, no. 19, pp. 3867–3875, 2011.

[9] R. A. Eeles, A. A. Olama, S. Benlloch et al., "Identification of 23 new prostate cancer susceptibility loci using the iCOGS custom genotyping array," *Nature Genetics*, vol. 45, no. 4, pp. 385–392, 2013.

[10] P. Gaj, N. Maryan, E. E. Hennig et al., "Pooled sample-based GWAS: a cost-effective alternative for identifying colorectal and prostate cancer risk variants in the Polish population," *PLoS ONE*, vol. 7, no. 4, Article ID e35307, 2012.

[11] E. M. Lange, A. M. Johnson, Y. Wang et al., "Genome-wide association scan for variants associated with early-onset prostate cancer," *PloS ONE*, vol. 9, no. 4, Article ID e93436, 2014.

[12] C. A. Haiman, Y. Han, Y. Feng et al., "Genome-wide testing of putative functional exonic variants in relationship with breast and prostate cancer risk in a multiethnic population," *PLoS Genetics*, vol. 9, no. 3, Article ID e1003419, 2013.

[13] D. Duggan, S. L. Zheng, M. Knowlton et al., "Two genome-wide association studies of aggressive prostate cancer implicate putative prostate tumor suppressor gene DAB2IP," *Journal of the National Cancer Institute*, vol. 99, no. 24, pp. 1836–1844, 2007.

[14] M. B. Cook, Z. Wang, E. D. Yeboah et al., "A genome-wide association study of prostate cancer in West African men," *Human Genetics*, vol. 133, no. 5, pp. 509–521, 2014.

[15] J. Shan, K. Al-Rumaihi, D. Rabah et al., "Genome scan study of prostate cancer in Arabs: identification of three genomic regions with multiple prostate cancer susceptibility loci in Tunisians," *Journal of Translational Medicine*, vol. 11, no. 1, article 121, 2013.

[16] Z. Xu, J. T. Bensen, G. J. Smith, J. L. Mohler, and J. A. Taylor, "GWAS SNP replication among African American and European American men in the North Carolina-Louisiana prostate cancer project (PCaP)," *The Prostate*, vol. 71, no. 8, pp. 881–891, 2011.

[17] N. J. Camp, J. M. Farnham, J. Wong, G. B. Christensen, A. Thomas, and L. A. Cannon-Albright, "Replication of the 10q11 and Xp11 prostate cancer susceptibility variants: results from a Utah pedigree-based study," *Cancer Epidemiology Biomarkers and Prevention*, vol. 18, no. 4, pp. 1290–1294, 2009.

[18] C. A. Haiman, G. K. Chen, W. J. Blot et al., "Characterizing genetic risk at known prostate cancer susceptibility loci in African Americans," *PLoS Genetics*, vol. 7, no. 5, Article ID e1001387, 2011.

[19] C. Robbins, J. B. Torres, S. Hooker et al., "Confirmation study of prostate cancer susceptibility variants at 8q24 in African Americans identifies a novel susceptibility locus," *Genome Research*, vol. 17, no. 12, pp. 1717–1722, 2007.

[20] C. A. Salinas, E. Kwon, C. S. Carlson et al., "Multiple independent genetic variants in the 8q24 region are associated with prostate cancer risk," *Cancer Epidemiology Biomarkers and Prevention*, vol. 17, no. 5, pp. 1203–1213, 2008.

[21] J. Sun, L. Purcell, Z. Gao et al., "Association between sequence variants at 17q12 and 17q24.3 and prostate cancer risk in European and African Americans," *Prostate*, vol. 68, no. 7, pp. 691–697, 2008.

[22] S. Hooker, W. Hernandez, H. Chen et al., "Replication of prostate cancer risk loci on 8q24, 11q13, 17q12, 19q33, and Xp11 in African Americans," *Prostate*, vol. 70, no. 3, pp. 270–275, 2010.

[23] J. Xu, A. S. Kibel, J. J. Hu et al., "Prostate cancer susceptibility associated loci in African Americans," *Cancer Epidemiology Biomarkers and Prevention*, vol. 18, no. 7, pp. 2145–2149, 2009.

[24] C. Bonilla, S. Hooker, T. Mason, C. H. Bock, and R. A. Kittles, "Prostate cancer susceptibility loci identified on chromosome 12 in african americans," *PLoS ONE*, vol. 6, no. 2, Article ID e16044, 2011.

[25] S. Lindstrom, F. Schumacher, A. Siddiq et al., "Characterizing associations and SNP-environment interactions for GWAS-identified prostate cancer risk markers—results from BPC3," *PLoS ONE*, vol. 6, no. 2, Article ID e17142, 2011.

[26] A. B. Murphy, F. Ukoli, V. Freeman et al., "8q24 risk alleles in West African and Caribbean men," *Prostate*, vol. 72, no. 12, pp. 1366–1373, 2012.

[27] Y.-R. Zhang, Y. Xu, M. Liu et al., "Association of six susceptibility loci with prostate cancer in Northern Chinese men," *Asian Pacific Journal of Cancer Prevention*, vol. 13, no. 12, pp. 6273–6276, 2012.

[28] J. Y. Chan, H. Li, O. Singh et al., "8q24 and 17q prostate cancer susceptibility loci in a multiethnic Asian cohort," *Urologic Oncology*, vol. 31, no. 8, pp. 1553–1560, 2013.

[29] E. A. Tindall, M. R. Bornman, S. Van Zyl et al., "Addressing the contribution of previously described genetic and epidemiological risk factors associated with increased prostate cancer risk and aggressive disease within men from South Africa," *BMC Urology*, vol. 13, article 74, 2013.

[30] Y. Han, L. B. Signorello, S. S. Strom et al., "Generalizability of established prostate cancer risk variants in men of African ancestry," *International Journal of Cancer*, vol. 136, no. 5, pp. 1210–1217, 2015.

[31] P. Fernandez, C. M. Zeigler-Johnson, E. Spangler et al., "Androgen metabolism gene polymorphisms, associations with prostate cancer risk and pathological characteristics: a comparative analysis between South African and Senegalese men," *Prostate Cancer*, vol. 2012, Article ID 798634, 8 pages, 2012.

[32] P. H. Westfall and S. S. Young, *Resampling-Based Multiple Testing*, Wiley, New York, NY, USA, 1993.

[33] J. J. Chen, P. K. Roberson, and M. J. Schell, "The false discovery rate: a key concept in large-scale genetic studies," *Cancer Control*, vol. 17, no. 1, pp. 58–62, 2010.

[34] H.-Y. Yeh, S.-W. Cheng, Y.-C. Lin, C.-Y. Yeh, S.-F. Lin, and V.-W. Soo, "Identifying significant genetic regulatory networks in the prostate cancer from microarray data based on transcription factor analysis and conditional independency," *BMC Medical Genomics*, vol. 2, article 70, 2009.

[35] D. J. Hazelett, S. K. Rhie, M. Gaddis et al., "Comprehensive functional annotation of 77 prostate cancer risk loci," *PLoS Genetics*, vol. 10, no. 1, Article ID e1004102, 2014.

[36] L. W. Harries, J. R. B. Perry, P. McCullagh, and M. Crundwell, "Alterations in LMTK2, MSMB and HNF1B gene expression are associated with the development of prostate cancer," *BMC Cancer*, vol. 10, article 315, 2010.

[37] L. Yang, C. Lin, C. Jin et al., "lncRNA-dependent mechanisms of androgen-receptor-regulated gene activation programs," *Nature*, vol. 500, no. 7464, pp. 598–602, 2013.

[38] S. Kastler, L. Honold, M. Luedeke et al., "*POU5F1P1*, a putative cancer susceptibility gene, is overexpressed in prostatic carcinoma," *The Prostate*, vol. 70, no. 6, pp. 666–674, 2010.

[39] M. M. Pomerantz, Y. Shrestha, R. J. Flavin et al., "Analysis of the 10q11 cancer risk locus implicates MSMB and NCOA4 in human prostate tumorigenesis," *PLoS Genetics*, vol. 6, no. 11, Article ID e1001204, 2010.

[40] C. Debiais-Delpech, J. Godet, N. Pedretti et al., "Expression patterns of candidate susceptibility genes HNF1β and CtBP2 in prostate cancer: association with tumor progression," *Urologic Oncology: Seminars and Original Investigations*, vol. 32, no. 4, pp. 426–432, 2014.

[41] A. Fujita, L. R. Gomes, J. R. Sato et al., "Multivariate gene expression analysis reveals functional connectivity changes between normal/tumoral prostates," *BMC Systems Biology*, vol. 2, article 106, 2008.

[42] H.-J. Ni, Y.-N. Chang, P.-H. Kao et al., "Depletion of SUMO ligase hMMS21 impairs G1 to S transition in MCF-7 breast cancer cells," *Biochimica et Biophysica Acta—General Subjects*, vol. 1820, no. 12, pp. 1893–1900, 2012.

[43] M. Brecht, A. C. M. Steenvoorden, S. Luf, C. R. Bartram, and J. W. G. Janssen, "Rearrangement and expression of myeov and hst in NIH/3T3 transfectants: a caveat for the interpretation of DNA transfection analyses," *Oncology Reports*, vol. 17, no. 5, pp. 1127–1131, 2007.

[44] South African National Cancer Registry (NCR) Reports, http://www.nioh.ac.za/assets/files/NCR_2009_FINAL.pdf.

[45] M. Daya, L. van der Merwe, P. D. van Helden, M. Möller, and E. G. Hoal, "The role of ancestry in TB susceptibility of an admixed South African population," *Tuberculosis*, vol. 94, no. 4, pp. 413–420, 2014.

[46] C. R. Ritch, B. F. Morrison, G. Hruby et al., "Pathological outcome and biochemical recurrence-free survival after radical prostatectomy in African-American, Afro-Caribbean (Jamaican) and Caucasian-American men: an international comparison," *BJU International*, vol. 111, no. 4, pp. E186–E190, 2013.

[47] N. Ahmadiyeh, M. M. Pomerantz, C. Grisanzio et al., "8q24 prostate, breast, and colon cancer risk loci show tissue-specific long-range interaction with *MYC*," *Proceedings of the National Academy of Sciences of the United States of America*, vol. 107, no. 21, pp. 9742–9746, 2010.

[48] M. M. Pomerantz, C. A. Beckwith, M. M. Regan et al., "Evaluation of the 8q24 prostate cancer risk locus and MYC expression," *Cancer Research*, vol. 69, no. 13, pp. 5568–5574, 2009.

[49] C. F. Heyns, S. Mathee, A. Isaacs, A. Kharwa, P. M. De Beer, and M. A. Pretorius, "Problems with prostate specific antigen screening for prostate cancer in the primary healthcare setting in South Africa," *BJU International*, vol. 91, no. 9, pp. 785–788, 2003.

6

Does Statin or ASA Affect Survival When Prostate Cancer Is Treated with External Beam Radiation Therapy?

J. Caon,[1] M. Paquette,[2] J. Hamm,[3] and T. Pickles[1,2]

[1] *BC Cancer Agency Radiation Therapy Program, BC Cancer Agency, Vancouver Centre, 600 West 10th Avenue, Vancouver, BC, Canada V5Z 4E6*
[2] *University of British Columbia, 2329 West Mall, Vancouver, BC, Canada V6T 1Z4*
[3] *Cancer Surveillance & Outcomes, Population Oncology, BC Cancer Agency, 600 West 10th Avenue, Vancouver, BC, Canada V5Z 4E6*

Correspondence should be addressed to J. Caon; jcaon-02@bccancer.bc.ca

Academic Editor: Katsuto Shinohara

Background. Prior studies evaluating the effect of statins or acetylsalicylic acid (ASA) on the survival of men receiving prostate cancer were treatment have reported conflicting results, and have not adjusted for comorbidity. Our aim is to investigate the influence of statins and ASA on prostate cancer survival, when comorbidity is adjusted for, in men treated with external beam radiation therapy (EBRT) for prostate cancer. *Methods.* A cohort of 3851 patients with prostate cancer treated with curative EBRT ± androgen deprivation therapy (ADT) between 2000 and 2007. Stage, treatment, medication use, and Charlson comorbidity index (CCI) scores were analyzed. *Results.* Median followup was 8.4 years. Mean age was 70.3 years. Neoadjuvant ADT was used in 67%. Statins were used in 23%, ASA in 24%, and both in 11%. Comorbidity scores were 0 in 65%, 1 in 25%, and ≥2 in 10% of patients. Statin and ASA use were associated with increased age and comorbidity. Although statin and ASA use were significantly associated with improved prostate cancer specific survival (PCSS) on univariate analysis, neither were on multivariate analysis. *Conclusion.* Neither statin nor ASA use impacted PCSS on multivariate competing risks analysis. Survival was impacted by increased comorbidity as well as statin and ASA use.

1. Introduction

As a medication class, 3-hydroxy-3-methyl-glutaryl-CoA reductase inhibitors, commonly known as statins, are prescribed to lower cholesterol and reduce the risk of death from cardiovascular disease [1]. However, statins may also modulate prostate cancer through alteration in the cholesterol levels required for signal transduction of prostate cancer cells [2, 3]. Statins may reduce androgen receptor expression and activity which could lead to reduced prostate cancer cell proliferation and increased apoptosis [4, 5] and a reduction in prostate specific antigen (PSA) release by such cells [4]. A number of other characteristics important to a neoplastic cell may also be altered in the presence of statin medications [6].

Acetylsalicylic acid (ASA) is an antiplatelet agent [7]. The effect on cancer is felt to be related to its properties as a nonsteroidal anti-inflammatory, particularly its effect on COX-2 receptors [8]. There is also a complex interplay between blood coagulation and cancer [9].

Studies evaluating the effect of statins or ASA on outcomes of men receiving curative intent treatment for prostate cancer have reported conflicting results. Acetylsalicylic acid has been associated with a decreased risk of prostate cancer [10]. In men with a preexisting diagnosis of prostate cancer, a prospective study did not show an association between this medication and prostate cancer death [11]; this is in contrast to a more recent study which found a lower risk of prostate cancer death in users of acetylsalicylic acid [12]. Some reports have suggested that statin use was associated with improved biochemical control [13, 14] but its effect in survival is less clear [13, 15, 16].

While differences in the health of users and nonusers of certain medications, such as statins, may impact survival outcomes [17], data accounting for comorbidity among patients with prostate cancer remains lacking. In 2010, an editorial by D'Amico [17] advocated for the inclusion of comorbidity in studies assessing the impact of such medications. This study investigates associations between prostate cancer survival and statin and/or ASA use in men treated with curative intent radiation therapy, after adjusting for comorbidity.

2. Methods and Materials

A retrospective electronic chart review was conducted of patients with newly diagnosed localized prostate cancer treated in British Columbia (BC) with curative intent external beam radiation therapy (EBRT) for prostate cancer from January 1, 2000, to December 31, 2007. The BC Cancer Agency (BCCA) is a provincial cancer care institution that managed five regional centres providing all of the radiation therapy in BC during the study era. The study period was chosen because statin use was relatively uncommon before this time. Data were obtained from electronic linkage to existing data sources, including tumor marker, cancer registry, and death registry records, supplemented by review of the electronic chart for comorbidity and medication use.

Of initial 6144 patients, 2091 were excluded because they were not treated with EBRT. 4053 charts were reviewed and additional 202 patients were excluded because they had nonadenocarcinoma histology, noncurative treatment intent, prior orchiectomy, postprostatectomy radiation, brachytherapy boost, incomplete radiation course, incomplete electronic records, or no information about medication use. The final cohort included 3851 subjects.

Patient characteristics analyzed were age at diagnosis, income level (generated from tables of average income by postal code), and comorbidity using the Charlson comorbidity index (CCI) which was collected retrospectively by review of charts. The CCI is the most widely used tool to measure comorbidity and is valid in predicting mortality risk in a number of conditions, including cancer [18]. Specific comorbid conditions, including myocardial infarction, congestive heart failure, peripheral vascular disease, cerebrovascular disease, dementia, chronic obstructive pulmonary disease, connective tissue disease, peptic ulcer disease, liver disease (mild to severe), diabetes (with or without end organ damage), hemiplegia, renal disease (moderate to severe), malignancy, leukemia, lymphoma, metastatic solid malignancy, and AIDS, are weighted with different scores [19]. As prostate cancer was present in all subjects, this was not included in the Charlson score generated.

Statin and ASA medication use was coded from documentation at the time of initial consultation, which included referring physician notes, consultation reports as well as the patients written list of medication provided at the time of treatment consultation. "Statins" included a range of different types: atorvastatin, rosuvastatin, pravastatin, simvastatin, lovastatin, pitavastatin, fluvastatin, and statin not otherwise specified (NOS). "ASA" included acetylsalicylic acid only. Duration of medication use was not analyzed.

Clinicopathologic characteristics analyzed were stage, Gleason score, and initial prostate specific antigen (iPSA), allowing classification into a National Comprehensive Cancer Network (NCCN) risk group (low, intermediate, and high risk). Treatment characteristics included EBRT dose, adjuvant androgen deprivation therapy (ADT) use, and ADT duration. The year of radiation treatment was stratified at the median (2004).

Prostate cancer specific survival (PCSS) and overall survival (OS) were the primary endpoints of this analysis. Biochemical control and metastasis-free endpoints were not feasible due to nonstandardized followup practices and nonuniform indications for imaging or intervention upon relapse.

Descriptive statistics with cross-tabulations were employed. Analysis of survival endpoints was completed using univariate Kaplan-Meier statistics; univariate and multivariate hazard ratio models using Fine and Gray's competing risks analysis [20]. Data analyses were completed using Statistical Package for Social Sciences version 17.0 (SPSS, Chicago, IL, USA) and the SAS statistical software package (SAS version 9.3; SAS Institute Inc., Cary, NC). Significance was defined as $P \leq 0.05$. The study was approved by the Research Ethics Board of the University of British Columbia.

3. Results

Clinicopathologic characteristics of the entire cohort and according to prostate cancer risk groups are summarized in Table 1. The mean age was 70.3 years (range 45 to 88 years). The mean EBRT dose was 70.9 Gy. Most patients (67%) received neoadjuvant ADT (mean duration 11.9 months). The distribution of prostate cancer risk groups was high risk in 44%, intermediate risk in 40%, and low risk in 14%. Charlson comorbidity scores were 0 in 65%, 1 in 25%, and ≥2 in 10% of subjects. Comorbidity indices were not associated with prostate cancer risk group ($P = 0.425$) or age ($P = 0.120$).

As expected there were significant differences ($P < 0.001$) between statin and ASA users and nonusers in regard to Charlson comorbidity scores (Table 1), with increasing comorbidity being associated with increased use of these medications. Overall, statins were used in 914 (24%) patients. Statin users were older ($P = 0.013$) and had a higher CCI score ($P < 0.001$) and a lower income level ($P = 0.04$). ASA medications were used in 917 (24%) patients. These patients were also older ($P < 0.001$) with higher CCI scores ($P < 0.001$).

Median followup for survival was 8.4 years. The association between statin or ASA use with PCSS and OS at 10 years is shown in Table 2. On Fine and Gray competing risks analysis, there was an improvement in PCSS with the use of statins (10-year survival 94.1% versus 91.2%, $P = 0.031$, Figure 1) and with ASA (93.4% versus 91.3%, $P = 0.004$). Neither statin nor ASA use was associated with OS ($P = 0.83$ and 0.37, resp.). As expected, those with higher risk prostate cancer had reduced PCSS and OS (both $P < 0.001$), and men with higher comorbidity had inferior 10-year OS: 67%, 56%, and 47% for CCI score 0, 1, and ≥2, respectively ($P < 0.001$).

Table 1: Patient, tumor, and treatment characteristics in the entire cohort and according to use of statin and ASA.

Characteristics	Entire cohort ($N = 3851$)	No statin/ASA ($n = 2428$)	Statin, no ASA ($n = 506$)	ASA, no statin ($n = 509$)	Statin + ASA ($n = 408$)
Median age	71 yrs	71 yrs	71 yrs	72 yrs	72 yrs
Charlson comorbidity index					
0	65% (2507)	73% (1773)	51% (260)	62% (313)	40% (161)
1	25% (961)	20% (473)	33% (166)	29% (145)	43% (177)
≥2	10% (383)	7.5% (182)	16% (80)	10% (51)	17% (70)
Low risk	14% (563)	14% (334)	15% (80)	14% (72)	17% (69)
Intermediate risk	39% (1534)	37% (900)	40% (201)	46% (236)	45% (182)
High risk	44% (1718)	47% (1141)	33% (217)	38% (191)	36% (146)
Null risk	2% (83)	2% (53)	2% (8)	2% (10)	2% (11)
Radiation dose Gy [a]Median (range)	70 Gy (50–80 Gy)	70 Gy (52.50–78 Gy)	70 Gy (52.50–78 Gy)	70 Gy (52.50–78 Gy)	70 Gy (52.50–78 Gy)
Radiation dose $BED_{1.5}$ [a]Median (range)	163 (126–201)	163 (126–201)	163 (133–201)	163 (128–195)	163 (140–182)
Frequency ADT[b] use	67%	71%	61%	63%	59%
Mean duration ADT[2] (if used)	16 mo	18 mo	18 mo	18 mo	1 mo

[a]RT: radiation therapy; [b]ADT: androgen deprivation therapy.

Table 2: Prostate cancer survival.

(a) Prostate cancer specific survival (PCSS) calculated using competing risk analysis by Fine and Gray

	Treatment	No treatment	P value
Statin	94.1%	91.2%	0.031
ASA	93.4%	91.3%	0.004

(b) Overall survival, Kaplan-Meier log rank analysis

	Treatment	No treatment	P value
Statin	63.1%	62.3%	0.827
ASA	61.8%	62.8%	0.371

The univariate and multivariate hazard ratio model using competing risks is reported for PCSS in Table 3. As expected, lower risk cancers (lower iPSA, T-stage, and Gleason score) were associated with improved PCSS on both univariate and multivariate analysis. However, increased comorbidity, as reflected by CCI score ≥2, had improved PCSS; this is likely due to the influence of competing risks. The improved PCSS seen on univariate analysis in statin and ASA users was not borne out in the multivariate model.

4. Discussion

This study is among the first to examine prostate cancer survival outcome relative to both statin and ASA use with comorbidity in a population-based cohort of men with localized prostate cancer treated with curative intent EBRT. When taking comorbidity into account using a multivariate completing risks analysis, neither statin nor ASA use was associated with PCSS.

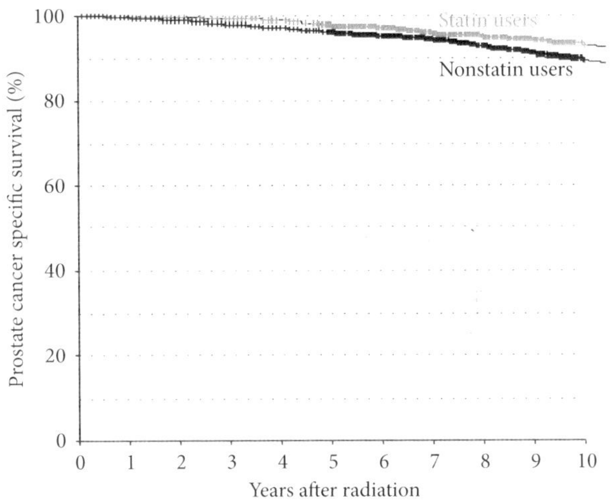

Figure 1: Prostate cancer specific survival between statin users and nonusers.

Population-based studies are typically undertaken to determine whether or not laboratory results are observed at a clinical level. Some studies suggest that statin use is associated with reduced risks of prostate cancer, especially with more aggressive disease [21–23], with larger benefits seen with longer duration [21, 23] and dose [23] of medication, but other studies have not been conclusive in this regard [24–26]. Tagalakis et al. [27] showed that, at a population level, men who used anticoagulants were less likely to be diagnosed with prostate cancer, a decrease in risk that was not seen for any other urogenital cancer and appeared to be related to the duration of medication use. Other studies have also reported a reduced risk of prostate cancer from the use of Warfarin

Table 3: Multivariate model for competing risk analysis using Fine and Gray's test [20] of significance of prostate cancer specific survival.

Variable	Univariate analysis				Multivariate analysis[a]		
	Hazard ratio	95% confidence interval	*P* value	10 yr PCSS %	Hazard ratio	95% confidence interval	*P* value
Statin (yes versus no)	0.656	0.478–0.898	0.0086	94.1 versus 91.1	0.769	0.548–1.08	NS
ASA (yes versus no)	0.728	0.537–0.985	0.040	93.4 versus 91.3	0.911	0.648–1.282	NS
Age	0.986	0.968–1.005	0.14	—	0.988	0.972–1.005	NS
Year of treatment (≥2004 versus ≤2003)	1.176	0.924–1.498	0.19	95.9 versus 98.5[b]	1.172	0.897–1.530	NS
Radiation dose	1.000	0.999–1.000	0.13	—	1.000	0.999–1.000	NS
ADT[c] (yes versus no)	1.789	1.418–2.500	0.0003	90.5 versus 94.5	0.710	0.481–1.049	0.085
iPSA[d]	2.764	1.988–3.843	<0.0001	—	1.59	1.13–2.24	0.0085
T stage				97.1			
(2 versus 1)	2.419	1.532–3.820	0.0002	93.5	2.10	1.33–3.33	0.0015
(3 versus 1)	5.916	3.766–9.924	<0.0001	85.6	3.83	2.41–6.08	<0.0001
(4 versus 1)	18.682	10.17–34.31	<0.0001	64.1	11.38	6.11–21.21	<0.0001
Charlson index				90.9			
(1 versus 0)	0.749	0.563–0.998	0.048	92.8	0.76	0.57–1.02	0.072
(≥2 versus 0)	0.495	0.298–0.823	0.0067	95.1	0.53	0.32–0.87	0.013
Gleason score				96.7			
(7 versus ≤6)	2.611	1.823–3.739	<0.0001	92.0	1.94	1.34–2.82	0.005
(≥8 versus ≤6)	5.718	3.987–8.202	<0.0001	83.2	3.21	2.16–4.78	<0.0001

NS: not significant ($P > 0.05$).

[a]Variables with P value ≤ 0.3 in univariate analysis were included in model for multivariate analysis.

[b]Year of treatment is 5-year survival.

[c]iPSA: initial pretreatment PSA.

[d]ADT: androgen deprivation therapy.

[28] and Aspirin [29] but again this has not been established unanimously [30].

If there is a potential benefit from statins or ASA in lowering the risk of prostate cancer, could the use of these medications affect outcomes in men with known prostate cancer? Several retrospective studies have examined this question with conflicting results. Some investigators [31], but not others [32–34], have reported improved biochemical control among men on statins who underwent radical prostatectomy. Others have observed better biochemical control with statin use in men treated with EBRT [13, 14] and have postulated that this may have been mediated through cholesterol or LDL [13]. Statin use was not associated with biochemical control among patients with prostate cancer treated with brachytherapy, perhaps because of the very high control rates achieved with this modality in comparison with EBRT [33]. Similarly studies, which included ASA with other anticoagulants, found improved biochemical control in prostate cancer patients for patients on such medication [12].

Statin use has been associated with better progression-free survival [16] and lower recurrence risk [15] among men with prostate cancer treated with curative intent on univariate but not multivariate analysis [16]. Gutt et al. [13] found statin use to be associated with better relapse-free survival and freedom from androgen deprivation therapy but not overall or cause-specific survival. The effect ASA may have on prostate cancer outcomes is similarly controversial. In 2012 alone, studies have been published and have found both no association [11] and reduced risk [12] of cancer specific mortalityin men who receive surgery or radiotherapy for prostate neoplasia.

Available studies examining prostate cancer specific and overall survival outcomes in association with statin or ASA use have been limited by a lack of information on subjects' comorbidity. The current study, which used the Charlson comorbidity index, a standardized and validated tool to examine comorbidity, demonstrated that men with a lower CCI had a lower risk of death compared to men with a higher CCI. Statin and ASA medication was used more commonly among men with higher CCI, particularly cardiovascular conditions, warranting the prescription of these medications.

There are several limitations of this study. It is a retrospective review and therefore the reporting of data, including medication use and comorbidities, may not have been complete. Medication use was obtained from the patient's written response to a question at the time of clinic admission and was then transcribed into the consultation record and may be subject to potential inaccuracy in reporting. Medication duration (prior and subsequent to treatment) and compliance was unknown. Our sample size, although large, might not have been enough to detect small difference in PCSS in those taking statins or ASA. Endpoints such as biochemical failure or metastasis-free survival were not reliably available. Death information was obtained from automated lists from BC Vital Statistics Agency, and annual updates from the Canadian national death registry are made. There is little outmigration from BC, but some men's vital statistics may be missing if they emigrated from BC or Canada. Despite these limitations, the current study's findings are of value in documenting the frequency of statin and ASA use among patients with localized prostate cancer and the associated survival outcomes stratified by comorbidity. These findings may be used to inform study design and sample estimates for future trials examining the use of these medications in the setting of prostate cancer [35].

5. Conclusion

Statin and ASA use were associated with improved PCSS on univariate analysis but not on multivariate analysis when assessed for competing risks. As expected, statin and ASA are used more often with increased comorbidity, which is significantly associated with worse survival.

Prospective evaluation of the impact of statin use in men with prostate cancer treated with radiation therapy is warranted because of the potential for reducing the mortality of prostate cancer, which remains the 3rd commonest cause of cancer death in the Western world.

Acknowledgment

This research was presented in poster form at CARO Conference in Winnipeg, MB, Canada, September 2011 and ASTRO Conference in Miami, FL, USA, October 2011.

References

[1] e-CPS English, "e-CPS : Drug Monographs : HMG-CoA Reductase Inhibitors (CPhA Monograph)," 2011, https://www.e-therapeutics.ca/cps.showMonograph.action?simpleMonographId=m250500.

[2] R. J. Hamilton, K. C. Goldberg, E. A. Platz, and S. J. Freedland, "The influence of statin medications on prostate-specific antigen levels," *Journal of the National Cancer Institute*, vol. 100, no. 21, pp. 1511–1518, 2008.

[3] H. Y. Oh, E. J. Lee, S. Yoon, B. H. Chung, K. S. Cho, and S. J. Hong, "Cholesterol level of lipid raft microdomains regulates apoptotic cell death in prostate cancer cells through EGFR-mediated Akt and ERK signal transduction," *The Prostate*, vol. 67, no. 10, pp. 1061–1069, 2007.

[4] L. Yang, M. Egger, R. Plattner, H. Klocker, and I. E. Eder, "Lovastatin causes diminished PSA secretion by inhibiting AR expression and function in LNCaP prostate cancer cells," *Urology*, vol. 77, no. 6, pp. 1508.e1–1508.e7, 2011.

[5] A. Yokomizo, M. Shiota, E. Kashiwagi et al., "Statins reduce the androgen sensitivity and cell proliferation by decreasing the androgen receptor protein in prostate cancer cells," *The Prostate*, vol. 71, no. 3, pp. 298–304, 2011.

[6] D. J. Mener, "Prostate specific antigen reduction following statin therapy: mechanism of action and review of the literature," *IUBMB Life*, vol. 62, no. 8, pp. 584–590, 2010.

[7] e-CPS English, "e-CPS : Drug Monographs : Aspirin," 2011, https://www.e-therapeutics.ca/cps.showMonograph.action?simpleMonographId=m069600.

[8] R. E. Harris, J. Beebe-Donk, H. Doss, and D. Burr Doss, "Aspirin, ibuprofen, and other non-steroidal anti-inflammatory drugs in cancer prevention: a critical review of non-selective COX-2 blockade (review)," *Oncology Reports*, vol. 13, no. 4, pp. 559–583, 2005.

[9] A. Falanga, M. Marchetti, A. Vignoli, and D. Balducci, "Clotting mechanisms and cancer: implications in thrombus formation and tumor progression," *Clinical Advances in Hematology & Oncology* , vol. 1, no. 11, pp. 673–678, 2003.

[10] T. Veitonmaki, T. L. Tammela, A. Auvinen, and T. J. Murtola, "Use of aspirin, but not other non-steroidal anti-inflammatory drugs is associated with decreased prostate cancer risk at the population level," *European Journal of Cancer*, vol. 49, no. 4, pp. 938–945, 2013.

[11] P. K. Dhillon, S. A. Kenfield, M. J. Stampfer, E. L. Giovannucci, and J. M. Chan, "Aspirin use after a prostate cancer diagnosis and cancer survival in a prospective cohort," *Cancer Prevention Research*, vol. 5, no. 10, pp. 1223–1228, 2012.

[12] K. S. Choe, D. Correa, A. B. Jani, and S. L. Liauw, "The use of anticoagulants improves biochemical control of localized prostate cancer treated with radiotherapy," *Cancer*, vol. 116, no. 7, pp. 1820–1826, 2010.

[13] R. Gutt, N. Tonlaar, R. Kunnavakkam, T. Karrison, R. R. Weichselbaum, and S. L. Liauw, "Statin use and risk of prostate cancer recurrence in men treated with radiation therapy," *Journal of Clinical Oncology*, vol. 28, no. 16, pp. 2653–2659, 2010.

[14] M. A. Kollmeier, M. S. Katz, K. Mak et al., "Improved biochemical outcomes with statin use in patients with high-risk localized prostate cancer treated with radiotherapy," *International Journal of Radiation Oncology, Biology, Physics*, vol. 79, no. 3, pp. 713–718, 2011.

[15] E. R. Mora, J. A. L. Garin, O. B. Gali, A. F. Comalat, L. F. Ciutat, and O. A. Toro, "The impact of statins use in clinically localized prostate cancer treated with radical prostatectomy," *Actas Urologicas Espanolas*, vol. 33, no. 4, pp. 351–355, 2009.

[16] D. E. Soto, S. Daignault, H. M. Sandler, and M. E. Ray, "No effect of statins on biochemical outcomes after radiotherapy for localized prostate cancer," *Urology*, vol. 73, no. 1, pp. 158–162, 2009.

[17] A. V. D'Amico, "Statin use and the risk of prostate-specific antigen recurrence after radiation therapy with or without hormone therapy for prostate cancer," *Journal of Clinical Oncology*, vol. 28, no. 16, pp. 2651–2652, 2010.

[18] M. Extermann, "Measuring comorbidity in older cancer patients," *European Journal of Cancer*, vol. 36, no. 4, pp. 453–471, 2000.

[19] M. E. Charlson, P. Pompei, K. A. Ales, and C. R. MacKenzie, "A new method of classifying prognostic comorbidity in longitudinal studies: development and validation," *Journal of Chronic Diseases*, vol. 40, no. 5, pp. 373–383, 1987.

[20] J. P. Fine and R. J. Gray, "A proportional hazards model for the subdistribution of a competing risk," *Journal of the American Statistical Association*, vol. 94, no. 446, pp. 496–509, 1999.

[21] R. H. Breau, R. J. Karnes, D. J. Jacobson et al., "The association between statin use and the diagnosis of prostate cancer in a population based cohort," *The Journal of Urology*, vol. 184, no. 2, pp. 494–499, 2010.

[22] E. A. Platz, M. F. Leitzmann, K. Visvanathan et al., "Statin drugs and risk of advanced prostate cancer," *Journal of the National Cancer Institute*, vol. 98, no. 24, pp. 1819–1825, 2006.

[23] J. Shannon, S. Tewoderos, M. Garzotto et al., "Statins and prostate cancer risk: a case-control study," *American Journal of Epidemiology*, vol. 162, no. 4, pp. 318–325, 2005.

[24] L. Blais, A. Desgagné, and J. LeLorier, "3-hydroxy-3-methylglutaryl coenzyme a reductase inhibitors and the risk of cancer: a nested case-control study," *Archives of Internal Medicine*, vol. 160, no. 15, pp. 2363–2368, 2000.

[25] S. Friis, A. H. Poulsen, S. P. Johnsen et al., "Cancer risk among statin users: a population-based cohort study," *International Journal of Cancer*, vol. 114, no. 4, pp. 643–647, 2005.

[26] M. R. Graaf, A. B. Beiderbeck, A. C. G. Egberts, D. J. Richel, and H.-J. Guchelaar, "The risk of cancer in users of statins," *Journal of Clinical Oncology*, vol. 22, no. 12, pp. 2388–2394, 2004.

[27] V. Tagalakis, H. Tamim, M. Blostein, J.-P. Collet, J. A. Hanley, and S. R. Kahn, "Use of warfarin and risk of urogenital cancer: a population-based, nested case-control study," *The Lancet Oncology*, vol. 8, no. 5, pp. 395–402, 2007.

[28] S. Schulman and P. Lindmarker, "Incidence of cancer after prophylaxis with warfarin against recurrent venous thromboembolism," *The New England Journal of Medicine*, vol. 342, no. 26, pp. 1953–1958, 2000.

[29] E. J. Jacobs, M. J. Thun, E. B. Bain, C. Rodriguez, S. J. Henley, and E. E. Calle, "A large cohort study of long-term daily use of adult-strength aspirin and cancer incidence," *Journal of the National Cancer Institute*, vol. 99, no. 8, pp. 608–615, 2007.

[30] L. R. Zacharski, W. G. Henderson, F. R. Rickles et al., "Effect of warfarin anticoagulation on survival in carcinoma of the lung, colon, head and neck, and prostate. Final report of VA Cooperative Study #75," *Cancer*, vol. 53, no. 10, pp. 2046–2052, 1984.

[31] R. J. Hamilton, L. L. Banez, W. J. Aronson et al., "Statin medication use and the risk of biochemical recurrence after radical prostatectomy: results from the Shared Equal Access Regional Cancer Hospital (SEARCH) Database," *Cancer*, vol. 116, no. 14, pp. 3389–3398, 2010.

[32] L. S. Krane, S. A. Kaul, H. J. Stricker, J. O. Peabody, M. Menon, and P. K. Agarwal, "Men presenting for radical prostatectomy on preoperative statin therapy have reduced serum prostate specific antigen," *The Journal of Urology*, vol. 183, no. 1, pp. 118–124, 2010.

[33] M. A. Moyad, G. S. Merrick, W. M. Butler et al., "Statins, especially atorvastatin, may favorably influence clinical presentation and biochemical progression-free survival after brachytherapy for clinically localized prostate cancer," *Urology*, vol. 66, no. 6, pp. 1150–1154, 2005.

[34] J. H. Ku, C. W. Jeong, Y. H. Park, M. C. Cho, C. Kwak, and H. H. Kim, "Relationship of statins to clinical presentation and biochemical outcomes after radical prostatectomy in Korean patients," *Prostate Cancer and Prostatic Diseases*, vol. 14, no. 1, pp. 63–68, 2011.

[35] T. J. Murtola, "Statin use is associated with improved prostate cancer survival: is it time for a clinical trial?" *Expert Review of Anticancer Therapy*, vol. 10, no. 10, pp. 1563–1567, 2010.

7

Androgen Deprivation Therapy Toxicity and Management for Men Receiving Radiation Therapy

Matthew E. Johnson and Mark K. Buyyounouski

Department of Radiation Oncology, Fox Chase Cancer Center, Philadelphia, PA 19111, USA

Correspondence should be addressed to Mark K. Buyyounouski, mark.buyyounouski@fccc.edu

Academic Editor: J. W. Moul

Androgen deprivation therapy is commonly used in combination with radiotherapy as part of the definitive treatment for men with clinically localized and locally advanced prostate cancer. Androgen deprivation has been associated with a wide range of iatrogenic effects impacting a variety of body systems including metabolic, musculoskeletal, cardiovascular, neurocognitive, and sexual. This review aims to provide the radiation oncology community with the knowledge to monitor and manage androgen deprivation therapy toxicity in an effort to provide the highest level of care for patients and to minimize the iatrogenic effects of androgen deprivation as much as possible.

1. Introduction

As a consequence of the benefits observed in several randomized trials comparing radiotherapy (RT) to RT with androgen deprivation therapy (ADT) [1–10], the use of ADT for the definitive treatment of clinically localized and locally advanced prostate cancer has become more commonplace [11], although recent declines in use have been observed in Canada [12]. With more widespread use of ADT, better awareness of the toxicities associated with ADT is required. This is especially true considering the metabolic effects of ADT and the possible increased cardiovascular risk to patients, highlighted by the Lupron prescribing information that warns "increased risk of heart attack, sudden death, and stroke can occur in men using Lupron Depot" [13]. Radiation oncologists will play an important role in the screening and management of these associated toxicities as advisory statements from the American Heart Association, American Cancer Society, and American Urological Association, endorsed by the American Society for Radiation Oncology, affirms "there is no clear indication for patients for whom ADT is believed to be beneficial to be referred to internists, endocrinologists, or cardiologists for evaluation before initiation of ADT" [14]. While new referrals are not needed, clinicians should be mindful to inform the patient's established physician team including the general practitioner, cardiologist, or endocrinologist regarding the modality and duration of ADT to both request their participation in side effect management and keep them informed as surveillance proceeds. Despite the radiation oncologist's important role, a comprehensive review for the radiation oncologist of ADT toxicity and its management is lacking. The purpose of this paper is to provide the radiation oncology community with the knowledge to monitor and manage ADT toxicity in order to provide the highest quality care for patients and to prevent as much as possible the iatrogenic effects linked to the use of ADT.

2. ADT Administration

Androgen deprivation may be attained through a variety of means when prescribed along with radiation therapy. These have historically included orchiectomy [7], luteinizing hormone-releasing hormone (LHRH) agonists [2, 6], antiandrogens [15], or combination of an anti-androgen and LHRH agonist [4, 10, 16, 17].

3. Metabolic Effects

The use of ADT has been associated with a wide range of metabolic alterations including weight gain, changes in lipid profile and worsening insulin resistance [18]. The impact and management of these alterations and their impact on cardiovascular morbidity and mortality are discussed here.

3.1. Weight Gain. Men on ADT often note an increase in body fat and redistribution of weight. As few as 48 weeks of ADT can increase BMI by 2.4% [19]. Small prospective studies have demonstrated an 11% increase in fat mass, 16.5% increase in total abdominal fat, and a 3.8% decrease in lean body mass with one year of ADT [20, 21]. The impact of weight gain alone may be significant: a large European prospective study has shown that increasing waist circumference and BMI have been associated with higher risk of death in the general population [22]. Men on ADT should be made aware of the possibility of weight gain so that they can monitor their weight and adjust their diet and activity level as needed during the course of therapy. The American Heart Association suggests at least 150 minutes per week of moderate exercise or 75 minutes per week of vigorous exercise. An example beginner exercise regimen may be walking 30 minutes a day, five days a week. The US Department of Health and Human Services and the US Department of Agriculture have jointly published the Dietary Guidelines every five years since 1980 [23]. Appropriate caloric intake with a diet high in fruits and vegetables while low in solid fats, sugars, and salts, is key to a healthy diet. Patients can estimate their dietary needs and learn more at ChooseMyPlate.gov.

3.2. Lipids. The effect of ADT on the lipid profile can also be significant. Less than one year of ADT can increase total cholesterol by 9%, increase LDL by 7.3%, and increase triglycerides by 26.5% [19]. The importance of lipid management has been seen in a meta-analysis of 900,000 people in the general population, where total cholesterol level has been directly associated with cardiovascular mortality at all blood pressure levels [24]. One management option for ADT-induced dyslipidemia is toremifene, which has been shown to significantly decrease total cholesterol, LDL, and triglyceride levels, as well as increase HDL levels in a phase III randomized trial [25]. The National Cholesterol Education Program Adult Treatment Panel III (NCEP ATP III) guidelines define the standard of care for lipid management in the general population and, as there are no guidelines specific to the population on ADT, these guidelines should generally be used to direct the management of ADT-induced dyslipidemia. Diet and lifestyle interventions, such as those discussed above, remain the first-line intervention, but statins should be initiated if needed to attain goals [26].

3.3. Insulin Resistance. Insulin resistance is associated with the use of ADT and can lead to an increase in the diagnosis of diabetes mellitus. Twelve weeks of ADT has been demonstrated to increase median serum insulin levels from 11.8 to 19.3 mU/L and reduce insulin sensitivity by 12.9% [27, 28]. An observational study of 37,000 men receiving ADT for prostate cancer noted an aHR of 1.28 for incident cases of diabetes mellitus [29]. This increased risk suggests a benefit to screening for diabetes in this population. The American Diabetes Association recommends screening at-risk populations with either a fasting plasma glucose test, hemoglobin A1c, or 2-hour oral glucose tolerance test. A baseline screening may help identify men with preexisting insulin resistance that may be at higher risk of diabetes during the course of ADT [30]. The most commonly used interventions for those with insulin resistance include lifestyle interventions and metformin. A randomized trial of 3,200 people with elevated glucose concentrations was randomized to lifestyle intervention, metformin (850 mg BID), or placebo. Lifestyle intervention reduced diabetes incidence by 58%, significantly more than metformin, which reduced it by 31% [31]. Once again, lifestyle intervention should be recommended to all patients receiving ADT, including education on diet, exercise, and weight loss.

4. Cardiovascular

The metabolic changes seen in men receiving ADT are concerning for their possible contribution to cardiovascular morbidity and mortality. Cardiovascular disease is already the leading cause of mortality in men with early stage prostate cancer [32], so any possible increase in this risk should be taken seriously. However, the existing literature on the relationship between ADT and cardiovascular morbidity is somewhat mixed. A large VA observational study demonstrated an aHR of 1.28 for myocardial infarction and 1.22 for sudden cardiac death for men on ADT [29], while another large retrospective study demonstrated a 20% increase in cardiovascular events with 12 months of ADT [14]. This increase has also been shown in men older than 65, who were noted to have a shorter time to fatal MI with a history of ADT use for as short as 3 months [33]. Other analyses have shown no correlation between ADT use and cardiovascular mortality. For example, the 8-year followup of RTOG 85-31 [34] and 10-year followup of EORTC 22863 [35] conclude that GnRH agonist use does not significantly increase cardiovascular mortality. Recently, a meta-analysis of over 4,000 patients was unable to show an increased risk of cardiovascular death regardless of ADT duration [36]. Nonetheless, the metabolic changes seen during the use of ADT have been demonstrated to confer excess cardiovascular risk in the general population, and close monitoring of modifiable cardiovascular risk factors is warranted. The science advisory statement from the American Heart Association, American Cancer Society, and American Urological Association recommends annual monitoring of blood pressure, lipid profile, and glucose level for men receiving ADT [14].

While lipid levels and glucose tolerance are adversely affected by ADT as described in the metabolic section, blood pressure is not known to be affected by ADT. Blood pressure, however, is a modifiable cardiovascular risk factor and should be tightly monitored during ADT use to minimize overall cardiovascular risk. Blood pressure should be managed similar to that recommended for the general population: prehypertension should be aggressively treated with lifestyle modification, while stage 1 hypertension should be managed with lifestyle modification and antihypertensive medication. Stage 2 hypertension is treated similarly to stage I with the addition of a diuretic [37].

5. Musculoskeletal

5.1. Muscle Loss. Patients receiving ADT often report loss of muscle mass and muscle weakness, and ADT has been demonstrated to be associated with a decrease in muscle strength and functional performance [38]. Lean body mass has also been shown to decrease by 3.8% with one year of ADT [21]. Two randomized controlled trials have reported on the utility of a structured exercise program to counteract this loss of muscle mass. One trial randomized patients to 12-weeks of a resistance exercise program, done 3 times per week [39]. A second trial reported on a 12 week program of twice per week combined aerobic and resistance exercise [40]. Aerobic exercise included 15–20 minutes of cycling, walking, or jogging at 65–80% maximum exertion. Resistance exercises included chest press, seated row, shoulder press, triceps extension, leg press, leg extension, leg curl, abdominal crunches, and flexibility exercises. Both trials found that participants in the exercise programs had improved muscle strength, muscle mass, quality of life, and reduced fatigue. At the time of the initiation of ADT, patients should be provided recommendations regarding an exercise program that can be used to maintain muscular fitness during the course of ADT.

5.2. Osteoporosis. Much has been published regarding the link between osteoporosis and ADT and subsequent fracture risk following therapy. ADT is used in a population where the baseline prevalence of osteopenia is as high as 46% and osteoporosis is 14% even prior to the initiation of any treatment [41]. Mechanistically, ADT has been shown to lead to microarchitectural decay in bone after 12 months of treatment [42]. An 8.5% decrease in bone mineral density (BMD) can be seen even after 48 weeks of ADT [43]. This has been linked to an increased risk for osteoporotic fracture during and after the use of ADT. A retrospective study of over 12,000 men demonstrated a relative risk of 1.21 for any fracture, 1.18 for vertebral fracture, and 1.76 for hip fracture for patients who had received ADT [44]. This increased risk has also been correlated to a number of doses of ADT administered [45]. Long-term ADT can increase the rate of osteoporosis to as high as 81% after 10 years of treatment [46].

Supplementation with 1200 mg calcium and 800 IU vitamin D daily has been shown to reduce the incidence of osteoporotic fractures in the general population over 50 years old [47], but calcium and vitamin D alone are not sufficient to prevent bone loss in men undergoing ADT [43]. The addition of a bisphosphonate—pamindronate [43, 48], alendronate [49], or zoledronic acid [50, 51]—has been shown to maintain or increase BMD during ADT and is generally well tolerated. Other agents have shown to be effective as well. A trial of 1,468 men receiving ADT randomized to denosumab, a RANKL inhibitor, given 60 mg SQ every 6 months versus placebo demonstrated a 5.6% gain in BMD at 2 years, versus a 1% loss in the placebo group, and was found to decrease the risk of vertebral fractures at 36 months to 1.5% from 3.9% in the placebo group [52]. Denosumab is currently FDA approved for both the prevention of ADT-induced bone loss and for the prevention of skeletal related events in patients with metastatic cancer, but is associated with severe hypocalcemia and osteonecrosis of the jaw [53, 54]. The selective estrogen receptor modulators raloxifene [55] and toremifene have also been used to improve BMD. A phase III randomized controlled trial of toremifene in 646 men demonstrated a reduction in new vertebral fractures from 4.9% in placebo group to 2.5% [56]. However, concern exists with hormonal agents for both their increased risk of venous thromboembolism and their modulation of hormone cascades, which has the potential to diminish the effectiveness of ADT.

Bone density can be assessed with dual-energy X-ray absorptiometry (DEXA). DEXA may be used at the start of ADT and monitored subsequently every 1-2 years as indicated. The National Osteoporosis Foundation recommends supplemental calcium (1,200 mg daily) and vitamin D3 (800–1,000 IU daily) for all men over age 50 years and an additional treatment for men when the 10-year probability of hip fracture is ≥3% or the 10-year probability of a major osteoporosisrelated fracture is ≥20% [57]. Encouragement of lifestyle measures (smoking cessation, moderating alcohol intake, and increasing weight-bearing exercise), along with calcium and vitamin D supplementation, should be routinely performed. Bisphosphonate use should be considered, especially for those men with osteoporosis or osteopenia at baseline [18, 58] or 10-year osteoporotic fracture risk of >20% by the FRAX model [59].

5.3. Hot Flushes. Hot flushes, also known as hot flashes or vasomotor flushing, are a common side effect of ADT, occurring in 80% of patients undergoing treatment. Up to 27% of patients receiving ADT report hot flushes to be the most troublesome treatment-related side effect [60]. Hot flushes are described as unpredictable episodes of intense warmth, most commonly occurring in the face and upper body that is often accompanied by diaphoresis that usually last less than 5 minutes [61]. Natural and complementary approaches to hot flushes have been tested with varying success. Herbal supplements, such as black cohosh, ginseng, licorice, and turmeric may have some benefit, but have not shown efficacy in randomized controlled trials. Weekly acupuncture for 12 weeks was able to demonstrate a 78% decrease in a hot flush symptom score and should be considered a reasonable treatment strategy [62]. Medical therapy with antidepressants and hormonal agents have also been studied. A small series examined transdermal estrogen, with 83% of men reporting an improvement in hot flushes, although an increase in breast swelling or nipple tenderness was reported [63]. Megestrol acetate given at 40 mg per day has also been shown to be effective at reducing the frequency of hot flushes [64]. A randomized controlled trial of patients having >14 hot flushes per week after 6 months of ADT was randomized to venlafaxine 75 mg daily, medroxyprogesterone acetate 20 mg daily, or cyproterone 100 mg daily. All three agents were able to decrease the frequency of hot flushes although both hormonal agents were more effective than venlafaxine [60]. However, there is a concern that hormonal agents may interact with the ADT and may even cause an increase in prostate specific antigen (PSA). As a result, venlafaxine, which is generally well tolerated, is more often considered the first-line treatment for ADT-induced hot flushes [65].

6. Neurocognitive

6.1. Memory. There has been some concern for the decline of memory and neurocognitive function during ADT although existing data on this topic is highly conflicted. One prospective Australian study utilized interval neurocognitive battery testing in 50 men treated with ADT and found that 48% demonstrated decline in one cognitive task and 14% in two or more tasks at one year [66], while a prospective trial of 244 patients was unable to demonstrate any evidence of neurocognitive function decline after ADT use for 12 months on a 12-test battery [67].

6.2. Depression. Depressive disorders have been reported to be more common in men receiving ADT. The proportion of men developing at least one depressive, cognitive, or constitutional disorder was 31.3% in men with prostate cancer undergoing ADT, compared to 23.7% in men with prostate cancer not receiving ADT, and 22.9% in a noncancer control group [68]. Men getting ADT should be informed of this potential side effect so that they can have increased awareness and seek rapid intervention. Radiation oncologists seeing men on ADT should be cognizant of mood disorders so that affected men can be appropriately referred for treatment.

Table 1: Suggested management for patients receiving androgen deprivation therapy.

At time of ADT[1] initiation
Patient education on spectrum of expected side effects
Education on initiation of exercise program
Patient resources at http://go4life.nia.nih.gov/
Education on diet and weight management
Obtain baseline weight
Patient resources at http://www.choosemyplate.gov/
Inform primary care physician of modality and duration of ADT
Baseline lipid panel
Blood pressure measurement
Insulin resistance screening
Smoking cessation
Baseline DEXA[2] scan
Assess fracture risk at http://www.shef.ac.uk/FRAX/
Year 1
Ensure continued followup with primary care physician
Blood pressure management
Lipid monitoring
Weight management
Diabetes screening
Ongoing screening for depression, sexual side effects, and hot flushes
Year 2-3
Ensure continued followup with primary care physician
Blood pressure management
Lipid monitoring
Weight management
Diabetes screening
Ongoing screening for depression, sexual side effects, and hot flushes
DEXA scan
Reassess fracture risk at http://www.shef.ac.uk/FRAX/

[1]Androgen deprivation therapy, [2]dual-energy X-ray absorptiometry.

7. Sexual

7.1. Erectile Dysfunction, Loss of Libido. Onset of loss of libido is frequently seen within the first few months of initiation of ADT and is often followed by erectile dysfunction. Up to 73% of men ceased engaging in sexual activity after initiation of treatment, and 38% of patients getting an LHRH agonist reported sexual function as a "moderate" or "big" problem [69]. As in the general population, first-line treatment for ADT induced erectile dysfunction is phosphodiesterase-5 inhibitors, although these agents have been shown to have a reduced response rate in men who have received ADT. 4 months of ADT reduce the response rate to sildenafil at 24 months from 61% to 47% [70]. Other options for the management of erectile dysfunction follow the same paradigm as that for the general population and include penile implants, vacuum devices, and intracavernosal injections [65].

7.2. Decreased Penile and Testicle Size, Thinning of Body Hair. Men receiving ADT often notice a decrease in both penile and testicle size, as well as a thinning of body hair. For some men, these findings have a significant impact on self-image and quality of life. There are currently no interventions to reverse these side effects, so pretreatment counseling on expected side effects remains important.

7.3. Gynecomastia and Breast Pain. ADT may lead to the development of gynecomastia and breast pain in as many as 70% of patients [71]. This can also have a significant effect on a patient's sense of self-image and their overall quality of life. Two approaches have been taken in the prophylactic setting: tamoxifen 10 mg daily for 24 weeks and breast irradiation, both of which have been shown to significantly decrease the incidence of gynecomastia [71, 72]. Radiotherapy may include either single fraction (9–12 Gy) or fractionated treatment (12–15 Gy given in 2-3 fractions) [73–75]. Once gynecomastia and breast pain have developed, the same two approaches have been used for treatment, but results in this setting favor the use of tamoxifen given 10–20 mg per day for 12 weeks [71, 72]. Although not studied, concern has been raised about the possibility of a synergistic neurocognitive impact of tamoxifen and ADT together. The aromatase inhibitor anastrozole has also been compared to tamoxifen for the treatment of gynecomastia and breast pain, with anastrozole having no significant reduction in symptoms and tamoxifen reducing gynecomastia from 73% to10% and breast pain from 39% to 6% [76].

8. Conclusion

The administration of ADT is associated with a diverse set of known side effects which, when compiled, have a significant impact on a prostate cancer patient's quality of life, overall health, and possibly mortality. While the impact of these side effects can be diminished by early diagnosis and treatment, many of the current management strategies discussed in this paper do not yet appear in consensus guidelines for the treatment of prostate cancer. A compilation of management suggestions can be found in Table 1. Radiation oncologists will serve an important role in advocating for the screening, diagnosis, and management of these side effects, as much of the current role for ADT is its concurrent use in combination with radiation therapy. Improved awareness of the far-reaching effects of ADT by radiation oncologists will lead to a better identification of these ADT side effects and improved multidisciplinary care and, as a result, will mitigate much of the short-term and long-term impact that they can have on the patient.

References

[1] M. V. Pilepich, K. Winter, M. J. John et al., "Phase III radiation therapy oncology group (RTOG) trial 86-10 of androgen deprivation adjuvant to definitive radiotherapy in locally advanced carcinoma of the prostate," *International Journal of Radiation Oncology Biology Physics*, vol. 50, no. 5, pp. 1243–1252, 2001.

[2] M. Bolla, L. Collette, L. Blank et al., "Long-term results with immediate androgen suppression and external irradiation in patients with locally advanced prostate cancer (an EORTC study): a phase III randomised trial," *The Lancet*, vol. 360, no. 9327, pp. 103–108, 2002.

[3] G. E. Hanks, T. F. Pajak, A. Porter et al., "Phase III trial of long-term adjuvant androgen deprivation after neoadjuvant hormonal cytoreduction and radiotherapy in locally advanced carcinoma of the prostate: the radiation therapy oncology group protocol 92-02," *Journal of Clinical Oncology*, vol. 21, no. 21, pp. 3972–3978, 2003.

[4] A. V. D'Amico, J. Manola, M. Loffredo, A. A. Renshaw, A. DellaCroce, and P. W. Kantoff, "6-Month androgen suppression plus radiation therapy vs radiation therapy alone for patients with clinically localized prostate cancer: a randomized controlled trial," *The Journal of the American Medical Association*, vol. 292, no. 7, pp. 821–827, 2004.

[5] J. Laverdière, A. Nabid, L. D. de Bedoya et al., "The efficacy and sequencing of a short course of androgen suppression on freedom from biochemical failure when administered with radiation therapy for T2-T3 prostate cancer," *Journal of Urology*, vol. 171, no. 3, pp. 1137–1140, 2004.

[6] M. V. Pilepich, K. Winter, C. A. Lawton et al., "Androgen suppression adjuvant to definitive radiotherapy in prostate carcinoma—long-term results of phase III RTOG 85-31," *International Journal of Radiation Oncology Biology Physics*, vol. 61, no. 5, pp. 1285–1290, 2005.

[7] T. Granfors, H. Modig, J. E. Damber, and R. Tomic, "Long-term followup of a randomized study of locally advanced prostate cancer treated with combined orchiectomy and external radiotherapy versus radiotherapy alone," *Journal of Urology*, vol. 176, no. 2, pp. 544–547, 2006.

[8] M. Bolla, T. M. de Reijke, G. van Tienhoven et al., "Duration of androgen suppression in the treatment of prostate cancer," *The New England Journal of Medicine*, vol. 360, no. 24, pp. 2516–2527, 2009.

[9] J. W. Denham, A. Steigler, D. S. Lamb et al., "Short-term neoadjuvant androgen deprivation and radiotherapy for locally advanced prostate cancer: 10-year data from the TROG 96.01 randomised trial," *The Lancet Oncology*, vol. 12, no. 5, pp. 451–459, 2011.

[10] C. U. Jones, D. Hunt, D. G. McGowan et al., "Radiotherapy and short-term androgen deprivation for localized prostate cancer," *The New England Journal of Medicine*, vol. 365, no. 2, pp. 107–118, 2011.

[11] V. B. Shahinian, Y. F. Kuo, J. L. Freeman, E. Orihuela, and J. S. Goodwin, "Increasing use of gonadotropin-releasing hormone agonists for the treatment of localized prostate carcinoma," *Cancer*, vol. 103, no. 8, pp. 1615–1624, 2005.

[12] M. Krahn, K. E. Bremner, G. Tomlinson, J. Luo, P. Ritvo, G. Naglie et al., "Androgen deprivation therapy in prostate cancer: are rising concerns leading to falling use?" *British Journal of Urology International*, vol. 108, no. 10, pp. 1588–1596, 2011.

[13] "Lupron depot prescribing information," http://www.lupron.com/prescribing-information.cfm.

[14] G. N. Levine, A. V. D'Amico, P. Berger et al., "Androgen-deprivation therapy in prostate cancer and cardiovascular risk: a science advisory from the American heart association, American cancer society, and American urological association: endorsed by the American society for radiation oncology," *CA: Cancer Journal for Clinicians*, vol. 60, no. 3, pp. 194–201, 2010.

[15] W. Shipley, "Initial report of RTOG, 9601, a phase III trial in prostate cancer: effect of anti-androgen therapy (AAT) with bicalutamide during and after radiation therapy (RT) on freedom from progression and incidence of metastatic disease in patients following radical prostatectomy (RP) with pT2-3, N0 disease and elevated PSA levels," *Journal of Clinical Oncology*, vol. 29, supplement 7, 2011, abstract no. 1.

[16] M. Roach III, K. Bae, J. Speight et al., "Short-term neoadjuvant androgen deprivation therapy and external-beam

radiotherapy for locally advanced prostate cancer: long-term results of RTOG 8610," *Journal of Clinical Oncology*, vol. 26, no. 4, pp. 585–591, 2008.

[17] A. Widmark, O. Klepp, A. Solberg et al., "Endocrine treatment, with or without radiotherapy, in locally advanced prostate cancer (SPCG-7/SFUO-3): an open randomised phase III trial," *The Lancet*, vol. 373, no. 9660, pp. 301–308, 2009.

[18] M. Grossmann, E. J. Hamilton, C. Gilfillan, D. Bolton, D. L. Joon, and J. D. Zajac, "Bone and metabolic health in patients with non-metastatic prostate cancer who are receiving androgen deprivation therapy," *Medical Journal of Australia*, vol. 194, no. 6, pp. 301–306, 2011.

[19] M. R. Smith, J. S. Finkelstein, F. J. McGovern et al., "Changes in body composition during androgen deprivation therapy for prostate cancer," *Journal of Clinical Endocrinology and Metabolism*, vol. 87, no. 2, pp. 599–603, 2002.

[20] M. R. Smith, H. Lee, F. McGovem et al., "Metabolic changes during gonadotropin-releasing hormone agonist therapy for prostate cancer: differences from the classic metabolic syndrome," *Cancer*, vol. 112, no. 10, pp. 2188–2194, 2008.

[21] M. R. Smith, "Changes in fat and lean body mass during androgen-deprivation therapy for prostate cancer," *Urology*, vol. 63, no. 4, pp. 742–745, 2004.

[22] T. Pischon, H. Boeing, K. Hoffmann et al., "General and abdominal adiposity and risk of death in Europe," *The New England Journal of Medicine*, vol. 359, no. 20, pp. 2105–2120, 2008.

[23] U.S. Department of Agriculture and U.S. Department of Health and Human Services, *Dietary Guidelines for Americans, 2010*, U.S. Government Printing Office, Washington, DC, USA, 7th edition, 2010.

[24] Prospective Studies Collaboration, "Blood cholesterol and vascular mortality by age, sex, and blood pressure: a meta-analysis of individual data from 61 prospective studies with 55,000 vascular deaths," *The Lancet*, vol. 370, no. 9602, pp. 1829–1839, 2007.

[25] M. R. Smith, S. B. Malkowicz, F. Chu et al., "Toremifene improves lipid profiles in men receiving androgen-deprivation therapy for prostate cancer: interim analysis of a multicenter phase III study," *Journal of Clinical Oncology*, vol. 26, no. 11, pp. 1824–1829, 2008.

[26] National Cholesterol Education Program, "Third report of the national cholesterol education program (NCEP) expert panel on detection, evaluation, and treatment of high blood cholesterol in adults (adult treatment panel III) final report," *Circulation*, vol. 106, no. 25, pp. 3143–3421, 2002.

[27] M. R. Smith, H. Lee, M. A. Fallon, and D. M. Nathan, "Adipocytokines, obesity, and insulin resistance during combined androgen blockade for prostate cancer," *Urology*, vol. 71, no. 2, pp. 318–322, 2008.

[28] J. C. Smith, S. Bennett, L. M. Evans et al., "The effects of induced hypogonadism on arterial stiffness, body composition, and metabolic parameters in males with prostate cancer," *Journal of Clinical Endocrinology and Metabolism*, vol. 86, no. 9, pp. 4261–4267, 2001.

[29] N. L. Keating, A. J. O'Malley, S. J. Freedland, and M. R. Smith, "Diabetes and cardiovascular disease during androgen deprivation therapy: observational study of veterans with prostate cancer," *Journal of the National Cancer Institute*, vol. 102, no. 1, pp. 39–46, 2010.

[30] American Diabetes Association, "Standards of medical care in diabetes—2012," *Diabetes Care*, vol. 35, supplement 1, pp. S11–S63, 2012.

[31] W. C. Knowler, E. Barrett-Connor, S. E. Fowler et al., "Reduction in the incidence of type 2 diabetes with lifestyle intervention or metformin," *The New England Journal of Medicine*, vol. 346, no. 6, pp. 393–403, 2002.

[32] M. Grossmann and J. D. Zajac, "Androgen deprivation therapy in men with prostate cancer: how should the side effects be monitored and treated?" *Clinical Endocrinology*, vol. 74, no. 3, pp. 289–293, 2011.

[33] A. V. D'Amico, J. W. Denham, J. Crook et al., "Influence of androgen suppression therapy for prostate cancer on the frequency and timing of fatal myocardial infarctions," *Journal of Clinical Oncology*, vol. 25, no. 17, pp. 2420–2425, 2007.

[34] J. A. Efstathiou, K. Bae, W. U. Shipley et al., "Cardiovascular mortality after androgen deprivation therapy for locally advanced prostate cancer: Rtog 85-31," *Journal of Clinical Oncology*, vol. 27, no. 1, pp. 92–99, 2009.

[35] M. Bolla, G. van Tienhoven, P. Warde et al., "External irradiation with or without long-term androgen suppression for prostate cancer with high metastatic risk: 10-year results of an EORTC randomised study," *The Lancet Oncology*, vol. 11, no. 11, pp. 1066–1073, 2010.

[36] P. L. Nguyen, Y. Je, F. A. B. Schutz et al., "Association of androgen deprivation therapy with cardiovascular death in patients with prostate cancer: a meta-analysis of randomized trials," *The Journal of the American Medical Association*, vol. 306, no. 21, pp. 2359–2366, 2011.

[37] A. V. Chobanian, G. L. Bakris, H. R. Black et al., "The seventh report of the joint national committee on prevention, detection, evaluation, and treatment of high blood pressure: the JNC 7 report," *The Journal of the American Medical Association*, vol. 289, no. 19, pp. 2560–2572, 2003.

[38] D. A. Galvão, D. R. Taaffe, N. Spry, D. Joseph, D. Turner, and R. U. Newton, "Reduced muscle strength and functional performance in men with prostate cancer undergoing androgen suppression: a comprehensive cross-sectional investigation," *Prostate Cancer and Prostatic Diseases*, vol. 12, no. 2, pp. 198–203, 2009.

[39] R. J. Segal, R. D. Reid, K. S. Courneya et al., "Resistance exercise in men receiving androgen deprivation therapy for prostate cancer," *Journal of Clinical Oncology*, vol. 21, no. 9, pp. 1653–1659, 2003.

[40] D. A. Galvão, D. R. Taaffe, N. Spry, D. Joseph, and R. U. Newton, "Combined resistance and aerobic exercise program reverses muscle loss in men undergoing androgen suppression therapy for prostate cancer without bone metastases: a randomized controlled trial," *Journal of Clinical Oncology*, vol. 28, no. 2, pp. 340–347, 2010.

[41] A. Berruti, L. Dogliotti, C. Terrone et al., "Changes in bone mineral density, lean body mass and fat content as measured by dual energy x-ray absorptiometry in patients with prostate cancer without apparent bone metastases given androgen deprivation therapy," *Journal of Urology*, vol. 167, no. 6, pp. 2361–2367, 2002.

[42] E. J. Hamilton, A. Ghasem-Zadeh, E. Gianatti et al., "Structural decay of bone microarchitecture in men with prostate cancer treated with androgen deprivation therapy," *Journal of Clinical Endocrinology and Metabolism*, vol. 95, no. 12, pp. E456–E463, 2010.

[43] M. R. Smith, F. J. McGovern, A. L. Zietman et al., "Pamidronate to prevent bone loss during androgen-deprivation therapy for prostate cancer," *The New England Journal of Medicine*, vol. 345, no. 13, pp. 948–955, 2001.

[44] M. R. Smith, S. P. Boyce, E. Moyneur, M. S. Duh, M. K. Raut, and J. Brandman, "Risk of clinical fractures after

gonadotropin-releasing hormone agonist therapy for prostate cancer," *Journal of Urology*, vol. 175, no. 1, pp. 136–139, 2006.

[45] V. B. Shahinian, Y. F. Kuo, J. L. Freeman, and J. S. Goodwin, "Risk of fracture after androgen deprivation for prostate cancer," *The New England Journal of Medicine*, vol. 352, no. 2, pp. 154–164, 2005.

[46] J. Morote, J. P. Morin, A. Orsola et al., "Prevalence of osteoporosis during long-term androgen deprivation therapy in patients with prostate cancer," *Urology*, vol. 69, no. 3, pp. 500–504, 2007.

[47] P. R. Ebeling, "Osteoporosis in men," *The New England Journal of Medicine*, vol. 358, no. 14, pp. 1474–1482, 2008.

[48] T. H. Diamond, J. Winters, A. Smith et al., "The antiosteoporotic efficacy of intravenous pamidronate in men with prostate carcinoma receiving combined androgen blockade: a double blind, randomized, placebo-controlled crossover study," *Cancer*, vol. 92, no. 6, pp. 1444–1450, 2001.

[49] S. L. Greenspan, J. B. Nelson, D. L. Trump, and N. M. Resnick, "Effect of once-weekly oral alendronate on bone loss in men receiving androgen deprivation therapy for prostate cancer: a randomized trial," *Annals of Internal Medicine*, vol. 146, no. 6, pp. 416–424, 2007.

[50] M. D. Michaelson, D. S. Kaufman, H. Lee et al., "Randomized controlled trial of annual zoledronic acid to prevent gonadotropin-releasing hormone agonist-induced bone loss in men with prostate cancer," *Journal of Clinical Oncology*, vol. 25, no. 9, pp. 1038–1042, 2007.

[51] M. R. Smith, J. Eastham, D. M. Gleason, D. Shasha, S. Tchekmedyian, and N. Zinner, "Randomized controlled trial of zoledronic acid to prevent bone loss in men receiving androgen deprivation therapy for nonmetastatic prostate cancer," *Journal of Urology*, vol. 169, no. 6, pp. 2008–2012, 2003.

[52] M. R. Smith, B. Egerdie, N. H. Toriz et al., "Denosumab in men receiving androgen-deprivation therapy for prostate cancer," *The New England Journal of Medicine*, vol. 361, no. 8, pp. 745–755, 2009.

[53] "Prolia prescribing information," http://pi.amgen.com/united_states/prolia/prolia_pi.pdf.

[54] "Xgeva prescribing information," http://pi.amgen.com/united_states/xgeva/xgeva_pi.pdf.

[55] M. R. Smith, M. A. Fallon, H. Lee, and J. S. Finkelstein, "Raloxifene to prevent gonadotropin-releasing hormone agonist-induced bone loss in men with prostate cancer: a randomized controlled trial," *Journal of Clinical Endocrinology and Metabolism*, vol. 89, no. 8, pp. 3841–3846, 2004.

[56] M. R. Smith, R. A. Morton, K. G. Barnette et al., "Toremifene to reduce fracture risk in men receiving androgen deprivation therapy for prostate cancer," *Journal of Urology*, vol. 184, no. 4, pp. 1316–1321, 2010.

[57] National Osteoporosis Foundation, *Clinician's Guide to Prevention and Treatment of Osteoporosis*, 2010, http://www.nof.org/professionals/clinical-guidelines.

[58] F. Saad, J. D. Adachi, J. P. Brown et al., "Cancer treatment-induced bone loss in breast and prostate cancer," *Journal of Clinical Oncology*, vol. 26, no. 33, pp. 5465–5476, 2008.

[59] N. B. Watts, E. M. Lewiecki, P. D. Miller, and S. Baim, "National osteoporosis foundation 2008 clinician's guide to prevention and treatment of osteoporosis and the world health organization fracture risk assessment tool (FRAX): what they mean to the bone densitometrist and bone technologist," *Journal of Clinical Densitometry*, vol. 11, no. 4, pp. 473–477, 2008.

[60] J. Irani, L. Salomon, R. Oba, P. Bouchard, and N. Mottet, "Efficacy of venlafaxine, medroxyprogesterone acetate, and cyproterone acetate for the treatment of vasomotor hot flushes in men taking gonadotropin-releasing hormone analogues for prostate cancer: a double-blind, randomised trial," *The Lancet Oncology*, vol. 11, no. 2, pp. 147–154, 2010.

[61] M. D. Michaelson, S. E. Cotter, P. C. Gargollo, A. L. Zietman, D. M. Dahl, and M. R. Smith, "Management of complications of prostate cancer treatment," *CA: Cancer Journal for Clinicians*, vol. 58, no. 4, pp. 196–213, 2008.

[62] J. Frisk, A. C. Spetz, H. Hjertberg, B. Petersson, and M. Hammar, "Two modes of acupuncture as a treatment for hot flushes in men with prostate cancer—a prospective multicenter study with long-term follow-up," *European Urology*, vol. 55, no. 1, pp. 156–163, 2009.

[63] G. S. Gerber, G. P. Zagaja, P. S. Ray, and D. B. Rukstalis, "Transdermal estrogen in the treatment of hot flushes in men with prostate cancer," *Urology*, vol. 55, no. 1, pp. 97–101, 2000.

[64] C. L. Loprinzi, J. C. Michalak, S. K. Quella et al., "Megestrol acetate for the prevention of hot flashes," *The New England Journal of Medicine*, vol. 331, no. 6, pp. 347–352, 1994.

[65] N. Sharifi, J. L. Gulley, and W. L. Dahut, "Androgen deprivation therapy for prostate cancer," *The Journal of the American Medical Association*, vol. 294, no. 2, pp. 238–244, 2005.

[66] E. Salminen, R. Portin, J. Korpela et al., "Androgen deprivation and cognition in prostate cancer," *British Journal of Cancer*, vol. 89, no. 6, pp. 971–976, 2003.

[67] S. Alibhai, "Impact of 12 months of androgen deprivation therapy (ADT) on cognitive function in men with non-metaastatic prostate cancer (PC): a matched cohort study," *Journal of Clinical Oncology*, abstract no. 9027, 2010.

[68] V. B. Shahinian, Y. F. Kuo, J. L. Freeman, and J. S. Goodwin, "Risk of the "androgen deprivation syndrome" in men receiving androgen deprivation for prostate cancer," *Archives of Internal Medicine*, vol. 166, no. 4, pp. 465–471, 2006.

[69] A. L. Potosky, K. Knopf, L. X. Clegg et al., "Quality-of-life outcomes after primary androgen deprivation therapy: results from the prostate cancer outcomes study," *Journal of Clinical Oncology*, vol. 19, no. 17, pp. 3750–3757, 2001.

[70] P. E. Teloken, M. Ohebshalom, N. Mohideen, and J. P. Mulhall, "Analysis of the impact of androgen deprivation therapy on sildenafil citrate response following radiation therapy for prostate cancer," *Journal of Urology*, vol. 178, no. 6, pp. 2521–2525, 2007.

[71] G. Di Lorenzo, S. Perdoná, S. de Placido et al., "Gynecomastia and breast pain induced by adjuvant therapy with bicalutamide after radical prostatectomy in patients with prostate cancer: the role of tamoxifen and radiotherapy," *Journal of Urology*, vol. 174, no. 6, pp. 2197–2203, 2005.

[72] S. Perdonà, R. Autorino, S. de Placido et al., "Efficacy of tamoxifen and radiotherapy for prevention and treatment of gynaecomastia and breast pain caused by bicalutamide in prostate cancer: a randomised controlled trial," *The Lancet Oncology*, vol. 6, no. 5, pp. 295–300, 2005.

[73] S. Cook and A. Rodríguez-Antunez, "Pre-estrogen irradiation of the breast to prevent gynecomastia," *The American Journal of Roentgenology, Radium Therapy, and Nuclear Medicine*, vol. 117, no. 3, pp. 662–663, 1973.

[74] D. Fass, A. Steinfeld, J. Brown, and A. Tessler, "Radiotherapeutic prophylaxis of estrogen-induced gynecomastia: a study of late sequela," *International Journal of Radiation Oncology Biology Physics*, vol. 12, no. 3, pp. 407–408, 1986.

8

The Role of Vascular Endothelial Growth Factor in Metastatic Prostate Cancer to the Skeleton

Emma Roberts,[1] Davina A. F. Cossigny,[1] and Gerald M. Y. Quan[1,2]

[1] *Spinal Biology Research Laboratory, University of Melbourne, Department of Surgery, Austin Health, P.O. Box 5555, Heidelberg, VIC 3084, Australia*
[2] *Department of Spinal Surgery, Austin Health, P.O. Box 5555, Heidelberg, VIC 3084, Australia*

Correspondence should be addressed to Gerald M. Y. Quan; gerald.quan@austin.org.au

Academic Editor: Manfred Wirth

Despite the clinical implication and high incidence of bone and spinal metastases, the molecular mechanisms behind prostate cancer metastasis to bone and spine are not well understood. In this review the molecular mechanisms that may contribute to the highly metastatic phenotype of prostate cancer are discussed. Proangiogenic factors such as vascular endothelial growth factor (VEGF) have been shown to not only aid in the metastatic capabilities of prostate cancer but also encourage the colonization and growth of prostate tumour cells in the skeleton. The importance of VEGF in the complex process of prostate cancer dissemination to the skeleton is discussed, including its role in the development of the bone premetastatic niche, metastatic tumour cell recognition of bone, and bone remodeling. The expression of VEGF has also been shown to be upregulated in prostate cancer and is associated with clinical stage, Gleason score, tumour stage, progression, metastasis, and survival. Due to the multifaceted effect VEGF has on tumour angiogenesis, tumour cell proliferation, and bone destruction, therapies targeting the VEGF pathways have shown promising clinical application and are being investigated in clinical trials.

1. Introduction

The five-year survival rate for prostate cancer is extremely high when confined to the prostate, but in the presence of metastatic disease it is reduced to 33% [1]. In Australia, prostate cancer contributes to almost 5% of all registered male deaths [2] of which more than 80% will have developed spinal metastases during the course of their disease [3–5]. Once cancer metastasizes to bone and the vertebral column, patients often experience intractable pain and neurological deficit due to pathological fractures, spinal instability, and metastatic epidural spinal cord compression. The neurological sequelae include sensory disturbance, motor weakness, paralysis, and incontinence, leading to decreased function, inability to ambulate and impaired quality of life [5]. Treatment options include radiotherapy, hormonal therapy, chemotherapeutic agents such as docetaxel, cabazitaxel, sipuleucel-T and abiraterone acetate, and decompression and stabilization surgery [6, 7]. These modalities may be able to extend survival rates but are all predominantly palliative, with median survival time limited from one to two years from the onset of metastases [5, 6]. Despite the clinical implication and high incidence of spinal metastasis, the molecular mechanisms behind prostate cancer metastasis to bone and the spine are not well understood. Vascular endothelial growth factor (VEGF) is well known to be potent stimulator of angiogenesis in both physiological and pathological conditions and is highly expressed in most solid tumours, including prostate cancer. This review discusses the role of VEGF in tumour angiogenesis and bone destruction in metastatic prostate cancer to the spine.

2. VEGF and Its Receptors

VEGF is a ligand of the VEGF tyrosine kinase receptor superfamily and includes VEGF-A, -B, -C and -D, with splice variants of VEGF-A resulting in several different isoforms [8, 9]. The VEGF family ligands bind to tyrosine kinase receptors VEGFR1, VEGFR2, and VEGFR3 (Figure 1), each receptor containing an extracellular domain of approximately 750 amino acid residues, arranged within seven

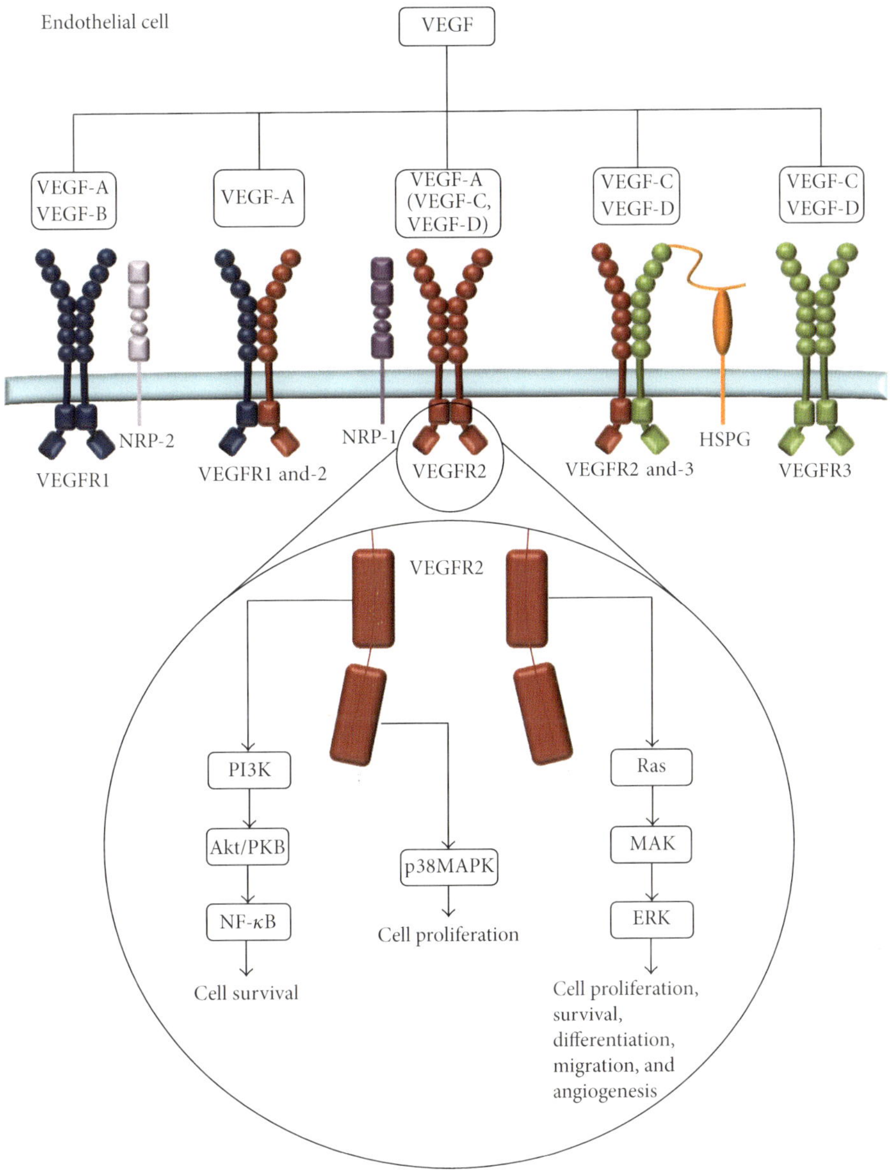

Figure 1: VEGF receptor binding. The five mammalian vascular endothelial growth factors (VEGF-A-D) bind to the receptor tyrosine kinases, VEGF receptor (VEGFR1-3 and co-receptors HSPG, NRP-1 and NRP-2). VEGFR-binding leads to the formation of homodimers and/or heterodimers. Proteolytic cleavage enables VEGF-C and -D to bind VEGFR-2 forming a homodimer. The binding and activation of VEGFR-2 lead to downstream signaling of the PI3 K, MAPK, and Ras pathways which promote cell survival, proliferation, differentiation, migration, and angiogenesis.

immunoglobulin-like folds [10]. Additionally, heparin sulphate proteoglycans (HSPGs) as well as neuropilins (NRP-1 and NRP-2) can act as coreceptors for VEGF and promote VEGFR activation [11, 12]. Each VEGF family member binds with differential affinity for their receptors; for example, VEGFR2 is primarily activated by VEGF-A and VEGFR3 is only activated by VEGF-C and -D. Upon specific VEGF binding, the three VEGF receptors induce receptor dimerization and autophosphorylation leading to downstream signaling via a number of secondary messengers including several protein kinases and phosphatases that support a proangiogenic phenotype [10–12]. Important pathways include the phosphoinositide 3-kinase/Protein Kinase B/NF-κB pathway that promotes cell survival, the mitogen-activated protein kinase (MAPK) pathway that promotes cell proliferation, and the Ras/extracellular signal-regulated kinase (ERK) pathway that promotes cell proliferation, survival, differentiation, migration, and angiogenesis. Through these signaling pathways each of the VEGF family provides different actions, with VEGF-A activation of VEGFR2 representing the major mediator of angiogenesis induction [13–15].

There are many factors that influence and regulate the VEGF/VEGFR pathway, including local environmental hypoxia and various hormones, growth factors, and cytokines. Hormones such as androgens upregulate stromal cell and malignant cell VEGF production and angiogenesis, enhancing prostate cancer growth [16–18]. As such, hormone withdrawal has been shown to inhibit VEGF expression as well as angiogenesis in prostate cancer patients while inducing apoptosis in these cells [19]. Growth factors such as PDGFs, TGF-β1, and IGFs also have a significant impact on the VEGF/VEGFR pathway by inducing the transcription and secretion of VEGF [18, 20, 21]. Cytokines such as TNF-α, IL-6, and IL-8 have also been shown to induce VEGF signalling to promote angiogenesis and tumourogenesis [22, 23]. IL-6 and IL-8 are also involved with the PI3 K/Akt/NF-κB pathways as well as the MAPK pathway of VEGF signalling [24, 25].

3. VEGF and Angiogenesis

Angiogenesis is the growth and development of new blood vessels and is necessary to supply nutrients and maintain homeostasis in the tissues of the body [12]. Normal angiogenesis is tightly regulated by inducers and inhibitors of endothelial growth and is established from preexisting vessels, which develop ordered and predictable vasculature [26]. The actions of VEGF affect numerous cell types, thus enabling a multifaceted response. Initial activation of VEGF promotes the secretion of proteolytic enzymes to degrade the basement membrane and extracellular matrix whilst also aiding in the proliferation and migration of endothelial cells to form immature vasculature [13, 26]. VEGF also maintains newly formed vessels by inducing the expression of Bcl-2 and A1 anti-apoptotic proteins that promote cell survival, whilst activating colony formation by attracting mature subsets of granulocyte macrophage progenitor cells [27, 28]. VEGF-A exhibits vast up-regulation under hypoxic conditions whereby hypoxia-inducible factors (HIFs) stabilize and bind to specific promoter elements present in the promoter region of VEGF-A [11]. VEGFR1 and VEGFR2 are also directly regulated by HIFs [11].

In cancer, alterations in this balance of inducers and inhibitors in favour of angiogenesis can stimulate an "angiogenic switch", via overexpresson of pro-angiogenic factors such as VEGF by tumour cells and tumour-associated stroma [26, 29]. Hypoxic conditions activate the uptake of VEGF and other growth factors and induce the growth of neovasculature, allowing the tumour cells to gain access to oxygen and nutrients [26, 29–31]. Indeed, the induction of angiogenesis has been shown to correlate with the invasive properties of tumours and is associated with poor prognosis [32]. Along with tumour vascularization, activation of genes governing the disruption of cell to cell adhesion and cell motility enables proliferation of primary tumour cells as well as allowing detached cells to disseminate throughout the circulatory system [28]. In benign prostate glands, VEGF expression is mainly confined to the basal cell layer and has weak levels of VEGF binding, while in prostate tumours VEGF is upregulated and found beyond this layer, including neoplastic secretory cells [33].

4. VEGF and Skeletal Metastasis

During the normal development of long bones and vertebrae or bone repair, growth and remodeling of bone formation occurs through osteogenesis [34]. A balanced state is created through the continuous and integrated processes of bone formation and deposition by osteoblasts and bone and mineralized matrix resorption by proteolytic enzymes and hydrochloric acid secreted by osteoclasts, derived from the haematopoietic stem cells of the bone marrow [35, 36]. It is a complex process dictated by growth factors and cytokines including fibroblast growth factors (FGFs), platelet-derived growth factor (PDGF), transforming growth factor-β (TGF-β), and bone morphogenetic proteins (BMPs) [34]. VEGF is expressed by osteoblasts and has autocrine and paracrine effects including chemotactic migration, proliferation, and differentiation of osteoblasts, as well as stimulating the formation, survival, and resorptive activity of osteoclasts. It is essential for normal angiogenesis and appropriate bone repair and mineralization in response to bone injury [37]. *In vivo*, absence of VEGF leads to impaired blood vessel invasion, cartilage remodeling, and skeletal growth [38–40]. Blood vessels serve as a way of transporting circulating osteoblasts [41] and osteoclast precursors [42] to sites undergoing active remodelling [43]. Cancer metastases to bone cause alterations in normal bone metabolism and the balance between osteoclasts and osteoblasts in favour of one or the other, resulting in destructive lytic or sclerotic lesions, or a combination of both [44]. Osteoclasts are primarily responsible for tumour induced bone destruction, and during the resorption of the bone matrix, embedded growth factors are released that produce a permissive microenvironment and further promote tumour growth [30, 45]. Of note, in human prostate cancer, bone metastases generally favour an osteoblastic phenotype, in contrast to other metastases such as those from renal cell carcinoma, which are often lytic [46, 47].

The spread of prostate cancer metastasis to bone is a complex process involving tumour cell migration from the primary tumour site, dissemination through the vascular system, extravasation, and finally establishment, growth, and invasion at the secondary bone site [4]. In a clinical trial of patients with metastatic prostate cancer, bone metastases were noted in 88.9% of patients, compared with soft tissue/lymph node metastases in 22.2% and visceral metastases in 16.7%, demonstrating the preferential homing capabilities of prostate metastasis to bone [48]; however the propensity of prostate cancer to metastasize to bone and the vertebral column remains largely unknown. Prior to the attachment of these cancer cells to bone, it is thought that a premetastatic niche may be created by nonmalignant bone marrow-derived cells that are stimulated by tumour-secreted proteins, which in combination with various bone-enriched growth factors, cytokines, proteases, and components of the extracellular matrix such as a high extracellular calcium concentration support the colonization and growth of prostate cancer cells in bone [49–51]. The actions of VEGF are thought to assist in tumour cell recognition of bone and encourage nesting of the tumour cells in bone [52]. Prior to attachment, VEGF via VEGFR2 modulates the migratory responses of tumour cells encouraging adhesion molecules such as fibronectin and bone sialoprotein within the extracellular matrix [53]. Additionally, VEGF and its cognate receptors may be able to regulate integrin activity, promoting recognition of the bone matrix [32]. Various tumour-expressed growth factors, endothelial markers, and cytokines attract and activate osteoclasts, which in turn disrupt the bone balance through overstimulation and discharge of bone-derived growth factors (Figure 2). Other factors which affect the progression of prostate cancer to bone are Dickkopf-1 (DKK-1), sclerostin, and Wnt signalling. Upregulation of DKK-1 and sclerostin enhances osteoclastic activity by suppressing Wnt signaling and is thought to be able to inhibit the advancement of bone cancer metastases [54, 55]. Whilst DKK-1 levels in patients with bone metastases decrease, Wnt levels rise [56]. This increase of Wnt signalling promotes osteoblast and inhibits osteoclast differentiation, leading to an osteoblastic tumour phenotype [56, 57]. Furthermore, in response to various hormonal, cellular, and cytokine signals, receptor activator of nuclear factor-k B ligand (RANKL), induces osteoclast formation and activation [58, 59]. Osteoprotegerin (OPG) may act as a decoy receptor for RANKL in order to inhibit osteoclastogenesis, which in turn increases osteoblast formation [60]. This RANK/RANKL/OPG axis therefore is important in determining the phenotype of the bone tumour [59]. These factors are deposited into the bone matrix and create a microenvironment that is favourable for cancer cells, leading to further proliferation of tumour cells and bone degradation through the secretion of osteolytic factors [61].

Expression levels of VEGF and VEGFRs have also been shown to be elevated at the site of bone metastases in comparison to primary prostate tumours, indicating that VEGF is an important factor in metastasis development, particularly to bone [53]. Increased VEGF plasma levels have been shown to correlate with skeletal metastasis and poor prognosis in prostate cancer patients and VEGF expression levels in many cancer types have been shown to correlate with poorer prognosis and metastatic potential [62]. However, other studies have shown that there is no correlation between VEGF serum levels and prognosis [63, 64]. The expression of VEGF is upregulated in prostate cancer and is associated with clinical stage, Gleason score, tumour stage, progression, metastasis and survival [65–67]. In prostate cancer VEGF-dependant autocrine stimulation activates the $\alpha V\beta 3$ integrin via the VEGFR2 receptor leading to cell proliferation, survival and recognition of extracellular matrix components, which may influence their metastatic capabilities [53]. Many prostate cancer cell lines known to produce osteoblastic metastases highly express VEGF [68].

Interactions of VEGF with markers such as TNF-α, IL-6, IL-8, and CCN3 have been linked to the pro-angiogenic activities of tumour cells [69–71]. High expression of VEGF has been observed in human metastatic prostate cancer cell lines PC-3, Du145, and line LNCaP-C4–2, where it has been shown to promote osteoblastic differentiation and activity *in vitro* [53, 71–73].

5. Current Treatment of Prostate Cancer and VEGF/VEGF-R Targeted Therapies

Traditionally, androgen ablation has been the main treatment for the prevention of metastases from prostate cancer. As prostate cancer cells are initially dependant on androgens, suppressing the levels of testosterone and dihydrotestosterone decreases the growth rate of prostate cancer cells [74]. However, after this initial response these cells can become castrate-resistant and develop a more aggressive phenotype, with increased VEGF expression and proliferative potential [74, 75]. The commonest conventional treatments for bone metastases secondary to prostate cancer are chemotherapy, radiation, and surgery. Although chemo- and radiotherapy has the potential ability to kill rapidly dividing cancer cells, they each have their own toxic side effects and there is little survival benefit in patients with metastatic cancer [76, 77]. Bisphosphonates such as zoledronic acid or Denosumab, a human monoclonal antibody that targets RANKL signalling, also have a therapeutic role in preventing skeletal-related events in bone metastases via inhibition of osteoclast-mediated bone resorption [78]. Patient morbidity and mortality due to local tumour recurrence, multimetastatic disease, loss of structural function of the bony skeleton destroyed by tumour, and metastatic epidural nerve or spinal cord compression remain important challenges.

Due to the multifaceted effect VEGF has on tumour angiogenesis, tumour cell proliferation, and bone destruction, antiangiogenic therapies targeting the VEGF pathways have shown promising early clinical application and are being investigated in clinical trials. These anti-VEGF therapies consist of VEGF-neutralizing antibodies and tyrosine kinase receptor inhibitors. Bevacizumab is a monoclonal IgG1 antibody that blocks the binding of VEGF-A to its receptors by neutralizing all VEGF isoforms and bioactive proteolytic fragments through the binding of the antibody Fab-ligand epitope to the Gly88 residue of VEGF [79]. Bevacizumab is currently in Phase II clinical trials in relapsed prostate cancer and is approved by the US Food and Drug Administration (FDA) for treatment of metastatic colorectal, renal, and breast cancer and other solid tumours [80, 81]. Similarly, Aflibercept is another antibody which neutralizes VEGF and is currently being used in Phase II clinical trials for patients with recurrent or metastatic urothelial cancer [82]. Tyrosine kinase inhibitors act on VEGF receptors inhibiting activation following ligand binding [83]. Ramucirumab is a human IgG1 monoclonal antibody which binds to the extracellular domain of VEGFR-2 and blocks the VEGF-A to VEGFR-2 interaction and subsequent downstream signaling [84]. Other small molecule tyrosine kinase receptor inhibitors include Semaxanib, which targets a single receptor (VEGFR2), and Sorafenib, which targets multiple tyrosine kinase receptors VEGFR1, -2 and -3, as well as platelet-derived growth factor receptor-β [83, 85]. Recently, studies have suggested that using anti-VEGF therapies such as Bevacizumab in concert with radiation therapy or chemotherapy may be able to increase the response to radiation therapy [86]. These synergistic actions have been reported in several preclinical studies and have been shown to improve the survival rates in patients with advanced cancers and decrease levels of radiation necrosis [86–88].

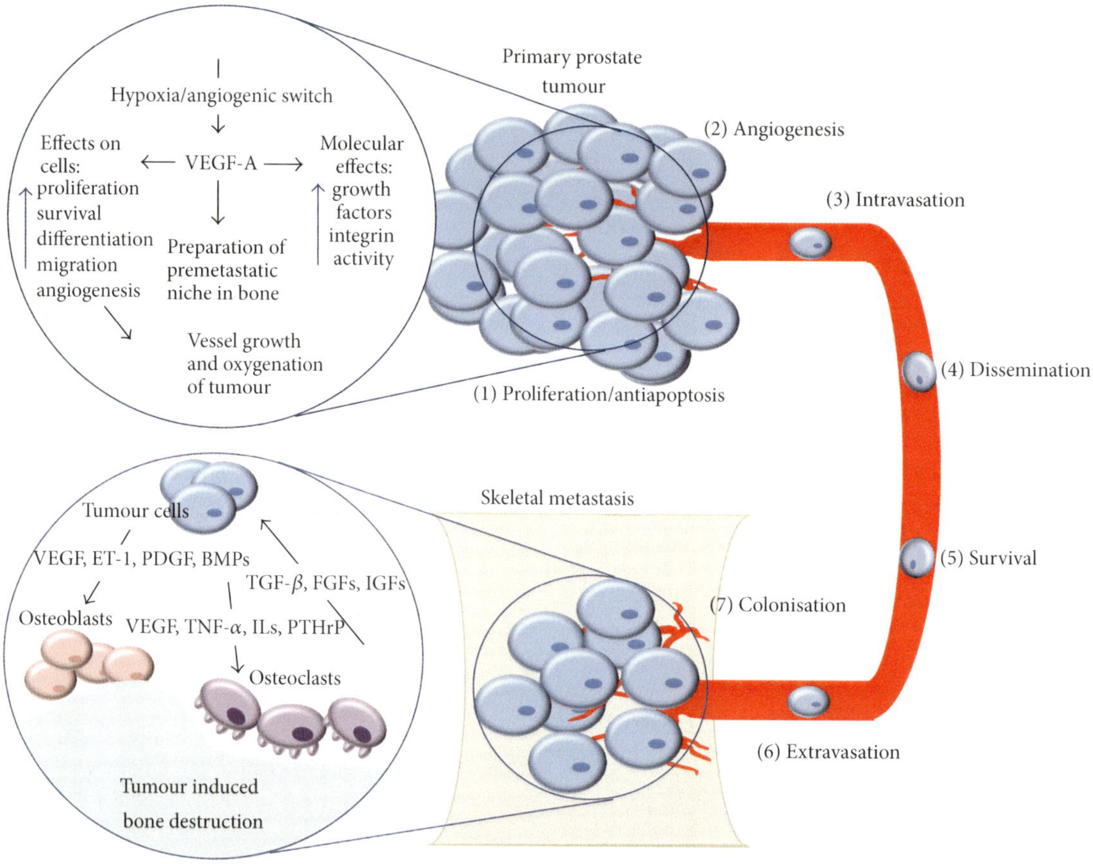

Figure 2: Tumour induced bone destruction. In the prostate, an angiogenic switch promotes the secretion of VEGF, leading to various effects on cells, increasing the release of growth factors and activating integrin activity. (1) Proliferation/antiapoptosis: the cells undergo a transformation that increases the proliferation, survival, differentiation, and migration of the tumour cells. (2) Angiogenesis: the actions of VEGF activate angiogenesis—allowing the tumour cells to access nutrients. (3) Intravasation: cells invade into the local stroma and then enter the local vasculature. (4) Dissemination: cancer cells travel to distant target organs. (5) Survival: Cells can undergo apoptosis or stop proliferation after dissemination and need to evade local immune surveillance. (6) Extravasation: invasion of target organ. (7) Colonisation: after surviving dissemination and extravasation of the target site, tumour cells invade the bone and undergo progressive growth. In metastatic bone disease, tumour cells secrete humoral factors that stimulate osteoclastic and osteoblastic recruitment and differentiation. Once these osteoclasts begin to break down bone, growth factors are released, stimulating growth of the tumour cells. This encourages the tumour cells to release factors that further increase bone resorption by osteoclast and stimulate bone formation through the activation of osteoblasts.

6. Conclusion

To date there have been many articles published suggesting the possible molecular mechanisms behind the propensity of prostate cancer to metastasize to bone and the vertebral column. VEGF has been implicated in many of these, including facilitating cancer cell migration to bone, induction of angiogenesis, and stimulating bone forming and resorbing cells of the bone marrow. Anti-angiogenic treatments targeting the VEGF/VEGF receptor pathway have shown promising early clinical application. Further research is required to determine whether this may be translated into better disease control, decreased morbidity, higher survival rates, and improved quality of life in patients with prostate cancer.

Acknowledgments

This work was supported by the National Health and Medical Research Council of Australia (Fellowship no. 558418), the Austin Health Medical Research Foundation, and the Victorian Orthopaedic Research Trust.

References

[1] "Statistics, A.B.o., 3303. 0 Causes of Death, Australia," 2012, http://www.abs.gov.au/ausstats/abs@.nsf/Products/E0BA9CC2096C3886CA25788400127C4C?opendocument.

[2] S. C. Gupta, J. H. Kim, S. Prasad, and B. B. Aggarwal, "Regulation of survival, proliferation, invasion, angiogenesis, and metastasis of tumor cells through modulation of inflammatory pathways by nutraceuticals," *Cancer and Metastasis Reviews*, vol. 29, no. 3, pp. 405–434, 2010.

[3] K. Pietras and A. Östman, "Hallmarks of cancer: interactions with the tumor stroma," *Experimental Cell Research*, vol. 316, no. 8, pp. 1324–1331, 2010.

[4] I. Roato, P. D'Amelio, E. Gorassini et al., "Osteoclasts are active in bone forming metastases of prostate cancer patients," *PLoS ONE*, vol. 3, no. 11, Article ID e3627, 2008.

[5] S. A. Meyer, H. Singh, and A. L. Jenkins, "Surgical treatment of metastatic spinal tumors," *Mount Sinai Journal of Medicine*, vol. 77, no. 1, pp. 124–129, 2010.

[6] E. J. Brown and E. Chow, "Bone biomarkers in research and clinical practice," in *Bone Metastases*, vol. 12 of *Cancer Metastasis—Biology and Treatment*, pp. 93–116, 2009.

[7] M. E. McGee-Lawrence and J. J. Westendorf, "Histone deacetylases in skeletal development and bone mass maintenance," *Gene*, vol. 474, no. 1-2, pp. 1–11, 2011.

[8] R. L. Clifford, K. Deacon, and A. J. Knox, "Novel regulation of vascular endothelial growth factor-A (VEGF-A) by transforming growth factor $\beta 1$: requirement for Smads, β-catenin, and GSK3β," *Journal of Biological Chemistry*, vol. 283, no. 51, pp. 35337–35353, 2008.

[9] F. Fan, J. S. Wey, M. F. McCarty et al., "Expression and function of vascular endothelial growth factor receptor-1 on human colorectal cancer cells," *Oncogene*, vol. 24, no. 16, pp. 2647–2653, 2005.

[10] A. K. Olsson, A. Dimberg, J. Kreuger et al., "VEGF receptor signalling—in control of vascular function," *Nature Reviews Molecular Cell Biology*, vol. 7, no. 5, pp. 359–371, 2006.

[11] N. Ferrara, H.-P. Gerber, and J. LeCouter, "The biology of VEGF and its receptors," *Nature Medicine*, vol. 9, no. 6, pp. 669–676, 2003.

[12] H. Takahashi and M. Shibuya, "The vascular endothelial growth factor (VEGF)/VEGF receptor system and its role under physiological and pathological conditions," *Clinical Science*, vol. 109, no. 3, pp. 227–241, 2005.

[13] T. L. Phung, K. Ziv, D. Dabydeen et al., "Pathological angiogenesis is induced by sustained Akt signaling and inhibited by rapamycin," *Cancer Cell*, vol. 10, no. 2, pp. 159–170, 2006.

[14] J. D. Hood, R. Frausto, W. B. Kiosses, M. A. Schwartz, and D. A. Cheresh, "Differential αv integrin-mediated Ras-ERK signaling during two pathways of angiogenesis," *Journal of Cell Biology*, vol. 162, no. 5, pp. 933–943, 2003.

[15] X. Jin, J. Yin, S.-H. Kim et al., "EGFR-AKT-Smad signaling promotes formation of glioma stem-like cells and tumor angiogenesis by ID3-driven cytokine induction," *Cancer Research*, vol. 71, no. 22, pp. 7125–7134, 2011.

[16] A. C. Levine, X.-H. Liu, P. D. Greenberg et al., "Androgens induce the expression of vascular endothelial growth factor in human fetal prostatic fibroblasts," *Endocrinology*, vol. 139, no. 11, pp. 4672–4678, 1998.

[17] M. W. Jackson, "A potential autocrine role for vascular endothelial growth factor in prostate cancer," *Cancer Research*, vol. 62, pp. 854–859, 2002.

[18] X. Li, Y. Feng, J. Liu et al., "Epigallocatechin-3-gallate inhibits IGF-I-stimulated lung cancer angiogenesis through downregulation of HIF-1alpha and VEGF expression," *Journal of Nutrigenetics and Nutrigenomics*, vol. 6, no. 3, pp. 169–178, 2013.

[19] R. K. Jain, N. Safabakhsh, A. Sckell et al., "Endothelial cell death, angiogenesis, and microvascular function after castration in an androgen-dependent tumor: role of vascular endothelial growth factor," *Proceedings of the National Academy of Sciences of the United States of America*, vol. 95, no. 18, pp. 10820–10825, 1998.

[20] J. Yu, C. Ustach, and H.-R. C. Kim, "Platelet-derived growth factor signaling and human cancer," *Journal of Biochemistry and Molecular Biology*, vol. 36, no. 1, pp. 49–59, 2003.

[21] K. Eisermann, C. J. Broderick, A. Bazarov et al., "Androgen up-regulates vascular endothelial growth factor expression in prostate cancer cells via an Sp1 binding site," *Molecular Cancer*, vol. 12, p. 7, 2013.

[22] T. Cohen, D. Nahari, L. W. Cerem, G. Neufeld, and B.-Z. Levin, "Interleukin 6 induces the expression of vascular endothelial growth factor," *Journal of Biological Chemistry*, vol. 271, no. 2, pp. 736–741, 1996.

[23] Z. Von Marschall, T. Cramer, M. Höcker, G. Finkenzeller, B. Wiedenmann, and S. Rosewicz, "Dual mechanism of vascular endothelial growth factor upregulation by hypoxia in human hepatocellular carcinoma," *Gut*, vol. 48, no. 1, pp. 87–96, 2001.

[24] B. Paule, S. Terry, L. Kheuang, P. Soyeux, F. Vacherot, and A. de Taille, "The NF-κB/IL-6 pathway in metastatic androgen-independent prostate cancer: new therapeutic approaches?" *World Journal of Urology*, vol. 25, no. 5, pp. 477–489, 2007.

[25] F. Luppi, A. M. Longo, W. I. de Boer, K. F. Rabe, and P. S. Hiemstra, "Interleukin-8 stimulates cell proliferation in non-small cell lung cancer through epidermal growth factor receptor transactivation," *Lung Cancer*, vol. 56, no. 1, pp. 25–33, 2007.

[26] B. I. Terman and K. V. Stoletov, "VEGF and tumor angiogenesis," *The Einstein Quarterly Journal of Biology and Medicine*, vol. 18, no. 2, 2001.

[27] S. P. Ivy, J. Y. Wick, and B. M. Kaufman, "An overview of small-molecule inhibitors of VEGFR signaling," *Nature Reviews Clinical Oncology*, vol. 6, no. 10, pp. 569–579, 2009.

[28] P. G. Tsoutsou and M. L. Koukourakis, "Angiogenesis and bone metastasis: implications for diagnosis, prevention and treatment," in *Bone Metastases*, vol. 12 of *Cancer Metastasis—Biology and Treatment*, pp. 51–76, 2009.

[29] D. Hanahan and R. A. Weinberg, "Hallmarks of cancer: the next generation," *Cell*, vol. 144, no. 5, pp. 646–674, 2011.

[30] G. Van Der Pluijm, B. Sijmons, H. Vloedgraven, M. Deckers, S. Papapoulos, and C. Löwik, "Monitoring metastatic behavior of human tumor cells in mice with species-specific polymerase chain reaction: elevated expression of angiogenesis and bone resorption stimulators by breast cancer in bone metastases," *Journal of Bone and Mineral Research*, vol. 16, no. 6, pp. 1077–1091, 2001.

[31] R. A. Cairns, I. S. Harris, and T. W. Mak, "Regulation of cancer cell metabolism," *Nature Reviews Cancer*, vol. 11, no. 2, pp. 85–95, 2011.

[32] S. De, J. Chen, N. V. Narizhneva et al., "Molecular pathway for cancer metastasis to bone," *Journal of Biological Chemistry*, vol. 278, no. 40, pp. 39044–39050, 2003.

[33] J. Köllermann and B. Helpap, "Expression of vascular endothelial growth factor (VEGF) and VEGF receptor Flk-1 in benign, premalignant, and malignant prostate tissue," *American Journal of Clinical Pathology*, vol. 116, no. 1, pp. 115–121, 2001.

[34] V. J. Mandracchia, S. C. Nelson, and E. A. Barp, "Current concepts of bone healing," *Clinics in Podiatric Medicine and Surgery*, vol. 18, no. 1, pp. 55–77, 2001.

[35] B. F. Boyce, E. Rosenberg, A. E. de Papp et al., "The osteoclast, bone remodelling and treatment of metabolic bone disease," *European Journal of Clinical Investigation*, vol. 42, no. 12, pp. 1332–1341, 2012.

[36] J. Street and B. Lenehan, "Vascular endothelial growth factor regulates osteoblast survival—evidence for an autocrine feedback mechanism," *Journal of Orthopaedic Surgery and Research*, vol. 4, no. 1, article 19, 2009.

[37] R. A. D. Carano and E. H. Filvaroff, "Angiogenesis and bone repair," *Drug Discovery Today*, vol. 8, no. 21, pp. 980–989, 2003.

[38] H.-P. Gerber, K. J. Hillan, A. M. Ryan et al., "VEGF is required for growth and survival in neonatal mice," *Development*, vol. 126, no. 6, pp. 1149–1159, 1999.

[39] H.-P. Gerber, V. Dixit, and N. Ferrara, "Vascular endothelial growth factor induces expression of the antiapoptotic proteins Bcl-2 and A1 in vascular endothelial cells," *Journal of Biological Chemistry*, vol. 273, no. 21, pp. 13313–13316, 1998.

[40] H.-P. Gerber, T. H. Vu, A. M. Ryan, J. Kowalski, Z. Werb, and N. Ferrara, "VEGF couples hypertrophic cartilage remodeling, ossification and angiogenesis during endochondral bone formation," *Nature Medicine*, vol. 5, no. 6, pp. 623–628, 1999.

[41] G. Z. Eghbali-Fatourechi, J. Lamsam, D. Fraser, D. Nagel, B. L. Riggs, and S. Khosla, "Circulating osteoblast-lineage cells in humans," *The New England Journal of Medicine*, vol. 352, no. 19, pp. 1959–1966, 2005.

[42] E. F. Eriksen, "Cellular mechanisms of bone remodeling," *Reviews in Endocrine and Metabolic Disorders*, vol. 11, no. 4, pp. 219–227, 2010.

[43] M. Kassem, L. Risteli, L. Mosekilde, F. Melsen, and E. F. Eriksen, "Formation of osteoblast-like cells from human mononuclear bone marrow cultures," *Acta Pathologica, Microbiologica et Immunologica Scandinavica*, vol. 99, no. 3, pp. 269–274, 1991.

[44] J.-K. Jin, F. Dayyani, and G. E. Gallick, "Steps in prostate cancer progression that lead to bone metastasis," *International Journal of Cancer*, vol. 128, no. 11, pp. 2545–2561, 2011.

[45] K. N. Weilbaecher, T. A. Guise, and L. K. McCauley, "Cancer to bone: a fatal attraction," *Nature Reviews Cancer*, vol. 11, no. 6, pp. 411–425, 2011.

[46] D. Cossigny and G. M. Y. Quan, "In vivo animal models of spinal metastasis," *Cancer and Metastasis Reviews*, vol. 31, no. 1, pp. 99–108, 2012.

[47] P. Curtin, H. Youm, and E. Salih, "Three-dimensional cancer-bone metastasis model using ex-vivo co-cultures of live calvarial bones and cancer cells," *Biomaterials*, vol. 33, no. 4, pp. 1065–1078, 2012.

[48] G. Sonpavde and C. N. Sternberg, "Satraplatin for the therapy of castration-resistant prostate cancer," *Future Oncology*, vol. 5, no. 7, pp. 931–940, 2009.

[49] B. Psaila and D. Lyden, "The metastatic niche: adapting the foreign soil," *Nature Reviews Cancer*, vol. 9, no. 4, pp. 285–293, 2009.

[50] C. Zhang, M. Soori, F. L. Miles et al., "Paracrine factors produced by bone marrow stromal cells induce apoptosis and neuroendocrine differentiation in prostate cancer cells," *Prostate*, vol. 71, no. 2, pp. 157–167, 2011.

[51] R. R. Langley and I. J. Fidler, "The seed and soil hypothesis revisited—the role of tumor-stroma interactions in metastasis to different organs," *International Journal of Cancer*, vol. 128, no. 11, pp. 2527–2535, 2011.

[52] J. A. Sterling, J. R. Edwards, T. J. Martin, and G. R. Mundy, "Advances in the biology of bone metastasis: how the skeleton affects tumor behavior," *Bone*, vol. 48, no. 1, pp. 6–15, 2011.

[53] J. Chen, S. De, J. Brainard, and T. V. Byzova, "Metastatic properties of prostate cancer cells are controlled by VEGF," *Cell Communication and Adhesion*, vol. 11, no. 1, pp. 1–11, 2004.

[54] M. P. Yavropoulou, A. H. van Lierop, N. A. Hamdy et al., "Serum sclerostin levels in Paget's disease and prostate cancer with bone metastases with a wide range of bone turnover," *Bone*, vol. 51, no. 1, pp. 153–157, 2012.

[55] D. Diarra, M. Stolina, K. Polzer et al., "Dickkopf-1 is a master regulator of joint remodeling," *Nature Medicine*, vol. 13, no. 2, pp. 156–163, 2007.

[56] J. L. Sottnik, C. L. Hall, J. Zhang et al., "Wnt and Wnt inhibitors in bone metastasis," *BoneKEy Reports*, vol. 1, p. 101, 2012.

[57] S. M. Tu, A. Som, B. Tu et al., "Effect of Paget's disease of bone (osteitis deformans) on the progression of prostate cancer bone metastasis," *British Journal of Cancer*, vol. 107, no. 4, pp. 646–651, 2012.

[58] Y. Li, D. Kong, A. Ahmad, B. Bao, and F. H. Sarkar, "Targeting bone remodeling by isoflavone and 3,3′-diindolylmethane in the context of prostate cancer bone metastasis," *PLoS ONE*, vol. 7, no. 3, Article ID e33011, 2012.

[59] D. L. Lacey, W. J. Boyle, W. S. Simonet et al., "Bench to bedside: elucidation of the OPG-RANK-RANKL pathway and the development of denosumab," *Nature Reviews Drug Discovery*, vol. 11, no. 5, pp. 401–419, 2012.

[60] L. Mercatali, M. Ricci, E. Scarpi et al., "RANK/RANK-L/OPG in patients with bone metastases treated with anticancer agents and zoledronic acid: a prospective study," *International Journal of Molecular Sciences*, vol. 14, no. 6, pp. 10683–10693, 2013.

[61] T. A. Guise, K. S. Mohammad, G. Clines et al., "Basic mechanisms responsible for osteolytic and osteoblastic bone metastases," *Clinical Cancer Research*, vol. 12, no. 20, pp. 6213s–6216s, 2006.

[62] J. L. F. Duque, K. R. Loughlin, R. M. Adam, P. W. Kantoff, D. Zurakowski, and M. R. Freeman, "Plasma levels of vascular endothelial growth factor are increased in patients with metastatic prostate cancer," *Urology*, vol. 54, no. 3, pp. 523–527, 1999.

[63] P. J. Saylor, K. R. Kozak, M. R. Smith et al., "Changes in biomarkers of inflammation and angiogenesis during androgen deprivation therapy for prostate cancer," *Oncologist*, vol. 17, no. 2, pp. 212–219, 2012.

[64] F. Botelho, F. Pina, P. Silva, G. Figueiredo, F. Cruz, and N. Lunet, "Vascular endothelial growth factor (VEGF) and prostate pathology," *International Brazilian Journal of Urology*, vol. 36, no. 4, pp. 430–438, 2010.

[65] E. K. Amankwah, T. A. Sellers, and J. Y. Park, "Gene variants in the angiogenesis pathway and prostate cancer," *Carcinogenesis*, vol. 33, no. 7, pp. 1259–1269, 2012.

[66] M. Borre, S. M. Bentzen, B. Nerstrøm, and J. Overgaard, "Tumor cell proliferation and survival in patients with prostate cancer followed expectantly," *Journal of Urology*, vol. 159, no. 5, pp. 1609–1614, 1998.

[67] T. T. Tomiá, H. Gustavsson, W. Wang, K. Jennbacken, K. Welén, and J.-E. Damber, "Castration resistant prostate cancer is associated with increased blood vessel stabilization and elevated levels of VEGF and Ang-2," *Prostate*, vol. 72, no. 7, pp. 705–712, 2012.

[68] N. K. Thudi, C. K. Martin, M. V. P. Nadella et al., "Zoledronic acid decreased osteolysis but not bone metastasis in a nude mouse model of canine prostate cancer with mixed bone lesions," *Prostate*, vol. 68, no. 10, pp. 1116–1125, 2008.

[69] G. Ligresti, A. C. Aplin, P. Zorzi, A. Morishita, and R. F. Nicosia, "Macrophage-derived tumor necrosis factor-α is an early component of the molecular cascade leading to angiogenesis in response to aortic injury," *Arteriosclerosis, Thrombosis, and Vascular Biology*, vol. 31, no. 5, pp. 1151–1159, 2011.

[70] C. Fischbach, J. K. Hyun, S. X. Hsiong, M. B. Evangelista, W. Yuen, and D. J. Mooney, "Cancer cell angiogenic capability is regulated by 3D culture and integrin engagement," *Proceedings of the National Academy of Sciences of the United States of America*, vol. 106, no. 2, pp. 399–404, 2009.

[71] V. Ouellet and P. M. Siegel, "CCN3 modulates bone turnover and is a novel regulator of skeletal metastasis," *Journal of Cell Communication and Signaling*, vol. 6, no. 2, pp. 73–85, 2012.

[72] Y. Takei, K. Kadomatsu, Y. Yuzawa, S. Matsuo, and T. Muramatsu, "A small interfering RNA targeting vascular endothelial growth factor as cancer therapeutics," *Cancer Research*, vol. 64, no. 10, pp. 3365–3370, 2004.

[73] S. Srinivasan, R. Kumar, S. Koduru, A. Chandramouli, and C. Damodaran, "Inhibiting TNF-mediated signaling: a novel therapeutic paradigm for androgen independent prostate cancer," *Apoptosis*, vol. 15, no. 2, pp. 153–161, 2010.

[74] E. Corey, "Androgen suppression: the good, the bad and the ugly," *Andrology*, vol. 1, Article ID e106, 2012.

[75] L. Pan, S. Baek, P. R. Edmonds et al., "Vascular endothelial growth factor (VEGF) expression in locally advanced prostate cancer: secondary analysis of radiation therapy oncology group (RTOG) 8610," *Radiation Oncology*, vol. 8, article 100, 2013.

[76] L. Yang, S. You, V. Kumar et al., "In vitro the behaviors of metastasis with suppression of VEGF in human bone metastatic LNCaP-derivative C4-2B prostate cancer cell line," *Journal of Experimental & Clinical Cancer Research*, vol. 31, article 40, 2012.

[77] T. Brabletz, D. Lyden, P. S. Steeg et al., "Roadblocks to translational advances on metastasis research," *Nature Medicine*, vol. 19, no. 9, pp. 1104–1109, 2013.

[78] N. Kamiya, H. Suzuki, T. Endo et al., "Additive effect of zoledronic acid on serum prostate-specific antigen changes for hormone-sensitive prostate cancer patients with bone metastasis treated by combined androgen blockade," *International Journal of Urology*, vol. 19, no. 2, pp. 169–173, 2012.

[79] A. F. Dawood, P. Lotfi, S. N. Dash, S. K. Kona, K. T. Nguyen, and M. I. Romero-Ortega, "VEGF release in multiluminal hydrogels directs angiogenesis from adult vasculature in vitro," *Cardiovascular Engineering and Technology*, vol. 2, no. 3, pp. 173–185, 2011.

[80] V. T. Labropoulou, A. D. Theocharis, A. Symeonidis, S. S. Skandalis, N. K. Karamanos, and H. P. Kalofonos, "Pathophysiology and pharmacological targeting of tumor-induced bone disease: current status and emerging therapeutic interventions," *Current Medicinal Chemistry*, vol. 18, no. 11, pp. 1584–1598, 2011.

[81] K. N. Syrigos, E. Karapanagiotou, P. Boura, C. Manegold, and K. Harrington, "Bevacizumab-induced hypertension: pathogenesis and management," *BioDrugs*, vol. 25, no. 3, pp. 159–169, 2011.

[82] P. Twardowski, W. M. Stadler, P. Frankel et al., "Phase II study of aflibercept (VEGF-Trap) in patients with recurrent or metastatic urothelial cancer: a California cancer consortium trial," *Urology*, vol. 76, pp. 923–926, 2010.

[83] S. M. Wilhelm, L. Adnane, P. Newell, A. Villanueva, J. M. Llovet, and M. Lynch, "Preclinical overview of sorafenib, a multikinase inhibitor that targets both Raf and VEGF and PDGF receptor tyrosine kinase signaling," *Molecular Cancer Therapeutics*, vol. 7, no. 10, pp. 3129–3140, 2008.

[84] A. Grothey and E. Galanis, "Targeting angiogenesis: progress with anti-VEGF treatment with large molecules," *Nature Reviews Clinical Oncology*, vol. 6, no. 9, pp. 507–518, 2009.

[85] A. O'Donnell, A. Padhani, C. Hayes et al., "A Phase I study of the angiogenesis inhibitor SU5416 (semaxanib) in solid tumours, incorporating dynamic contrast MR pharmacodynamic end points," *British Journal of Cancer*, vol. 93, no. 8, pp. 876–883, 2005.

[86] A. Narayana, D. Gruber, S. Kunnakkat et al., "A clinical trial of bevacizumab, temozolomide, and radiation for newly diagnosed glioblastoma: clinical article," *Journal of Neurosurgery*, vol. 116, no. 2, pp. 341–345, 2012.

[87] H. I. Hurwitz, N. C. Tebbutt, F. Kabbinavar et al., "Efficacy and safety of bevacizumab in metastatic colorectal cancer: pooled analysis from seven randomized controlled trials," *Oncologist*, vol. 18, no. 9, pp. 1004–1012, 2013.

[88] M. Furuse, N. Nonoguchi, S. Kawabata et al., "Bevacizumab treatment for symptomatic radiation necrosis diagnosed by amino acid PET," *Japanese Journal of Clinical Oncology*, vol. 43, no. 3, pp. 337–341, 2013.

9

Cellular Plasticity in Prostate Cancer Bone Metastasis

Dima Y. Jadaan,[1] Mutaz M. Jadaan,[2] and John P. McCabe[2]

[1]University College Dublin, Belfield, Dublin, Ireland
[2]Department of Orthopaedic Surgery, Galway University Hospitals, Galway, Ireland

Correspondence should be addressed to Dima Y. Jadaan; dima.jadaan@gmail.com

Academic Editor: Craig Robson

Purpose. Experimental data suggest that tumour cells can reversibly transition between epithelial and mesenchymal states (EMT and MET), a phenomenon known as cellular plasticity. The aim of this review was to appraise the clinical evidence for the role of cellular plasticity in prostate cancer (PC) bone metastasis. *Methods.* An electronic search was performed using PubMed for studies that have examined the differential expression of epithelial, mesenchymal, and stem cell markers in human PC bone metastasis tissues. *Results.* The review included nineteen studies. More than 60% of the studies used ≤20 bone metastasis samples, and there were several sources of heterogeneity between studies. Overall, most stem cell markers analysed, except for CXCR4, were positively expressed in bone metastasis tissues, while the expression of EMT and MET markers was heterogeneous between and within samples. Several EMT and stemness markers that are involved in osteomimicry, such as Notch, Met receptor, and Wnt/β pathway, were highly expressed in bone metastases. *Conclusions.* Clinical findings support the role of cellular plasticity in PC bone metastasis and suggest that epithelial and mesenchymal states cannot be taken in isolation when targeting PC bone metastasis. The paper also highlights several challenges in the clinical detection of cellular plasticity.

1. Introduction

Despite advances in the early diagnosis and management of prostate cancer (PC), bone metastasis of PC cells causes significant morbidity and is associated with four to six times higher mortality rates than localized PC [1, 2]. Furthermore, it is not uncommon for PC patients with bone metastasis who initially respond to androgen deprivation therapy to progress to castration resistant PC (CRPC) [3, 4]. It has been recently recognised that the development of successful therapeutic targets against metastasis is challenged by the presence of a subpopulation of cells within tumours characterised by increased resistance to standard radiotherapy, chemotherapy, and hormonal therapy. These cells, referred to as cancer stem cells (CSCs), have tumour-initiating and self-renewal abilities and are believed to be critical drivers of tumour progression [5].

CSCs have first been described in human leukaemia [6] and subsequently demonstrated in solid tumours, such as those of the breast, brain, and prostate [7–9]. Prostate cancer stem cells have been characterised by a $CD44^{+}/\alpha_2\beta_1{}^{hi}/CD133^{+}$ phenotype [9]. Importantly, studies have indicated a connection between CSCs and the transition from epithelial to mesenchymal state (EMT) [10–12]. In EMT, polarized immobile epithelial cells convert into spindle-shaped motile mesenchymal cells. This process facilitates detachment of cancer cells from the primary tumour via loss of intercellular adhesion and acquisition of migratory and invasive characteristics. One of the hallmarks of EMT is loss of the transmembrane cell adhesion glycoprotein E-cadherin and an increase in the expression of the mesenchymal markers N-cadherin and vimentin [13, 14]. Several transcription factors have been shown to regulate E-cadherin expression including Snail1, Snail2, Slug, TWIST1, ZEB1, and ZEB2 [13–16]. In addition, maintenance of cellular adhesion between epithelial cells requires the proper interaction between the intracellular domain of E-cadherin and the β-catenin protein. Disruption of this E-cadherin/β-catenin complex in EMT results in translocation of β-catenin into the nuclear compartment and activation of the Wingless (Wnt) signalling pathway [13, 15]. Preclinical models have shown that activation of the Wnt pathway and other signalling pathways such as Notch and transforming growth factor-β (TGFβ) induces EMT and generates stem cell-like phenotypes [17–21].

There is evidence that a transition from a mesenchymal to an epithelial (MET) state, which is the reverse process of EMT, occurs when tumour cells colonise distant sites [22]. The reexpression of E-cadherin facilitates intercellular adhesion between metastatic cells and subsequent tumour growth. This ability of cancer cells to switch between epithelial and mesenchymal phenotypes is referred to as cellular plasticity [23]. An emerging paradigm, based mostly on experimental evidence, proposes that cellular plasticity plays a critical role during the metastatic process, where EMT is critical in the initial invasive and migratory stages, while MET enhances the latter stages of metastatic colonization and growth [22, 24].

The role of cellular plasticity in PC bone metastasis formation is not yet fully understood [25]. In two experimental studies, interaction between the androgen refractory cancer of the prostate (ARCaP) cell lines and bone stromal cells resulted in a mesenchymal phenotype with a switch from E-cadherin to N-cadherin expression [26, 27]. While in another study, similar interactions resulted in an epithelial phenotype with increased expression of E-cadherin [28]. In addition, there have been inconclusive data from experimental studies on the connection between EMT/MET and cancer stem cell states in PC. In one report, pluripotent PC stem cells that express SOX2 and OCT3/4 were found to express E-cadherin [29], while, in two other studies, an EMT phenotype was associated with reduced E-cadherin expression and increased expression of stem cell markers Sox2, Nanog, Oct4, Lin28B, CD44, and/or Notch-1 [12, 30].

These, and other preclinical studies for other types of cancers, suggest that the relation between mesenchymal, epithelial, and CSC states may be more complex than previously viewed and that an epithelial phenotype could promote tumour aggressiveness. For example, breast CSCs have been demonstrated to have the ability to reversibly transition between mesenchymal-like and epithelial-like stem cell states, and it has been shown that the colonization of breast CSCs in bone induces a phenotypic switch from $CD44^+/CD24^-$ to $CD44^-/CD24^+$ cells and co-expression of both epithelial and mesenchymal markers [31, 32]. This ability of CSCs to dynamically transition between epithelial, mesenchymal, and intermediate states facilitates their adaptation to altered microenvironmental stimuli [30]. Hypoxia seems to have a central role in promoting phenotypic transitions and cellular plasticity [33], and E-cadherin has been recently reported to play a role in regulating the response of cancer cells to hypoxia by inducing the expression of hypoxia-inducible factor-1α (HIF-1α) [34]. These experimental data support a context-dependent role for the epithelial phenotype in enhancing the survival of cancer cells. In addition, E-cadherin has been shown to have a central function in establishing and maintaining the pluripotent and self-renewal properties of prostate CSCs and metastatic tumour-initiating cells [29, 35, 36]. Taken together, these experimental data demonstrate that both epithelial and mesenchymal phenotypes endow metastatic cells with structural and functional properties that allow their survival and growth within the altered environment.

Despite the wealth of *in vitro* and experimental data suggesting the plasticity of cancer cells, it has been difficult to validate cellular plasticity of metastatic tumours in the clinical setting. This is in part because samples taken from patients represent tumour status at a static point in time and do not capture the dynamic phenotypic alterations that have been demonstrated in experimental studies. However, it is imperative that these findings be clinically validated before their translation into potential therapeutic approaches is considered. Therefore, this paper focuses on the clinical evidence of the role of cellular plasticity in PC bone metastasis by reviewing studies that have analysed the differential expression of epithelial, mesenchymal, and stem cell markers in clinical PC bone metastasis tissues compared to primary PC or nonskeletal metastasis tissues.

2. Methods

2.1. Literature Search and Eligibility Criteria. A search of the PubMed database for English language studies published up to June 2014 was conducted using the following search algorithms for keywords in the title/abstract: (1) ("prostate cancer" OR "prostate carcinoma") AND ("bone" OR "skeletal" OR "skeleton" OR "osseous") AND ("metastasis" OR "metastases") AND ("cadherin" OR "catenin" OR "vimentin" OR "stem" OR "progenitor" OR "tumor initiating" OR "EMT") and (2) ("prostate cancer" OR "prostate carcinoma") AND ("bone" OR "skeletal" OR "skeleton" OR "osseous") AND ("metastasis" OR "metastases") AND ("tissue" OR "specimen"). Only studies of human bone metastasis tissues were reviewed. Studies based solely on the use of cell lines or animal models, reviews, case reports, letters to editors, and abstracts with no full reports were excluded. The reference lists from included articles were examined to identity further relevant studies.

2.2. Data Extraction. The following data were extracted from eligible studies: first author and year of publication, number of tissue specimens analysed and their type, tumour grade or Gleason score, treatment status at time of biopsy, marker(s) studied, method of marker detection, criteria used to score marker expression, differential pattern of expression in bone metastasis tissues, and statistical significance of results. Online supplementary files were used to extract relevant data when they were not available in main article.

2.3. Data Synthesis. Descriptive characteristics for studies were summarised. No formal quantitative synthesis (meta-analysis) of the data was performed due to heterogeneity between studies with regard to markers investigated, study population (tumour grade and treatment status), criteria used to score marker expression, and quantitative analysis methods employed.

3. Results

3.1. Literature Search Results. The electronic search identified a total of 720 studies. Of these, 660 were excluded and 60

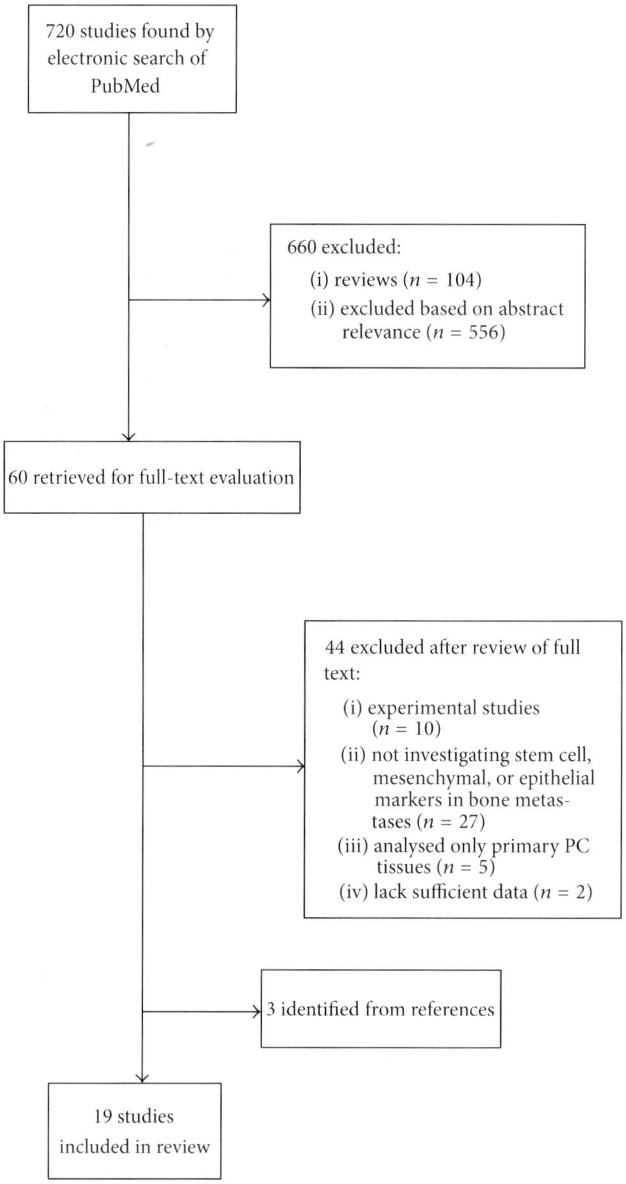

FIGURE 1: Flow chart of search strategy and study selection.

studies were retrieved based on abstract relevance. Following full-text assessment, 16 studies were deemed eligible, and three additional relevant studies were identified from reference lists. Thus, a total of 19 studies were included in this review. A flowchart of the search and study selection process is shown in Figure 1.

3.2. Study Characteristics. Table 1 summarises the descriptive characteristics of included studies. More than 60% of the studies were published after 2007. Eight studies [37–44] investigated the differential expression of stem cell markers in bone metastasis tissues, and eleven studies [45–55] analysed the differential expression of epithelial markers (mostly E-cadherin) and/or mesenchymal markers (mostly vimentin). Most studies (74%) compared marker expression between primary PC and bone metastasis tissue samples, and only 7 studies used matched tissue samples from the same patients [37, 39, 41, 42, 46, 51, 52].

The median number of bone samples analysed was 17, and around 63% of the studies used ≤20 bone samples. All studies used immunohistochemistry (IHC) for protein detection in bone metastasis samples, except for one study [46], which used *in situ* hybridisation (ISH) for mRNA detection. The study by Armstrong et al. [52] used IHC for marker staining in bone tissues and the FDA-approved CellSearch system for detecting circulating tumour cells. Not all studies reported the tumour grade or Gleason score of the primary or metastasis tissues examined or the treatment status of patients at time of bone biopsy, and among those that did, there was wide heterogeneity in the patient population (details provided in Supplementary Tables 1 and 2) (see Supplementary Material available online at http://dx.doi.org/10.1155/2015/651580).

TABLE 1: Descriptive characteristics of included studies.

Year of publication	Number of studies
1999	1
2000	1
2002	3
2004	1
2005	1
2008	3
2010	3
2011	3
2012	2
2013	1
Sample size	Median (range)
Number of BM specimens	17 (2–184)
Number of primary PC specimens	22 (6–112)
Number of nonskeletal specimens	23 (7–97)
Tissue comparisons	Number of studies
Studies that used matched samples	7
Comparisons between BM and primary PC	14
Comparisons between BM and nonskeletal metastases	7
Comparisons between different BM tissues	2
Markers analysed	Number of studies
Stem cell markers	8
EMT/MET markers	11
Main method of marker detection	Number of studies
Immunohistochemistry (IHC)	18
In situ hybridisation (ISH)	1
Tumour grade and treatment status	Number of studies
Studies that reported tumour grade	12
Studies that reported treatment status	9
Criteria used to score expression	Number of studies
Pattern of distribution of staining across cell	6
Percentage of positive cells in each specimen	5
Staining intensity scoring	2
Staining intensity multiplied by % of positive cells	5
Quantitative analysis of % of positive staining areas using Image Pro Plus 6.2 software	1
Did not report a scoring method	2
Reporting of results	Number of studies
Statistical analysis of differential expression	11

Note: BM: bone metastasis.

In general, different criteria were used to score marker expression patterns. Although only two studies did not report scoring criteria, there were variations in the criteria used to categorise positive staining, staining intensity, and staining pattern. Details of these are provided in Supplementary Tables 1 and 2. Eleven studies (58%) reported statistical analysis results of differences in pattern of marker expression between bone metastasis tissues and other tissues, all of which showed statistically significant results. Five out of these eleven studies (45%) used $\leq$20 bone metastasis specimens.

3.3. Expression Pattern of Stem Cell Markers. Table 2 and supplementary Table 1 show details from eight studies that analysed the differential expression of different stem cell markers in bone metastasis tissues compared to primary PC [37, 38, 40–44] and nonskeletal metastasis [38, 39, 43, 44].

TABLE 2: Details of studies analysing expression of stem cell markers in PC bone metastases.

Study	Marker	No. of BM specimens	Comparison tissue (No. of specimens)	Results	Significance
Gu et al., 2000 [37]	PSCA	9	Normal (25) Primary PC (112, 3 matched)	All normal tissues were negative. PSCA expression was positive in 105/112 (94%) primary and in 9/9 (100%) BM	NR
Knudsen et al., 2002 [38]	Met receptor	45	Primary PC (90) LN (35) Other soft tissues (8)	High Met expression in 52% of primary, 83% of BM, and 54% of LN metastases	$P = 0.0003$ for BM versus LN
Lam et al., 2005 [39]	PSCA	47	LN (6, 5 matched) Matched liver (3)	PSCA staining intensity was higher in BM (87%) compared with LN (67%) and liver (67%) metastases	$P = 0.014$ for BM versus LN. No statistical analysis for liver metastases due to small sample size
Wiesner et al., 2008 [40]	c-kit, SCF	20	Primary PC (21) BPH (22)	Positive staining for c-kit in 5% of BPH, 14% of primary PC, and 40% of BM Positive SCF staining in 95% of BPH and primary PC and in 85% of BM specimens	$P = 0.0077$ for BM versus BPH
Eaton et al., 2010 [41]	CD133, CD44, $\alpha 2\beta 1$ integrin, CXCR4, c-met, $\alpha 6$ integrin	11	Matched primary PC (11)	50% of samples positive for CD133. >70% positive for CD44, $\alpha 2\beta 1$, c-met, and $\alpha 6$ integrin. No difference in expression between primary and BM samples for all markers except for CD44. Higher expression of CD44 in BM, with positive staining in bone stoma. Low staining for CXCR4 in both BM and primary samples	NR
van den Hoogen et al., 2010 [42]	ALDH isoforms	10	Matched primary PC (10)	No staining for ALDH1 in BM or primary PC ALDH7A1 in 7/10 primary PC and 8/10 BM with no staining in bone stroma	NR
Castellón et al., 2012 [43]	CD133, CD44	5	Primary PC (34) LN (7)	BM and LN showed lower expression of both CD133 and CD44 compared with primary tissues	$P < 0.05$ for BM and LN versus medium Gleason grade
Sottnik et al., 2013 [44]	$\alpha 2\beta 1$	184	BPH (43) Primary PC (76) LN (61) Liver (36)	Higher expression in BM compared to primary PC and nonskeletal metastases	$P < 0.042$ for BM versus LN

ALDH: aldehyde dehydrogenase, BM: bone metastasis, BPH: benign prostatic hyperplasia, LN: lymph node, No.: number, NR: not reported, PSCA: prostate stem cell antigen, and SCF: stem cell factor.

The prostate stem cell antigen (PSCA) was found to be overexpressed in bone metastases compared to both primary PC tissues [37] and nonskeletal (lymph node and liver) metastases [39]. C-kit was found to be overexpressed in bone metastases compared to primary PC tissues [40]. A study that analysed the expression of aldehyde dehydrogenase (ALDH) isoforms in 10 PC tissues and their matched bone metastases found positive staining for the ALDH7A1 isoform in both tissues, with absent staining for ALDH1 [42].

Two studies [41, 43] reported different results in relation to the expression of the stem cells markers CD133 and CD44. Castellón et al. [43] found significantly lower expression of both CD133 and CD44 in bone metastases compared to primary tissues. While in the study by Eaton et al. [41], CD44 expression was more frequent in bone metastasis tissues than in primary cancers and CD133 was detected in half of the bone metastases samples. Eaton et al. also found that >70% of bone specimens displayed positive staining for $\alpha 2\beta 1$ integrin, c-met, and $\alpha 6$ integrin, but the staining for CXCR4 was low in both primary and metastases tissues [41]. Sottnik et al. [44] and Knudsen et al. [38] also reported significant overexpression of $\alpha 2\beta 1$ and Met receptor, respectively, in bone metastases compared to lymph node metastases.

3.4. Expression Pattern of EMT/MET Markers. Table 3 and supplementary Table 2 show data extracted from eleven studies that analysed the expression pattern of EMT and MET markers. Only two studies analysed the expression of both epithelial and mesenchymal markers. Sethi et al. [54] found no significant difference in the pattern of expression of E-cadherin or vimentin between primary and bone metastasis tissues. However, in both PC and bone metastasis tissues, reduced expression of E-cadherin was found at the invasive front of the tumour, while it was highly expressed within the tumour centre. Vimentin expression, on the other hand,

Table 3: Details of studies analysing expression of EMT/MET markers in PC bone metastases.

Study	Marker	No. of BM specimens	Comparison tissue (No. of specimens)	Results	Significance for differential expression
Bryden et al., 1999 [45]	E-Cadherin	20	Different grades of BM tissues	Decrease in expression with increasing tumour grade	NR
Bryden et al., 2002 [46]	E-Cadherin, β-catenin	14	Matched primary PC (14)	mRNA for both markers was expressed uniformly in 9/14 primary PC. In BM, 6/14 showed negative mRNA for one or both markers and 6/14 expressed both heterogeneously	NR
Lang et al., 2002 [47]	Vimentin	8	Primary (54)	16/54 of primary expressed vimentin with ≤50% staining cells. 7/8 BM expressed vimentin with 100% of cells staining positive in 5 specimens	NR
Chen et al., 2004 [48]	Wnt-1/β-catenin	23 (from 9 patients)	Primary PC (62, from 49 patients) LN (23, from 9 patients)	High Wnt-1/β-catenin in 85% of BM and 77% of LN. Highest expression was observed in BM	$P < 0.05$ for BM (& for LN) versus normal tissues
Saha et al., 2008 [49]	E-Cadherin, β-catenin	17	Primary PC (22) BPH (11)	BM tissues showed higher frequency of homogenous expression of both markers compared to primary PC	$P < 0.001$ for BM versus primary PC
Saha et al., 2008 [50]	E-Cadherin	15	Primary PC (20) BPH (11)	Higher expression of unmethylated gene and homogenous protein in BM compared to primary tissues	$P < 0.001$ for BM versus primary PC
Pontes et al., 2010 [51]	E-Cadherin, β-catenin	28	Matched primary PC (6)	For E-cadherin & β-catenin, respectively, there was abnormal expression in 86% and 82% of 28 BM specimens. In matched specimens, normal expression was seen in 5/6 and 3/6 of primary PC and abnormal expression was seen in 5/6 of BM for both markers	NR
Armstrong et al., 2011 [52]	Vimentin, CK	2	CTCs (10, 2 matched)	Coexpression of vimentin and CK in 10/10 of CTCs Absent vimentin expression in 2/2 of CK-positive BM. Strong vimentin expression in bone stroma	NR
Putzke et al., 2011 [53]	E-Cadherin	109	LN (30) Liver (18) Other (8)	Higher expression in BM compared to all soft tissue metastases	$P < 0.01$ for BM versus all soft tissue metastases
Sethi et al., 2011 [54]	E-Cadherin, Vimentin, PDGF-D, NF-kB, Notch-1, ZEB1	10	Primary PC (10)	Higher expression of Notch-1 in BM compared to primary PC. No quantitative difference in expression for other markers. In primary and BM, EMT markers (vimentin & NF-kB) had higher expression at invasive tumour front than within tumour centre. The opposite pattern was observed for E-cadherin	For BM versus primary PC: $P = 1$ for E-cadherin, vimentin, PDGF-D, NF-kB, $P = 0.057$ for Notch-1, NR for ZEB1
Wan et al., 2012 [55]	β-catenin	27	Association with AR expression in BM tissues	Nuclear localization of β-catenin in 10/27 BM specimens. Localization was inversely associated with AR expression	$P = 0.056$ for inverse association between nuclear localization of β-catenin and AR expression

AR: androgen receptor, BM: bone metastasis, BPH: benign prostatic hyperplasia, CK: cytokeratin, CTCs circulating tumour cells, ISH: *in situ* hybridisation, LN: lymph node, MS-PCR: methylation specific polymerase chain reaction, No.: number, and NR: not reported.

showed an opposite pattern, where it was overexpressed at the invasive front of the tumour and downexpressed within the tumour centre. In this study, only Notch-1 expression was found to be statistically significantly higher in bone metastasis tissues compared to primary PC [54]. Armstrong et al. [52], on the other hand, found that circulating tumour cells in men with castration resistant prostate cancer (CRPC) coexpress both vimentin and CK (an epithelial marker), while bone metastasis lesions lose vimentin expression and maintain the positive expression of CK. Expression of vimentin was examined in another study [47] and was found to be higher in bone metastasis tissues than in primary PC tissues.

Six studies [45, 46, 49–51, 53] investigated the differential expression of E-cadherin in PC bone metastases. Two of these reported lower expression of E-cadherin in bone metastasis tissues compared to matched primary PC tissues [46, 51]. In contrast, two studies by Saha et al. [49, 50] demonstrated significant upregulation of E-cadherin expression in bone metastases compared to unmatched primary tissue samples, and another study [53] found significantly increased E-cadherin expression in bone compared to soft tissue metastases. Bryden et al. [45] compared different grades of bone metastasis tissues and found an inverse correlation between E-cadherin expression and degree of tumour differentiation, where it was highest in well-differentiated tumours and declined with increasing grade.

Five studies examined changes in the expression of β-catenin in bone metastases [46, 48, 49, 51, 55]. Bryden at al. [46] and Pontes et al. [51] found lower β-catenin expression in bone metastasis tissues compared to matched primary PC tissues, while Saha et al. [49] demonstrated significantly higher membranous β-catenin expression in bone metastases compared to unmatched primary PC samples. It is important to note that in the studies by Pontes et al. [51] and Saha et al. [49], nuclear expression of β-catenin (which would indicate EMT) was considered to be negative, while in the study by Bryden et al. [46] the location of β-catenin could not be evaluated as mRNA was detected using ISH. Chen et al. [48] reported higher nuclear staining for β-catenin and Wnt 1 in bone metastases compared to primary PC and lymph node tissues, with 85% of bone metastases showing strong expression of nuclear β-catenin and Wnt 1. In the study by Wan et al. [55], on the other hand, the proportion of bone metastasis tissues that displayed positive nuclear staining for β-catenin was lower than that reported by Chen et al. (85% versus 37%). Both studies demonstrated an inverse association between nuclear β-catenin expression and androgen receptor status [48, 55].

4. Discussion

4.1. Summary and Interpretations of Findings. At present, the role of cellular plasticity in bone metastasis formation is not fully clear. Recent preclinical models indicate that the relationship between EMT/MET and CSCs is complex and dynamic. In this paper, we focused on the clinical importance of cellular plasticity in PC bone metastasis by reviewing studies that have comparatively analysed different stemness and EMT/MET markers in bone metastasis and primary tissue samples. We identified methodological limitations and sources of heterogeneity among studies. Sample size in most studies was small, and not all studies used matched primary and metastasis samples from the same patients. In addition, different scoring criteria for defining positive marker expression were used. The study population analysed was heterogeneous with respect to tumour grades and treatment status, which makes direct comparisons between patients difficult. For example, many studies did not report the androgen receptor (AR) status of the tissues analysed. This is important because two studies here showed an inverse association between nuclear β-catenin localization and androgen receptor (AR) status, suggesting that reduced AR expression enables Wnt/b-catenin signalling [48, 55]. This is in line with data from the literature that suggests that low AR expression levels are required for EMT in PC cells [56]. Thus, the heterogeneity in expression of EMT and MET markers observed between studies in this review might be partially attributed to differences in AR status in bone metastasis tissues.

Despite these methodological difference between studies reviewed, in general, most stem cell markers analysed, except for CXCR4, were positively expressed in bone metastasis tissues, with an expression level either similar to or higher than primary PC tissues and soft tissue metastases. On the other hand, the expression levels of EMT and MET markers in bone metastasis tissues showed variability within and between samples. This variation does not simply imply that studies are providing conflicting results but highlights the dynamic and transient nature of cellular plasticity that has been reported by preclinical studies and the challenges in capturing this clinically. Pathological samples represent observations of established masses taken at static points in time and are not capable of reflecting the dynamic plasticity of cancer cells. For example, the expression of markers belonging to the metastasis initiating cell population may gradually decrease as foci progress and the metastatic mass becomes more established [41].

Data from studies in this review and others confirm that temporal and spatial factors as well as degree of metastasis differentiation and metastasis size play a critical role in influencing marker expression status at distant sites. The low expression of CXCR4 in bone metastases reported by Eaton et al. [41] suggests that this marker (with its ligand SDF-1) could be important for cancer cell homing to bone and stem cell trafficking [57, 58], but not for distant tumour growth [41]. Thus, as metastases grow, this marker loses its expression. Bryden et al. [45] reported an inverse link between E-cadherin expression and level of tumour differentiation in bone metastases, where E-cadherin expression was highest in well-differentiated tumours and lowest in poorly differentiated ones. Sethi et al. [54] showed evidence for heterogeneity in the expression of EMT and MET markers within bone metastases, where expression of E-cadherin was reduced at the tumour invasive front and was high within the tumour centre, while the expression pattern for vimentin was the opposite. Armstrong et al. [52] provided evidence

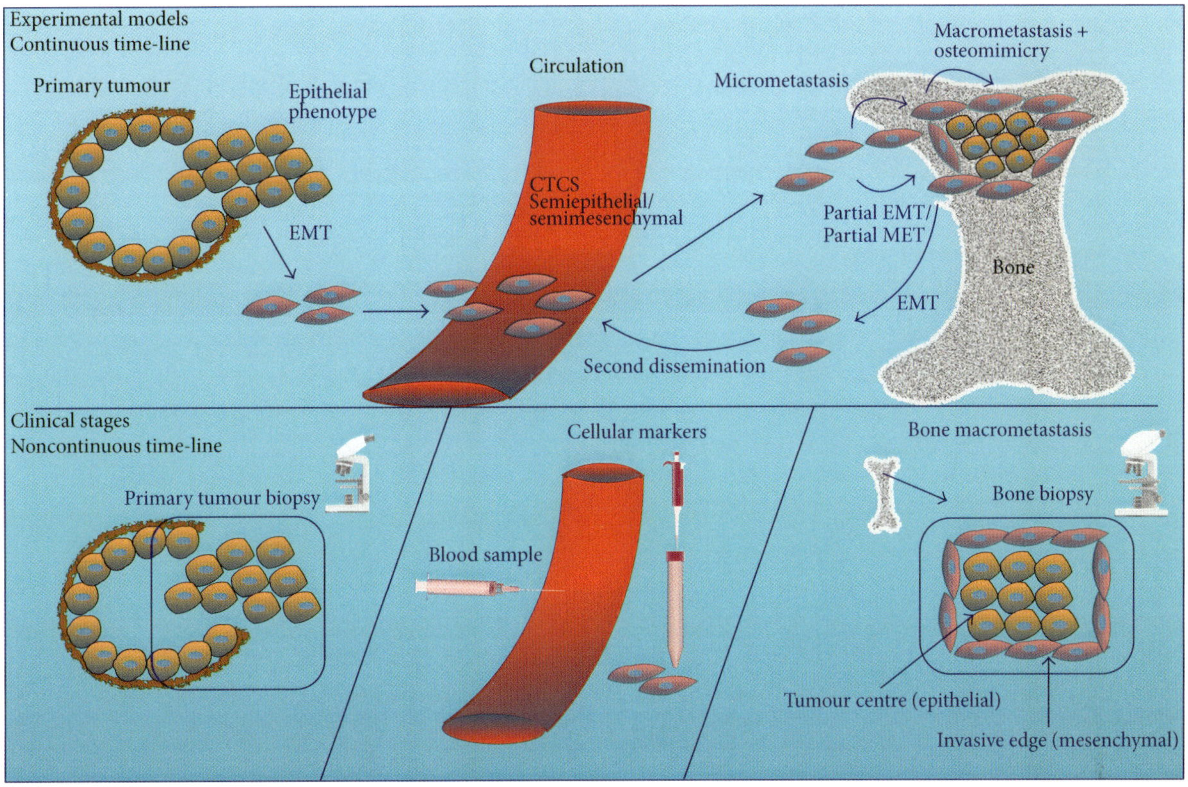

Figure 2: Cellular plasticity of prostate cancer cells over time. The plasticity of cancer cells over time can be delineated from experimental animal and *in vitro* models. Cells in the primary tumour undergo EMT, which enhances their migratory and invasive potential. These invasive cells enter the circulation and may exist as mesenchymal, epithelial, or semimesenchymal/semiepithelial circulating tumour cells (CTCs). Extravasation of CTCs into the bone gives rise to micrometastases. As the metastatic tumour cells colonise the bone and grow into macrometastasis, cells within the tumour centre undergo MET to enable tumour growth and survival under hypoxia, while cells at the invasive edge retain their mesenchymal phenotype to enable invasiveness and osteomimicry. It is suggested that these phenotypic changes are partial and that metastatic cells can dynamically transition between these two states to allow for adaptation to altered microenvironmental stimuli and for further invasion and secondary dissemination. Clinical samples, on the other hand, represent observations of established primary masses and macrometastases at static points in time. Therefore, they cannot capture the dynamic nature of cellular plasticity. Furthermore, current CTC-detection techniques are epithelial-based and cannot capture CTCs that are mostly mesenchymal and have reduced expression of epithelial markers, which would result in missing a significant fraction of CTCs that are predominantly in the mesenchymal state.

that circulating tumour cells can exist in an intermediate state expressing both epithelial and mesenchymal markers. In addition, Chao et al. [59] reported an inverse correlation between E-cadherin expression and metastasis size, where E-cadherin expression decreases as tumour mass gets bigger. Taken together, these data suggest that EMT and MET could be partial and reversible and that an increase in epithelial markers in metastasis tissues does not mean a full reversal into an epithelial state. Chao et al. hypothesise that a second EMT can occur at the distant site allowing for further dissemination into other sites [59] (Figure 2).

This plasticity and ability to dynamically transition between epithelial, mesenchymal, and intermediate states facilitates adaptation to altered microenvironmental stimuli [30]. One type of plasticity that allows adaptation in the bone microenvironment is osteomimicry [23]. Several clinical studies in this review found increased expression of markers implicated in osteomimicry. In osteomimicry, PC cells acquire an osteoblast-like phenotype [60] and express bone-related markers, such as osteocalcin, bone sialoprotein [61], osteoprotegerin, and RANKL [62]. Expression of Runx2, a major transcription factor of osteoblast differentiation, is a crucial element in the acquisition of osteomimicry [63]. Several experimental studies demonstrated a positive role for EMT and stemness pathways (e.g., TWIST and Notch) in osteomimicry by promoting the expression of Runx2 [64–66]. In addition, interaction between the hepatocyte growth factor (HGF) and its receptor, Met, has been shown to enhance osteomimicry through activation of the Wnt/β-catenin pathway [67, 68]. In this review, positive expression of Met (the stem cell marker and receptor for HGF) in PC bone metastases was demonstrated in two studies [38, 41]; another study reported significant overexpression of the Wnt/nuclear β-catenin pathway in bone metastases [48], and Notch expression was found to be significantly higher expression in bone metastasis tissues compared to primary PC tissues [54].

4.2. Clinical Challenges and Therapeutic Implications. As noted previously, cellular plasticity is difficult to capture clinically. A clear insight into the dynamics of cellular plasticity in time and space in the clinical context would require comparisons between a large number of matched samples that are serially obtained from primary tumour, circulating cancer cells, bone metastasis, and tumour-associated normal tissues at several points in time and space. This could prove extremely difficult and inconvenient. Furthermore, the currently approved technology for the detection of circulating tumour cells (CTCs) poses some limitations. CellSearch, the only FDA-cleared tool for identifying CTCs relies on the antibodies against the epithelial cell adhesion molecule (EpCAM) for capturing these cells and on the epithelial marker CK for their identification. As this is an epithelial-based detection technique, it cannot capture CTCs that are mostly mesenchymal and have reduced expression of EpCAM. Thus, this method would miss a significant fraction of CTCs that are predominantly in the mesenchymal state [69–71] (Figure 2).

The dynamic phenotypic switching of CSCs in bone metastasis tissues poses important therapeutic implications. The link between EMT and stem cell traits previously reported in the literature has motivated suggestions that counteracting the EMT phenotype could hold promise by targeting cells that are resistant to conventional treatments [25, 70, 72]. However, the evidence for the positive expression of both epithelial and mesenchymal markers in bone metastases implies that therapeutic approaches targeting one of those states might result in an unfavourable activation of the other [73, 74]. Thus, cellular plasticity entails that it may be necessary to target both mesenchymal-like and epithelial-like states in order to eliminate these cells [25]. For example, Bitting et al. [23] propose combining antiepithelial drugs, such as AR antagonists, with drugs against mesenchymal targets such as anti-N-cadherin antibodies in the treatment against metastasis.

Targeting the cancer stem cell phenotype might prove to be better than targeting epithelial and mesenchymal states. Emerging insights into the role of microRNAs in cellular plasticity could provide novel therapeutic approaches. MicroRNAs are small noncoding RNAs that mediate post-transcriptional gene regulation. These molecules have been implicated in the network regulating cellular plasticity and stemness in PC progression [75, 76]. For example, Liu et al. [75] demonstrated that microRNA-34a could be a potential therapeutic target against PC stems cells. In addition, microRNA-143 and microRNA-145 have been shown by three studies [77–79] to potentially play a role in PC bone metastasis by targeting the EMT regulator HEF1 [79] and the stem cell markers CD133, CD44, Oct-4, c-myc, and Klf4 [78]. Nevertheless, the microRNA-detection methods employed in these studies were not cell type-specific, and it is yet to be determined whether these microRNAs were expressed by tumour cells or by the surrounding bone stroma [80].

In conclusion, although findings suggest a potential role of CSCs in PC bone metastasis and stemness as a mediator of cellular plasticity, there are major challenges in detecting cellular plasticity in the clinical setting and questions remain unanswered as to whether phenotypic transitions are full or partial, whether nonstem cancer cells undergo phenotypic switching as well, and when and how do these phenotypic transitions occur.

References

[1] M. Nørgaard, A. Ø. Jensen, J. B. Jacobsen, K. Cetin, J. P. Fryzek, and H. T. Sørensen, "Skeletal related events, bone metastasis and survival of prostate cancer: a population based cohort study in Denmark (1999 to 2007)," *Journal of Urology*, vol. 184, no. 1, pp. 162–167, 2010.

[2] N. Sathiakumar, E. Delzell, M. A. Morrisey et al., "Mortality following bone metastasis and skeletal-related events among men with prostate cancer: a population-based analysis of US Medicare beneficiaries, 1999–2006," *Prostate Cancer and Prostatic Diseases*, vol. 14, no. 2, pp. 177–183, 2011.

[3] B. J. Feldman and D. Feldman, "The development of androgen-independent prostate cancer," *Nature Reviews Cancer*, vol. 1, no. 1, pp. 34–45, 2001.

[4] B. I. Rini and E. J. Small, "Hormone-refractory prostate cancer," *Current Treatment Options in Oncology*, vol. 3, no. 5, pp. 437–446, 2002.

[5] F. Li, B. Tiede, J. Massagué, and Y. Kang, "Beyond tumorigenesis: cancer stem cells in metastasis," *Cell Research*, vol. 17, no. 1, pp. 3–14, 2007.

[6] D. Bonnet and J. E. Dick, "Human acute myeloid leukemia is organized as a hierarchy that originates from a primitive hematopoietic cell," *Nature Medicine*, vol. 3, no. 7, pp. 730–737, 1997.

[7] M. Al-Hajj, M. S. Wicha, A. Benito-Hernandez, S. J. Morrison, and M. F. Clarke, "Prospective identification of tumorigenic breast cancer cells," *Proceedings of the National Academy of Sciences of the United States of America*, vol. 100, no. 7, pp. 3983–3988, 2003.

[8] S. K. Singh, I. D. Clarke, M. Terasaki et al., "Identification of a cancer stem cell in human brain tumors," *Cancer Research*, vol. 63, no. 18, pp. 5821–5828, 2003.

[9] A. T. Collins, P. A. Berry, C. Hyde, M. J. Stower, and N. J. Maitland, "Prospective identification of tumorigenic prostate cancer stem cells," *Cancer Research*, vol. 65, no. 23, pp. 10946–10951, 2005.

[10] S. A. Mani, W. Guo, M.-J. Liao et al., "The epithelial-mesenchymal transition generates cells with properties of stem cells," *Cell*, vol. 133, no. 4, pp. 704–715, 2008.

[11] A.-P. Morel, M. Lièvre, C. Thomas, G. Hinkal, S. Ansieau, and A. Puisieux, "Generation of breast cancer stem cells through epithelial-mesenchymal transition," *PLoS ONE*, vol. 3, no. 8, Article ID e2888, 2008.

[12] D. Kong, S. Banerjee, A. Ahmad et al., "Epithelial to mesenchymal transition is mechanistically linked with stem cell signatures in prostate cancer cells," *PLoS ONE*, vol. 5, no. 8, Article ID e12445, 2010.

[13] J. P. Thiery and J. P. Sleeman, "Complex networks orchestrate epithelial-mesenchymal transitions," *Nature Reviews Molecular Cell Biology*, vol. 7, no. 2, pp. 131–142, 2006.

[14] J. P. Thiery, H. Acloque, R. Y. J. Huang, and M. A. Nieto, "Epithelial-mesenchymal transitions in development and disease," *Cell*, vol. 139, no. 5, pp. 871–890, 2009.

[15] K. Polyak and R. A. Weinberg, "Transitions between epithelial and mesenchymal states: acquisition of malignant and stem cell traits," *Nature Reviews Cancer*, vol. 9, no. 4, pp. 265–273, 2009.

[16] H. Peinado, D. Olmeda, and A. Cano, "Snail, Zeb and bHLH factors in tumour progression: an alliance against the epithelial phenotype?" *Nature Reviews Cancer*, vol. 7, no. 6, pp. 415–428, 2007.

[17] T.-C. He, A. B. Sparks, C. Rago et al., "Identification of c-MYC as a target of the APC pathway," *Science*, vol. 281, no. 5382, pp. 1509–1512, 1998.

[18] V. J. M. Wielenga, R. Smits, V. Korinek et al., "Expression of CD44 in Apc and Tcf mutant mice implies regulation by the WNT pathway," *The American Journal of Pathology*, vol. 154, no. 2, pp. 515–523, 1999.

[19] J.-H. Zhao, Y. Luo, Y.-G. Jiang, D.-L. He, and C.-T. Wu, "Knockdown of β-catenin through shRNA cause a reversal of EMT and metastatic phenotypes induced by HIF-1α," *Cancer Investigation*, vol. 29, no. 6, pp. 377–382, 2011.

[20] J. Zavadil, L. Cermak, N. Soto-Nieves, and E. P. Böttinger, "Integration of TGF-β/Smad and Jagged1/Notch signalling in epithelial-to-mesenchymal transition," *The EMBO Journal*, vol. 23, no. 5, pp. 1155–1165, 2004.

[21] N. Takebe, P. J. Harris, R. Q. Warren, and S. P. Ivy, "Targeting cancer stem cells by inhibiting Wnt, Notch, and Hedgehog pathways," *Nature Reviews Clinical Oncology*, vol. 8, no. 2, pp. 97–106, 2011.

[22] C. L. Chaffer, J. P. Brennan, J. L. Slavin, T. Blick, E. W. Thompson, and E. D. Williams, "Mesenchymal-to-epithelial transition facilitates bladder cancer metastasis: role of fibroblast growth factor receptor-2," *Cancer Research*, vol. 66, no. 23, pp. 11271–11278, 2006.

[23] R. L. Bitting, D. Schaeffer, J. A. Somarelli, M. A. Garcia-Blanco, and A. J. Armstrong, "The role of epithelial plasticity in prostate cancer dissemination and treatment resistance," *Cancer Metastasis Reviews*, vol. 33, no. 2-3, pp. 441–468, 2014.

[24] M. Ksiąkiewicz, A. Markiewicz, and A. J. Zaczek, "Epithelial-mesenchymal transition: a hallmark in metastasis formation linking circulating tumor cells and cancer stem cells," *Pathobiology*, vol. 79, no. 4, pp. 195–208, 2012.

[25] G. van der Pluijm, "Epithelial plasticity, cancer stem cells and bone metastasis formation," *Bone*, vol. 48, no. 1, pp. 37–43, 2011.

[26] J. Xu, R. Wang, Z. H. Xie et al., "Prostate cancer metastasis: role of the host microenvironment in promoting epithelial to mesenchymal transition and increased bone and adrenal gland metastasis," *Prostate*, vol. 66, no. 15, pp. 1664–1673, 2006.

[27] H. E. Zhau, V. Odero-Marah, H.-W. Lue et al., "Epithelial to mesenchymal transition (EMT) in human prostate cancer: lessons learned from ARCaP model," *Clinical and Experimental Metastasis*, vol. 25, no. 6, pp. 601–610, 2008.

[28] S. Josson, S. Sharp, S.-Y. Sung et al., "Tumor-stromal interactions influence radiation sensitivity in epithelial- versus mesenchymal-like prostate cancer cells," *Journal of Oncology*, vol. 2010, Article ID 232831, 10 pages, 2010.

[29] K.-M. Bae, Z. Su, C. Frye et al., "Expression of pluripotent stem cell reprogramming factors by prostate tumor initiating cells," *The Journal of Urology*, vol. 183, no. 5, pp. 2045–2053, 2010.

[30] G. Deep, A. K. Jain, A. Ramteke et al., "SNAI1 is critical for the aggressiveness of prostate cancer cells with low E-cadherin," *Molecular Cancer*, vol. 13, article 37, 2014.

[31] S. Liu, Y. Cong, D. Wang et al., "Breast cancer stem cells transition between epithelial and mesenchymal states reflective of their normal counterparts," *Stem Cell Reports*, vol. 2, no. 1, pp. 78–91, 2014.

[32] L. D'Amico, S. Patanè, C. Grange et al., "Primary breast cancer stem-like cells metastasise to bone, switch phenotype and acquire a bone tropism signature," *British Journal of Cancer*, vol. 108, no. 12, pp. 2525–2536, 2013.

[33] S. J. Conley, E. Gheordunescu, P. Kakarala et al., "Antiangiogenic agents increase breast cancer stem cells via the generation of tumor hypoxia," *Proceedings of the National Academy of Sciences of the United States of America*, vol. 109, no. 8, pp. 2784–2789, 2012.

[34] K. Chu, K. M. Boley, R. Moraes, S. H. Barsky, and F. M. Robertson, "The paradox of E-cadherin: role in response to hypoxia in the tumor microenvironment and regulation of energy metabolism," *Oncotarget*, vol. 4, no. 3, pp. 446–462, 2013.

[35] T. Celià-Terrassa, Ó. Meca-Cortés, F. Mateo et al., "Epithelial-mesenchymal transition can suppress major attributes of human epithelial tumor-initiating cells," *The Journal of Clinical Investigation*, vol. 122, no. 5, pp. 1849–1868, 2012.

[36] K. M. Bae, N. N. Parker, Y. Dai, J. Vieweg, and D. W. Siemann, "E-cadherin plasticity in prostate cancer stem cell invasion," *The American Journal of Cancer Research*, vol. 1, no. 1, pp. 71–84, 2011.

[37] Z. Gu, G. Thomas, J. Yamashiro et al., "Prostate stem cell antigen (PSCA) expression increases with high gleason score, advanced stage and bone metastasis in prostate cancer," *Oncogene*, vol. 19, no. 10, pp. 1288–1296, 2000.

[38] B. S. Knudsen, G. A. Gmyrek, J. Inra et al., "High expression of the Met receptor in prostate cancer metastasis to bone," *Urology*, vol. 60, no. 6, pp. 1113–1117, 2002.

[39] J. S. Lam, J. Yamashiro, I. P. Shintaku et al., "Prostate stem cell antigen is overexpressed in prostate cancer metastases," *Clinical Cancer Research*, vol. 11, no. 7, pp. 2591–2596, 2005.

[40] C. Wiesner, S. M. Nabha, E. B. D. Santos et al., "C-kit and its ligand stem cell factor: potential contribution to prostate cancer bone metastasis," *Neoplasia*, vol. 10, no. 9, pp. 996–1003, 2008.

[41] C. L. Eaton, M. Colombel, G. van der Pluijm et al., "Evaluation of the frequency of putative prostate cancer stem cells in primary and metastatic prostate cancer," *Prostate*, vol. 70, no. 8, pp. 875–882, 2010.

[42] C. van den Hoogen, G. van der Horst, H. Cheung et al., "High aldehyde dehydrogenase activity identifies tumor-initiating and metastasis-initiating cells in human prostate cancer," *Cancer Research*, vol. 70, no. 12, pp. 5163–5173, 2010.

[43] E. A. Castellón, R. Valenzuela, J. Lillo et al., "Molecular signature of cancer stem cells isolated from prostate carcinoma and expression of stem markers in different Gleason grades and metastasis," *Biological Research*, vol. 45, no. 3, pp. 297–305, 2012.

[44] J. L. Sottnik, S. Daignault-Newton, X. Zhang et al., "Integrin alpha$_2$beta$_1$ ($\alpha_2\beta_1$) promotes prostate cancer skeletal metastasis," *Clinical and Experimental Metastasis*, vol. 30, no. 5, pp. 569–578, 2013.

[45] A. A. G. Bryden, A. J. Freemont, N. W. Clarke, and N. J. R. George, "Paradoxical expression of E-cadherin in prostatic bone metastases," *BJU International*, vol. 84, no. 9, pp. 1032–1034, 1999.

[46] A. A. G. Bryden, J. A. Hoyland, A. J. Freemont, N. W. Clarke, D. Schembri Wismayer, and N. J. R. George, "E-cadherin and β-catenin are down-regulated in prostatic bone metastases," *BJU International*, vol. 89, no. 4, pp. 400–403, 2002.

[47] S. H. Lang, C. Hyde, I. N. Reid et al., "Enhanced expression of vimentin in motile prostate cell lines and in poorly differentiated and metastatic prostate carcinoma," *Prostate*, vol. 52, no. 4, pp. 253–263, 2002.

[48] G. Chen, N. Shukeir, A. Potti et al., "Up-regulation of Wnt-1 and β-catenin production in patients with advanced metastatic prostate carcinoma: potential pathogenetic and prognostic implications," *Cancer*, vol. 101, no. 6, pp. 1345–1356, 2004.

[49] B. Saha, A. Arase, S. S. Imam et al., "Overexpression of E-cadherin and beta-catenin proteins in metastatic prostate cancer cells in bone," *Prostate*, vol. 68, no. 1, pp. 78–84, 2008.

[50] B. Saha, P. Kaur, D. Tsao-Wei et al., "Unmethylated E-cadherin gene expressionis significantly associated with metastatic human prostate cancer cells in bone," *The Prostate*, vol. 68, no. 15, pp. 1681–1688, 2008.

[51] J. Pontes Jr., M. Srougi, P. M. Borra, M. F. Dall'Oglio, L. A. Ribeiro-Filho, and K. R. Leite, "E-cadherin and β-catenin loss of expression related to bone metastasis in prostate cancer," *Applied Immunohistochemistry & Molecular Morphology*, vol. 18, no. 2, pp. 179–184, 2010.

[52] A. J. Armstrong, M. S. Marengo, S. Oltean et al., "Circulating tumor cells from patients with advanced prostate and breast cancer display both epithelial and mesenchymal markers," *Molecular Cancer Research*, vol. 9, no. 8, pp. 997–1007, 2011.

[53] A. P. Putzke, A. P. Ventura, A. M. Bailey et al., "Metastatic progression of prostate cancer and E-cadherin: regulation by ZEB1 and Src family kinases," *American Journal of Pathology*, vol. 179, no. 1, pp. 400–410, 2011.

[54] S. Sethi, J. Macoska, W. Chen, and F. H. Sarkar, "Molecular signature of epithelial-mesenchymal transition (EMT) in human prostate cancer bone metastasis," *American Journal of Translational Research*, vol. 3, no. 1, pp. 90–99, 2011.

[55] X. Wan, J. Liu, J.-F. Lu et al., "Activation of β-catenin signaling in androgen receptor-negative prostate cancer cells," *Clinical Cancer Research*, vol. 18, no. 3, pp. 726–736, 2012.

[56] M.-L. Zhu and N. Kyprianou, "Role of androgens and the androgen receptor in epithelial-mesenchymal transition and invasion of prostate cancer cells," *The FASEB Journal*, vol. 24, no. 3, pp. 769–777, 2010.

[57] R. S. Taichman, C. Cooper, E. T. Keller, K. J. Pienta, N. S. Taichman, and L. K. McCauley, "Use of the stromal cell-derived factor-1/CXCR4 pathway in prostate cancer metastasis to bone," *Cancer Research*, vol. 62, no. 6, pp. 1832–1837, 2002.

[58] M. Kucia, R. Reca, K. Miekus et al., "Trafficking of normal stem cells and metastasis of cancer stem cells involve similar mechanisms: pivotal role of the SDF-1-CXCR4 axis," *Stem Cells*, vol. 23, no. 7, pp. 879–894, 2005.

[59] Y. Chao, Q. Wu, M. Acquafondata, R. Dhir, and A. Wells, "Partial mesenchymal to epithelial reverting transition in breast and prostate cancer metastases," *Cancer Microenvironment*, vol. 5, no. 1, pp. 19–28, 2012.

[60] K. S. Koeneman, F. Yeung, and L. W. K. Chung, "Osteomimetic properties of prostate cancer cells: a hypothesis supporting the predilection of prostate cancer metastasis and growth in the bone environment," *Prostate*, vol. 39, no. 4, pp. 246–261, 1999.

[61] W.-C. Huang, Z. Xie, H. Konaka, J. Sodek, H. E. Zhau, and L. W. K. Chung, "Human osteocalcin and bone sialoprotein mediating osteomimicry of prostate cancer cells: role of cAMP-dependent protein kinase A signaling pathway," *Cancer Research*, vol. 65, no. 6, pp. 2303–2313, 2005.

[62] J. M. Brown, E. Corey, Z. D. Lee et al., "Osteoprotegerin and rank ligand expression in prostate cancer," *Urology*, vol. 57, no. 4, pp. 611–616, 2001.

[63] K. D. Brubaker, R. L. Vessella, L. G. Brown, and E. Corey, "Prostate cancer expression of runt-domain transcription factor Runx2, a key regulator of osteoblast differentiation and function," *Prostate*, vol. 56, no. 1, pp. 13–22, 2003.

[64] H.-F. Yuen, W.-K. Kwok, K.-K. Chan et al., "TWIST modulates prostate cancer cell-mediated bone cell activity and is upregulated by osteogenic induction," *Carcinogenesis*, vol. 29, no. 8, pp. 1509–1518, 2008.

[65] M. Zayzafoon, S. A. Abdulkadir, and J. M. McDonald, "Notch signaling and ERK activation are important for the osteomimetic properties of prostate cancer bone metastatic cell lines," *The Journal of Biological Chemistry*, vol. 279, no. 5, pp. 3662–3670, 2004.

[66] N. Sethi and Y. Kang, "Notch signaling: mediator and therapeutic target of bone metastasis," *BoneKEy Reports*, vol. 1, article 3, 2012.

[67] S. Previdi, P. Maroni, E. Matteucci, M. Broggini, P. Bendinelli, and M. A. Desiderio, "Interaction between human-breast cancer metastasis and bone microenvironment through activated hepatocyte growth factor/Met and β-catenin/Wnt pathways," *European Journal of Cancer*, vol. 46, no. 9, pp. 1679–1691, 2010.

[68] M. Q. Hassan, Y. Maeda, H. Taipaleenmaki et al., "miR-218 directs a Wnt signaling circuit to promote differentiation of osteoblasts and osteomimicry of metastatic cancer cells," *Journal of Biological Chemistry*, vol. 287, no. 50, pp. 42084–42092, 2012.

[69] N. Bednarz-Knoll, C. Alix-Panabières, and K. Pantel, "Plasticity of disseminating cancer cells in patients with epithelial malignancies," *Cancer and Metastasis Reviews*, vol. 31, no. 3-4, pp. 673–687, 2012.

[70] J. H. Tsai and J. Yang, "Epithelial-mesenchymal plasticity in carcinoma metastasis," *Genes & Development*, vol. 27, no. 20, pp. 2192–2206, 2013.

[71] H. Liu, X. Zhang, J. Li, B. Sun, H. Qian, and Z. Yin, "The biological and clinical importance of epithelial–mesenchymal transition in circulating tumor cells," *Journal of Cancer Research and Clinical Oncology*, vol. 141, no. 2, pp. 189–201, 2015.

[72] P. Li, R. Yang, and W.-Q. Gao, "Contributions of epithelial-mesenchymal transition and cancer stem cells to the development of castration resistance of prostate cancer," *Molecular Cancer*, vol. 13, no. 1, article 55, 2014.

[73] J. H. Tsai, J. L. Donaher, D. A. Murphy, S. Chau, and J. Yang, "Spatiotemporal regulation of epithelial-mesenchymal transition is essential for squamous cell carcinoma metastasis," *Cancer Cell*, vol. 22, no. 6, pp. 725–736, 2012.

[74] D. Gao, L. T. Vahdat, S. Wong, J. C. Chang, and V. Mittal, "Microenvironmental regulation of epithelial-mesenchymal transitionsin cancer," *Cancer Research*, vol. 72, no. 19, pp. 4883–4889, 2012.

[75] C. Liu, K. Kelnar, B. Liu et al., "The microRNA miR-34a inhibits prostate cancer stem cells and metastasis by directly repressing CD44," *Nature Medicine*, vol. 17, no. 2, pp. 211–216, 2011.

[76] C. Liu and D. G. Tang, "MicroRNA regulation of cancer stem cells," *Cancer Research*, vol. 71, no. 18, pp. 5950–5954, 2011.

[77] X. Peng, W. Guo, T. Liu et al., "Identification of miRs-143 and -145 that is associated with bone metastasis of prostate cancer and involved in the regulation of EMT," *PLoS ONE*, vol. 6, no. 5, Article ID e20341, 2011.

[78] S. Huang, W. Guo, Y. Tang, D. Ren, X. Zou, and X. Peng, "miR-143 and miR-145 inhibit stem cell characteristics of PC-3 prostate cancer cells," *Oncology Reports*, vol. 28, no. 5, pp. 1831–1837, 2012.

[79] W. Guo, D. Ren, X. Chen et al., "HEF1 promotes epithelial mesenchymal transition and bone invasion in prostate cancer under the regulation of microRNA-145," *Journal of Cellular Biochemistry*, vol. 114, no. 7, pp. 1606–1615, 2013.

[80] O. A. Kent, M. N. McCall, T. C. Cornish, and M. K. Halushka, "Lessons from miR-143/145: the importance of cell-type localization of miRNAs," *Nucleic Acids Research*, vol. 42, no. 12, pp. 7528–7538, 2014.

10

Robotic Radical Prostatectomy in Patients with Previous Prostate Surgery and Radiotherapy

Ömer Acar[1] and Tarık Esen[1,2]

[1] *Department of Urology, VKF American Hospital, 34365 Istanbul, Turkey*
[2] *School of Medicine, Koc University, 34450 Istanbul, Turkey*

Correspondence should be addressed to Ömer Acar; omer_acar_@hotmail.com

Academic Editor: Katsuto Shinohara

Herein, we will review the available literature about robot-assisted radical prostatectomy in patients who have undergone prostate surgery or radiotherapy. Current data about this topic consists of small case series with limited follow-up. Despite being technically demanding, robot-assisted radical prostatectomy (RARP) can be considered feasible in either setting. Prostate surgery or prostatic irradiation should not be considered as a contraindication for robot-assisted radical prostatectomy. Nevertheless, patient counseling about the possible complications and the need for reintervention is of extreme importance in this patient population. Early oncologic and functional results of RARP performed in case of radiorecurrent prostate cancer look promising. Regarding postprostate surgery RARP, some series have reported comparable results, while some have demonstrated more inferior outcomes than those of naive cases. In order to assess the exact functional and oncologic outcome of RARP in patients with previous prostate surgery and radiotherapy, studies enrolling higher number of patients and providing longer follow-up data are needed.

1. Introduction

Radical prostatectomy (RP) after previous treatments to the prostate such as transurethral resection of the prostate (TURP), photoselective vaporization (PVP), external-beam radiotherapy (EBRT), and brachytherapy (BT) is widely considered to be a more challenging task than in a prostate that has not been manipulated surgically or affected by radiotherapy. It is considered that previous prostatic resection or irradiation may hinder optimal results for radical prostatectomy in several ways. Most importantly, perioperative difficulties in defining correct surgical planes will increase the likelihood of significant complications and positive surgical margins. Additionally, functional outcomes related to erectile function and continence are at risk, due to the relative inability to identify and preserve neurovascular structures.

With increasing experience and the proven efficacy of robot-assisted radical prostatectomy (RARP), more complex cases such as those with previous TURP or radiotherapy (RT) are also being investigated using this technique. This review will focus on the perioperative, functional, and oncologic outcomes of robot-assisted radical prostatectomy, performed after prostate surgery or radiotherapy.

2. Robot-Assisted Radical Prostatectomy after Radiation Failure

2.1. Radiotherapy for Prostate Cancer. In localized prostate cancer (T1c-T2 N0 M0), three-dimensional (3D) conformal radiotherapy, with or without intensity modulated radiotherapy (IMRT), is recommended even for young patients who refuse surgical intervention. Irradiation offers the same long-term survival results as radical prostatectomy; moreover, EBRT provides a quality of life (QoL) at least as good as that provided by surgery [1]. Transperineal low-dose rate BT is another safe and effective technique that might be used to treat low-risk prostate cancer [2]. The eligibility criteria are stage cT1-T2a N0 M0, a Gleason score of 6 or lower assessed on a sufficient number of random biopsies, an initial PSA level of 10 ng/mL or lower, 50% or fewer of biopsy cores involved with cancer, a prostate volume of 50 mL or less, and a good IPSS. Recurrence-free survival after 5 and 10 years has been reported to range from 71% to 93% and from 65% to 85% [2].

According to the American Society for Therapeutic Radiology and Oncology (ASTRO) criteria, biochemical failure is defined as a PSA rise of 2 ng/mL above the posttreatment nadir, whether or not the patient received hormonal therapy in conjunction with radiation therapy [3].

Routine prostate biopsy should not be ordered for the evaluation of PSA-only recurrences, according to an ASTRO consensus recommendation [3]. On the other hand, prostate biopsy documenting local recurrence represents the main cornerstone in the decision-making process for salvage RP in patients with rising PSA levels following a nadir after radiation therapy. It is a general recommendation to wait about 18 months after radiation therapy or seed implantation [4]. Patients with rising PSA and viable cancer on biopsy 2 years after radiation therapy have true locally recurrent disease and might be candidates for salvage RP.

2.2. Therapeutic Options after Radiation Failure. In case of radiorecurrent PCa, treatment options include salvage radical prostatectomy (SRP), cryotherapy, high-intensity focused ultrasound (HIFU), and salvage BT [4, 5]. According to data from the Cancer of the Prostate Strategic Urological Research Endeavor (CaPSURE) database, 5277 men with PCa underwent RP (4342 men) or RT (935 men). In the latter group, 587 patients (63%) developed recurrent disease or received secondary treatment after a mean follow-up of 38 months [6]. Ninety-two percent of the patients in the CaPSURE database, who had radiorecurrent prostate cancer, received systemic ADT while only 2% of the patients underwent salvage RP [6]. Thus, more than 90% of the patients were placed on salvage hormonal therapy which is noncurative, indefinite, and associated with its own side effects and quality of life concerns such as hot flashes, sexual dysfunction, reduction in muscle mass, increased fracture risk, insulin resistance, and cardiovascular morbidity. The underutilization of salvage RP may be explained by its technically demanding nature and the fact that RT-induced cystitis, fibrosis, and tissue plane obliteration can increase the probability of complications with rectal injury, urinary incontinence, erectile dysfunction, and anastomotic contracture being reported in a substantial proportion of the cases [7–9]. However, in well-selected patients, the procedure may result in long-term disease-free survival.

2.3. General Considerations about Salvage Radical Prostatectomy. A candidate for salvage RP should fulfill the following requirements: surgically curable disease at initial radiation, no evidence of metastatic disease, a postradiation biopsy confirming PCa, and a life expectancy long enough (≥10 years) to benefit from intervention. Presurgical PSA (<10 ng/mL) and Gleason score of the postradiation biopsy (≤7) should also be considered when selecting a patient for salvage therapy [4, 10]. The first series of salvage RP and cystoprostatectomy following radiation failure was published in 1985 by Mador et al. [11]. The initial series reporting on salvage RP have included patients treated in the pre-PSA era without modern radiotherapeutic techniques, when local recurrences were usually detected at a late stage. Consequently, as high as 65% of the patients suffered from treatment-related morbidities. Up to 60% of patients who underwent salvage RP had to undergo anterior or total exenteration for locally extensive disease, associated with a high rate of local recurrences and a mean time of progression of only 1.3 years [4, 12]. Since then, salvage surgery has been used with increasing relative success.

Reports that have been published in the era of modern radiotherapy have described far more optimistic outcomes after salvage RP. In the recent literature review analyzing the currently available data on salvage RP, Chade et al. [10] reported that positive surgical margins varied from 43% to 70% in the earlier series and from 0% to 36% in the later studies (publication date before or after 2000). Pathologic organ-confined disease was reported in 22–53% and 25–81% of studies, respectively. At 10 years, biochemical recurrence-free probability ranged from 28% to 53%. Series from single centers reported probabilities of cancer-specific survival (CSS) from 70% to 79% at 10 years, while the multi-institutional study reported an 83% CSS at 10 years. Overall survival (OS) varied from 54% to 89% at 10 years [10].

Before SRP, PSA may be considered as the strongest prognostic factor predicting the oncologic outcome after salvage RP, because it was shown to significantly predict progression-free survival (PFS), CSS, and OS in most of the series [13–16]. Clinical stage before the commencement of RT [17], Gleason score prior to salvage RP, percentage of positive cores at biopsy, PSA doubling time, and low-dose brachytherapy were the other reported variables that have the potential to influence the oncologic outcome [18–20].

Regarding perioperative results and surgical complications, rectal injury ranged from 0% to 28% in patients and anastomotic stricture from 7% to 41%. Major complications (Clavien 3–5) occurred in 0–25% of patients, and estimated blood loss (EBL) varied between 119 mL and 1 L. Blood transfusion rates were found to be similar to the standard RP procedures [10].

Post-SRP erectile function sufficient for sexual intercourse ranged from 0% to 20% which led to the recommendation for oral medication or surgical treatment for ED in at least 80% of patients. Post-SRP urinary continence, defined by zero pads after SRP, ranged from 21% to 90% [10].

2.4. Salvage Laparoscopic Radical Prostatectomy. The feasibility of performing salvage prostatectomies has been extended into laparoscopy and more recently into robotic platforms [21, 22]. In 2003, Vallancien et al. were the first to report the outcome of laparoscopic SRP in seven cases with radiorecurrent PCa. Average operating time was 190 min (170–210 min). Two patients had positive surgical margins (PSM). At follow-up of 7, 12, 15, and 21 months, four patients were free of disease. No complications were reported. Five patients were continent and two patients who were potent before surgery became impotent [21]. Stolzenburg et al. investigated the feasibility of salvage endoscopic extraperitoneal RP for locally recurrent PCa in 9 patients. Regarding complications, only one patient with urinary retention was reported. Biochemical recurrence was recognized in only one patient 12 months postoperatively. Seven patients were completely continent [23]. Liatsikos et al. reported the outcome of another series of 12 patients who underwent salvage endoscopic extraperitoneal RP. Average operative time was 153 min, and mean blood loss was 238 mL. No intraoperative complications were reported. Biochemical recurrence was observed in one patient 12 months post-operatively. 10 patients were completely continent, but 3 preoperatively potent patients became impotent after the operation [24].

2.5. Salvage Robot-Assisted Radical Prostatectomy. Robot-assisted radical prostatectomy (RARP) is the most commonly performed surgical procedure for the treatment of patients with clinically localized prostate cancer in the United States. The robot offers several advantages, such as 3D vision, wristed instrumentation, motion scaling, image magnification, and tremor filtration. Hence, it may theoretically overcome the major limitations of salvage radical prostate surgery, such as the inability to identify correct surgical planes and neurovascular protection and therefore improve the oncologic and functional outcomes.

Avoidance of bladder neck contracture is very important after salvage RARP and, as a result of either the contracture or the treatment itself, these patients are at very high risk for incontinence. Watertight anastomosis with a running barbed suture may decrease the risk of anastomotic leakage and rate of bladder neck contractures.

Pneumoperitoneum may contribute to reduced blood loss compared to open salvage prostatectomy with EBL and transfusion requirements that do not appear to exceed that of primary (nonsalvage) robotic prostatectomy. However, all of these advantages may be offset by the lack of tactile feedback which is a major concern in this setting. Future improvements in haptic feedback technology are especially important in salvage surgeries where tissue planes are harder to discern.

In 2008, Jamal et al. reported a case of salvage robot-assisted radical prostatectomy (sRARP) [25]. The patient previously underwent 70 Gy of conformal EBRT and 3 months of antiandrogen treatment for a Gleason 6 tumor. He presented 2 years later due to hemospermia when he had a PSA of 0.7 ng/mL. Prostatic biopsy showed residual tumor and he underwent sRARP. After 3 months, the patient was continent, and his PSA was less than 0.03 ng/mL. After this initial report, several case-series have been published to date (Tables 1 and 2).

The first robotic series was reported by Kaouk et al. in which four patients underwent sRARPs with a mean operative time and EBL of 125 minutes and 117 mL, respectively. All patients had obturator lymph node dissection, and none showed any lymph node metastasis. The intraoperative courses were uneventful, but PSM occurred in two patients. At 1-month follow-up, 75% of the patients were dry on most days [22].

Subsequently, Boris et al. reported 11 patients who underwent sRARP with pelvic lymph node dissection. The mean operative time was 183 minutes, while the mean EBL was 113 mL. There were no intraoperative complications; however, an anastomotic leak developed in one patient necessitating extended catheterization, while an anastomotic stricture developed in another patient. Eight (72.7%) patients were continent (0-1 pad/d), of which six were pad free. Two patients had erections adequate for sexual intercourse. After a mean follow-up of 20.5 months, 3 patients had biochemical recurrence. They also supported the feasibility of sRARP [26].

Eandi et al. have reported their series of sRARPs consisting of 18 patients. Median operative time, EBL, and length of stay were, respectively, 2.6 h, 150 mL, and 2 days. Neither significant complications (rectal or ureteral injuries) nor need for blood transfusion was reported. Anastomotic extravasation was present in six (33%) cases, of which an anastomotic stricture developed in three. Five (28%) patients had a PSM, of whom two had organ-confined disease. One patient had lymph node metastasis. Six (33%) patients were completely continent, while all patients had ED after surgery. At a median follow-up of 18 months, 12 (67%) patients were free of biochemical recurrence [27].

Strope et al. reported the results of six patients who underwent RARP after definitive RT. The mean preoperative PSA level and the mean operative time were 9.3 ng/mL and 356 minutes, respectively. No rectal injuries or other intra-operative complications were experienced. Mean estimated blood loss was 280 mL. None received blood transfusion. Mean duration of hospitalization was 2 days. At 1 year, 2.3 pads per day were being used in the four patients who had eligible data regarding functional status. In three patients with available data at 1 year, all reported erectile dysfunction. Margins were negative in all but one patient and none of the patients had lymph node involvement. All except for 2 patients remained free of biochemical recurrence at a mean follow-up of 15 months [28].

Recently, Chauhan et al. retrospectively identified 15 patients who underwent sRARP in three academic institutions over a 20-month period with biopsy-proven prostate cancer after definitive radiotherapy. The median operative time, the median estimated blood loss, and the median length of hospital stay were 140.5 min, 75 mL, and 1 day, respectively. There were no rectal injuries. Two patients had a PSM. Of the patients, 71.4% were continent. At a median follow-up of 4.6 months, four (28.6%) patients presented with biochemical recurrence after sRARP [29].

Kaffenberger et al. reported their series of sRARP consisting of 34 patients who had surgery after the failure of prior definitive ablative therapy. Median time from primary therapy to sRARP was 48.5 months with a median preoperative PSA of 3.86 ng/mL. There were 2 Clavien grade 2 and higher complications. Postoperatively, 39% of patients were continent (0-1 pad/day). After a median follow-up of 16 months, 18% of patients had biochemical failure. The PSM rate was 26%, of which 33% had biochemical failure after surgery. On univariable analysis, PSA doubling time and Gleason score at original diagnosis were found to be significantly associated with biochemical failure. They highlighted the advantages of sRARP as superior visualization of the posterior prostatic

TABLE 1: Perioperative outcomes in sRARP series.

Series	Patients, n	Type of radiation	Mean follow-up, mos	Mean EBL, mL	Mean OR time, min	Mean days on catheter, d	Mean hospital stay, d	Nerve sparing, n
Jamal et al. [25]	1	1 XRT	3	100	150	14	1	0
Kaouk et al. [22]	4	2 BT, 2 XRT + BT	5	117	125	15	2.7	0/4
Boris et al. [26]	11	6 BT, 4 XRT, 1 XRT + BT	20.5	113	183	10.4	1.4	NA
Eandi et al. [27]	18	8 BT, 8 XRT, 2 PBT	18	150	156	14	2	NA
Strope et al. [28]	6	4 XRT, 2 BT	>12	280	356	NA	2	1
Chauhan et al. [29]	15	5 XRT, 3 XRT + BT, 2 PBT, 5 BT	4.6	75	138	NA	1	2/15
Kaffen-berger et al. [30]	34	13 BT, 11 XRT, 6 BT + XRT, 4 HIFU	16.1	NA (88% had EBL ≤ 250 mL)	176	NA	NA (94% discharged on day 1)	NA
Yuh et al. [32]	51	22 BT, 18 XRT, 6 PBT, 3 Cryo, 1 HIFU, 1 XRT + BT	36	175	179	14	2	NA

EBL: estimated blood loss; OR: operative; XRT: external-beam radiation therapy; NA: not available; BT: brachytherapy; PBT: proton beam therapy; HIFU: high intensity focused ultrasound; and Cryo: cryotherapy.

TABLE 2: Oncologic and functional outcomes in sRARP series.

Series	Patients, n	Overall complications, n	Rectal injury, n	+LN, n	Continence, n	Potency, n	PSM, n	BCR during follow-up, n
Jamal et al. [25]	1	0	0	0	1/1	NA	0/1	0
Kaouk et al. [22]	4	1	0	0	3/4	NA	2/4	NA
Boris et al. [26]	11	3	0	2	8/11	2/11	3/11	3
Eandi et al. [27]	18	7	0	1	6/18	0/18	5/18	6
Strope et al. [28]	6	4	0	0	0/6	0/6	1/6	2
Chauhan et al. [29]	15	4	0	1	10/14	0/15	2/15	4
Kaffen-berger et al. [30]	34	13	1	0	12/33	5/33	9/34	6
Yuh et al. [32]	51	24	1	3	23/51	6/13	16/51	10

EBL: estimated blood loss; OR: operative; LN: lymph node; PSM: positive surgical margin; BCR: biochemical recurrence; and NA: not available.

plane, modest blood loss, low complication rates, and short length of stay [30].

Zugor et al. have reported the data of 13 patients who have undergone sRARP after failed external-beam radiotherapy ($n = 7$) or brachytherapy ($n = 6$). Neurovascular bundle preservation was performed in 3 patients (23.1%). Interestingly, they did not report any major intraoperative or postoperative complication. At 12 months, 7 patients were continent (53.8%), and 3 patients (23.1%) were potent. During the follow-up period, only 3 patients (23.1%) exhibited BCR [31].

The largest sRARP series has recently been published by Yuh et al. They reported the outcome of 51 consecutive patients who underwent sRARP after previous failed local therapy. Median age at surgery was 68 years and a median of 68 months has elapsed since primary treatment. Median operative time and estimated blood loss amount were 179 minutes and 175 mL, respectively. Half of the patients had extracapsular disease on eventual histopathologic assessment and the positive surgical margin rate was 31%. After a median follow-up of 36 months, their estimated 3-year biochemical recurrence or progression-free survival was 57%. Noteworthy, they reported significant complications (47%), incontinence, and erectile dysfunction rates. However, potency was maintained in 23% of preoperatively potent men and spontaneous return of urinary continence was achieved in 23 patients (45%) with a median time to continence of 6 months. Nevertheless, they emphasized the importance of proper patient counseling and selection before sRARP [32].

2.6. *Summary.* Salvage RP is a surgically challenging but effective secondary local treatment of PCa that recurred after radiotherapy with curative intent. Recommended criteria and identified predictive factors may help to select patients who are most suitable for salvage RP with long-term cure and good functional outcome. Extensive counseling regarding possible side effects of the procedure are mandatory.

In sRARP for radiorecurrent prostate cancer, tissue planes are often obscured and there is adherence of adjacent structures such as the rectum, pubic bone, and bladder. Healing and recovery are also delayed following energy destruction of tissue. Despite the fact that complications were not reported in a standardized categorical manner, the majority of them were of high importance as they required procedural intervention for bladder neck contracture, artificial urinary sphincter, or penile prosthesis.

Available data is consisting of small case series with limited follow-up. Larger series with a longer follow-up are necessary to make definitive conclusions about the oncologic and functional outcomes.

3. Robot-Assisted Radical Prostatectomy after Prostate Surgery

3.1. General Considerations. It is not uncommon for men to be diagnosed of cancer on TURP chips or to develop prostate cancer later after having undergone TURP for benign prostatic obstruction. Such men may have different outcomes on radical prostatectomy compared to those who have no such previous intervention. The relative paucity of the number of patients who underwent a previous TURP makes any comparative analysis difficult and also is a reflection of the few available studies on this subject in the literature (Tables 3 and 4).

There are several important factors which may affect the outcome of post-TURP RARP. The vesicourethral anastomosis may be technically difficult as a result of the rigidity of the bladder neck and the loss of elasticity of the urethra. Previous resection of the bladder neck could also distort the position of the ureteral orifices and thus increase the risk of ureteral injury. Increased periprostatic adhesions may increase the amount of blood lost and the risk of rectal injury during RARP.

The need for bladder neck reconstruction is increased because the bladder neck is wide, which may impact anastomotic urinary leakage and continence outcomes. TURP renders the internal sphincter mechanism deficient and also places the external sphincter at risk if the proper technique is not used which may increase the cumulative risk of postprocedural incontinence. Neurovascular bundle identification may be difficult as a result of periprostatic adhesions and therefore the risk of erectile dysfunction may be increased. Urethral manipulation and catheterization during TURP may result in anterior urethral stricture formation, a fact which may lead to infravesical obstruction and cause lower urinary tract symptoms after RARP.

Moreover, lymph nodes may be enlarged secondary to reactional changes post-TURP and may be difficult to interpret on preoperative imaging. There may be an increased risk of metastatic spread of disease because of the opening of lymphovascular channels during TURP along with continuous fluid irrigation.

3.2. Open and Laparoscopic Series. Most studies comparing the oncologic and functional outcomes in patients with and without previous TURP involve perineal, retropubic, laparoscopic, and endoscopic extraperitoneal RP series, data that ignore the advantages of the robotic technique. Colombo et al. evaluated the outcome of retropubic RP after TURP. They found a mean operative time from 135 to 105 minutes in the TURP group versus from 125 to 85 minutes in the control group. Complications were encountered in up to 50% of the patients. They reported that 74% and 86% of patients were dry at 6 and 12 months, respectively, and that 28% of patients were potent at 6 months. They considered RP to be feasible in patients after TURP [33].

Jaffe et al. compared the operative and postoperative outcomes of 119 patients who underwent laparoscopic RP after TURP to that of a randomized matched control group. Mean estimated blood loss, transfusion rate, and reoperation rates were statistically similar between the 2 groups. Postoperative length of stay (6.5 versus 5.2 days) and operative time (179 versus 171 minutes) were statistically higher in the TURP group. Positive surgical margin rate was significantly higher in the TURP group compared to the non-TURP group (21.8% versus 12.6%). Complications were observed in 64 patients in the TURP group compared to 34 in the non-TURP group ($p < 0.01$). Five (4.2%) and 2 (1.7%) men in the TURP and non-TURP groups, respectively, underwent reoperation during the postoperative period ($P = 0.13$) [34].

In a study by Teber et al., the authors evaluated the effect of previous TURP on surgical, functional, and oncologic outcomes after laparoscopic RP in comparison with a control group. The positive surgical margin rates were 14.5% and 16.3%, and the long-term continence rates were similar; however, previous TURP was associated with a lower continence rate (49.1%) at 3 months compared with 61.8% for the control group. There was no significant difference in the potency rates between the two groups at 12 months [35].

3.3. Robotic Series. Martin et al. were the first to investigate the effect of previous prostatic surgery on the outcome of robot-assisted RP. They evaluated the data of 24 patients who underwent RARP with a history of at least one previous treatment to the prostate including TURP, transurethral incision of the prostate (TUIP), transurethral microwave thermotherapy (TUMT), transurethral needle ablation (TUNA), photoselective vaporization of the prostate (PVP), simple prostatectomy, and open bladder neck reconstruction (group 1) and compared that of 486 patients with no treatment prior to RARP (group 2). Mean estimated blood loss, length of hospital stay, and operative duration were not statistically significantly different. However, the catheter time was significantly longer in group 1 (12 versus 8 days, $P = 0.028$). Complication rates were comparable (8.3% versus 6.8%). There were no bowel injuries in either group. The combined, overall PSM rate was 20.8% and 22.6% in groups 1 and 2, respectively ($P = 1.0$). Overall, there was no statistically

Table 3: Perioperative outcomes in clinical series consisting of patients who underwent RARP after prostate surgery.

Series	Study population	Mean follow-up, mos	Mean EBL, mL	Mean OR time, min	Mean days on catheter, d	Mean hospital stay, d	Nerve sparing, n
Zugor et al. [38]	80 pts with TURP before RARP versus 80 pts with RARP	13.5	165 versus 144	189 versus 149	6.8 versus 5.2	NA	42 versus 54
Martin et al. [36]	24 pts with previous treatment to the prostate and RARP versus 486 with no previous treatment and RARP	NA	155 versus 137	200 versus 186	12 versus 8 ($P = 0.028$)	2.2 versus 1.5	14 versus 403
Gupta et al. [37]	18 pts with TURP before RARP versus 8 pts with pT1b CaP and RARP versus 132 pts with RARP	15.3	4941 versus 358.3 versus 324.2 ($P = 0.03$)	189.1 versus 162.5 versus 166	15.5 versus 14.2 versus 13.3	4.4 versus 4.1 versus 3.2	NA
Martin-schek et al. [39]	19 pts with previous TURP and RARP versus 19 pts with previous TURP and RRP	NA	333 versus 1103 ($P < 0.001$)	217 versus 174 ($P = 0.02$)	7.9 versus 11.7 ($P = 0.001$)	8.5 versus 11.7 ($P = 0.003$)	14 versus 13

TURP: transurethral resection of the prostate; RARP: robot-assisted radical prostatectomy; CaP: prostate cancer; EBL: estimated blood loss; OR: operating; and NA: not available.

Table 4: Oncologic and functional outcomes in clinical series consisting of patients who underwent RARP after prostate surgery.

Series	Study population	Transfusion, n	Rectal injury, n	+LN, n	Continence, n	Potency, n	PSM, n	BCR during f/u, n
Zugor et al. [38]	80 pts with TURP before RARP versus 80 pts with RARP	1 versus 0	1 versus 0	2 versus 0	70 versus 73	38 versus 58	6 versus 4	NA
Martin et al. [36]	24 pts with previous treatment to the prostate and RARP versus 486 with no previous treatment and RARP	0 versus 0	0 versus 0	NA	NA	NA	5 versus 110	NA
Gupta et al. [37]	18 pts with TURP before RARP versus 8 pts with pT1b CaP and RARP versus 132 pts with RARP	2 versus 1 versus 9	0 versus 0 versus 0	0 versus 0 versus 3	6/8 versus 5/6 versus 78/85	1/5 versus 1/3 versus 20/61	4 versus 1 versus 17	3 versus 1 versus 9 ($P = 0.04$)
Martinschek et al. [39]	19 pts with previous TURP and RARP versus 19 pts with previous TURP and RRP	0 versus 2 ($P < 0.001$)	0 versus 0	NA	NA	NA	3 versus 3	NA

TURP: transurethral resection of the prostate; RARP: robot-assisted radical prostatectomy; CaP: prostate cancer; LN: lymph node; PSM: positive surgical margin; BCR: biochemical recurrence; and NA: not available.

significant difference in perioperative outcomes between the groups [36].

In the subsequent study conducted by Gupta et al., 158 cases of RARP for clinically localized prostate cancer, including 26 cases that had undergone previous TURP and 132 cases without TURP were analyzed in terms of surgical, oncological, and functional outcomes. The TURP cases were further subclassified into those who were found to have cancer after the histopathologic examination of TURP chips and those who had benign histopathology on TURP chips but developed cancer on subsequent follow-up. Post-TURP patients were found to have significantly greater blood loss (494 versus 324 mL) and a need for bladder neck reconstruction (26.7% versus 9.7%) compared to the non-TURP group. Conversion rates were also higher in TURP group (7.7%; 2/26) compared to non-TURP group (3%; 4/132). Importantly, all conversions in TURP were noted in those who had cT1b disease. Surgical time (189 versus 166 min), margin positivity rate, and biochemical recurrence rate were also higher in the TURP group. Regarding functional outcomes, incontinence rates in TURP group were higher both at 6 (14% versus 11.8%) and 12 (25% versus 8%) months follow-up than that of non-TURP group [37].

Zugor et al. compared the perioperative, oncologic, and functional outcomes of the patients who had undergone TURP before RARP ($n = 80$) and those who underwent

RARP without a history of TURP ($n = 80$). Groups had equivalent clinicopathologic characteristics in this matched-pair analysis. Regarding preoperative characteristics, the only statistically significant difference was between potency rates (67.5% in TURP group versus 83.75% in non-TURP group, $P = 0.056$). The need for bladder neck reconstruction and operative time was significantly higher in the TURP group compared to the non-TURP group (58.7% versus 2.5%, $P = 0.073$ and 189 min versus 149 min, $P = 0.069$, respectively). The PSM rate did not exhibit statistical significance between two groups (6.25% versus 5%). Continence and potency rates in 12 months were similar (87.5%/91.25% and 70.3%/86.5%, respectively) [38].

Martinschek et al. compared the surgical outcome of robot-assisted radical prostatectomy and radical retropubic prostatectomy (RRP) in patients who underwent TURP. Mean operative time was 217 minutes for RARP and 174 minutes for RRP ($P < 0.05$). The overall positive surgical margin rate was 15.8% in both groups. Mean estimated blood loss was 33 mL in RARP patients and 1103 mL in RRP patients ($P < 0.001$). The RARP and RRP groups also differed in terms of hospital stay (8.58 versus 11.74 days; $P = 0.0037$), duration of catheterization (7.95 versus 11.78 days; $P = 0.0016$), postoperative complications according to the Clavien classification system (6 versus 15 patients; $P = 0.0027$), and transfusion rate (0% versus 10.5%; $P < 0.001$). They concluded that robot-assisted radical prostatectomy may be more feasible while dealing with prostate cancer patient who had undergone TURP [39].

Several newer modifications of TURP (e.g., transurethral vaporization resection of the prostate, bipolar TURP) and several types of laser prostatectomy (e.g., photoselective vaporization, holmium laser enucleation of the prostate, etc.) are available with each having its advantages and disadvantages. It may be possible that that these different technologies produce different degrees of prostatic, periprostatic, and bladder neck changes and may, therefore, have different degrees of impact on the outcomes of RARP. A recent study has reported on the feasibility of RARP after holmium laser enucleation of the prostate [40]. Apart from the technology used to resect the prostate, there are several other factors that may influence the final outcome. These include the size of the prostate gland, resection time, depth and completeness of resected prostate, presence of prostatitis, infection, surgeon's technique, and an individual's immune response. These factors directly affect the degree of inflammatory response in and around the prostate after TURP and may play important roles with respect to individual patient outcome.

3.4. Summary. The existing literature deals mainly with the post-TURP open and laparoscopic radical prostatectomies. Data is relatively scarce about the outcomes of RARP performed after prostate surgery. Some of the papers suggest that relatively poorer outcomes are achieved in men with previous pelvic or prostatic surgery. There are also suggestions that although surgery may be technically more difficult, overall morbidity, complications, and long-term functional or oncological outcomes are not different between these groups.

In conclusion, RARP is feasible after TURP, with good overall results being achieved. However, previous prostate surgery can cause difficulties for the surgical team during radical prostatectomy. Although previous TURP should not be considered as a contraindication for RARP, patients should be made aware of the above facts before undergoing RARP.

References

[1] F. J. Fowler Jr., M. J. Barry, G. Lu-Yao, J. H. Wesson, and L. Bin, "Outcomes of external-beam radiation therapy for prostate cancer: a study of medicare beneficiaries in three surveillance, epidemiology, and end results areas," *Journal of Clinical Oncology*, vol. 14, no. 8, pp. 2258–2265, 1996.

[2] A. Heidenreich, J. Bellmunt, M. Bolla et al., "EAU guidelines on prostate cancer. Part 1: screening, diagnosis, and treatment of clinically localised disease," *European Urology*, vol. 59, no. 1, pp. 61–71, 2011.

[3] M. Roach III, G. Hanks, H. Thames Jr. et al., "Defining biochemical failure following radiotherapy with or without hormonal therapy in men with clinically localized prostate cancer: recommendations of the RTOG-ASTRO Phoenix Consensus Conference," *International Journal of Radiation Oncology Biology Physics*, vol. 65, no. 4, pp. 965–974, 2006.

[4] N. Mottet, J. Bellmunt, M. Bolla et al., "EAU guidelines on prostate cancer. Part II. Treatment of advanced, relapsing, and castration-resistant prostate cancer," *European Urology*, vol. 59, no. 4, pp. 572–583, 2011.

[5] M. Kimura, V. Mouraviev, M. Tsivian, J. M. Mayes, T. Satoh, and T. J. Polascik, "Current salvage methods for recurrent prostate cancer after failure of primary radiotherapy," *BJU International*, vol. 105, no. 2, pp. 191–201, 2010.

[6] G. D. Grossfeld, Y. Li, D. P. Lubeck, J. M. Broering, S. S. Mehta, and P. R. Carroll, "Predictors of secondary cancer treatment in patients receiving local therapy for prostate cancer: data from cancer of the prostate strategic urologic research endeavor," *Journal of Urology*, vol. 168, no. 2, pp. 530–535, 2002.

[7] B. T. Chen and D. P. Wood Jr., "Salvage prostatectomy in patients who have failed radiation therapy or cryotherapy as primary treatment for prostate cancer," *Urology*, vol. 62, supplement, pp. 69–78, 2003.

[8] M. Garzotto and Z. Wajsman, "Androgen deprivation with salvage surgery for radiorecurrent prostate cancer: results at 5-year followup," *Journal of Urology*, vol. 159, no. 3, pp. 950–955, 1998.

[9] E. Rogers, M. Ohori, V. S. Kassabian, T. M. Wheeler, and P. T. Scardino, "Salvage radical prostatectomy: outcome measured by serum prostate specific antigen levels," *Journal of Urology*, vol. 153, no. 1, pp. 104–110, 1995.

[10] D. C. Chade, J. Eastham, M. Graefen et al., "Cancer control and functional outcomes of salvage radical prostatectomy for radiation-recurrent prostate cancer: a systematic review of the literature," *European Urology*, vol. 61, no. 5, pp. 961–971, 2012.

[11] D. R. Mador, R. P. Huben, Z. Wajsman, and J. E. Pontes, "Salvage surgery following radical radiotherapy for adenocarcinoma of

the prostate," *The Journal of Urology*, vol. 133, no. 1, pp. 58–60, 1985.

[12] N. J. Touma, J. I. Izawa, and J. L. Chin, "Current status of local salvage therapies following radiation failure for prostate cancer," *Journal of Urology*, vol. 173, no. 2, pp. 373–379, 2005.

[13] L. Cheng, T. J. Sebo, J. Slezak et al., "Predictors of survival for prostate carcinoma patients treated with salvage radical prostatectomy after radiation therapy," *Cancer*, vol. 83, no. 10, pp. 2164–2171, 1998.

[14] C. L. Amling, S. E. Lerner, S. K. Martin, J. M. Slezak, M. L. Blute, and H. Zincke, "Deoxyribonucleic acid ploidy and serum prostate specific antigen predict outcome following salvage prostatectomy for radiation refractory prostate cancer," *Journal of Urology*, vol. 161, no. 3, pp. 857–863, 1999.

[15] F. J. Bianco Jr., P. T. Scardino, A. J. Stephenson, C. J. DiBlasio, P. A. Fearn, and J. A. Eastham, "Long-term oncologic results of salvage radical prostatectomy for locally recurrent prostate cancer after radiotherapy," *International Journal of Radiation Oncology Biology Physics*, vol. 62, no. 2, pp. 448–453, 2005.

[16] K. M. Sanderson, D. F. Penson, J. Cai et al., "Salvage radical prostatectomy: quality of life outcomes and long-term oncological control of radiorecurrent prostate cancer ," *Journal of Urology*, vol. 176, no. 5, pp. 2025–2032, 2006.

[17] E. L. Gheiler, M. V. Tefilli, R. Tiguert et al., "Predictors for maximal outcome in patients undergoing salvage surgery for radio-recurrent prostate cancer," *Urology*, vol. 51, no. 5, pp. 789–795, 1998.

[18] A. Heidenreich, S. Richter, D. Thüer, and D. Pfister, "Prognostic parameters, complications, and oncologic and functional outcome of salvage radical prostatectomy for locally recurrent prostate cancer after 21st-century radiotherapy," *European Urology*, vol. 57, no. 3, pp. 437–445, 2010.

[19] G. T. Gotto, L. H. Yunis, K. Vora, J. A. Eastham, P. T. Scardino, and F. Rabbani, "Impact of prior prostate radiation on complications after radical prostatectomy," *Journal of Urology*, vol. 184, no. 1, pp. 136–142, 2010.

[20] E. Rogers, M. Ohori, V. S. Kassabian, T. M. Wheeler, and P. T. Scardino, "Salvage radical prostatectomy: Outcome measured by serum prostate specific antigen levels," *Journal of Urology*, vol. 153, no. 1, pp. 104–110, 1995.

[21] G. Vallancien, R. Gupta, X. Cathelineau, H. Baumert, and F. Rozet, "Initial results of salvage laparoscopic radical prostatectomy after radiation failure," *The Journal of Urology*, vol. 170, no. 5, pp. 1838–1840, 2003.

[22] J. H. Kaouk, J. Hafron, R. Goel, G. Haber, and J. S. Jones, "Robotic salvage retropubic prostatectomy after radiation/brachytherapy: initial results," *BJU International*, vol. 102, no. 1, pp. 93–96, 2008.

[23] J. Stolzenburg, B. Bynens, M. Do, R. Rabenalt, P. F. Katsakiori, and E. Liatsikos, "Salvage laparoscopic extraperitoneal radical prostatectomy after failed high-intensity focused ultrasound and radiotherapy for localized prostate cancer," *Urology*, vol. 70, no. 5, pp. 956–960, 2007.

[24] E. Liatsikos, B. Bynens, R. Rabenalt, P. Kallidonis, M. Do, and J. Stolzenburg, "Treatment of patients after failed high intensity focused ultrasound and radiotherapy for localized prostate cancer: salvage laparoscopic extraperitoneal radical prostatectomy," *Journal of Endourology*, vol. 22, no. 10, pp. 2295–2298, 2008.

[25] K. Jamal, B. Challacombe, O. Elhage, R. Popert, R. Kirby, and P. Dasgupta, "Successful salvage robotic-assisted radical prostatectomy after external beam radiotherapy failure," *Urology*, vol. 72, no. 6, pp. 1356–1358, 2008.

[26] R. S. Boris, A. Bhandari, L. S. Krane, D. Eun, S. Kaul, and J. O. Peabody, "Salvage robotic-assisted radical prostatectomy: initial results and early report of outcomes," *BJU International*, vol. 103, no. 7, pp. 952–956, 2009.

[27] J. A. Eandi, B. A. Link, R. A. Nelson et al., "Robotic assisted laparoscopic salvage prostatectomy for radiation resistant prostate cancer," *Journal of Urology*, vol. 183, no. 1, pp. 133–137, 2010.

[28] S. A. Strope, M. Coelho, D. P. Wood, and B. K. Hollenbeck, "Robot-assisted salvage prostatectomy: evaluation of initial patient-reported outcomes," *Journal of Endourology*, vol. 24, no. 3, pp. 425–427, 2010.

[29] S. Chauhan, M. B. Patel, R. Coelho et al., "Preliminary analysis of the feasibility and safety of salvage robot-assisted radical prostatectomy after radiation failure: multi-institutional perioperative and short-term functional outcomes," *Journal of Endourology*, vol. 25, no. 6, pp. 1013–1019, 2011.

[30] S. D. Kaffenberger, K. A. Keegan, N. K. Bansal et al., "Salvage robotic assisted laparoscopic radical prostatectomy: a single institution, 5-year experience," *Journal of Urology*, vol. 189, no. 2, pp. 507–513, 2013.

[31] V. Zugor, A. P. Labanaris, D. Porres, A. Heidenreich, and J. H. Witt, "Robot-assisted radical prostatectomy for the treatment of radiation-resistant prostate cancer: surgical, oncological and short-term functional outcomes," *Urologia Internationalis*, vol. 92, no. 1, pp. 20–26, 2014.

[32] B. Yuh, N. Ruel, S. Muldrew et al., "Complications and outcomes of robot-assisted salvage radical prostatectomy—a single institution experience," *BJU International*, vol. 113, no. 5, pp. 769–776, 2014.

[33] R. Colombo, R. Naspro, A. Salonia et al., "Radical prostatectomy after previous prostate surgery: clinical and functional outcomes," *The Journal of Urology*, vol. 176, no. 6, part 1, pp. 2459–2463, 2006.

[34] J. Jaffe, O. Stakhovsky, X. Cathelineau, E. Barret, G. Vallancien, and F. Rozet, "Surgical outcomes for men undergoing laparoscopic radical prostatectomy after transurethral resection of the prostate," *Journal of Urology*, vol. 178, no. 2, pp. 483–487, 2007.

[35] D. Teber, J. Cresswell, M. Ates et al., "Laparoscopic radical prostatectomy in clinical T1a and T1b prostate cancer: oncologic and functional outcomes—a matched-pair analysis," *Urology*, vol. 73, no. 3, pp. 577–581, 2009.

[36] A. D. Martin, P. J. Desai, R. N. Nunez et al., "Does a history of previous surgery or radiation to the prostate affect outcomes of robot-assisted radical prostatectomy?" *BJU International*, vol. 103, no. 12, pp. 1696–1698, 2009.

[37] N. P. Gupta, P. Singh, and R. Nayyar, "Outcomes of robot-assisted radical prostatectomy in men with previous transurethral resection of prostate," *BJU International*, vol. 108, no. 9, pp. 1501–1505, 2011.

[38] V. Zugor, A. P. Labanaris, D. Porres, and J. H. Witt, "Surgical, oncologic, and short-term functional outcomes in patients undergoing robot-assisted prostatectomy after previous transurethral resection of the prostate," *Journal of Endourology*, vol. 26, no. 5, pp. 515–519, 2012.

[39] A. Martinschek, K. Heinzelmann, M. Ritter, E. Heinrich, and L. Trojan, "Radical prostatectomy after previous transurethral

resection of the prostate: robot-assisted laparoscopic versus open radical prostatectomy in a matched-pair analysis," *Journal of Endourology*, vol. 26, no. 9, pp. 1136–1141, 2012.

[40] N. Suardi, V. Scattoni, A. Briganti et al., "Nerve-sparing radical retropubic prostatectomy in patients previously submitted to Holmium laser enucleation of the prostate for bladder outlet obstruction due to benign prostatic enlargement," *European Urology*, vol. 53, no. 6, pp. 1180–1185, 2008.

11

Role of *p73* Dinucleotide Polymorphism in Prostate Cancer and p73 Protein Isoform Balance

L. Michael Carastro,[1] Hui-Yi Lin,[2] Hyun Y. Park,[3] Donghwa Kim,[4] Selina Radlein,[3] Kaia K. Hampton,[1] Ardeshir Hakam,[5] Babu Zachariah,[6] Julio Pow-Sang,[7] and Jong Y. Park[3]

[1] *Department of Chemistry, Biochemistry & Physics, University of Tampa, Tampa, FL 33606, USA*
[2] *Department of Biostatistics, Moffitt Cancer Center, Tampa, FL 33612, USA*
[3] *Department of Cancer Epidemiology, Moffitt Cancer Center, 12902 Magnolia Drive, Tampa, FL 33612, USA*
[4] *Department of Molecular Oncology, Moffitt Cancer Center, Tampa, FL 33612, USA*
[5] *Department of Anatomic Pathology, Moffitt Cancer Center, Tampa, FL 33612, USA*
[6] *Genitourinary Program, James Haley VA Hospital, Tampa, FL 33612, USA*
[7] *Genitourinary Program, Moffitt Cancer Center, Tampa, FL 33612, USA*

Correspondence should be addressed to Jong Y. Park; jong.park@moffitt.org

Academic Editor: Scott E. Eggener

Background. Molecular markers for prostate cancer (PCa) risks are currently lacking. Here we address the potential association of a dinucleotide polymorphism (DNP) in exon 2 of the *p73* gene with PCa risk/progression and discern any disruption of p73 protein isoforms levels in cells harboring a *p73* DNP allele. *Methods.* We investigated the association between *p73* DNP genotype and PCa risk/aggressiveness and survival by fitting logistic regression models in 1,292 incident cases and 682 controls. *Results.* Although we detected no association between *p73* DNP and PCa risk, a significant inverse relationship between *p73* DNP and PCa aggressiveness (AT/AT + GC/AT versus GC/GC, OR = 0.55, 95%Cl = 0.31–0.99) was detected. Also, *p73* DNP is marginally associated with overall death (dominant model, HR = 0.76, 95%Cl = 0.57–1.00, $P = 0.053$) as well as PCa specific death (HR = 0.69, 95%Cl = 0.45–1.06, $P = 0.09$). Western blot analyses for p73 protein isoforms indicate that cells heterozygous for the *p73* DNP have lower levels of △Np73 relative to TAp73 ($P < 0.001$). *Conclusions.* Our findings are consistent with an association between *p73* DNP and low risk for PCa aggressiveness by increasing the expressed TAp73/△Np73 protein isoform ratio.

1. Introduction

Prostate cancer is the most common nonskin malignancy among men worldwide. In the US, incidence rate in 2014 is 147.8 per 100,000 men per year [1]. One of the clinical challenges of prostate cancer (PCa) is distinguishing indolent from aggressive disease. This distinction is important to facilitate clinical treatment decision-making. For instance, patients with indolent disease can be classified as low risk and provided with conservative management and treatment, while patients with aggressive disease may be classified as high risk and provided with immediate therapy (surgery, radiation, and/or chemotherapy).

In the present prostate specific antigen (PSA) era, the majority of PCa cases are now diagnosed at an early stage when the tumor is confined to the prostate. Radical prostatectomy is the treatment of reference for organ-confined prostate tumors with good outcome in a large series of patients. However, about 20–30% of patients who undergo radical prostatectomy develop tumor recurrence within 10 years after surgery [2]. Currently, the level of PSA, clinical stage, and Gleason score are used to estimate prognosis and inform treatment modalities [3, 4]. Although these features are extremely useful, they do not fully account for the varied interindividual outcomes associated with treatment [5]. Therefore, there is a strong need for biomarkers that can distinguish aggressive from non-aggressive disease which is therefore of paramount importance.

Several lines of evidence support an association between a dinucleotide polymorphism (DNP) (rs1801173) in the *p73* gene and risk for several cancer types, but some studies reported conflicting results [38–41]. This particular *p73* DNP is a G4C14-to-A4T14 (*p73* DNP) (rs1801173) linked pair of transition changes located in the 5′-UTR portion of exon 2. In a meta-analysis of 8,017 various cancer patients and 10,610 controls from 27 epidemiological studies focusing on potential associations between various cancer risk and *p73* DNP, it was reported that *p73* DNP was associated with an increased risk for colorectal and head and neck cancers, but not lung, gastric, and oesophageal cancers, and PCa was not addressed [40]. In another combined analysis of 8,148 cancer patients and 8,150 controls from 26 studies, some of which overlapped with the meta-analysis, a positive association was detected between the *p73* DNP and cervical, colorectal, head and neck, and other cancers, including breast, endometrial, non-Hodgkin's lymphoma, and ovarian cancers, but PCa was not addressed [5]. Up to this point, only one small study ($n = 177$ cases) of a population in northern India reported no association of *p73* DNP with risk of PCa [37]. Therefore, we investigated the potential for an association between risk/aggressiveness and survival of PCa and the *p73* DNP using 1,292 PCa patients, surgically treated at the Moffitt Cancer Center from 1986 to 2003, and 682 age-matched healthy male controls.

The *p73* gene is a member of the p53 tumor suppressor family. The biology of the p73 tumor suppressor gene expression is complex and not completely understood. At least 14 isoforms of the p73 protein are translated from multiple mRNA variants transcribed from the *p73* gene [42]. These p73 protein isoforms are grouped into two major categories, TAp73 and ΔNp73, which differ in their N-termini and are transcribed from two different promoters, designated P1 and P2 (see Supplemental Figure 1 in Supplementary Material available online at http://dx.doi.org/10.1155/2014/129582). The transcriptionally active TAp73 isoforms are transcribed from the P1 promoter and include the full-length N-terminal sequence encompassing exons 1 through 3. However, the ΔNp73 isoforms are transcribed from promoter P2, which begins transcription at exon 4 (Supplemental Figure 1) and does not contain the N-terminal transactivation (TA) domain. Therefore, the ΔNp73 protein isoform acts in a dominate negative manner toward TAp73 because ΔNp73 isoforms are able to form tetramers with TAp73, as well as p53, but are not capable of activating transcription of p73- or p53-target genes [43]. This ΔNp73 dominate negative mechanism explains the observation of higher ΔNp73 levels, relative to TAp73, detected in human cancers [42, 44, 45].

The exact molecular consequences of the presence of the *p73* DNP allele are not known. Likewise, the mechanism by which the *p73* DNP influences cancer risks is also unknown. Because the *p73* DNP is located in exon 2 within the 5′-UTR of the *p73* gene and lies between the two *p73* gene promoters (Supplemental Figure 1), we speculated that this *p73* DNP might have an effect on the p73 N-terminal protein isoform balance, possibly due to the *p73* gene promoter utilization and/or stability or translational efficiency of the TAp73 mRNA or some other heretofore unknown molecular mechanism. Therefore, we investigated the relative p73 isoform protein levels in cancer cell lines and then discerned any correlation between the TAp73/ΔNp73 protein isoform ratios and the p73 DNP (rs1801173) genotype status.

2. Patients and Methods

2.1. Study Participants and Data Collection. The study population consisted of 1,292 prostatectomy cases (1,232 Caucasians and 60 African Americans) treated at the Moffitt Cancer Center from 1986 to 2003. Cases were PCa patients aged 36–84 at diagnosis with pathologically confirmed primary invasive PCa and treated with radical prostatectomy. Demographic and clinical information including age at diagnosis, Gleason score, TNM stage, and length of followup were obtained from the Moffitt Tumor Registry and medical records. Date of death, cause of death, and vital status information through September 30, 2011 were obtained from the medical records and the Moffitt Tumor Registry, which follows cases diagnosed or initially treated at the Moffitt Cancer Canter. Additional information on pretreatment serum PSA level, prostatic capsular invasion, surgical margin status, seminal vesicle invasion, and lymph node status was obtained from medical records. Recurrence was defined as elevated PSA level (>0.2 ng/mL), clinical metastasis, or PCa related death. The study was approved by the Institutional Review Board of the University of South Florida (Tampa, FL) and all participants gave a written informed consent.

Healthy controls consisted of 682 subjects (595 Caucasians and 87 African Americans) who were visiting Moffitt's Lifetime Cancer Screening Center or the James A. Haley VA Hospital (Tampa, FL). All control subjects were male and had no previous diagnosis of cancer.

2.2. Genomic DNA Preparation and Genotyping for p73 DNP. Genomic DNA was prepared from either blood/buccal samples (control) or formalin-fixed paraffin embedded normal prostate tissue blocks (cases) obtained from the Tissue Core Facility at the Moffitt Cancer Center. DNA was extracted using the DNeasy tissue kit (Qiagen, Valencia, CA) according to the manufacturer's recommendations. Genomic DNA samples from cultured cell lines were extracted from cell cultures using a PureLink Genomic DNA Isolation Kit (Invitrogen-Life Technologies) according to the manufacturer's recommendations. Genomic DNA samples were quantified using a NanoDrop (Thermo Scientific). All genomic DNA samples, from patient samples and cell lines, were stored at −80°C.

The *p73* DNP was determined using a commercially available TaqMan Real-Time PCR allelic discrimination assay (Life Technologies; Assay ID number C_16180356_10) and TaqMan Gene Expression Assay Master Mix (Applied Biosystems-Life Technologies; part number 4369016) according to the manufacturer's protocol. Genotyping assays (20 μL reaction volume) included 20 ng of genomic DNA and were performed using a 7900HT Fast Real-Time PCR System (Applied Biosystems-Life Technologies).

2.3. Cell Lines. Tissue culture cell lines HepG2, HCT116, H1299, CaCO-2, HEK293, JEKO-1, Jurkat, and BEAS-2B were acquired from ATCC. Other tissue culture cell lines used HeLa, MCF7, and H460 were kindly provided (DK). All cell lines, except H460, Jurkat, and JEKO-1, were maintained in DMEM supplemented with 10% FBS, 100 U penicillin, and 100 μg/mL streptomycin. The H460, Jurkat, and JEKO-1 cell lines were maintained in RPMI supplemented with 10% heat-inactivated FBS, 100 U penicillin, and 100 μg/mL streptomycin. All cell lines were cultured at 37°C and 5% CO_2.

2.4. Western Analyses. Total protein samples were harvested from tissue culture cells by lysing in RIPA (Thermo Scientific) buffer supplemented with Halt Protease Inhibitor Cocktail (Thermo Scientific) according to the manufacturer's protocol. Protein samples were quantified using a BCA protein assay kit (Thermo Scientific) resolved on 10% SDS-PAGE and then electrotransferred onto Immunoblot PVDF (Bio-Rad, Hercules, CA) membranes in 1XTris-Glycine (Bio-Rad, Hercules, CA)/20% MeOH. Blotted membranes were blocked in 1XPBS/5% nonfat milk/0.1% Tween-20/0.02% NaN_3. Blocked membranes were probed with a p73 isoform-specific primary monoclonal antibody in blocking solution at 1 : 200 (v/v) dilution or a primary polyclonal antibody against actin at 1 : 1000 (v/v) dilution for 1 hr and then were washed with three changes of blocking solution without NaN_3 for 10 min. Primary antibodies were detected by secondary antibody-horseradish peroxidase (HRP) conjugates at 1 : 5000 dilution in blocking solution without NaN_3 for 1 hr. After probing with secondary antibody-HRP conjugate, membranes were washed five times in 1XPBS/0.1% Tween-20 for 10 min. Immunoreactive proteins were detected by chemiluminescence using Amersham ECL Prime Western Blotting Detection reagent (GE Healthcare Life Sciences) and visualized by fluorography. The p73 isoform and actin protein bands detected by western analyses were quantified using ImageJ64 (http://rsbweb.nih.gov/ij/docs/install/osx.html), and these values were used to calculate TAp73/ΔNp73 relative expression level ratios using the formula: TAp73/ΔNp73 = ((TAp73/actin)/(ΔNp73/actin)).

2.5. Antibodies. Primary antibodies used to detect p73 protein isoforms were monoclonal antibody against ΔNp73 (clone 38C674; Calbiochem, Merck KGaA, Darmstadt, Germany) and monoclonal antibody against full-length TAp73 (clone 5B429; Santa Cruz Biotechnologies, Dallas, TX, USA). A goat primary polyclonal antibody was used to detect actin (I-19; Santa Cruz Biotechnologies, Dallas, TX, USA). Secondary antibody-HRP conjugates were utilized for detection of p73 isoform-specific monoclonal antibodies (Sigma-Aldrich, St Louis, MO, USA) and goat polyclonal antibody against actin (Rockland Immunochemicals, Gilbertsville, PA, USA).

2.6. Statistical Analysis. Descriptive statistics were used to summarize participants' demographic and clinical characteristics. The *p73* DNP genotype (rs1801173) was summarized using descriptive statistics by disease status (risk and recurrence), survival (prostate cancer specific survival and overall survival), and characteristics (Gleason score and clinical stage), the patients' outcome. Logistic regressions were applied to evaluate the *p73* DNP genotype associated with the binary outcomes, including prostate cancer risk (yes/no), recurrence (yes/no), Gleason score (8–10 versus ≤7), and TNM stage (III-IV versus I-II).

For cases, overall survival and prostate cancer specific survival were evaluated. Overall survival was defined as the time from date of surgical treatment to date of death due to any cause. For patients who do not die, time to death was censored at the time of last contact. For evaluating the DNP associated with overall survival, the overall survival curves by the genotype category were generated using the Kaplan-Meier method. The Cox proportional hazard model was used to examine the association after adjusting for age. The hazard ratios and their 95% confidence intervals will be calculated.

The competing risks approach was applied to analyze the *p73* DNP genotype associated with prostate cancer specific death. Time to prostate cancer specific death was defined as time from date of surgical treatment to date of prostate cancer specific death. Death due to other causes was treated as a competing risk. The plot of cumulative incidence of disease-specific deaths was generated. Cumulative incidence is the probability of observing a specific event at a given time-point for the individual who did not experience any event prior to this time-point. The DNP genotype associated with disease-specific death adjusting for age at diagnosis was evaluated using the competing risks regression [46]. The major allele was considered as the reference allele and all models were adjusted for age, which was age at diagnosis for cases and at enrolment for controls. Different inheritance models (log-additive and dominant) were taken into consideration. Due to a limited sample size of African Americans, we did not evaluate the recessive model.

Sample size was decided based on feasibility. The significant level of 0.05 and power of 80% were applied. With a sample size of 1,827 Caucasians (1,232 cases and 595 controls), the minimum detectable OR was 1.2. With a sample size of 147 African Americans (60 cases and 87 controls), the minimum detectable OR was 1.6.

We have assessed the potential association between p73 protein isoform ratios and the *p73* DNP genotype of cancer cell lines using the *t*-test. Deviation of genotype distribution from Hardy-Weinberg equilibrium in controls was tested using the exact test. Statistical tests were two-sided with an alpha level <0.05 considered statistically significant. All statistical analyses were performed using SAS 9.2 (SAS Institute, Cary, NC) and the cmprsk R package for the competing risk approach.

3. Results

Table 1 provides descriptive characteristics of the PCa patients and controls. African American patients tended

Table 1: Characteristics of study subjects by disease status and data source.

		Caucasians, N (%)		African Americans, N (%)	
		Cases, (n = 1232)	Controls, (n = 595)	Cases, (n = 60)	Controls, (n = 87)
Age[1]	Mean ± SD	60.0 ± 7.4	61.3 ± 9.6	56.4 ± 7.4	57.3 ± 9.2
Gleason score	≤6	628 (60.6)	N/A	34 (60.6)	N/A
	7	348 (33.6)		19 (33.9)	
	8–10	60 (5.8)		3 (5.3)	
Stage	1	55 (4.5)	N/A	2 (3.4)	N/A
	2	955 (78.3)		48 (81.4)	
	3	201 (16.5)		9 (15.2)	
	4	9 (0.7)		0 (0.0)	
PSA level		7.5 ± 9.1	1.1 ± 1.1	5.1 ± 3.1	1.3 ± 1.4
Recurrence	No	905 (73.6)	N/A	43 (71.7)	N/A
	Yes	325 (26.4)		17 (28.3)	
Death	Alive	975 (79.9)		54 (90.0)	
	PCa death	106 (8.7)		2 (3.3)	
	Other death cases	139 (11.4)		4 (6.7)	
Marital status	Divorced	80 (6.6)		5 (8.3)	
	Married	1057 (87.0)		49 (81.7)	
	Separated	4 (0.3)		1 (1.7)	
	Widowed	21 (1.7)		0 (0)	
	Single	53 (4.4)		5 (8.3)	
Weight (kg)		88.4 ± 14.6	93.6 ± 21.6	90.5 ± 14.2	92.5 ± 18.7
Height (m)		1.76 ± 0.07	1.76 ± 0.18	1.77 ± 0.06	1.75 ± 0.21

[1] Age at diagnosis for cases and age at enrolment for controls.

to be younger than Caucasian patients ($P < 0.001$). The distribution of Gleason score, clinical stage, and proportion of recurrent cases are similar in both racial groups. As expected, means of PSA level among cases are significantly higher than controls in both races ($P < 0.001$).

3.1. p73 DNP and Prostate Cancer Susceptibility and Progression. The genotype distributions of *p73* DNP among controls were consistent with Hardy-Weinberg equilibrium with a P value of 0.903 for Caucasians and 1.0 for African Americans using the exact test. The minor allelic frequency (MAF) of this DNP among Caucasians was similar in the public data (Table 2). A racial difference in the MAFs of *p73* DNP (rs1801173) was observed among the controls: 22% versus 11% for Caucasians versus African Americans, respectively ($P < 0.001$) (Table 2).

To determine whether this genetic variant was associated with increased risk for PCa, we compared genotype frequencies between PCa cases and controls. In both racial groups, PCa risk was not modified for subjects with *p73* DNP (additive model per AT/AT genotype, Caucasians: OR = 1.02, 95%CI = 0.86–1.21, African Americans: OR = 1.00, 95%CI = 0.49–2.07) after adjusting for age at diagnosis (Table 2).

We investigate a role of *p73* DNP in prostate cancer progression and aggressiveness. The *p73* DNP was significantly associated with high Gleason score [37, 40, 41] (dominant model, odds ratio (OR) = 0.55, 95% confidence interval (CI) = 0.31–0.99) among Caucasians (Table 2). The similar association was not observed in African American patients. Interestingly, *p73* DNP is marginally associated with overall death (dominant model, hazard ratio (HR) = 0.76, 95%CI = 0.57–1.00, $P = 0.053$) as well as PCa specific death (HR = 0.69, 95%CI = 0.45–1.06, $P = 0.09$, Table 2 and Figure 1). The survival analyses were not performed for African American patients due to a small sample size.

3.2. p73 DNP Genotype and the p73 Protein Isoforms Ratios in Cancer Cell Lines. We assessed the potential for a correlation between p73 protein isoform ratios and the *p73* DNP genotype of cancer cell lines observed in cultured cancer cell lines. Genomic DNA samples were isolated from eleven cultured cell lines and the *p73* DNP genotype was determined (Table 3). Total cellular protein samples were isolated from these cancer cell lines and subjected to p73 protein N-terminal isoform-specific western analyses for TAp73 and for ΔNp73, while blotting for actin in parallel as a protein loading control (Figures 2(a) and 2(b)). The TAp73 isoform, ΔNp73 isoform, and actin western blotting data were quantified using the ImageJ64 program. These values were used to calculate p73 protein N-terminal isoform ratios, in the form of TAp73/ΔNp73, relative to the actin control. Cancer cell line data were consistent with higher levels of TAp73 protein relative to ΔNp73 in the heterozygous cell lines compared to the wild type (Table 3 and Figure 3, $P < 0.001$). It was noteworthy that the only cancer cell line analyzed that was homozygous polymorphic for the *p73* DNP, CaCO-2, contained no detectable p73 protein (Figure 2(b)).

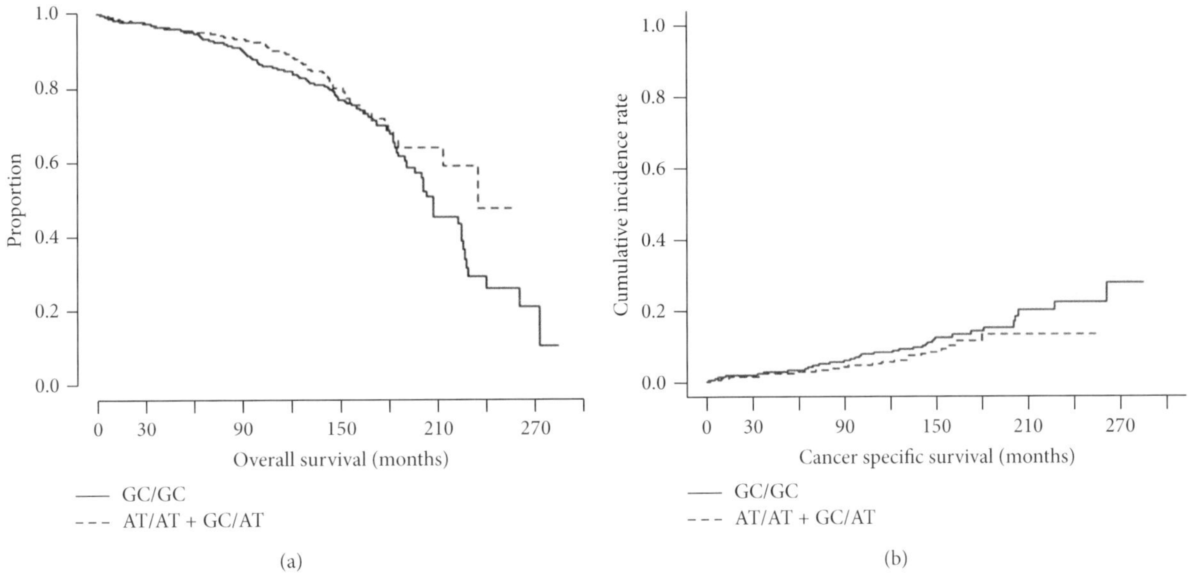

FIGURE 1: Association between rs1801173 and overall survival (a) and prostate cancer specific survival (b). A role of *p73* DNP in prostate cancer progression and aggressiveness was investigated. p73 DNP is marginally associated with overall death (dominant model, hazard ratio (HR) = 0.76, 95%CI = 0.57–1.00, $P = 0.053$ by Cox regression adjusted for age) as well as PCa specific death (HR = 0.69, 95%CI = 0.45–1.06, $P = 0.09$ by the competing risk regression adjusted for age).

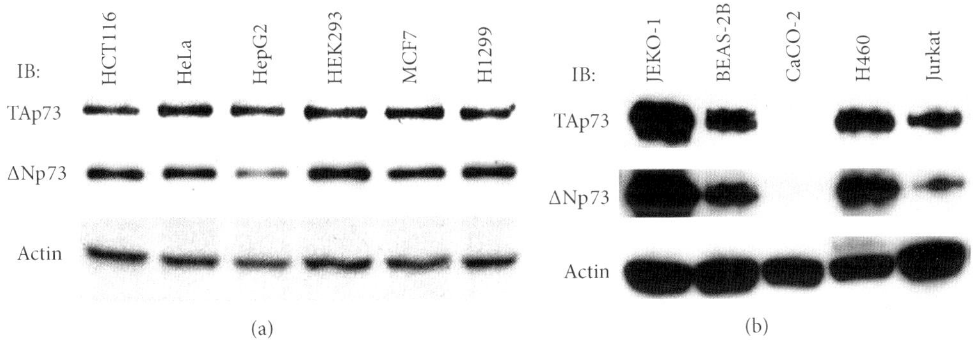

FIGURE 2: Western analyses of p73 protein N-terminal isoforms in cancer cell lines. Proteins from cancer cell line lysates in Figure 2(a) (1.25 μg/well) and Figure 2(b) (7.50 μg/well) were resolved on 10% SDS-PAGE gels and the resolved proteins were electrotransferred onto PVDF membranes and then immunoblotted (IB) with a p73 isoform-specific monoclonal antibody against TAp73 or ΔNp73. As a positive loading control, actin was immunoblotted with a goat polyclonal antibody. Primary antibodies were detected using appropriate secondary antibody-horseradish peroxidase conjugates and an enhanced chemoluminescence method followed by fluorography (IB = primary western antibody).

4. Discussion

In this study, we investigate whether the *p73* DNP is associated with modified *p73* gene expression, as well as to ascertain any association with risk/progression of PCa (Table 2). We observed that the *p73* DNP is significantly associated with high Gleason score among Caucasian men. In addition, data from our analysis of TAp73 and ΔNp73 protein isoforms in cancer cell lines is consistent with a relative increase in the ratio of TAp73/ΔNp73 protein isoforms expressed in cell lines heterozygous for the *p73* DNP compared to cell lines wild type for *p73* DNP (Table 3, Figure 3).

Multiple studies have identified the *p73* DNP as a risk factor for multiple cancer sites, including bladder [6], breast [8], cervical [12], colorectal [15], liver [26], lung [27, 28, 32], lymphoma [34], and head and neck cancers [20, 23, 24]. However, other studies have reported a decreased risk in lung [29] and head and neck cancers [19]. In addition, many studies reported no association in breast [7, 9, 10], cervical [11], colorectal [13, 14, 16], endometrial [17], head and neck [13, 18, 19, 21, 22], gastric [13, 25], ovarian [36], melanoma [35], and lung [30, 31, 33] cancers (Table 4). Recent meta-analyses have shown that the *p73* DNP is associated with various cancer risks in general [38–41]. These inconsistent results may be due to different MAFs in different ethnic populations and environmental factors. Currently, only one study (n = 177 cases) reported no association between PCa risk and *p73* DNP [37]. This is the first study to address the potential role

Table 2: Associations of genotypes with prostate cancer risk, aggressiveness, and survival.

Factors	Race	GC/GC	GC/AT	AT/AT	Dom[1] OR (95% CI)[2]	P value	Additive[1] OR (95% CI)[2]	P value
Case/control	White	750/357	417/202	65/27	1.00 (0.82–1.23)	0.995	1.02 (0.86–1.21)	0.82
	Black	49/68	9/16	2/1	0.87 (0.37–2.04)	0.75	1.00 (0.49–2.07)	0.99
Recurrence Y/N	White	205/544	100/316	20/45	0.86 (0.66–1.12)	0.25	0.92 (0.74–1.15)	0.48
	Black	14/35	3/6	0/2	0.97 (0.21–4.36)	0.97	0.76 (0.22–2.69)	0.68
Gleason 8–10/≤7	White	44/589	14/336	2/51	**0.55 (0.31–0.99)**	**0.04**	0.61 (0.37–1.02)	0.06
	Black	2/43	1/8	0/2	2.16 (0.17–26.99)	0.55	1.36 (0.19–9.92)	0.76
Stage 3 & 4/1 & 2	White	129/615	70/342	11/53	0.97 (0.71–1.31)	0.83	0.98 (0.76–1.26)	0.85
	Black	8/40	1/8	0/2	0.46 (0.05–4.63)	0.51	0.43 (0.06–3.07)	0.40
					HR (95% CI)[3]	P value	HR (95% CI)[3]	P value
Overall death Death/alive	White	160/590	68/348	17/48	**0.76 (0.57–1.00)**	**0.05**	0.87 (0.68–1.10)	0.24
	Black	5/44	1/8	0/2	—	—	—	—
Specific death Other/PCa/alive	White	88/72/590	40/28/338	11/6/47	0.84 (0.58–1.21)[4]	0.35	0.93 (0.67–1.28)[4]	0.64
					0.69 (0.45–1.06)[5]	0.09	0.81 (0.55–1.20)[5]	0.29
	Black	3/2/44	1/0/8	0/0/2	—	—	—	—

[1]Dom: dominant (AT/AT + GC/AT versus GC/GC); add: log-additive (per AT/AT).
[2]OR: odds ratio; CI: confidence interval; logistic model adjusted for age.
[3]HR: hazard ratio; for overall death, Cox model; for specific death, competing risk regression; all models adjusted for age.
[4]Other death cases versus alive.
[5]PCa death versus alive.

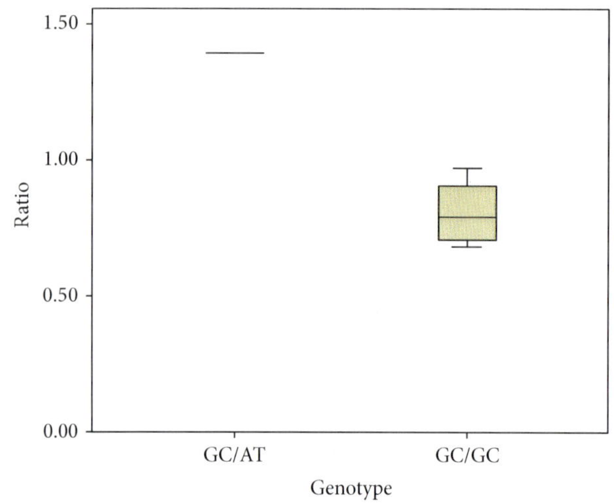

Figure 3: Relative TAp73/ΔNp73 protein isoform ratios in cancer cell line lysates with GC/GC and GC/AT genotype. The TAp73/ΔNp73 protein isoform levels were determined from the western blotting data in Figures 2(a) and 2(b). These p73 protein isoform levels were used to calculate the relative ratio values reported in Table 3. The mean of TAp73/ΔNp73 protein isoform ratio values is box-plotted.

Table 3: *p73* DNP genotypes and *p73* isoform expression ratios for cancer cell lines.

Cell line	*p73* DNP genotype	TAp73/ΔNp73*
HCT116	GC/GC	0.68
HeLa	GC/GC	0.95
H460	GC/GC	0.74
HEK293	GC/GC	0.72
MCF7	GC/GC	0.97
H1299	GC/GC	0.69
JEKO-1	GC/GC	0.84
BEAS-2B	GC/GC	0.86
Jurkat	GC/AT	1.40
HepG2	GC/AT	1.39
CaCO-2	AT/AT	N/A

Cell lines were used for genotyping for *p73* DNP status and western analyses for *p73* protein N-terminal isoforms and beta-actin. *TAp73/ΔNp73 protein isoform levels were determined from the western data in Figures 2(a) and 2(b) by quantifying protein bands using ImageJ64. Relative TAp73/ΔNp73 protein isoform ratios were corrected for using actin levels as loading controls and were calculated using the formula: TAp73/ΔNp73 = ((TAp73/actin)/(ΔNp73/actin)).

for an association between aggressiveness of PCa and the *p73* DNP.

Several studies have detected a disruption in the relative abundance of the two major p73 N-terminal isoforms in tumor tissues and tumor derived cell lines when compared to normal tissues [47, 48]. The balance between TAp73 and ΔNp73 expression is altered in many cancer types due to relatively higher levels of ΔNp73 [44]. The transcriptionally inactive ΔNp73 acts in a dominate negative fashion towards TAp73 transcriptional activity and against p53 as well [44]. This dominate negative effect is thought to underlie the tumor-promoting properties associated with ΔNp73. Some reports have detected an alteration in the ratio of TAp73/ΔNp73 expression through real-time PCR analysis of mRNA and immunohistochemical staining in tumor tissues as compared to normal tissues [48, 49]. Thus, we addressed

Table 4: Summary of association studies of *p73* DNP in various cancer sites[1].

Site	Population	Case/control	OR (95% CI)	Reference
Bladder	Indian	200/200	**1.54 (1.02–2.33)**	[6]
Breast	Chinese	170/178	0.77 (0.50–1.19)	[7]
Breast	Chinese	170/0	**2.76 (1.17–6.49)**[2]	[8]
Breast	Japanese	200/282	0.82 (0.57–1.19)	[9]
Breast	France white	59/34	2.46 (0.92–6.58)	[10]
Cervical	Portuguese	176/141	1.01 (0.63–1.62)	[11]
Cervical	Japanese	112/442	**1.51 (1.00–2.30)**	[12]
Colorectal	Japanese	147/235	0.85 (0.56–1.29)	[13]
Colorectal	Tunisian	150/204	1.09 (0.71–1.66)	[14]
Colorectal	Korean	383/469	**1.50 (1.14–1.96)**	[15]
Colorectal	Swedish	179/260	0.92 (0.53–1.53)	[16]
Endometrial	Japanese	114/442	1.36 (0.90–2.06)	[17]
Esophageal	Chinese	348/630	1.02 (0.78–1.34)	[18]
Esophageal	Japanese	102/235	0.64 (0.40–1.04)	[13]
Esophageal	UK whites	84/152	0.90 (0.53–1.53)	[19]
H&N	US white	708/1229	**1.31 (1.09–1.58)**	[20]
H&N	Italian	283/295	1.36 (0.95–1.93)	[21]
H&N	US whites	326/349	1.06 (0.78–1.45)	[22]
Oral	Indian	303/319	**2.38 (1.73–3.29)**	[23]
Oropharyngeal	US mixed	309/0	**2.10 (1.20–3.80)**[2,3]	[24]
Gastric	Italian	114/295	0.94 (0.58–1.54)	[25]
Gastric	Japanese	144/235	0.88 (0.58–1.34)	[13]
Liver	Chinese	476/526	**2.19 (1.25–3.83)**[4]	[26]
Lung	Chinese	293/380	**1.48 (1.08–2.02)**	[27]
Lung	US white	1054/1139	**1.34 (1.13–1.59)**	[28]
Lung	Chinese	425/588	**0.67 (0.52–0.86)**	[29]
Lung	Korean	582/582	1.13 (0.90–1.43)	[30, 31]
Lung	US white	863/852	**1.34 (1.10–1.64)**	[32]
Lung	Japanese	189/235	0.91 (0.62–1.34)	[33]
Lymphoma	Japanese	103/440	**1.61 (1.04–2.47)**	[34]
Melanoma	Whites	805/838	1.05 (0.86–1.28)	[35]
Ovary	Chinese	257/257	0.81 (0.95–1.18)	[36]
Prostate	Indian	177/265	1.21 (0.80–1.86)	[37]

[1]Analysis is based on dominant model (AT/AT + GC/AT versus GC/GC).
[2]Cases only.
[3]HPV16+ versus HPV16−.
[4]HbsAg-positive individuals.

the potential for an association between *p73* DNP genotype and p73 protein isoform expression ratios through analyses of several cancer cell lines known to be p73-positve.

The *p73* DNP, a putative functional polymorphism in exon 2, may theoretically affect a putative stem-loop structure and thereby affect p73 protein expression. Several studies have reported significant associations between the *p73* DNP (rs1801173) and various cancer types including prostate [47]. Arvanitis et al. [47] reported that the p73 protein isoform balance is disrupted in benign prostatic hyperplasia (BPH) and PCa. These results suggested that disrupted balance of p73 protein isoforms may be critical carcinogenesis in prostate.

One of the suggested biological mechanisms for the inverse relationship between the *p73* DNP allele and PCa aggressiveness comes from our p73 protein isoform molecular data. Our western analyses (Figures 2(a) and 2(b)) of multiple cancer cell lines indicate that ΔNp73 is decreased relative to TAp73 in cell lines heterozygous for *p73* DNP (Table 3 and Figure 3). Therefore, it is plausible that presence of the *p73* DNP allele causes a relative decrease in ΔNp73 protein levels in PCa tissues, which could be predicted to decrease risk for PCa aggressiveness or recurrence. Although the only cell line (CaCO-2) determined to be homozygous polymorphic for the *p73* DNP (Table 3) contained no detectable p73 protein in our western analyses (Figure 2(b)), we cannot eliminate the possibility that the CaCO-2 cell line harbors other aberrations in the *p73* alleles, such as a partial homozygous deletion as that one present in the p53-negative NCI-H1299 cell line. Further molecular studies would be needed to gain a full understanding of the molecular mechanism(s) by which the *p73* DNP genetic variant might result in lower expression levels of ΔNp73 relative to TAp73 in PCa.

The limitations of the current study are a small sample size of African American population and cancer cell lines. Therefore, a larger study is necessary to confirm this observed association between protein expression and risk/progression of PCa and *p73* DNP is real and not a chance finding. Additionally, future studies of p73 protein isoform ratios in cancer cell lines derived from prostate cancer tissues may provide further insight into the relationship between *p73* DNP genotype and p73 protein isoform expression levels.

In summary, *p73* DNP may influence aggressiveness of prostate cancer and p73 protein expression. These novel findings warrant a larger study to investigate their significance. The identification of the *p73* DNP allele as a protective factor for aggressiveness of PCa could lead to personalized intervention strategies, which can be applied that are appropriate for the level of risk.

Acknowledgments

This study was supported, in part, by the National Cancer Institute (R01CA128813, PI: Jong Y. Park) and by a University of Tampa David Delo Research Professor Grant (PI: L. Michael Carastro).

References

[1] Institute NC. Surveillance, Epoidemiology, and End Results program, 2014.

[2] S. A. Siddiqui, B. A. Inman, S. Sengupta et al., "Obesity and survival after radical prostatectomy: a 10-year prospective cohort study," *Cancer*, vol. 107, no. 3, pp. 521–529, 2006.

[3] A. E. Teeter, J. C. Presti Jr., W. J. Aronson et al., "Do nomograms designed to predict biochemical recurrence (BCR) do a better job of predicting more clinically relevant prostate cancer outcomes than BCR? A report from the SEARCH database group," *Urology*, vol. 82, no. 1, pp. 53–58, 2013.

[4] Y. M. Cho, S. J. Jung, N. Cho et al., "Impact of international variation of prostate cancer on a predictive nomogram for biochemical recurrence in clinically localised prostate cancer," *World Journal of Urology*, pp. 1–7, 2013.

[5] V. Iremashvili, M. S. Soloway, L. Pelaez, D. L. Rosenberg, and M. Manoharan, "Comparative validation of nomograms predicting clinically insignificant prostate cancer," *Urology*, vol. 81, no. 6, pp. 1202–1208, 2013.

[6] P. K. Jaiswal, V. Singh, and R. D. Mittal, "Polymorphism at P21 codon 31 and dinucleotide polymorphism of P73 gene and susceptibility to bladder cancer in individuals from North India," *Indian Journal of Human Genetics*, vol. 19, no. 3, pp. 293–300, 2013.

[7] X. Zhou and C. Wu, "Association of p73 G4C14-A4T14 polymorphisms with genetic susceptibilities to breast cancer: a case-control study," *Medical Oncology*, vol. 29, no. 5, pp. 3216–3221, 2012.

[8] X. Zhou, "P73 G4C14-to-A4T14 polymorphisms are positively correlated with triple-negative breast cancer in southwestern China," *Medical Oncology*, vol. 30, no. 2, article 515, 2013.

[9] X.-E. Huang, N. Hamajima, N. Katsuda et al., "Association of p53 Codon Arg72Pro and p73 G4C 14-to-A4T14 at exon 2 genetic polymorphisms with the risk of Japanese breast cancer," *Breast Cancer*, vol. 10, no. 4, pp. 307–311, 2003.

[10] J. C. Ahomadegbe, S. Tourpin, M. Kaghad et al., "Loss of heterozygosity, allele silencing and decreased expression of p73 gene in breast cancers: prevalence of alterations in inflammatory breast cancers," *Oncogene*, vol. 19, no. 47, pp. 5413–5418, 2000.

[11] R. Craveiro, I. Bravo, R. Catarino et al., "The role of p73 G4C14-to-A4T14 polymorphism in the susceptibility to cervical cancer," *DNA and Cell Biology*, vol. 31, no. 2, pp. 224–229, 2012.

[12] Y. Niwa, N. Hamajima, Y. Atsuta et al., "Genetic polymorphisms of p73 G4C14-to-A4T14 at exon 2 and p53 Arg72Pro and the risk of cervical cancer in Japanese," *Cancer Letters*, vol. 205, no. 1, pp. 55–60, 2004.

[13] N. Hamajima, K. Matsuo, T. Suzuki et al., "No associations of p73 G4C14-to-A4T14 at exon 2 and p53 Arg72Pro polymorphisms with the risk of digestive tract cancers in Japanese," *Cancer Letters*, vol. 181, no. 1, pp. 81–85, 2002.

[14] A. T. Arfaoui, L. B. M. Kriaa, O. E. A. El Hadj et al., "Association of a p73 exon 2 GC/AT polymorphism with colorectal cancer risk and survival in Tunisian patients," *Virchows Archiv*, vol. 457, no. 3, pp. 359–368, 2010.

[15] K. E. Lee, Y. S. Hong, B. G. Kim et al., "P73 G4C14 to A4T14 polymorphism is associated with colorectal cancer risk and survival," *World Journal of Gastroenterology*, vol. 16, no. 35, pp. 4448–4454, 2010.

[16] D. Pfeifer, G. Arbman, and X. F. Sun, "Polymorphism of the p73 gene in relation to colorectal cancer risk and survival," *Carcinogenesis*, vol. 26, no. 1, pp. 103–107, 2005.

[17] Y. Niwa, K. Hirose, K. Matsuo et al., "Association of p73 G4C14-to-A4T14 polymorphism at exon 2 and p53 Arg72Pro polymorphism with the risk of endometrial cancer in Japanese subjects," *Cancer Letters*, vol. 219, no. 2, pp. 183–190, 2005.

[18] H. Ge, Y. M. Wang, Y. Y. Cao et al., "The p73 polymorphisms are not associated with susceptibility to esophageal squamous cell carcinoma in a high incidence region of China," *Diseases of the Esophagus*, vol. 20, no. 4, pp. 290–296, 2007.

[19] B. M. Ryan, R. McManus, J. S. Daly et al., "A common p73 polymorphism is associated with a reduced incidence of oesophageal carcinoma," *British Journal of Cancer*, vol. 85, no. 10, pp. 1499–1503, 2001.

[20] G. Li, E. M. Sturgis, L. E. Wang et al., "Association of a p73 exon 2 G4C14-to-A4T14 polymorphism with risk of squamous cell carcinoma of the head and neck," *Carcinogenesis*, vol. 25, no. 10, pp. 1911–1916, 2004.

[21] P. Gallì, G. Cadoni, M. Volante et al., "A case-control study on the combined effects of p53 and p73 polymorphisms on head and neck cancer risk in an Italian population," *BMC Cancer*, vol. 9, article 137, 2009.

[22] X. Chen, E. M. Sturgis, A. K. El-Naggar, Q. Wei, and G. Li, "Combined effects of the p53 codon 72 and p73 G4C14-to-A4T14 polymorphisms on the risk of HPV16-associated oral cancer in never-smokers," *Carcinogenesis*, vol. 29, no. 11, pp. 2120–2125, 2008.

[23] C. Misra, M. Majumder, S. Bajaj, S. Ghosh, B. Roy, and S. Roychoudhury, "Polymorphisms at p53, p73, and MDM2 loci modulate the risk of tobacco associated leukoplakia and oral cancer," *Molecular Carcinogenesis*, vol. 48, no. 9, pp. 790–800, 2009.

[24] Z. Wang, E. M. Sturgis, W. Guo et al., "Association of combined p73 and p53 genetic variants with tumor HPV16-positive oropharyngeal cancer," *PLoS ONE*, vol. 7, no. 4, Article ID e35522, 2012.

[25] E. De Feo, R. Persiani, A. La Greca et al., "A case-control study on the effect of p53 and p73 gene polymorphisms on gastric cancer risk and progression," *Mutation Research*, vol. 675, no. 1-2, pp. 60–65, 2009.

[26] B. Deng, F. Liu, Y. Wei et al., "Association of a p73 exon 2 G4C14-to-A4T14 polymorphism with risk of hepatocellular carcinoma in a Chinese population," *Tumor Biology*, vol. 34, no. 1, pp. 293–299, 2013.

[27] X. Zhang, X. Li, Z. Wu, F. Lin, and H. Zhou, "The p73 G4C14-to-A4T14 polymorphism is associated with risk of lung cancer in the Han nationality of North China," *Molecular Carcinogenesis*, vol. 52, no. 5, pp. 387–391, 2013.

[28] G. Li, L. E. Wang, R. M. Chamberlain, C. I. Amos, M. R. Spitz, and Q. Wei, "p73 G4C14-to-A4T14 polymorphism and risk of lung cancer," *Cancer Research*, vol. 64, no. 19, pp. 6863–6866, 2004.

[29] Z. Hu, X. Miao, H. Ma et al., "Dinucleotide polymorphism of p73 gene is associated with a reduced risk of lung cancer in a Chinese population," *International Journal of Cancer*, vol. 114, no. 3, pp. 455–460, 2005.

[30] J. E. Choi, H. G. Kang, M. H. Chae et al., "No association between p73 G4C14-to-A4T14 polymorphism and the risk of lung cancer in a Korean population," *Biochemical genetics*, vol. 44, no. 11-12, pp. 543–550, 2006.

[31] H. J. Jun, S. H. Park, W. K. Lee et al., "Combined effects of p73 and MDM2 polymorphisms on the risk of lung cancer," *Molecular Carcinogenesis*, vol. 46, no. 2, pp. 100–105, 2007.

[32] M. B. Schabath, X. Wu, Q. Wei, G. Li, J. Gu, and M. R. Spitz, "Combined effects of the p53 and p73 polymorphisms on lung cancer risk," *Cancer Epidemiology Biomarkers and Prevention*, vol. 15, no. 1, pp. 158–161, 2006.

[33] A. Hiraki, K. Matsuo, N. Hamajima et al., "Different risk relations with smoking for non-small-cell lung cancer: comparison of TP53 and TP73 genotypes," *Asian Pacific Journal of Cancer Prevention*, vol. 4, no. 2, pp. 107–112, 2003.

[34] A. Hishida, K. Matsuo, K. Tajima et al., "Polymorphisms of p53 Arg72Pro, p73 G4C14-to-A4T14 at exon 2 and p21 Ser31Arg and the risk of non-Hodgkin's lymphoma in Japanese," *Leukemia and Lymphoma*, vol. 45, no. 5, pp. 957–964, 2004.

[35] C. Li, K. Chen, Z. Liu et al., "Polymorphisms of TP53 Arg72Pro, but not p73 G4C14>A4TA4 and p21 Ser31Arg, contribute to risk of cutaneous melanoma," *Journal of Investigative Dermatology*, vol. 128, no. 6, pp. 1585–1588, 2008.

[36] S. Kang, D. J. Wang, W. S. Li et al., "Association of p73 and MDM2 polymorphisms with the risk of epithelial ovarian cancer in Chinese women," *International Journal of Gynecological Cancer*, vol. 19, no. 4, pp. 572–577, 2009.

[37] R. D. Mittal, G. P. George, J. Mishra, T. Mittal, and R. Kapoor, "Role of functional polymorphisms of P53 and P73 genes with the risk of prostate cancer in a case-control study from Northern India," *Archives of Medical Research*, vol. 42, no. 2, pp. 122–127, 2011.

[38] L. Wang, R. Gao, and L. Yu, "Combined analysis of the association between p73 G4C14-to-A4T14 polymorphisms and cancer risk," *Molecular Biology Reports*, vol. 39, no. 2, pp. 1731–1738, 2012.

[39] X. J. Yu, F. Fang, and J. Xie, "Relationship between TP73 polymorphism (G4C14-A4T14) and cancer risk: a meta-analysis based on literatures," *Gene*, vol. 484, no. 1-2, pp. 42–46, 2011.

[40] F. Liu, L. Liu, B. Li et al., "p73 G4C14-A4T14 polymorphism and cancer risk: a meta-analysis based on 27 case-control studies," *Mutagenesis*, vol. 26, no. 4, pp. 573–581, 2011.

[41] Y. Hu, L. Jiang, J. Zheng, Y. You, Y. Zhou, and S. Jiao, "Association between the p73 exon 2 G4C14-to-A4T14 polymorphism and cancer risk: a meta-analysis," *DNA and Cell Biology*, vol. 31, no. 2, pp. 230–237, 2012.

[42] F. Murray-Zmijewski, D. P. Lane, and J.-C. Bourdon, "p53/p63/p73 isoforms: an orchestra of isoforms to harmonise cell differentiation and response to stress," *Cell Death and Differentiation*, vol. 13, no. 6, pp. 962–972, 2006.

[43] M. Marabese, F. Vikhanskaya, and M. Broggini, "p73: a chiaroscuro gene in cancer," *European Journal of Cancer*, vol. 43, no. 9, pp. 1361–1372, 2007.

[44] S. G. Bailey, M. S. Cragg, and P. A. Townsend, "Family friction as Δnp73 antagonises p73 and p53," *International Journal of Biochemistry and Cell Biology*, vol. 43, no. 4, pp. 482–486, 2011.

[45] A. I. Zaika, N. Slade, S. H. Erster et al., "δNp73, a dominant-negative inhibitor of wild-type p53 and TAp73, is up-regulated in human tumors," *Journal of Experimental Medicine*, vol. 196, no. 6, pp. 765–780, 2002.

[46] J. P. Fine and R. J. Gray, "A proportional hazards model for the subdistribution of a competing risk," *Journal of the American Statistical Association*, vol. 94, no. 446, pp. 496–509, 1999.

[47] D. A. Arvanitis, E. Lianos, N. Soulitzis, D. Delakas, and D. A. Spandidos, "Deregulation of p73 isoform equilibrium in benign prostate hyperplasia and prostate cancer," *Oncology Reports*, vol. 12, no. 5, pp. 1131–1137, 2004.

[48] M. Guan and Y. Chen, "Aberrant expression of ΔNp73 in benign and malignant tumours of the prostate: correlation with Gleason score," *Journal of Clinical Pathology*, vol. 58, no. 11, pp. 1175–1179, 2005.

[49] A. T. Arfaoui, L. K. B. Mahmoud, A. B. Hmida et al., "Relationship between p73 polymorphism and the immunohistochemical profile of the full-length (TAp73) and NH2-truncated (ΔNp73) isoforms in Tunisian patients," *Applied Immunohistochemistry and Molecular Morphology*, vol. 18, no. 6, pp. 546–554, 2010.

12

Urologic Characteristics and Sexual Behaviors Associated with Prostate Cancer in an African-Caribbean Population in Barbados, West Indies

Anselm J. M. Hennis,[1,2,3,4] Suh-Yuh Wu,[2] Barbara Nemesure,[2] and M. Cristina Leske[2]

[1] *Chronic Disease Research Centre, The University of the West Indies, Jemmott's Lane, St. Michael, BB11115, Barbados*
[2] *Department of Preventive Medicine, Stony Brook University, Stony Brook, NY 11794-8036, USA*
[3] *Ministry of Health, Frank Walcott Building, Culloden Road, St. Michael, BB14001, Barbados*
[4] *Faculty of Medical Sciences, Cave Hill Campus, The University of the West Indies, St. Michael, BB11000, Barbados*

Correspondence should be addressed to Anselm J. M. Hennis; anselm.hennis@cavehill.uwi.edu

Academic Editor: Katsuto Shinohara

Prostate cancer (PC) is the principal malignancy affecting African descent men in the Caribbean and the USA. Disparities in incidence, prevalence, and mortality in these populations are poorly understood. We evaluated the urologic characteristics and sexual behaviors of men with histologically confirmed PC (cases) and age-matched controls in the nationwide Prostate Cancer in a Black Population (PCBP) study conducted in Barbados. Cases were around 1.5 to 3 times more likely to report symptoms of prostatic enlargement, hematuria/hematospermia, and previous prostatitis. Sexually transmitted infections (STIs) were similar among cases (24.5%) and controls (26.7%). First sexual intercourse before the age of 16 was associated with an increased likelihood of both low- (Gleason score < 7; OR 1.63; 95% CI: 1.03–1.66) and high-grade PC (Gleason score ≥ 7; OR 1.82; 1.11–2.99). PC risk decreased with later age of sexual debut (P-trend $= 0.004$). More lifetime sexual partners was associated with increased odds of high grade PC (P-trend $= 0.02$). The contribution of sexual behaviors to the development and the outcomes of PC is likely due to multiple mechanisms, and further study will be necessary to elucidate the underlying pathophysiologic mechanisms in this and similar populations.

1. Introduction

Prostate cancer (PC) rates and mortality are highest among African American men globally [1]. PC is also the most frequent malignancy affecting African-Caribbean men [2–5], a group which shares a common heredity with African Americans as a historical consequence of the West African slave trade. The reasons for the high PC risk and poor outcomes in African-derived populations remain unknown and are likely multifactorial.

Among environmental factors associated with PC, various investigators have described associations between increased PC risk and sexual behaviors [6–8]. In spite of the high burden of PC in the Caribbean, there are few data on disease manifestations or environmental risk factors, particularly sexual behaviors [9, 10]. While some urologic signs and symptoms are commonly observed among persons with PC, this information remains largely unreported in African-Caribbean populations. This paper describes urologic characteristics of men diagnosed with prostate cancer and presents new information about sexual behaviors and PC risk in a national case-control study conducted in Barbados, West Indies.

2. Materials and Methods

2.1. Study Population. The Prostate Cancer in a Black Population (PCBP) study was a nationwide case-control study of Barbadian men with histologically confirmed newly diagnosed primary PC. Study methods have been described in detail elsewhere [11]. In summary, cases were identified from histological specimens of confirmed prostate cancer evaluated at the country's only Pathology Department, located at the Queen Elizabeth Hospital, Bridgetown. Cases were recruited from men identified with PC between July, 2002 and January, 2011. Age-matched controls (by 5-year age group) were randomly selected from an electronic database of Barbadian citizens and permanent residents and were frequency matched to cases. Of the 1,260 and 1,333 eligible cases and controls, 80% (1,007) and 75% (1,005) participated, respectively. There were no significant age differences between participants and eligible nonparticipants. All study subjects provided informed consent and study protocols conformed to the Declaration of Helsinki. Ethical approval was granted by the Barbados Ministry of Health Medical Ethics Committee and the Stony Brook University's Committee on Research Involving Human Subjects (CORIHS).

2.2. Data Collection. Data collection was conducted by trained certified nurse interviewers, masked to the case-control status of participants. They administered a comprehensive standardized study questionnaire, which sought information about participant demographic details, medical and family history, and lifestyle factors prior to the date of PC diagnosis for the cases (and a similarly assigned date for the matched controls). Anthropometric, blood pressure, and pulse rate measurements were also performed by nurse interviewers, and blood samples were collected for assay of HbA1c, PSA, Duffy blood groups, and relevant genetic markers.

The PCBP study was funded by the National Human Genome Research Institute and the Office of Minority Health, with subsequent funding provided by the National Cancer Institute of the National Institutes of Health. The study's organizational structure comprised a Coordinating Center (Stony Brook Medicine, Stony Brook, NY, USA), a Clinical Center and Local Laboratory Center (Ministry of Health and The University of the West Indies, Bridgetown, Barbados), a Collaborating Center at the National Human Genome Research Institute (Bethesda, MD, USA), and a Gene Discovery Center (Translational Genomics Research Institute, Phoenix, AZ, USA).

2.3. Statistical Analyses. Urologic characteristics and sexual risk behaviors investigated in this study were based on self-reported history. Urologic characteristics included previous vasectomy, prostatectomy, and benign prostatic hyperplasia (BPH, and related symptoms of nocturia, urinary retention, dysuria, hesitancy, urgency, frequency, and weak urinary stream), as well as symptoms of painful ejaculation, hematuria, and hematospermia. Sexual risk behaviors were assessed according to the reported history of sexually transmitted infection (STI), age at first sexual intercourse, and lifetime number of sexual partners. Tumors were histologically graded according to Gleason score as low grade disease (score < 7), and high-grade disease (score ≥ 7). Differences between cases and controls were evaluated using t-tests (for continuous variables) and chi-square tests (for categorical variables). Odds ratios (ORs) and 95% confidence intervals (CIs) were determined by logistic regression analyses adjusted for demographic and other factors associated with PC in this population (e.g., age, marital status, religion, lifetime occupation, family history of PC, and waist-hip ratio) [11]. The Statistical Analysis System (SAS Institute Inc., Cary, NC, USA) was used to conduct the analyses.

Table 1: Urologic characteristics among PCBP African-Barbadian men.

	Cases (n = 963)	Controls (n = 941)	Multivariate adjusted OR (95% CI)*
Vasectomy, %	1.5	0.7	1.67 (0.65, 4.31)
Prostatitis hx, %	7.8	2.4	3.16 (1.92, 5.19)*
BPH hx, %	44.4	19.8	3.05 (2.46, 3.79)*
Nocturia, %	58.1	36.1	2.41 (1.99, 2.93)*
Urinary retention, %	15.4	6.6	2.60 (1.88, 3.59)*
Dysuria, %	28.0	18.5	1.77 (1.41, 2.22)*
Hesitancy, %	33.9	21.2	1.80 (1.46, 2.23)*
Painful ejaculation,%	4.7	3.1	1.70 (1.03, 2.81)*
Blood in the urine/semen, %	14.9	10.0	1.58 (1.18, 2.11)*
Urgent need to void, %	45.1	33.1	1.64 (1.35, 1.99)*
Frequent urination, %	56.7	41.8	1.72 (1.43, 2.08)*
Weak flow	34.8	21.5	1.85 (1.49, 2.28)*

*OR: odds ratio; CI: confidence interval. $P < 0.05$, based on logistic regression analyses adjusted for age, marital status, religion, lifetime occupation, family history of PC, and waist-hip ratio.

3. Results

Of the total 2,012 PCBP participants, 95% (n = 1904) self-reported their race as black or black/white mixed. Due to the small number of white/other participants in the study, this report is based on the 963 incident cases and 941 age-matched controls of African origin. The mean (±SD) ages of the cases and controls were similar: 67.2 (±9.0) years and 67.0 (±9.2) years, respectively [11].

Table 1 presents urologic characteristics of African-Barbadian cases and controls. Vasectomy was rare in both groups and reported by 1.5% and 0.7% of cases and controls, respectively. Multivariate-adjusted odds ratios showed statistically significant differences between cases and controls for symptoms consistent with prostatic enlargement. Cases were between one and a half to three times more likely to report a history of benign prostatic hyperplasia (BPH), nocturia, urinary retention, hesitancy, urgency, frequency of urination, or poor urinary stream. Men with PC were also three times more likely than age-matched controls to report a history of prostatitis (OR; 95% confidence interval: 3.16; 1.92–5.19). Similarly symptoms of dysuria, painful ejaculation, and hematuria/hematospermia were higher in cases than controls, with adjusted odds around 1.7.

Table 2 presents data about sexual activity reported by cases and controls. Around a quarter of cases (25.4%) and controls (26.7%) reported a previous sexually transmitted

TABLE 2: Sexual behaviors among African-Barbadian men.

	Cases (n = 963)	Controls (n = 941)	P value*
Sexually transmitted infection, %	25.4	26.7	0.54
First sexual intercourse age (years),			
mean ± SD (median)	17.3 ± 3.5 (17.0) (n = 825)	17.8 ± 4.2 (17.0) (n = 808)	0.01
<16, %	29.3	24.9	
16–18, %	41.0	41.3	0.01
19–21, %	20.8	21.8	
>21, %	8.8	12.0	
Lifetime no. of sexual partners,			
mean ± SD (median)	12.0 ± 29.0 (6.0) (n = 707)	10.5 ± 19.5 (6.0) (n = 708)	0.28
0–3, %	25.0	27.0	
4–9, %	40.7	41.8	0.12
10–20, %	23.5	23.0	
>20, %	10.8	8.2	

*Chi-square test for categorical variables; t-test for continuous variables.

TABLE 3: Association between prostate cancer grade and sexual behaviors.

	Multivariate-adjusted OR (95% CI)		
	Low-grade PC OR (95% CI)	High-grade PC OR (95% CI)	All PC cases OR (95% CI)
Age at first sexual intercourse (years)[a]			
<16	1.63 (1.03, 2.60)*	1.82 (1.11, 2.99)*	1.74 (1.20, 2.54)*
16–18	1.28 (0.82, 2.00)	1.66 (1.04, 2.66)*	1.43 (1.00, 2.05)*
19–21	1.25 (0.84, 2.18)	1.50 (0.90, 2.49)	1.36 (0.92, 2.00)
>21	1.0 (reference)	1.0 (reference)	1.0 (reference)
	P-trend = 0.06	P-trend = 0.02	P-trend = 0.004
Lifetime no. of sexual partners[b]			
0–3	1.0 (reference)	1.0 (reference)	1.0 (reference)
4–9	1.04 (0.74, 1.46)	1.05 (0.74, 1.48)	1.00 (0.76, 1.31)
10–20	1.21 (0.82, 1.78)	1.16 (0.78, 1.73)	1.14 (0.83, 1.56)
>20	1.09 (0.64, 1.87)	1.74 (1.06, 2.85)*	1.35 (0.89, 2.04)
	P-trend = 0.65	P-trend = 0.02	P-trend = 0.10
Sexually transmitted infection[c]	1.00 (0.76, 1.31)	1.01 (0.77, 1.33)	1.01 (0.82, 1.26)

OR: odds ratio; CI: confidence interval.
*$P < 0.05$, based on logistic regression analyses adjusted for age, marital status, religion, lifetime occupation, family history of PC, and waist-hip ratio.
[a]Sample size for low-grade PC: 412; high-grade PC: 373; all PC cases: 825; controls: 808.
[b]Sample size for low-grade PC: 349; high-grade PC: 327; all PC cases: 707; controls: 708.
[c]Sample size for low-grade PC: 476; high-grade PC: 426; all PC cases: 948; controls: 930.

infection (STI). While the median age of first sexual intercourse was 17 years in both groups, more men with PC reported their sexual debut at a younger age (P = 0.01). The overall number of lifetime sexual partners reported by cases and controls were similar (means of 12 and 10.5, resp.; P = 0.28; median of 6).

Table 3 presents logistic regression results of associations between PC grade and sexual behaviors. Gleason scores were available for 914 cases (data were not located for 49 individuals). A total of 480 men with PC (52.5%) had low-grade disease, and 434 (47.5%) had high-grade disease. For men diagnosed with low-grade PC, first sexual activity before age 16 was associated with a more than 60% increased risk of PC (OR 1.63; 1.03–2.60). Odds ratios for risk of low-grade PC tended to decrease with older age at first sexual intercourse (P-trend = 0.06). A stronger relationship was evident for age at first sexual encounter and risk of high-grade PC. First coitus before age 16 was associated with an increased likelihood of high-grade PC (OR 1.82; 1.11–2.99), with a clear trend to a reduced risk with older age at the first intercourse (P-trend = 0.02). As expected, the same associations were also evident for analyses based on combined tumor grade (P-trend = 0.004).

With regards to tumor grade and lifetime number of sexual partners, there was no observable trend between number of partners and odds of low-grade PC. There was, however, a statistically significant positive trend between the lifetime number of sexual partners and odds of high-grade PC ($P = 0.02$). The relationship between combined (low and high grade) PC tumors and the number of sexual partners was not found to be statistically significant (P-trend = 0.10). Of note, a past history of STI was also not associated with PC tumor grade.

4. Discussion

In this population, cases were between one and a half to three times more likely to report a history of benign prostatic hyperplasia (BPH), nocturia, urinary retention, hesitancy, urgency, frequency of urination, and a poor urinary stream. Men with PC were also three times more likely than age-matched controls to report a history of prostatitis (OR; 95% confidence interval: 3.16; 1.92–5.19). Symptoms of dysuria, painful ejaculation, and hematuria/hematospermia were similarly higher in cases than controls, with the adjusted odds being around 1.7. Approximately 25% of both cases and controls reported a past STI, while more men with PC reported an earlier age at first sexual activity. Men aged less than 16 years at first sexual activity were at an increased risk of both low- and high-grade PC, with a similar relationship evident for high-grade PC in men aged 16–18 years at their sexual debut. There was also a statistically significant trend to a decreased risk of high-grade PC with older age at first coitus. Similarly, higher numbers of lifetime sexual partners was associated with an increased likelihood of high-grade PC.

4.1. Urologic Characteristics. Compared to controls, cases reported more symptoms indicative of prostatic enlargement (frequency, urgency, incontinence, poor stream, and urinary retention), as well as features associated with prostate tumors, such as blood in the urine or semen.

Data from NHANES (2005-2006 and 2007-2008 cycles) indicated that around 1 in 5 American men reported nocturia, a symptom associated with both BPH and PC [12]. The frequency of this symptom was higher in non-Hispanic black men than in other racial/ethnic groups (30.2%, CI 26.7–34.1 versus 20.1%, CI 18.1–22.1, $P < 0.001$). In adjusted models, black race remained an independent predictor of nocturia. An earlier assessment of genitourinary symptoms in the US population carried out in NHANES III assessed lower urinary tract symptoms of nocturia, incomplete emptying, and hesitancy in men aged 30 years and older, as well as symptoms of weak stream and noncancer prostate surgery in men aged 60+. Interestingly, rates of at least 3 symptoms or surgery were similar in black and white men [13]. We report a similar frequency of nocturia (single event nightly) in Barbadian control subjects and the US population (36.1% versus 35.6%), but higher rates in Barbadian men with PC (58.1%). Rates of urinary hesitancy were much higher in Barbadian men with PC compared to control subjects (33.9% versus 21.1%). These frequencies are in contrast with a reported 7.5% prevalence of hesitancy in US men. Barbadian men with PC were approximately 60% more likely to report hematospermia/hematuria compared to controls ($P < 0.05$). While hematospermia is a rare symptom at PC screening in populations with a frequency of 0.5%, around 14% of affected men were later discovered to have PC [14]. This observation highlights the clinical relevance of this symptom.

Few Barbadian men underwent vasectomy, and this procedure was not associated with PC risk. Early studies had suggested possible associations between vasectomy and PC risk [15, 16], but this relationship was likely due to confounding [17].

4.2. Sexual Behaviors and PC Risk. Around 30% of Barbadian men with PC reported a first sexual encounter before age 16. This frequency is similar to the experience of cohorts of UK men since 1960, with a "universally reported" median age of first coitus at 16 years, and who also demonstrate a trend to an earlier age of sexual debut over time [18]. The median age of sexual debut in 6 sub-Saharan African countries was somewhat higher and ranged from around 17 to 20 years [19]. The median age of sexual debut among control Barbadian men was 17.8 years, similar to that reported in African populations. Of note, Barbadian men with PC reported their sexual debut at an earlier age ($P = 0.01$). While this finding is suggestive of a possible hormonal etiology [20], there is an evidence that earlier age at first coitus may be associated with more sexual partners, increased risk of STI, and riskier lifestyle behaviors [7, 19, 21, 22], factors all potentially associated with higher risk of PC.

Our investigation also found statistically significant associations between the lifetime number of sexual partners and high-grade PC among Barbadian men. The relationship between number of sexual partners and PC is not straightforward. Some authors have reported associations between multiple sexual partners and increased risk of PC [7, 8], but this association has not been demonstrated by others [6]. A meta-analysis of case-control studies which investigated PC risk and the number of sexual partners found that PC risk steadily increased from 4% for five sexual partners to 8% for 10 partners and 27% for 30 partners, respectively [10]. PC risk also increased with frequency of sexual activity, such that men who were sexually active once a week had a 6% increased risk, in contrast to a 53% increased risk for men reporting daily activity. In a study of younger men (aged 40–64 years), Rosenblatt et al. [7] also reported increased PC risk associated with multiple female sexual partners. Stratifying by tumor aggressiveness ("aggressive PC" was defined as tumors with a Gleason grade of 8–10 or regional or metastatic disease), this relationship appeared to be stronger for men with nonaggressive tumors. A marginally significant trend of increasing risk was found in men with aggressive PC, which could have been a matter of statistical imprecision due to a smaller sample size than that of the group with nonaggressive tumors.

Hayes et al. [6] examined PC risk factors in a case-control study of black and white Americans. Consistent with national data, they documented higher self-reported rates of syphilis or gonorrhea in African American men with PC compared to white men (18.7% versus 2.5%). The odds of self-reported STI were similar in black (OR = 1.7; 95% CI: 1.2–2.2) and white men (OR = 1.6; 95% CI: 0.8–3.2) with PC, compared to racially matched controls. Encounters with prostitutes and lack of condom use were also associated with increased PC risk. Serological evidence of previous syphilis was also positively associated with increased PC risk.

STIs are postulated to increased PC risk through inflammatory changes, with chronic *in situ* inflammation thought to underpin prostate carcinogenesis [23]. Associations with sexually transmitted diseases and/or specific diseases such as syphilis and gonorrhea have been reported in some studies [6, 7]. We however, did not note any differences in self-reported frequency of STI and PC among cases and controls (24.5% and 26.7%, resp.) in the PCBP study. Under reporting of STIs, however, is a possibility in this population. Participants were asked whether they "have or had a sexually transmitted disease (e.g., gonorrhea, syphilis, chlamydia, etc.)" but the occurrence of specific diseases was not recorded. Therefore, although data were collected to evaluate associations between PC and exposure to infectious agents, it was not possible to evaluate individual exposures in this investigation. It should be noted that while there were no differences between cases and controls in self-reported STIs, we did not measure serological markers of disease. As such, it might be possible that true differences in STI distributions, if present, would not have been detected.

The positive associations between earlier age of sexual debut as well as higher numbers of sexual partners and risk of high-grade prostate cancer might be due to multifactorial exposures such as hormonal factors, chemical and physical injury, inflammatory, and infectious agents leading to cellular injury and later malignant change. However, more research is needed to elucidate these potential risk factors.

4.3. Strengths and Limitations. This large case-control study represents a nationwide investigation that identified all cases of PC occurring in a predominantly African descent Caribbean population, with cases age matched to population-based controls. The study followed standardized protocols and achieved high participation among cases and controls. We described the urologic characteristics reported by cases and matched controls and evaluated the likelihood of cases reporting symptoms compared with controls for the first time in an African-Caribbean population. Men with prostatic disease or symptoms are more likely to seek medical care and to be screened for PC than men who are asymptomatic. In view of this potential for bias, we did not evaluate associations between PC and urologic characteristics. It is also likely that a proportion of men in the control group would have had undiagnosed PC. The net effect of this misclassification would have been to attenuate true associations between risks and observed PC outcomes. While there may be causal relationships, associations between sexual activity and PC risk are invariably subject to recall bias, response bias, and interviewer bias, as well as confounding by factors related to both PC risk and sexual behaviors. For example, persons who practice high-risk sexual activities are less likely to attend routine health exams and are less socially integrated [17]. Questions about a history of prostate symptoms elicited very few "unknown" responses (ranging from 0.1% for urinary retention to 0.5% for weak flow and STI), but a higher percentage of such replies were noted for questions about age at first sexual intercourse and the lifetime number of sexual partners (approximately 15% and 25%, resp.). While recall difficulties and/or cultural concerns might underlie these response limitations, it is difficult to discern whether they would under- or overestimate the associations documented in this study. Nonetheless, we found no differences in the reporting of "unknown" between cases and controls, suggesting that the likelihood of bias would be small, if indeed present.

5. Conclusion

This paper provides the first data about urologic characteristics and sexual behaviors associated with prostate cancer in a Caribbean population. Our findings of increased risk of PC associated with an earlier age at onset of sexual activity and an increased risk of high-grade disease with a larger number of lifetime partners are suggestive of multiple mechanisms contributing to the development of PC in this population. It remains unclear, however, how these underlying processes influence the development of PC and subsequent clinical outcomes. To our best knowledge, this is the first time that such associations have been reported in an African-origin Caribbean population. Further study will be necessary to elucidate the role of potential factors and agents in the pathogenesis of PC in this and similar populations.

Acknowledgments

Prostate Cancer in a Black Population Group: investigators: Coordinating Center: M. C. Leske, M.D., M.P.H.; B. Nemesure, Ph.D.; S.-Y. Wu, M.A.; Department of Preventive Medicine, Stony Brook Medicine, Stony Brook, NY, USA. Clinical Center: A. Hennis, M.B.B.S., Ph.D., F.R.C.P.; Winston Scott Polyclinic, Bridgetown, Barbados. Local Laboratory Center: Lyndon Waterman, Ph.D.; University of the West Indies, Bridgetown, Barbados. Gene Discovery Center: John Carpten, Ph.D.; Jeffrey Trent, Ph.D.; Translational Genomics Research Institute, Phoenix, AZ, USA. NHGRI: Joan Bailey-Wilson, Ph.D.; National Human Genome Research Institute, Bethesda, M.D.: Nutritional Collaborator: Sangita Sharma, Ph.D.; University of Alberta, Canada. Scientific Advisory Committee: Agnes Baffoe-Bonnie, Merck Corporation, Philadelphia, PA, USA; Louise Brinton, National Cancer Institute, Bethesda, M.D.; Olufunmilayo Olopade, University of Chicago Medical Center, Chicago, IL, USA; Tim Rebbeck,

University of Pennsylvania School of Medicine, Philadelphia, PA, USA; Duncan Thomas, University of Southern California, Los Angeles, CA, USA. Barbados Advisory Committee: Professor Trevor A. Hassell, G.C.M., M.B.B.S., F.R.C.P., F.A.C.C.; Professor Henry Fraser, G.C.M., M.B.B.S., F.R.C.P., F.A.C.P.; Dr. Jerry Emtage, M.B.B.S., F.R.C.S.(C); Mr. Selwyn Ferdinand M.B.B.S., F.R.C.S.(Ed); The Honourable Mr. Justice W. Leroy Inniss QC; Professor Timothy Roach M.B.B.S., F.R.C.P.; Dr. Gina Watson (PAHO); Dr. Joy St. John (CMO). Consultant Urologists: Dr. Jerry Emtage, MBBS, FRCS(C); Dr. Dave Padmore, M.B.B.S., F.R.C.S.(C); Mr. Irving Smith, M.B.B.S., F.R.C.S. Departments of Urology, Surgery, Pathology and Radiotherapy of the Queen Elizabeth Hospital, Bridgetown Barbados. This project was supported by the Intramural Research Program of the NIH, National Human Genome Research Institute (Contract no. N01HG25487), and the National Cancer Institute (Grant no. RO1CA114379).

References

[1] A. Jemal, M. M. Center, C. DeSantis, and E. M. Ward, "Global patterns of cancer incidence and mortality rates and trends," *Cancer Epidemiology Biomarkers and Prevention*, vol. 19, no. 8, pp. 1893–1907, 2010.

[2] A. J. Hennis, I. R. Hambleton, S. Y. Wu et al., "Prostate cancer incidence and mortality in Barbados, West Indies," *Prostate Cancer*, vol. 2011, Article ID 565230, 10 pages, 2011.

[3] T. N. Gibson, B. Hanchard, N. Waugh, and D. McNaughton, "Thirty-year trends in incidence and age-distribution of prostate cancer in Kingston and St Andrew, Jamaica, 1978–2007," *West Indian Medical Journal*, vol. 60, no. 1, pp. 9–12, 2011.

[4] C. H. Bunker, A. L. Patrick, B. R. Konety et al., "High prevalence of screening-detected prostate cancer among Afro-Caribbeans: the Tobago prostate cancer survey," *Cancer Epidemiology Biomarkers and Prevention*, vol. 11, no. 8, pp. 726–729, 2002.

[5] M. Dieye, J. Veronique-Baudin, C. Draganescu, and H. Azaloux, "Cancer incidence in Martinique: a model of epidemiological transition," *European Journal of Cancer Prevention*, vol. 16, no. 2, pp. 95–101, 2007.

[6] R. B. Hayes, L. M. Pottern, H. Strickler et al., "Sexual behaviour, STDs and risks for prostate cancer," *British Journal of Cancer*, vol. 82, no. 3, pp. 718–725, 2000.

[7] K. A. Rosenblatt, K. G. Wicklund, and J. L. Stanford, "Sexual factors and the risk of prostate cancer," *American Journal of Epidemiology*, vol. 153, no. 12, pp. 1152–1158, 2001.

[8] A. V. Sarma, J. C. McLaughlin, L. P. Wallner et al., "Sexual behavior, sexually transmitted diseases and prostatitis: the risk of prostate cancer in black men," *Journal of Urology*, vol. 176, no. 3, pp. 1108–1113, 2006.

[9] L. Fernández, Y. Galán, R. Jiménez et al., "Sexual behaviour, history of sexually transmitted diseases, and the risk of prostate cancer: a case-control study in Cuba," *International Journal of Epidemiology*, vol. 34, no. 1, pp. 193–197, 2005.

[10] L. K. Dennis and D. V. Dawson, "Meta-analysis of measures of sexual activity and prostate cancer," *Epidemiology*, vol. 13, no. 1, pp. 72–79, 2002.

[11] B. Nemesure, S. Y. Wu, A. Hennis et al., "Central adiposity and prostate cancer in a black population," *Cancer Epidemiology, Biomarkers & Prevention*, vol. 21, no. 5, pp. 851–858, 2012.

[12] A. D. Markland, C. P. Vaughan, T. M. Johnson, P. S. Goode, D. T. Redden, and K. L. Burgio, "Prevalence of nocturia in United States men: results from the national health and nutrition examination survey," *Journal of Urology*, vol. 185, no. 3, pp. 998–1002, 2011.

[13] E. A. Platz, E. Smit, G. C. Curhan, L. M. Nyberg, and E. Giovannucci, "Prevalence of and racial/ethnic variation in lower urinary tract symptoms and noncancer prostate surgery in U.S. men," *Urology*, vol. 59, no. 6, pp. 877–883, 2002.

[14] M. Han, R. E. Brannigan, J. A. V. Antenor, K. A. Roehl, and W. J. Catalona, "Association of hemospermia with prostate cancer," *Journal of Urology*, vol. 172, no. 6, pp. 2189–2192, 2004.

[15] G. D. Honda, L. Bernstein, R. K. Ross, S. Greenland, V. Gerkins, and B. E. Henderson, "Vasectomy, cigarette smoking, and age at first sexual intercourse as risk factors for prostate cancer in middle-aged men," *British Journal of Cancer*, vol. 57, no. 3, pp. 326–331, 1988.

[16] L. Rosenberg, J. R. Palmer, A. G. Zauber et al., "The relation of vasectomy to the risk of cancer," *American Journal of Epidemiology*, vol. 140, no. 5, pp. 431–438, 1994.

[17] S. Sutcliffe, I. Kawachi, J. F. Alderete et al., "Correlates of sexually transmitted infection histories in a cohort of American male health professionals," *Cancer Causes and Control*, vol. 20, no. 9, pp. 1623–1634, 2009.

[18] K. Wellings, K. Nanchahal, W. Macdowall et al., "Sexual behaviour in Britain: early heterosexual experience," *The Lancet*, vol. 358, no. 9296, pp. 1843–1850, 2001.

[19] M. Marston, E. Slaymaker, I. Cremin et al., "Trends in marriage and time spent single in sub-Saharan Africa: a comparative analysis of six population-based cohort studies and nine Demographic and Health Surveys," *Sexually Transmitted Infections*, vol. 85, supplement 1, pp. i64–i71, 2009.

[20] M. S. Golub, G. W. Collman, P. M. D. Foster et al., "Public health implications of altered puberty timing," *Pediatrics*, vol. 121, no. 3, pp. S218–S230, 2008.

[21] J. S. Santelli, N. D. Brener, R. Lowry, A. Bhatt, and L. S. Zabin, "Multiple sexual partners among U.S. Adolescents and young adults," *Family Planning Perspectives*, vol. 30, no. 6, pp. 271–275, 1998.

[22] C. E. Kaestle, C. T. Halpern, W. C. Miller, and C. A. Ford, "Young age at first sexual intercourse and sexually transmitted infections in adolescents and young adults," *American Journal of Epidemiology*, vol. 161, no. 8, pp. 774–780, 2005.

[23] F. M. E. Wagenlehner, J. E. Elkahwaji, F. Algaba et al., "The role of inflammation and infection in the pathogenesis of prostate carcinoma," *BJU International*, vol. 100, no. 4, pp. 733–737, 2007.

13

Variation in *HNF1B* and Obesity May Influence Prostate Cancer Risk in African American Men

Ganna Chornokur,[1,2] Ernest K. Amankwah,[1] Stacy N. Davis,[3] Catherine M. Phelan,[1,2] Jong Y. Park,[1] Julio Pow-Sang,[4] and Nagi B. Kumar[1,2]

[1] *Department of Cancer Epidemiology, Moffitt Cancer Center, Tampa, FL 33612, USA*
[2] *The Center for Equal Health, Tampa, FL 33612, USA*
[3] *Department of Health Outcomes and Behavior, Moffitt Cancer Center, Tampa, FL 33612, USA*
[4] *Department of Genitourinary Oncology, Moffitt Cancer Center, Tampa, FL 33612, USA*

Correspondence should be addressed to Ganna Chornokur; ganna.chornokur@moffitt.org

Academic Editor: James L. Gulley

Background. Prostate cancer (PCa) racial disparity is multifactorial, involving biological, sociocultural, and lifestyle determinants. We investigated the association between selected potentially functional polymorphisms (SNPs) and prostate cancer (PCa) risk in Black (AAM) and White (EAM) men. We further explored if these associations varied by the body mass index (BMI) and height. *Methods.* Age-matched DNA samples from 259 AAM and 269 EAM were genotyped for 10 candidate SNPs in 7 genes using the TaqMan allelic differentiation analysis. The dominant, recessive, and additive age-adjusted unconditional logistic regression models were fitted. *Results.* Three SNPs showed statistically significant associations with PCa risk: in AAM, *HNF1B* rs7501939 (OR = 2.42, $P = 0.0046$) and rs4430796 (OR = 0.57, $P = 0.0383$); in EAM, *CTBP2* rs4962416 (OR = 1.52, $P = 0.0384$). In addition, high BMI in AAM (OR = 1.06, $P = 0.022$) and height in EAM (OR = 0.92, $P = 0.0434$) showed significant associations. Interestingly, *HNF1B* rs7501939 was associated with PCa exclusively in obese AAM (OR = 2.14, $P = 0.0103$). *Conclusion.* Our results suggest that variation in the *HNF1B* may influence PCa risk in obese AAM.

1. Introduction

Prostate cancer (PCa) remains the most common type of solid malignancy and the second-leading cause of all cancer death in US men [1]. However, the burden of PCa is not the same across all racial and ethnic groups, as African American/Black men (AAM) consistently demonstrate 1.6 times higher incidence and 2-3 times higher mortality rates of PCa, compared to their nonhispanic white (EAM) counterparts [2]. In addition, AAM are more likely to be diagnosed at an earlier age and have more aggressive tumors and higher recurrence rates following definite treatments [2, 3]. The etiology of racial disparity in PCa is thought to be multifactorial, involving biological, sociocultural, and lifestyle determinants [4]. Although genome-wide association studies (GWAS) have identified more than a dozen PCa risk loci [5], elucidating the biological basis for these associations is challenging [6]. Identified risk loci include the noncoding variants, such as those located in the 8q24 region [7], as well as polymorphisms in the coding regions (genes) that either alter, or are predicted to alter, the protein expression (such as HNF1B [8], TERT [5], and RNASEL [9]). The post-GWAS studies are increasingly suggestive of the interaction between genetic variants and environmental risk factors [10] for which our understanding is still largely inadequate [11].

Established risk factors for PCa are increasing age, race, and family history of the disease [2–4]. Obesity (which affects 35% of all US adults [12] and is more prevalent in African American population [13]) is linked to a plethora of diseases including cardiovascular problems, type II diabetes, gallbladder disease, and osteoarthritis [14], and an array of human cancers such as breast, uterine, and pancreas [15, 16]. Furthermore, obesity alters the individual's biochemical and hormonal profile [17], which may facilitate cancer growth

[18]. However, obesity has been inconsistently associated with PCa risk [19], and the inconsistency may be due to an interaction with genetic variants [20, 21]. In an attempt to elucidate the connection between PCa health disparity, genetic variation, and obesity, we hypothesized that genetic variation differentially alters the PCa risk in obese and nonobese AAM and EAM. Given the extremely high burden of PCa and staggering rates of obesity, elucidating the links between the individual's genetic variation, race, PCa risk, and obesity is likely to have a major positive impact on the public health of the US population. Thus, our hypothesis-generating study may open new venues for tackling the PCa disparity from a new perspective.

2. Methods

2.1. Study Participants. Study participants were recruited from various clinics in the Tampa Bay area in Florida, including the Moffitt Cancer Center, Tampa Bay Radiation Oncology centers, Moffitt Cancer Center affiliated-Lifetime Cancer Screening & Prevention Center, James A. Haley Veteran Affairs (VA), and the 30th Street Medical Associates (a community clinic). All recruitment protocols were approved by the University of South Florida Institutional Review Board (IRB), while the VA protocol was approved by the VA IRB. The study population comprised of AAM and EAM aged 30–85 years and enrolled between 2006 and 2012. The cases and controls were recruited during the initial PCa screening of all consecutive, unselected patients. Cases were histologically confirmed PCa patients and controls were men with low PSA and/or no evidence of PCa on biopsy. The AAM or EAM ancestry was self-reported. Men were excluded if they did not self-identify as either AAM or EAM, were outside of the 30–85 year old range, were in poor physical or mental health, were diagnosed with other cancers (excluding nonmelanoma skin cancer), or did not speak English well enough to read and understand the informed consent. The response rates in all studies were high, at or above 90%.

2.2. Single Nucleotide Polymorphism (SNP) Selection and Genotyping. Literature search using PubMed and Google scholar databases was performed to identify potentialSNPs of interest. The following criteria were set to guide the SNP search (all inclusive): (1) confer increased PCa risk in AAM; (2) confer increased PCa risk in EAM; (3) demonstrate potential for functional significance (i.e., located in or close to a gene with a known function); (4) reported minor allele frequency (MAF) $\geq$ 15% in AAM and EAM. Based on these criteria, 10 SNPs in 7 genes were selected: rs4430796; rs7501939; rs1859962 in *HNF1B*; rs10993994 in *MSMB*; rs822396 in *ADIPOQ*; rs4263970; rs4612601 in *EPHB2*; rs4962416 in *CTBP2*; rs627839 in *RNASEL*; rs2070874 in *IL4*. All these SNPs have reported functional significance (actual or hypothesized). DNA was extracted from blood or buccal cell samples using commercially available extraction kits and TaqMan genotyping was conducted at the Moffitt Cancer Center on the DNA samples from 259 (136 cases and 123 controls) AAM and 269 (147 cases and 142 controls) EAM, matched on age at diagnosis.

2.3. Statistical Analyses. Descriptive statistics were used to summarize participants' demographic and clinical characteristics. Genotypes among participants were used to estimate allele frequencies and departure from Hardy-Weinberg equilibrium (HWE) was assessed among control subjects using Chi-squared test. The association between each SNP and PCa risk was estimated with odds ratios (OR) and 95% confidence intervals (CI) using unconditional logistic regression adjusted for age at diagnosis. Three inheritance genetic models (log-additive, dominant, and recessive) were tested for each SNP and the model with the minimum P value was considered as the best fitting model. Separate analyses were performed for each race and all men combined. We conducted exploratory subgroup analyses for different strata based on BMI and height within each race. Statistical tests were two sided with an alpha level <0.05 considered statistically significant. All statistical analyses were performed with SAS/Genetics version 9.2 (SAS Institute, NC, USA).

3. Results

Selected characteristics of the study participants by case/control status are shown in Table 1. For both ethnic groups, men were likely to be between 50 to 64 years of age and between 68 and 72 inches tall. AAM were more likely to be obese than EAM (47% and 35.5% obese men in each group, resp.). AAM were also more likely to be taller. Within each ethnic group, cases were more likely to be older, although there was no significant difference in the age of cases and controls between races. In addition, AAM cases were more likely to be obese than AAM controls. In contrast, EAM controls were more likely to be obese than EAM cases.

The results for association analyses between SNP and risk are shown in Table 2. The MAF of the SNPs ranged from 0.15–0.49 and none of the SNPs deviated from HWE (all $P >$ 0.05). In AAM, we observed an increased PCa risk at *HNF1B* rs7501939 (recessive model: OR = 2.42, 95% CI = 1.31–4.47, $P = 0.0046$; additive model: OR = 1.56, 95% CI = 1.08–2.27, $P = 0.0193$) and a decreased PCa risk at *HNF1B* rs4430796 (dominant model: OR = 0.57, 95% CI = 0.34–0.97, $P =$ 0.0383; additive model: OR = 0.67, 95% CI = 0.46–0.99, $P = 0.0431$). These SNPs were not significantly associated with PCa risk in EAM. In EAM, we observed an increased PCa risk at the *CTBP2* rs4962416 (dominant model: OR = 1.69, 95% CI = 1.02–2.80, $P = 0.0415$; additive model: OR = 1.52, 95% CI = 1.02–2.26, $P = 0.0384$). This association was not confirmed in AAM. We attempted to analyze for the interaction between SNPs and race in multivariable model. None of SNP and race interaction is significant ($P > 0.05$).

Age-adjusted association between selected anthropometric variables and PCa are shown in Table 3. We observed an increased PCa risk in obese, compared to nonobese AAM (OR = 1.06, 95% CI = 1.01–1.11, $P = 0.022$) and decreased PCa risk in the tallest group of EAM compared to all other EAM (OR = 0.92, CI = 0.85–0.99, $P = 0.0434$). Since our results indicated that BMI might be positively associated with PCa in AAM, we decided to examine the SNP-associations stratified by obesity for SNPs that were significant for AAM: rs7501939 and rs4430796.

TABLE 1: Selected characteristics of the study participants by case/control status.

	AAM: 259 total		EAM: 269 total		Total sample combined	
	No. of cases (%) 136 (52.5)	No. of controls (%) 123 (47.5)	No. of cases (%) 147 (54.6)	No. of controls (%) 122 (45.4)	No. of cases (%) 283 (53.6)	No. of controls (%) 245 (46.4)
Age						
<50	11 (8)	12 (8)	19 (16)	30 (24)	30 (12)	42 (16)
50–64	74 (54)	80 (54)	85 (70)	73 (59)	159 (62)	153 (56.5)
≥65	51 (38)	55 (38)	18 (14)	17 (14)	69 (26)	72 (26)
Missing	NA	NA	NA	3 (3)	NA	3 (1.5)
BMI						
≤24.9 normal weight	9 (7)	25 (17)	28 (23)	26 (21)	37 (15)	51 (19)
25.0–29.9 overweight	47 (34.5)	70 (48)	47 (38)	46 (37)	94 (36)	116 (42.5)
≥30.0 obese	71 (52)	48 (33)	46 (38)	51 (42)	58.5 (45)	49.5 (37.5)
Missing	9 (6.5)	4 (2)	1 (1)	NA	10 (3.5)	4 (1)
Height						
≤67	30 (22)	26 (17.5)	22 (18)	21 (17)	52 (20)	47 (17)
68–72	65 (48)	98 (66.5)	79 (65)	74 (60)	144 (56.5)	172 (63)
≥73	32 (23.5)	19 (13)	21 (17)	28 (23)	53 (20)	47 (18)
Missing	9 (6.5)	4 (3)	NA	NA	9 (3)	4 (1.5)

Results for SNP-associations stratified by obesity in AAM are shown in Table 4. Interestingly, when stratified by obesity status, rs7501939 at *HNF1B* only increased PCa risk in obese AAM (OR = 2.14, 95%CI = 1.2–3.8, $P = 0.01$) but not in the nonobese AAM ($P = 0.76$) or EAM of any BMI ($P = 0.3$ in obese, and $P = 0.8$ in nonobese EAM). No differential association with obesity status was observed at rs4430796 in AAM ($P = 0.18$ in obese and $P = 0.51$ in the nonobese AAM). There were no significant associations with PCa risk at these SNP in EAM regardless of obesity status ($P > 0.05$).

Finally, we used the SNP Annotation and Proxy Search (SNAP) software (Broad Institute) to elucidate whether there are other SNPs in linkage disequilibrium (LD) with our significant SNPs. The results are shown in Table 5. There are no SNPs in the LD ($r^2 \geq 0.8$) with either of the *HNF1B* SNPs significant in AAM. While there are several SNPs in weak LD ($r^2 \geq 0.5$) with rs7501939, they were not found to be associated with PCa or any other disease. In EAM, while a number of SNPs are reported to be in LD with the CTBP2 rs4962416, only one of those SNPs (rs12769019) was linked to a marginally increased PCa risk in EAM (OR = 1.1, 95% CI, 0.99–1.25) [22].

4. Discussion

We observe that the *HNF1B* SNPs (rs7501939 and rs4430796) identified in PCa GWAS [23, 24] are associated with PCa risk in AAM and that the *CTBP2* SNP rs4962416, also identified in PCa GWAS [23], is associated with PCa risk in EAM. Our novel finding is that the association of rs7501939 with PCa risk in AAM may be modified by obesity.

In this study we observed that the *HNF1B* SNPs (rs7501939 and rs4430796) identified in PCa GWAS [23, 24] are associated with PCa risk in AAM and that the *CTBP2* SNP (rs4962416), also identified in PCa GWAS [23], are associated with PCa risk in EAM. Our novel finding is that the association of rs7501939 with PCa risk in AAM may be modified by obesity.

Gudmundsson et al. [24] reported mixed results regarding the association of PCa risk and *HNF1B* SNPs in EAM (largely living in Europe). Similar to our findings, *HNF1B* SNP rs4430796 was not significantly associated with PCa in the EAM; however, *HNF1B* SNP rs7501939 was significantly associated with PCa in the EAM in their sample. The authors also reported that the same SNPs were significantly inversely associated with type II diabetes. Stevens et al. [8] reported that *HNF1B* SNPs (rs7501939 and rs4430796) were both significantly inversely associated with PCa risk in their cohorts of EAM. However, unlike Gudmundsson et al. [24], the authors did not observe a statistically significant association with diabetes. Liu et al. [25] conducted a meta-analysis of all PCa-related GWA studies. The authors have found that in combined analysis, *HNF1B* SNPs (rs7501939 and rs4430796) were significantly associated with PCa. However, when stratified by ethnicity, neither of the two SNPs attained statistical significance when analysis was restricted to AAM. Sun et al. [26] analyzed a diverse cohort of men (2139 EAM and 717 AAM) and reported significant associations with PCa risk and both SNPs in EAM. However, when analysis was restricted to AAM, only SNP rs4430796 retained statistical significance. This may be due to Sun et al. who used major alleles as risk alleles (T for rs4430796 and G for rs75001939), while our study and other cited studies used minor alleles as risk alleles. Ahn et al. [27] reported that SNP rs4430796 was not associated with risk for metastatic prostate cancer and recurrence.

TABLE 2: Age-adjusted odds ratios (OR) and 95% confidence intervals (95% CI) for PCa in AAM and EAM and combined.

Rs# and gene; minor allele and its frequency	Dominant model OR (CI); *P* value	Recessive model OR (CI); *P* value	Additive model OR (CI); *P* value
rs4612601; EPHB2	AAM: 1.09 (0.63–1.9); 0.749	0.86 (0.46–1.61); 0.638	0.99 (0.69–1.41); 0.951
AA: 0.49 (G)	EAM: 1.18 (0.67–2.10); 0.564	0.9 (0.52–1.56); 0.709	1.02 (0.73–1.43); 0.912
EA: 0.45 (A)	All: 1.13 (0.76–1.69); 0.537	0.89 (0.59–1.34); 0.565	1.00 (0.79–1.28); 0.969
rs4263970; EPHB2	AAM: 0.98 (0.57–1.68); 0.932	0.88 (0.44–1.75); 0.711	0.95 (0.66–1.38); 0.797
AA: 0.47 (T)	EAM: 1.08 (0.61–1.9); 0.795	0.76 (0.44–1.33); 0.334	0.93 (0.66–1.30); 0.665
EA: 0.45 (C)	All: 1.02 (0.69–1.5); 0.918	0.81 (0.53–1.25); 0.343	0.94 (0.73–1.21); 0.630
rs822396; ADIPOQ	AAM: 0.89 (0.52–1.52); 0.671	1.64 (0.37–7.21); 0.511	0.96 (0.6–1.54); 0.878
AA: 0.2 (G)	EAM: 0.75 (0.44–1.27); 0.288	1.1 (0.29–4.09); 0.094	0.82 (0.53–1.29); 0.392
EA: 0.15 (G)	All: 0.82 (0.56–1.19); 0.285	1.29 (0.49–3.48); 0.601	0.88 (0.64–1.22); 0.456
rs10993994; MSMB	AAM: 0.82 (0.48–1.4); 0.472	1.04 (0.51–2.10); 0.919	0.92 (0.63–1.33); 0.657
AA: 0.2 (C)	EAM: 1.04 (0.54–2.00); 0.899	0.61 (0.36–1.05); 0.077	0.81 (0.56–1.17); 0.258
EA: 0.34 (T)	All: 0.9 (0.6–1.35); 0.611	0.75 (0.49–1.14); 0.177	0.87 (0.67–1.11); 0.261
rs1859962; HNF1B	AAM: 1.03 (0.61–1.74); 0.905	1.23 (0.54–2.81); 0.626	1.06 (0.72–1.56); 0.752
AA: 0.49 (G)	EAM: 1.38 (0.77–2.45); 0.278	1.00 (0.57–1.76); 0.997	1.13 (0.79–1.6); 0.508
EA: 0.2 (G)	All: 1.16 (0.8–1.69); 0.431	1.06 (0.67–1.69); 0.790	1.09 (0.85–1.4); 0.503
rs7501939; HNF1B	AAM: 1.34 (0.73–2.47); 0.343	**2.42 (1.31–4.47); 0.0046**	**1.56 (1.08–2.27); 0.0193**
AA: 0.48 (C)	EAM: 0.82 (0.5–1.35); 0.439	1.13 (0.54–2.38); 0.742	0.93 (0.65–1.33); 0.692
EA: 0.49 (T)	All: 0.99 (0.68–1.45); 0.981	**1.76 (1.11–2.79); 0.0167**	1.18 (0.92–1.52); 0.187
rs4430796; HNF1B	AAM: **0.57 (0.34–0.97); 0.0383**	0.64 (0.29–1.42); 0.272	**0.67 (0.46–0.99); 0.0431**
AA: 0.34 (A)	EAM: 1.27 (0.7–2.3); 0.439	0.98 (0.57–1.68); 0.946	1.07 (0.76–1.51); 0.689
EA: 0.47 (A)	All: 0.81 (0.55–1.18); 0.273	0.86 (0.59–1.33); 0.500	0.87 (0.69–1.12); 0.279
rs2070874; IL4	AAM: 0.94 (0.54–1.64); 0.824	1.45 (0.7–3.0); 0.314	1.08 (0.73–1.59); 0.700
AA: 0.45 (T)	EAM: 0.65 (0.38–1.11); 0.115	0.92 (0.22–3.93); 0.916	0.72 (0.45–1.14); 0.161
EA: 0.2 (T)	All: 0.82 (0.57–1.17); 0.275	1.32 (0.7–2.49); 0.386	0.94 (0.71–1.24); 0.649
rs627839; RNASEL	AAM: 1.2 (0.7–2.06); 0.511	1.63 (0.78–3.42); 0.192	1.24 (0.85–1.83); 0.252
AA: 0.46 (T)	EAM: 0.86 (0.5–1.47); 0.571	0.99 (0.55–1.8); 0.986	0.94 (0.67–1.32); 0.710
EA: 0.45 (T)	All: 1.01 (0.69–1.48); 0.952	1.21 (0.76–1.91); 0.427	1.06 (0.83–1.37); 0.632
rs4962416; CTBP2	AAM: 0.9 (0.5–1.59); 0.709	5.65 (0.62–51.7); 0.125	1.05 (0.63–1.74); 0.861
AA: 0.23 (C)	**EAM: 1.69 (1.02–2.8); 0.0415**	1.72 (0.68–4.31); 0.251	**1.52 (1.02–2.26); 0.0384**
EA: 0.23 (C)	All: 1.28 (0.88–1.85); 0.198	2.12 (0.92–4.9); 0.0784	1.31 (0.97–1.78); 0.083

Bolded values denote statistically significant associations.

TABLE 3: Age-adjusted association between selected anthropometric variables and PCa in men stratifying by race and combined.

	AAM OR (95% CI); *P* value	EAM OR (95% CI); *P* value
Height (inches)	0.98 (0.9–1.05); 0.54	**0.92 (0.85–0.99); 0.0434**
BMI (kg/m^2)	**1.06 (1.01–1.11); 0.022**	0.98 (0.93–1.023); 0.33
<30 (nonobese)	1.0	1.0
≥30 (obese)	**2.07 (1.21–3.55); 0.008**	0.90 (0.54–1.51); 0.69

Bold denotes statistically significant associations.

TABLE 4: rs7501939 and rs4430796 as PCa risk factors in AAM stratified by BMI.

	Nonobese AAM	Obese AAM	All AAM
rs7501939	1.09 (0.65–1.83); 0.75	**2.13 (1.20–3.81); 0.01**	**1.56 (1.08–2.27); *P* = 0.019**
rs4430796	0.84 (0.49–1.43); 0.52	0.67 (0.37–1.20); 0.18	**0.67 (0.46–0.99); 0.043**

Statistically significant associations are shown in bold. Data is age adjusted.

TABLE 5: SNPs reported to be in LD regions with our SNPs of interest.

SNP of interest	$r^2 \geq 0.8$	$r^2 \geq 0.5$	Disease and comments
rs7501939 in AAM	None	rs11657964 (r^2 = 0.61) rs8064454 (r^2 = 0.549)	None reported to be associated with prostate cancer or any other disease
rs4430796 in AAM	None	None	NA
rs4962416 in EAM	rs4962720 (r^2 = 1.00) rs4962419 (r^2 = 1.00) rs12771627 (r^2 = 1.00) rs12769019 (r^2 = 0.92) rs11598549 (r^2 = 0.92) rs12782469 (r^2 = 0.83)	14 additional SNPs	rs12769019: slightly increased risk for prostate cancer in EAM (OR = 1.1) [19]

Studies that investigated PCA risk and *HNF1B* SNPs within large AAM cohorts also found similar mixed results. Chang et al. [28] could not validate the association of PCa risk and *HNF1B* SNPs (rs7501939 and rs4430796) in their large cohort of 4,040 AAM PCa cases and 3,748 healthy AAM controls. Haiman et al. [29] also reported no association in their large cohort of 3,621 AAM PCa cases and 3,652 AAM controls. Hooker et al. [30] found mixed results in their attempts to replicate the PCa SNPs identified in the GWAS studies. In a cohort of 755 unrelated AAM, *HNF1B* rs7501939 was not associated with PCa risk, while HNF1B rs4430796 conferred significant increased PCa risk.

None of the aforementioned studies controlled for BMI in the association between PCa risk and *HNF1B* SNPs (rs7501939 and rs4430796). However, Lindstrom et al. [31] investigated the modifying effects of BMI on PCA risk and different SNPs in EAM. Lindstrom et al. found that BMI does not have modifying effects on the SNP-PCa associations in EAM; similar analysis was not performed in AAM.

As can be concluded from the referenced studies, there is significant discordance between the published studies on the effects of the two aforementioned *HNF1B* SNPs on PCa risk. While the authors presented high-quality studies with large sample sizes, the majority did not report controlling for the environmental confounders, including BMI. To our knowledge, we are the first group to report that the association of the *HNF1B* SNPs with PCa risk may be modified by the level of adiposity and racial/ethnic background. Importantly, BMI was associated with PCa risk in our sample of AAM independently of genetic variation (OR = 1.06, P = 0.022) (Table 3). Our hypothesis-generating data may be even more intriguing in light of the ongoing debate surrounding the relationship between obesity and PCa risk. At present, there appears to be a consensus that obese men experience slightly reduced overall PCa incidence, at the expense of an increase in aggressive, "clinically significant" disease. The overall decreased PCa risk, therefore, is mainly due to reduction in the "clinically insignificant," potentially indolent PCa [17]. While several hypotheses aimed to explain that this observation have been proposed [32], neither has been widely accepted by scientific or medical communities. Additionally, because the data were obtained in EAM, the effect of obesity on PCa risk in AAM remains unknown. Our pilot study adds information to close this knowledge gap and serve as a basis for future sufficiently powered studies involving larger numbers of AA participants, as well as more extensive epidemiological data analysis.

Mutations in the *HNF1B* cause MODY5 (maturity-onset of diabetes, type 5) that may be accompanied by urinary tract disorders, including renal disease and/or undeveloped/malformed kidneys and atrophic pancreas [33, 34]. Some men with the *HNF1B* mutations have malformations in the reproductive tract including epididymal cysts, agenesis of the vas deferens, or infertility due to abnormal spermatozoa [35]. More recently, genetic variants in the *HNF1B* were implicated in the prostate [36, 37] and endometrial [38, 39] cancer risks. It was reported [40] that different *HNF1B* isoforms were expressed in prostate tumors versus normal prostate tissue, thus providing functional evidence for a potential role of this gene in PCa. However, the functional studies to examine whether *HNF1B* variants influence PCa risk and/or prognosis are lacking. *HNF1B* variants were implicated in a slightly reduced risk of type II diabetes mellitus in AAM and EAM [24]. Interestingly, PCa risk seems to be attenuated in men with diabetes [41], although the latter was only reported in people of EA descent and the biological basis for this association remains to be elucidated. At this time, the relationship between obesity, diabetes, and PCa is poorly understood, and so is the contribution of the *HNF1B* variants to the risk. However, since obesity as a risk factor for breast cancer differs in AA and EA women [42, 43], it is plausible that a similar effect may be observed with obesity and PCa in AAM and EAM. Additionally, our data suggests that *HNF1B* variants may be implicated in the risk. Future epidemiological, genetic, and functional tumor biology studies are required to address this provocative hypothesis.

In EAM, our results replicate a previously reported finding that the *CTBP2* rs4962416 confers increased PCa risk: OR = 1.69, P = 0.0415 in our study versus the overall GWAS data: OR = 1.25, P = 0.004 [25]. *CTBP2* encodes a transcriptional corepressor that is activated under stress condition and can mediate stress-induced migration of tumor cells [44]. *CTBP2* expression is detected in the prostate and has been linked to decreased *PTEN* expression and activation of the phosphatidylinositol 3-kinase pathway [45] which may support or promote PCa growth. rs4962416 was not previously implicated in PCa risk in AAM [25] which is also in agreement with our data.

The main strength of our study is inclusion of equal proportions of age-matched AA and EA men with high rates of obese men in both populations, allowing us to tease out the interaction of obesity with genetic variants. Our results should be interpreted in light of limitations of a small sample size and inability to access relevant information such as smoking/drinking behavior and diabetes history. However, given the increased PCa burden in AAM, alarming obesity rates, and limited number of studies that involve AAM, our results are novel, timely, and as such, deserve dissemination.

In summary, our results suggest that germline genetic variation in *HNF1B* and *CTBP2* differentially contribute to PCa risk in men of different races and adiposities. Future sufficiently powered studies involving a larger proportion of AAM are needed to elucidate the potential connection between the race, PCa, obesity, diabetes, and *HNF1B*. In addition, functional tumor biology studies are warranted to elucidate the effects of obesity on PCa in carriers and noncarriers of different races and ethnicities.

Authors' Contribution

Conception and design: G. Chornokur; N. Kumar; C. Phelan; J. Park. Data collection and analysis: G. Chornokur; E. Amankwah; S. Davis. Writing and editing of the paper: G. Chornokur; E. Amankwah; S. D Davis. Study supervision: J. Pow-Sang; N. Kumar.

Acknowledgments

This research is supported by the Department of Defense, Prostate Cancer Research Program (DoD PCRP): W81XWH-11-1-0376 (G. Chornokur), W81XWH-06-1-0034 (C. Phelan), and W81XWH-12-1-0113 (J. Park); the National Institute of Health (NIH): P20 MD003375-01 (C. Phelan, N. Kumar) and 5R25 CA090314 (S. Davis); the National Cancer Institute (NCI): R25T CA147832 (E. Amankwah) and R01CA128813 (J. Park). The sponsors had no role in the conception, execution, data analysis, or reporting of these results.

References

[1] American Cancer Society, *Cancer Facts & Figures for African Americans 2011-2012*, American Cancer Society, Atlanta, Ga, USA, 2011.

[2] G. Chornokur, K. Dalton, M. E. Borysova, and N. B. Kumar, "Disparities at presentation, diagnosis, treatment, and survival in African American men, affected by prostate cancer," *Prostate*, vol. 71, no. 9, pp. 985–997, 2011.

[3] I. J. Powell, "Epidemiology and pathophysiology of prostate cancer in African-American men," *Journal of Urology*, vol. 177, no. 2, pp. 444–449, 2007.

[4] E. D. Crawford, "Epidemiology of prostate cancer," *Urology*, vol. 62, no. 6, pp. 3–12, 2003.

[5] Z. Kote-Jarai, A. A. A. Olama, G. G. Giles et al., "Seven prostate cancer susceptibility loci identified by a multi-stage genome-wide association study," *Nature Genetics*, vol. 43, no. 8, pp. 785–791, 2011.

[6] M. L. Freedman, A. N. A. Monteiro, S. A. Gayther et al., "Principles for the post-GWAS functional characterization of cancer risk loci," *Nature Genetics*, vol. 43, no. 6, pp. 513–518, 2011.

[7] C. A. Haiman, N. Patterson, M. L. Freedman et al., "Multiple regions within 8q24 independently affect risk for prostate cancer," *Nature Genetics*, vol. 39, no. 5, pp. 638–644, 2007.

[8] V. L. Stevens, J. Ahn, J. Sun et al., "HNFIB and JAZFI genes, diabetes, and prostate cancer risk," *Prostate*, vol. 70, no. 6, pp. 601–607, 2010.

[9] M. M. Shen and C. Abate-Shen, "Molecular genetics of prostate cancer: new prospects for old challenges," *Genes and Development*, vol. 24, no. 18, pp. 1967–2000, 2010.

[10] C. Kooperberg, M. LeBlanc, J. Y. Dai, and I. Rajapakse, "Structures and assumptions: strategies to harness gene × gene and gene × environment interactions in GWAS," *Statistical Science*, vol. 24, no. 4, pp. 472–488, 2009.

[11] M. C. Cornelis, A. Agrawal, J. W. Cole et al., "The gene, environment association studies consortium (GENEVA): maximizing the knowledge obtained from GWAS by collaboration across studies of multiple conditions," *Genetic Epidemiology*, vol. 34, no. 4, pp. 364–372, 2010.

[12] D. S. Michaud, K. Augustsson, E. B. Rimm, M. J. Stampfer, W. C. Willet, and E. Giovannucci, "A prospective study on intake of animal products and risk of prostate cancer," *Cancer Causes and Control*, vol. 12, no. 6, pp. 557–567, 2001.

[13] R. Sinha, Y. Park, B. I. Graubard et al., "Meat and meat-related compounds and risk of prostate cancer in a large prospective cohort study in the United States," *American Journal of Epidemiology*, vol. 170, no. 9, pp. 1165–1177, 2009.

[14] E. L. Giovannucci, Y. Liu, M. F. Leitzmann, M. J. Stampfer, and W. C. Willett, "A prospective study of physical activity and incident and fatal prostate cancer," *Archives of Internal Medicine*, vol. 165, no. 9, pp. 1005–1010, 2005.

[15] C. M. Friedenreich and I. Thune, "A review of physical activity and prostate cancer risk," *Cancer Causes and Control*, vol. 12, no. 5, pp. 461–475, 2001.

[16] C. M. Friedenreich, S. E. McGregor, K. S. Courneya, S. J. Angyalfi, and F. G. Elliott, "Case-control study of lifetime total physical activity and prostate cancer risk," *American Journal of Epidemiology*, vol. 159, no. 8, pp. 740–749, 2004.

[17] S. J. Freedland and E. A. Platz, "Obesity and prostate cancer: making sense out of apparently conflicting data," *Epidemiologic Reviews*, vol. 29, no. 1, pp. 88–97, 2007.

[18] C. L. Ogden, M. M. Lamb, M. D. Carroll, and K. M. Flegal, "Obesity and socioeconomic status in adults: United States, 2005–2008," *NCHS Data Brief*, no. 50, pp. 1–8, 2010.

[19] CDC, *Health United States, 2011*, 2012, http://www.cdc.gov/nchs/data/hus/hus11.pdf.

[20] M. A. Kirschner, N. Ertel, and G. Schneider, "Obesity, hormones, and cancer," *Cancer Research*, vol. 41, no. 9, pp. 3711–3717, 1981.

[21] A. G. Renehan, M. Tyson, M. Egger, R. F. Heller, and M. Zwahlen, "Body-mass index and incidence of cancer: a systematic review and meta-analysis of prospective observational studies," *The Lancet*, vol. 371, no. 9612, pp. 569–578, 2008.

[22] K. M. Waters, L. Le Marchand, L. N. Kolonel et al., "Generalizability of associations from prostate cancer genome-wide association studies in multiple populations," *Cancer Epidemiology Biomarkers and Prevention*, vol. 18, no. 4, pp. 1285–1289, 2009.

[23] R. A. Eeles, Z. Kote-Jarai, G. G. Giles et al., "Multiple newly identified loci associated with prostate cancer susceptibility," *Nature Genetics*, vol. 40, no. 3, pp. 316–321, 2008.

[24] J. Gudmundsson, P. Sulem, V. Steinthorsdottir et al., "Two variants on chromosome 17 confer prostate cancer risk, and the one in TCF2 protects against type 2 diabetes," *Nature Genetics*, vol. 39, no. 8, pp. 977–983, 2007.

[25] H. Liu, B. Wang, and C. Han, "Meta-analysis of genome-wide and replication association studies on prostate cancer," *Prostate*, vol. 71, no. 2, pp. 209–224, 2011.

[26] J. Sun, L. Purcell, Z. Gao et al., "Association between sequence variants at 17q12 and 17q24.3 and prostate cancer risk in European and African Americans," *Prostate*, vol. 68, no. 7, pp. 691–697, 2008.

[27] J. Ahn, A. S. Kibel, J. Y. Park et al., "Prostate cancer predisposition loci and risk of metastatic disease and prostate cancer recurrence," *Clinical Cancer Research*, vol. 17, no. 5, pp. 1075–1081, 2011.

[28] B.-L. Chang, E. Spangler, S. Gallagher et al., "Validation of genome-wide prostate cancer associations in men of african descent," *Cancer Epidemiology Biomarkers and Prevention*, vol. 20, no. 1, pp. 23–32, 2011.

[29] C. A. Haiman, G. K. Chen, W. J. Blot et al., "Characterizing genetic risk at known prostate cancer susceptibility loci in African Americans," *PLoS Genetics*, vol. 7, no. 5, Article ID e1001387, 2011.

[30] S. Hooker, W. Hernandez, H. Chen et al., "Replication of prostate cancer risk loci on 8q24, 11q13, 17q12, 19q33, and Xp11 in African Americans," *Prostate*, vol. 70, no. 3, pp. 270–275, 2010.

[31] S. Lindstrom, F. Schumacher, A. Siddiq et al., "Characterizing associations and SNP-environment interactions for GWAS-identified prostate cancer risk markers-results from BPC3," *PLoS ONE*, vol. 6, no. 2, Article ID e17142, 2011.

[32] A. W. Hsing, L. C. Sakoda, and S. Chua Jr., "Obesity, metabolic syndrome, and prostate cancer," *The American Journal of Clinical Nutrition*, vol. 86, no. 3, pp. s843–s857, 2007.

[33] C. Bingham and A. T. Hattersley, "Renal cysts and diabetes syndrome resulting from mutations in hepatocyte nuclear factor-1β," *Nephrology Dialysis Transplantation*, vol. 19, no. 11, pp. 2703–2708, 2004.

[34] I. S. Haldorsen, M. Vesterhus, H. Ræder et al., "Lack of pancreatic body and tail in HNF1B mutation carriers," *Diabetic Medicine*, vol. 25, no. 7, pp. 782–787, 2008.

[35] M. Nakayama, K. Nozu, Y. Goto et al., "HNF1B alterations associated with congenital anomalies of the kidney and urinary tract," *Pediatric Nephrology*, vol. 25, no. 6, pp. 1073–1079, 2010.

[36] S. I. Berndt, J. Sampson, M. Yeager et al., "Large-scale fine mapping of the HNF1B locus and prostate cancer risk," *Human Molecular Genetics*, vol. 20, no. 16, pp. 3322–3329, 2011.

[37] J. Sun, S. L. Zheng, F. Wiklund et al., "Evidence for two independent prostate cancer risk-associated loci in the HNF1B gene at 17q12," *Nature Genetics*, vol. 40, no. 10, pp. 1153–1155, 2008.

[38] V. W. Setiawan, J. Haessler, F. Schumacher et al., "HNF1B and endometrial cancer risk: results from the page study," *PLoS ONE*, vol. 7, no. 1, Article ID e30390, 2012.

[39] A. B. Spurdle, D. J. Thompson, S. Ahmed et al., "Genome-wide association study identifies a common variant associated with risk of endometrial cancer," *Nature Genetics*, vol. 43, no. 5, pp. 451–455, 2011.

[40] L. W. Harries, J. R. B. Perry, P. McCullagh, and M. Crundwell, "Alterations in LMTK2, MSMB and HNF1B gene expression are associated with the development of prostate cancer," *BMC Cancer*, vol. 10, article 315, 2010.

[41] E. Weiderpass, W. Ye, H. Vainio, R. Kaaks, and H.-O. Adami, "Reduced risk of prostate cancer among patients with diabetes mellitus," *International Journal of Cancer*, vol. 102, no. 3, pp. 258–261, 2002.

[42] P. Berstad, R. J. Coates, L. Bernstein et al., "A case-control study of body mass index and breast cancer risk in white and African-American women," *Cancer Epidemiology Biomarkers and Prevention*, vol. 19, no. 6, pp. 1532–1544, 2010.

[43] M. Sarkissyan, Y. Wu, and J. V. Vadgama, "Obesity is associated with breast cancer in African-American women but not Hispanic women in South Los Angeles," *Cancer*, vol. 117, no. 16, pp. 3814–3823, 2011.

[44] S. Paliwal, R. C. Kovi, B. Nath, Y.-W. Chen, B. C. Lewis, and S. R. Grossman, "The alternative reading frame tumor suppressor antagonizes hypoxia-induced cancer cell migration via interaction with the COOH-terminal binding protein corepressor," *Cancer Research*, vol. 67, no. 19, pp. 9322–9329, 2007.

[45] G. Thomas, K. B. Jacobs, M. Yeager et al., "Multiple loci identified in a genome-wide association study of prostate cancer," *Nature Genetics*, vol. 40, no. 3, pp. 310–315, 2008.

14

Single High Intensity Focused Ultrasound Session as a Whole Gland Primary Treatment for Clinically Localized Prostate Cancer: 10-Year Outcomes

Ksenija Limani,[1] Fouad Aoun,[1,2] Serge Holz,[2] Marianne Paesmans,[3] Alexandre Peltier,[1,2] and Roland van Velthoven[1,2]

[1] *Department of Urology, Jules Bordet Institute, 1 Rue Héger-Bordet, 1000 Brussels, Belgium*
[2] *Université Libre de Bruxelles, 50 Franklin Roosevelt Avenue, 1050 Brussels, Belgium*
[3] *Department of Data Management, Jules Bordet Institute, 1 Rue Héger-Bordet, 1000 Brussels, Belgium*

Correspondence should be addressed to Fouad Aoun; fouad.aoun@bordet.be

Academic Editor: Katsuto Shinohara

Objectives. To assess the treatment outcomes of a single session of whole gland high intensity focused ultrasound (HIFU) for patients with localized prostate cancer (PCa). *Methods.* Response rates were defined using the Stuttgart and Phoenix criteria. Complications were graded according to the Clavien score. *Results.* At a median follow-up of 94months, 48 (44.4%) and 50 (46.3%) patients experienced biochemical recurrence for Phoenix and Stuttgart definition, respectively. The 5- and 10-year actuarial biochemical recurrence free survival rates were 57% and 40%, respectively. The 10-year overall survival rate, cancer specific survival rate, and metastasis free survival rate were 72%, 90%, and 70%, respectively. Preoperative high risk category, Gleason score, preoperative PSA, and postoperative nadir PSA were independent predictors of oncological failure. 24.5% of patients had self-resolving LUTS, 18.2% had urinary tract infection, and 18.2% had acute urinary retention. A grade 3b complication occurred in 27 patients. Pad-free continence rate was 87.9% and the erectile dysfunction rate was 30.8%. *Conclusion.* Single session HIFU can be alternative therapy for patients with low risk PCa. Patients with intermediate risk should be informed about the need of multiple sessions of HIFU and/or adjuvant treatments and HIFU performed very poorly in high risk patients.

1. Introduction

During the last decade, proactive screening for prostate cancer (PCa) led to a dramatic stage migration resulting in proportionally more men being diagnosed at early stages while the tumour is still organ confined [1]. Conventional established treatment options for organ confined PCa range from active surveillance to whole gland radical therapy [2]. Both radical prostatectomy (RP) and external-beam radiotherapy (EBRT) have undergone significant technical developments during the last decade and excellent long term cancer control data are available to support their clinical use [1]. However, these modalities are often associated with significant risk of treatment related complications that detrimentally affect quality of life [3, 4].

These facts have contributed to the development of "minimal invasive procedures" as an alternative option to standard therapies. Among these therapies, high intensity focused ultrasound (HIFU) emerged as a valid mini-invasive therapy for localised prostate cancer, using focused ultrasound to generate areas of intense heat to induce tissue necrosis. The ability of HIFU to achieve thermoablation of prostatic lesion was proven histologically on operative specimen [5], on MRI imaging [6], and on posttreatment biopsies [7, 8].

Oncological outcomes were first reported in 1995 [9] and 1996 [10] and subsequently the use of HIFU therapy has expanded. Nowadays, the available evidence on HIFU is comprised of case series with a significant overlap of patients among series. The median follow-up time is short with the longest series reporting data after a mean follow-up of 76.8 months [11, 12].

Another major problem is that most of the published case series included the results of retreatment in their efficacy rates. In the present single-centre study, we evaluated, at a median follow-up of 92 months, the oncological outcomes of single-session whole gland HIFU treatment of localised PCa in a unique case series of 110 patients treated between September 2001 and December 2012. The morbidity and urological after care were also analysed and discussed.

2. Patients and Methods

The study involved a cohort of 110 consecutive patients with clinically localized PCa primarily treated with whole gland HIFU at the Jules Bordet Institute between September 2001 and December 2012. Pooled prospectively collected data were retrospectively analyzed. Ethics approval in our institute covers the use of prospectively collected clinical information for clinical and prognostic studies.

Inclusion criteria were whole gland primary therapy with curative intent for localized PCa, prostate specific antigen (PSA) <20 ng/mL, clinical stage T1N0M0-T2N0M0, no previous radical therapy for PCa, and a follow-up >12 months. Baseline physical examination and PSA measurements were obtained for all patients. Extracapsular tumour extension and lymph node status were assessed using pelvic CT or MRI. Staging included a bone scan in patients with PSA ≥ 10 ng/mL, and laparoscopic lymphadenectomy was recommended in patients with PSA > 20 ng/mL. Exclusion criteria included clinically advanced PCa, evidence of metastatic or nodal disease on bone scan or cross-sectional imaging, prior significant rectal surgery, any contraindication for anaesthesia, and presence of prostatic calcification and cysts. All patients were unsuitable for surgery because of age, comorbidities, or patient refusal and were unwilling to undergo radiotherapy. All patients were treated by a single experienced surgeon, with Ablatherm HIFU devices (EDAP-TMS, Vaulx-en-Velin, France). From September 2001 to March 2006, patients were treated with the first commercially available device from Ablatherm (EDAP-Technomed, Lyon, France) and since April 2006 with Ablatherm Integrated Imaging (EDAP, Lyon, France). In our institution the upper volume limit for HIFU procedures is set to 40 cc and patients with prostates exceeding this threshold are offered androgen deprivation therapy (ADT) which was always discontinued at the time of therapy. All patients undergo a limited transurethral resection of prostate (TURP) at the end of the procedure, to prevent sloughing and acute urinary retention or prolonged need for indwelling catheter and to reduce the rate of urinary tract infection [5]. Complications were prospectively recorded and retrospectively graded according to the Clavien-Dindo score [13, 14]. Postoperatively, patients were followed with serial serum PSA determinations and DRE at 1, 3, 6, 12, 18, and 24 months and yearly thereafter. Oncological outcomes were evaluated using the D'Amico tumour recurrence risk group classification system [15]. Response rates were defined using the American Society for Therapeutic Radiology and Oncology (ASTRO)/Phoenix criteria (nadir + 2 ng/mL) (2005) [16]. Random systematic TRUS guided biopsies were offered only for a cause (phoenix criteria and/or suspicious DRE and/or PSA doubling time < 6 months). An individual PSA nadir was identified in each patient. PSA nadir was defined as the lowest PSA value reached during follow-up. Urinary functional outcomes were reported using physician reported rates. Stress incontinence was graduated according to Stamey into three grades [17]. Patients that were able to penetrate their partner without mechanical or pharmacological support were rated potent. Cause of death was identified from physician correspondence and all PCa specific deaths were verified. Overall QOL and costs were not reported in this study. The follow-up period was defined as the interval between HIFU treatment and last available monitoring data or the date of death. Only patients with complete data have been included in the final analysis (multivariate analysis, survival curves). A statistical analysis was performed with SPSS v.20 (IBM Corp., Armonk, NY, USA). Survival curves were based on the Kaplan-Meier method, and the log-rank test and a Cox regression model were used for univariate and multivariate analysis of the prognostic relevance of age, risk group, Gleason score, ADT, clinical stage, pretherapeutic PSA, and postoperative nadir PSA on biochemical recurrence, distant metastasis, and cancer specific survival. Actuarial survival rates were based on life table methods. A P value <0.05 was considered to indicate statistical significance.

3. Results

Baseline and tumour characteristics of the study population are summarized in Tables 1 and 2. Overall, a total of 110 patients (average age 76 years) were enrolled in this study with a median follow-up of 94 months. The mean (median) [range] PSA nadir was 0.55 ± 1.34 (0.71) [0–8.29] ng/mL and the mean (median) [range] time to achieve PSA nadir was 16.3 ± 8.2 (14.0) [4–46] weeks. A PSA nadir < 0.5 ng/mL was noted in 72/110 (65.5%) and 89/110 (80.9%) patients had a PSA nadir < 1 ng/mL. In spite of a good initial response to HIFU and a PSA nadir observation, two patients followed at distant centres were lost for evaluation and long term cancer control data were available for 108 patients (98.2%). During follow-up, 48/108 (44.4%) patients exhibited PSA elevation ≥2.00 ng/mL above nadir; they were offered a new set of bilateral biopsies, accordingly. Of the 35 (72.9%) patients who accepted control biopsy 22 were positive (62.9%). Of the 22 patients who experienced biochemical recurrence with a positive biopsy 12 patients were treated with a second HIFU session. Patients with negative biopsy or who refused biopsy were treated as follows: hormonal therapy (14 patients), second session HIFU (1 patient), and surveillance (11 patients). We evaluated retrospectively biochemical recurrence rate according to the definition of Stuttgart (nadir + 1.2 ng/mL): 50 (46.3%) patients experienced biochemical recurrence with a mean time to failure of 48 months.

Metastases were detected in 10 patients (seven with bone metastases and 3 with lymph node involvement) after PSA relapse including 6 patients with a positive biopsy, 2 patients with a negative biopsy, and 2 patients who refused control biopsy. 20 patients died during follow-up, of which 8 patients died of cancer specific cause. The 5- and 10-year actuarial

TABLE 1: Baseline and tumour characteristics of 110 patients with localized prostate cancer who were treated by a single session of high intensity focused ultrasound.

Mean age, years [range]	76.1 ± 6.2 [61–86]
Mean preoperative PSA, ng/mL [range]	12.1 ± 4.1 [0.55–49.0]
Mean prostate volume, mL [range]	29.3 ± 6.0 [18–39]
Hormone, *n* (%)	
Yes	37 (33.6)
No	73 (66.4)
Gleason score, *n* (%)	
≤6	69 (62.7)
=7	24 (21.8)
≥8	17 (15.5)
Stage, *n* (%)	
T1	51 (46.4)
T2	59 (53.6)
D'Amico risk group*, *N* (%)	
Low	40 (36.4)
Intermediate	49 (44.5)
High	21 (19.1)

*Risk group based on D'Amico definition (according to Stage, Gleason, and PSA).

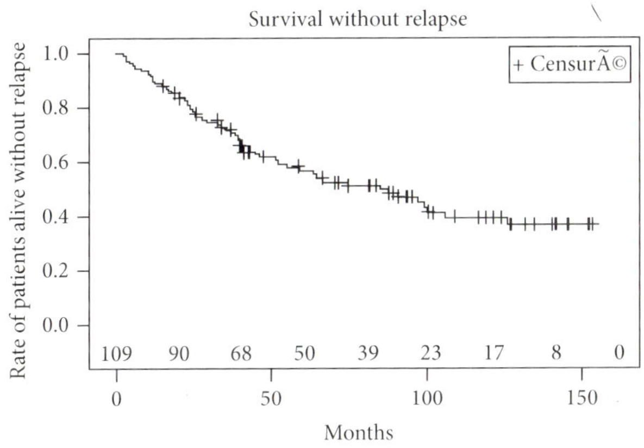

FIGURE 1: Kaplan-Meier curve of biochemical recurrence free survival using Phoenix definition (nadir + 2 ng/mL).

BRFS rates were 57% (CI 95%: 47–67%) and 40% (CI 95%: 29–51%), respectively (Figure 1). The median (range) time to oncological failure was 52 months (95% CI: 33–87 months). BRFS was significantly higher in patients in the low risk group compared to patients in the intermediate and high risk group (Figure 2). The 10-year estimated overall survival rate, cancer specific survival rate, and metastasis free survival rate were 72%, 90%, and 70%, respectively (Figures 3, 4, and 5). Preoperative high risk category, Gleason score, pPSA, and postoperative nadir PSA were independent predictors of oncological failure in univariate and multivariate analysis (Table 3).

The incidences of the most frequent complications were reported in Table 4. Regarding grade 1 and grade 2 complications, 27 patients (24.5%) had self-resolving hematuria and LUTS, 7 patients had storing LUTS treated by

TABLE 2: Intraoperative and postoperative results with high intensity focused ultrasound.

Anesthesia used	
Spinal anesthesia	109
General anesthesia	1
Ablatherm device	
EDAP-Technomed Ablatherm	59
Ablatherm Integrated Imaging	51
Preoperative complications	0
Concomitant TURP, *n* (%)	
Yes	79 (71.8)
No	31 (28.2)
Hospital stays in days, median (range)	4 (2–7)
Catheterization time in days, median (range)	6 (2–30)
Postoperative prostatic volume in mL, median (range)	14 (6–22)
Time to PSA nadir in weeks, mean (range)	16.3 ± 8.2 (4–46)
PSA nadir in ng/mL, mean (range)	0.55 ± 1.34 (0–8.29)
PSA < 0.5 ng/mL, *n* (%)	72 (65.5)
PSA 0.5–1 ng/mL, *n* (%)	17 (15.5)
PSA 1–4 ng/mL, *n* (%)	19 (17.2)
PSA > 4 ng/mL, *n* (%)	2 (1.8)
Follow-up in months, median (range)	94 (13–139)
Lost to follow-up, *n* (%)	2 (1.8)

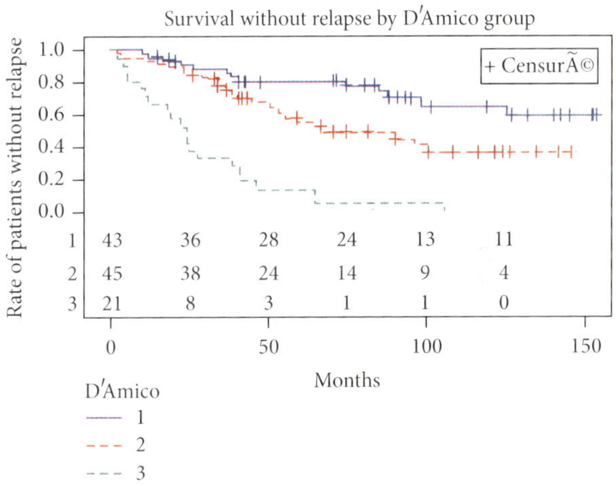

FIGURE 2: Kaplan-Meier curves of biochemical recurrence free survival using Phoenix definition (nadir + 2 ng/mL) according to D'Amico risk classification.

anticholinergics (6.4%), 4 patients had chronic pelvic pain, and 20 patients (18.2%) had urinary tract infection. A grade 3a complication occurred in 20 patients (18.2%) who had acute urinary retention. A grade 3b complication occurred in 26 patients who had bladder outlet obstruction or urethral stricture managed by optical urethrotomy and in one man (0.9%) who had developed a rectourethral fistula managed surgically. No patient presented any grade 4 or died from the procedure. Urinary functional outcomes were reported using physicians reported rates. Grade 1 stress urinary incontinence

TABLE 3: Univariate and multivariable analysis of factors affecting biochemical recurrence free survival in 108 patients.

	Univariate			Multivariate		
	OR	95% CI	*P* value	OR	95% CI	*P* value
Age (per 10 years)	0.95	0.51–1.76	0.87	—	—	—
Gleason score (<7; ≥7)	2.01	1.15–3.51	0.01	1.79	1.04–3.08	0.01
Prostate volume (per 10 mL)	1.29	0.74–2.22	0.37	—	—	—
Pretherapeutic PSA (per ng/mL)	1.06	1.04–1.09	<0.0001	1.08	1.05–1.11	<0.0001
PSA nadir (per ng/mL)	1.92	1.58–2.33	<0.0001	1.87	1.54–2.27	<0.0001
ADT before HIFU (yes v/s no)	1.56	0.92–2.62	0.1	—	—	—
D'Amico risk group (low v/s intermediate)	1.64	0.83–3.24	0.15	—	—	—
D'Amico risk group (low v/s high)	3.36	1.61–7.03	0.001	2.9	1.43–5.89	0.003

OR: odds ratio; CI: confidence interval; PSA: prostate-specific antigen; ADT: androgen deprivation therapy; HIFU: high intensity focused ultrasound.

TABLE 4: Adverse events.

	EDAP-Technomed Ablatherm (*N* = 59)	Ablatherm integrated imaging (*N* = 50)
Acute urinary retention (%)	15 (25.4%)	5 (10.0%)
Urinary tract infection (%)	16 (27.1%)	4 (8.0%)
Lower urinary tract Symptom (%)	16 (27.1%)	11 (22.0%)
Chronic pelvic pain (%)	4 (6.8%)	0 (0.0%)
Bladder outlet Obstruction (%)	18 (30.5%)	8 (16.0%)
Recto-Urethral Fistula (%)	1 (1.7%)	0 (0.0%)

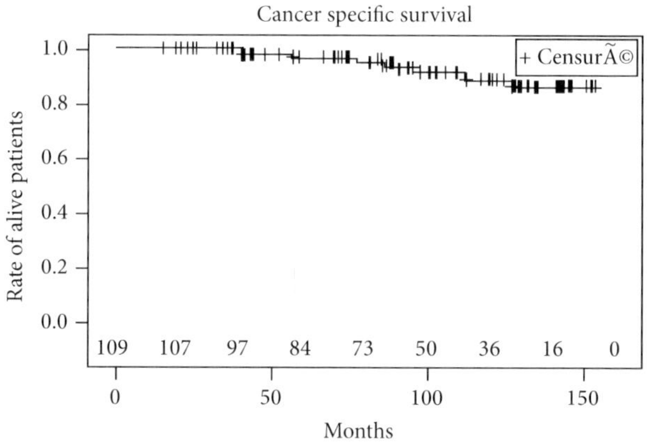

FIGURE 4: Cancer specific survival.

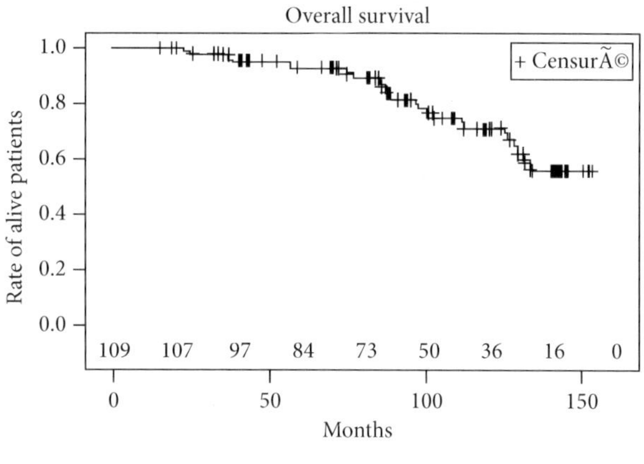

FIGURE 3: Overall survival.

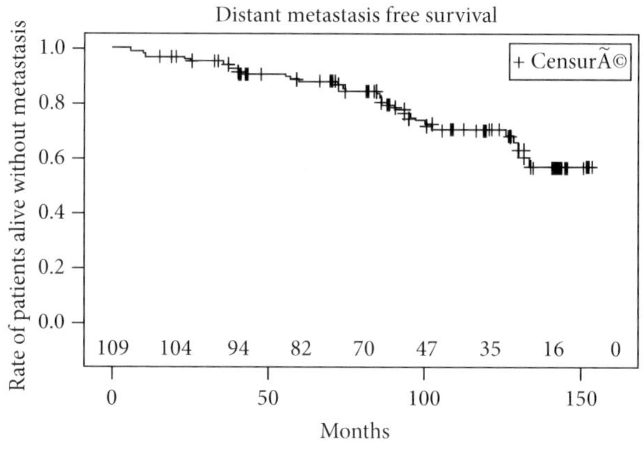

FIGURE 5: Distant metastasis free survival.

was reported in 8 patients (7.4%) and 5 patients (4.6%) had grade 2 stress urinary incontinence. The long term pad free continence rate was 87.9%. In preoperatively potent patients ($n = 68$), 7 men (10.3%) had documented post whole gland ablation erectile dysfunction (ED), 47 men (69.1%) had erections satisfactory for sexual intercourse with ($n = 16$) or without pharmacotherapy ($n = 31$), and data were lacking in 14 patients. The mean age of patients with postoperative ED was 77.3 years. If we consider the 14 patients with lacking data to have ED after treatment, the ED rate for this cohort post treatment would be 30.8% (21/68) and 45.6% (31/68) had erectile function sufficient for penetration without pharmacotherapy.

4. Discussion

Despite the fact that HIFU has been used in PCa for over 15 years [10], the European Association of Urology, the American Urological Association, and the National Comprehensive Cancer Network do not recommend the routine use of HIFU in the primary treatment of PCa. Disapproval is mainly due to the absence of prospective randomised controlled trials comparing HIFU with conventional treatment options and to the paucity of long term oncological follow-up data. Long term results on the efficacy and safety of HIFU have rarely been reported [12–20]. In the present study, only patients with a minimal follow-up of 1 year were included. With a median follow-up of 92 months, a well-founded oncologic, safety, and functional evaluation of whole gland ablation HIFU as a therapy for PCa was possible.

Assessment of oncologic efficacy was performed by serial PSA testing and random systematic TRUS guided biopsies were offered only for a cause in order to minimise burden on the patient. Furthermore, performance of systematic biopsies in all patients may increase the cancer detection rates during follow-up but the clinical implication of such a protocol is unknown because it may simply reveal small foci of low grade low volume PCa. In our opinion, the only valid endpoint with a follow-up >1 year is the PSA nadir and the biopsy should be offered routinely in case of a PSA elevation, a suspicious lesion on DRE and/or multiparametric MRI and/or contrast ultrasound. As a surrogate, although PSA testing is accepted as a valid outcome in standard therapies, the clinical utility of PSA kinetics in HIFU is yet to be determined. We acknowledge that the use of Phoenix criteria is a shortcoming of the present analysis and the need for a specific definition of treatment failure to evaluate the clinical outcome after HIFU.

In our series, there was a 95.4% decrease in PSA levels from baseline and a PSA nadir <0.5 ng/mL was noted in 65.5% of patients which indicate successful ablation of the prostate. The early achievement (between 3 and 6 months) of a PSA nadir not only provides immediate feedback on treatment efficacy but also identifies quickly patients with residual cancer. This rapid proof of a response to the treatment provides also stringent information about potential cure. The maintenance of a PSA < 0.5 ng/mL was noted in 50% (36/72) of these patients at 10 years of follow-up; only 12.5% (9/72) of these patients experienced biochemical failure according to the Phoenix criteria during the follow-up. The PSA nadir was, in our study, an independent predictor factor of oncologic failure (cancer specific survival, BRFS) in multivariable analysis. The PSA nadir, in most contemporary series, was found to be a surrogate for predicting treatment failure [21, 22]; however, a cut-off has not been yet standardized [23]. Furthermore, PSA nadir correlated strongly, in these studies, with preoperative baseline PSA and prostate volume. In our study, preoperative PSA was also an independent predictor factor to estimate the risk of treatment failure. This could be explained by the high likelihood of extraprostatic disease with increasing PSA level. Larger prostate volume remnants will produce a greater amount of PSA. In our study, cytoreductive ADT and the high percentage of TURP had led to small prostate remnants (mean 14 cc) and the prostate volume was not found to be an independent predictor of treatment failure.

A durable response was also seen in 68% of patients with low risk disease at 10 years of follow-up. All patients classified as D'Amico high risk experienced biochemical recurrence and were treated by second HIFU, salvage treatment, or palliative ADT. Intermediate risk disease presented an unacceptable risk of biochemical relapse when treated with a single session of HIFU (BCR free survival of 40% at 10 years) but with HIFU retreatment a biochemical recurrence free survival of 53% was achieved at 10 years of follow-up. HIFU delivered with intention to treat performs very poorly in high risk groups and should be indicated only for patients with localised PCa at low and intermediate risk of progression. Patients with intermediate risk of progression should be informed about the further need of multiple sessions of HIFU and/or adjuvant treatments. Some authors advocated HIFU plus ADT as an alternative to ADT plus EBRT in high risk PCa [24]. ADT, in the presented series, was not shown to be an independent predictor of oncologic outcomes but it was given for a short period of time, in a small percentage of patients, and according to prostate volume and not to the risk of progression. In routine practice, these prognostic factors should serve to the establishment of nomograms and would be useful for the clinician in informing patient regarding the likelihood of requiring salvage treatment. HIFU as a minimal invasive procedure appears to be one of the most attractive options for the treatment of localized PCa because of its low morbidity rates [21]. In our study, early self-resolving LUTS due to sloughing of necrotic tissue from the coagulated gland were the most common complications. Elimination of debris through micturition and swelling of the prostate due to thermal injury were the principle cause of acute urinary retention. Another important complication linked also to necrotic tissue is the high risk of urinary tract infection. Bladder outlet obstruction and urethral stricture are two long term complications occurring in 3.6% to 24.5% of patients [12–22] (24% in our study). The introduction of real time monitoring had dramatically decreased the incidence rate and the severity of these complications. Our study shows a good gastrointestinal tolerance with no late onset toxicity and no rectal toxicities were reported when real time monitoring was introduced. An urethrorectal fistula occurred in only one patient in a retreated gland with no monitoring of the rectal wall. Experience with the procedure, the addition of a cooling system, and safety monitoring with good margins has dramatically decreased the incidence of fistula which now ranges between 0.5 and 1.2% [21]. The procedure could possibly be delivered in an ambulatory care setting; the long stay of 4 days in our series is related to local reimbursement practice, preoperative anaesthetic evaluation, and transurethral partial resection of the prostate. Stress urinary incontinence occurred in 12% of patients, which is comparable to the rates reported in the literature [22–25].

In the current study, 30.8% of initially potent patients exhibited erectile dysfunction after HIFU therapy witch is in the range of 20–49.8% of the rates reported in the literature [26]. Generally the preservation of the lateral edges of the prostate permits to spare erectile function but should always be balanced with the risk of oncologic failure. Recently, we have reported better stress urinary incontinence and erectile function rates with hemi-ablation HIFU but validated questionnaire and further experience is therefore needed to confirm this important conclusion [27].

To our knowledge, our study is the first to report on a unique cohort of patients primarily treated by a single session of whole gland ablation HIFU for a clinically localised PCa with a median follow-up of 92 months. Moreover, a very limited number of patients were lost to follow up (1.8%) and all patients were treated by the same experienced surgeon.

Meanwhile we acknowledge several limitations to our study. First, the safety, functional, and oncologic outcomes are the results of a single centre with a long experience with whole gland HIFU and cannot be generalized. The outcomes could be variable in less experienced hands because HIFU is a dynamic therapy with real time feedback which is difficult to master while assessing quality control [28]. Second, the study reported retrospectively on a small cohort of patients. Well-designed, multicenter, prospective, and randomized controlled studies are required to assess collateral damage, functional and oncologic outcomes. Third, technological improvements (real time monitoring) and changes in surgical protocol (TURP, prophylactic antibiotics) may have confounded some of the outcome analyses. Fourth, a direct comparison of outcomes with other conventional PCa therapies is not possible due to differences in selection criteria, study design, and adjuvant/salvage therapies. Fifth, bias could have been introduced by including heterogeneous patient population with variations in prognostic factors and neoadjuvant ADT but the latter is unlikely to confound PSA outcomes especially when it is given for a short duration and the follow-up is long. In addition, neoadjuvant ADT was not a significant predictor of survival in the univariate analysis.

5. Conclusions

Our study, with a median follow-up of 92 months, has provided evidence that HIFU can be an alternative treatment for patients with low risk localised PCa who are not eligible or refuse conventional therapy. Patients with intermediate risk should be informed about the further need of multiple sessions of HIFU and/or adjuvant treatments. HIFU delivered with intention to treat performed very poorly in high risk patients, and those patients should probably be offered a more conventional treatment, such as radical surgery or radiation therapy. Patients should also be informed that whole gland HIFU ablation, though being a mini-invasive energy based modality, has a side effect profile that cannot be negligible and is offered in a study setting. Preoperative high risk category, Gleason score, pretherapeutic PSA, and postoperative nadir PSA were independent predictors of oncological failure and should serve the establishment of nomograms and could be useful for the clinician in informing patient regarding the likelihood of requiring salvage treatment.

References

[1] A. Heidenreich, J. Bellmunt, M. Bolla et al., "EAU guidelines on prostate cancer. Part 1: screening, diagnosis, and treatment of clinically localised disease," *European Urology*, vol. 59, no. 1, pp. 61–71, 2011.

[2] Y. Shao, P. C. Albertsen, C. B. Roberts et al., "Risk profiles and treatment patterns among men diagnosed as having prostate cancer and a prostate-specific antigen level below 4.0 ng/mL," *Archives of Internal Medicine*, vol. 170, no. 14, pp. 1256–1261, 2010.

[3] S. A. Boorjian, J. A. Eastham, M. Graefen et al., "A critical analysis of the long-term impact of radical prostatectomy on cancer control and function outcomes," *European Urology*, vol. 61, no. 4, pp. 664–675, 2012.

[4] M. J. Resnick, T. Koyama, K. Fan et al., "Long-term functional outcomes after treatment for localized prostate cancer," *The New England Journal of Medicine*, vol. 368, no. 5, pp. 436–445, 2013.

[5] H. P. Beerlage, G. J. L. H. van Leenders, G. O. N. Oosterhof et al., "High-intensity focused ultrasound (HIFU) followed after one to two weeks by radical retropubic prostatectomy: results of a prospective study," *Prostate*, vol. 39, no. 1, pp. 41–46, 1999.

[6] L. Dickinson, Y. Hu, H. U. Ahmed et al., "Image-directed, tissue-preserving focal therapy of prostate cancer: a feasibility study of a novel deformable magnetic resonance-ultrasound (MR-US) registration system," *BJU International*, vol. 112, no. 5, pp. 594–601, 2013.

[7] K. Biermann, R. Montironi, A. Lopez-Beltran, S. Zhang, and L. Cheng, "Histopathological findings after treatment of prostate cancer using high-intensity focused ultrasound (HIFU)," *Prostate*, vol. 70, no. 11, pp. 1196–1200, 2010.

[8] P. Ryan, A. Finelli, N. Lawrentschuk et al., "Prostatic needle biopsies following primary high intensity focused ultrasound (HIFU) therapy for prostatic adenocarcinoma: histopathological features in tumour and non-tumour tissue," *Journal of Clinical Pathology*, vol. 65, no. 8, pp. 729–734, 2012.

[9] S. Madersbacher, M. Pedevilla, L. Vingers, M. Susani, and M. Marberger, "Effect of high-intensity focused ultrasound on human prostate cancer in vivo," *Cancer Research*, vol. 55, no. 15, pp. 3346–3351, 1995.

[10] A. Gelet, J. Y. Chapelon, R. Bouvier et al., "Treatment of prostate cancer with transrectal focused ultrasound: early clinical experience," *European Urology*, vol. 29, no. 2, pp. 174–183, 1996.

[11] A. Blana, F. J. Murat, B. Walter et al., "First analysis of the long-term results with transrectal HIFU in patients with localised prostate cancer," *European Urology*, vol. 53, no. 6, pp. 1194–1203, 2008.

[12] S. Crouzet, J. Y. Chapelon, O. Rouviére et al., "Whole-gland ablation of localized prostate cancer with high-intensity focused ultrasound: oncologic outcomes and morbidity in 1002 patients," *European Urology*, vol. 65, no. 5, pp. 907–914, 2013.

[13] D. Dindo, N. Demartines, and P. Clavien, "Classification of surgical complications: A new proposal with evaluation in a cohort of 6336 patients and results of a survey," *Annals of Surgery*, vol. 240, no. 2, pp. 205–213, 2004.

[14] D. Mitropoulos, W. Artibani, M. Graefen, M. Remzi, M. Rouprêt, and M. Truss, "Reporting and grading of complications after urologic surgical procedures: an ad hoc EAU guidelines panel assessment and recommendations," *European Urology*, vol. 61, no. 2, pp. 341–349, 2012.

[15] A. V. D'Amico, R. Whittington, S. Bruce Malkowicz et al., "Biochemical outcome after radical prostatectomy, external beam

radiation therapy, or interstitial radiation therapy for clinically localized prostate cancer," *Journal of the American Medical Association*, vol. 280, no. 11, pp. 969–974, 1998.

[16] M. Roach III, G. Hanks, and H. Thames Jr., "Defining biochemical failure following radiation therapy with or without hormonal therapy in men with clinically localized prostate cancer: recommendation of the RTOG-ASTRO Phoenix Consensus Conference," *International Journal of Radiation Oncology∗Biology∗Physics*, vol. 65, pp. 965–974, 2006.

[17] T. A. Stamey, "Endoscopic suspension of the vesical neck for urinary incontinence," *Surgery Gynecology and Obstetrics*, vol. 136, no. 4, pp. 547–554, 1973.

[18] T. Uchida, S. Shoji, M. Nakano et al., "Transrectal high-intensity focused ultrasound for the treatment of localized prostate cancer: eight-year experience," *International Journal of Urology*, vol. 16, no. 11, pp. 881–886, 2009.

[19] D. Pfeiffer, J. Berger, and A. J. Gross, "Single application of high-intensity focused ultrasound as a first-line therapy for clinically localized prostate cancer: 5-year outcomes," *BJU International*, vol. 110, no. 11, pp. 1702–1708, 2012.

[20] T. Ripert, M. Azémar, J. Ménard et al., "Six years' experience with high-intensity focused ultrasonography for prostate cancer: oncological outcomes using the new "Stuttgart" definition for biochemical failure," *BJU International*, vol. 107, no. 12, pp. 1899–1905, 2011.

[21] E. R. Cordeiro, X. Cathelineau, S. Thüroff, M. Marberger, S. Crouzet, and J. J. M. C. H. de La Rosette, "High-intensity focused ultrasound (HIFU) for definitive treatment of prostate cancer," *BJU International*, vol. 110, no. 9, pp. 1228–1242, 2012.

[22] A. Blana, J. Hierl, S. Rogenhofer et al., "Factors predicting for formation of bladder outlet obstruction after high-intensity focused ultrasound in treatment of localized prostate cancer," *Urology*, vol. 71, no. 5, pp. 863–867, 2008.

[23] T. Uchida, R. O. Illing, P. J. Cathcart, and M. Emberton, "To what extent does the prostate-specific antigen nadir predict subsequent treatment failure after transrectal high-intensity focused ultrasound therapy for presumed localized adenocarcinoma of the prostate?" *BJU International*, vol. 98, no. 3, pp. 537–539, 2006.

[24] V. Ficarra, S. Z. Antoniolli, G. Novara et al., "Short-term outcome after high-intensity focused ultrasound in the treatment of patients with high-risk prostate cancer," *BJU International*, vol. 98, no. 6, pp. 1193–1198, 2006.

[25] L. Poissonnier, J. Chapelon, O. Rouvière et al., "Control of prostate cancer by transrectal HIFU in 227 patients," *European Urology*, vol. 51, no. 2, pp. 381–387, 2007.

[26] X. Rebillard, M. Soulié, E. Chartier-Kastler et al., "High-intensity focused ultrasound in prostate cancer; a systematic literature review of the French Association of Urology," *BJU International*, vol. 101, no. 10, pp. 1205–1213, 2008.

[27] R. van Velthoven, F. Aoun, K. Limani, K. Narahari, M. Lemort, and A. Peltier, "Primary zonal high intensity focused ultrasound for prostate cancer: results of a prospective phase IIa feasibility study," *Prostate Cancer*, vol. 2014, Article ID 756189, 6 pages, 2014.

[28] D. Baumunk, C. Andersen, U. Heile et al., "High-intensity focussed ultrasound in low-risk prostate cancer—oncological outcome and postinterventional quality of life of an inexperienced therapy centre in comparison with an experienced therapy centre," *Aktuelle Urologie*, vol. 44, no. 4, pp. 285–292, 2013.

15

Long-Term Efficacy and Tolerability of Abdominal Once-Yearly Histrelin Acetate Subcutaneous Implants in Patients with Advanced Prostate Cancer

Sean Woolen,[1] Cameron Holzmeyer,[1] Emily Nesbitt,[1] and Paul F. Siami[2]

[1] *Research Institute of Deaconess Clinic, 421 Chestnut Street, Evansville, IN 47713, USA*
[2] *Department of Urology, Deaconess Clinic, 421 Chestnut Street, Evansville, IN 47713, USA*

Correspondence should be addressed to Sean Woolen; swoolen@iupui.edu

Academic Editor: James L. Gulley

Objectives. Long-term assessment of the efficacy and tolerability of subcutaneous abdominal histrelin acetate implants that have been inserted for more than two years. *Materials and Methods.* Retrospective data collected over a six-year period at a single center from charts of 113 patients who received the subcutaneous abdominal histrelin acetate implant. *Results.* Following insertion of the first implant, 92.1% and 91.8% of patients had a serum testosterone level of ≤30 ng/dL at 24 and 48 weeks, respectively. Serum testosterone levels remained at <30 ng/dL for 96% of patients at two years and for 100% of patients at 3, 4, and 5 years. The testosterone levels remained significantly less than baseline ($P < 0.05$). Six patients (5.3%) had androgen-independent progression when followed up on the long term, increasing the mean serum PSA at 3, 4, and 5 years to 35.0 μg/L ($n = 22$), 30.7 μg/L ($n = 13$), and 132.9 μg/L ($n = 8$), respectively. The mean serum PSA was significantly greater than baseline during these years ($P < 0.05$). Eight patients (7.1%) experienced minor, but not serious, adverse events from the histrelin acetate. *Conclusion.* Subcutaneous abdominal histrelin acetate implants are an effective long-term and well-tolerated administration method for treating patients with advanced prostate cancer.

1. Introduction

Prostate cancer is a leading cancer among men in the United States (US). The American Cancer Society estimates that, in 2014, there will be over 233,000 new cases of prostate cancer (representing 27% of new cancer cases in men in the US) and over 29,480 deaths caused by the disease (representing 10% of cancer-related deaths) [1]. However, despite the high prevalence and death rates associated with prostate cancer, survival statistics are favorable for patients; the 5-year survival rate of prostate cancer has reached 99.8%, and the cause of death in the majority (87.4%) of patients is due to other disease etiologies [2]. These favorable survival statistics can be attributed to the slow progression of prostate adenocarcinoma as well as its therapeutic management. Currently, disease management options available for low-stage prostate cancer include active surveillance, radical prostatectomy, radiotherapy, and cryotherapy [3].

The management of metastatic and high-risk locally advanced prostate cancer often includes adjuvant therapy with androgen deprivation therapy (ADT) [4]. Testosterone stimulates prostate cancer growth and decreasing androgen hormone levels may slow disease progression [5]. A serum testosterone level <35–50 ng/dL is considered adequate for patients with prostate cancer [6]. The initiation of ADT should be decided individually for each patient based on risks and benefits of treatment [7]. ADT may be achieved surgically (bilateral orchiectomy) or by medical means, including the administration of luteinizing hormone-releasing hormone (LHRH) antagonist or agonist [5, 6, 8].

LHRH agonists are the mainstay therapy for patients with advanced prostate cancer [9]. Following the initial dose, the LHRH agonist stimulates Leydig cells within the interstitium of the gonads to cause a transient increase in testosterone level referred to as the flare phenomenon [5, 10]. Because of the flare phenomenon, LHRH agonist is typically started with an antiandrogen medication, which is subsequently stopped approximately 1 to 3 weeks after commencing therapy. After 1 to 3 weeks, LHRH receptors become desensitized and castration level of testosterone is achieved [5, 10]. LHRH agonists are available in the US as leuprolide, goserelin acetate, triptorelin acetate, and histrelin acetate.

The LHRH agonist histrelin acetate is the only available sustained-release hydrogel implant for once-yearly administration [11]. The once-yearly implant allows patients to receive fewer cycles of implanting and replanting to maintain continuous ADT therapy. The histrelin acetate implant is 3.5 cm long, is 3 mm in diameter, and is administered subcutaneously into the inner aspect of the upper arm or abdomen [12, 13]. The inner aspect of the upper arm can clinically be difficult for the surgeon as it is a mobile insertion site and difficult for elderly patients limited by strength/arthritis to maintain the necessary abducted and extended arm position. Thus, the arm compared to the abdomen site is more difficult for surgeon and is less tolerated by patients.

The long-term efficacy and tolerability of the once-yearly histrelin implant via arm insertion have previously been reported, but the abdomen insertion site has not yet been followed up on the long term to our knowledge. In the pivotal arm implant study, which consisted of an open-label, single-arm study in 138 patients with advanced adenocarcinoma, >99% of patients were observed to have reduced testosterone (<50 ng/dL) during a 52-week period [13]. In an extension of this clinical trial, testosterone levels were maintained at <50 ng/dL for up to 234 weeks in patients who received once-yearly histrelin acetate implants [14]. In a single center retrospective chart review, two-year efficacy and tolerability were demonstrated in 64 patients receiving abdominal histrelin acetate implants; testosterone levels were maintained at <50 ng/dL for 96 weeks in these patients [12]. Thus, long-term efficacy in the arm implantation site and two-year efficacy for the abdominal implant have been observed.

The long-term efficacy of histrelin acetate implants in the abdomen has not been formally evaluated. This study is an extension of the original retrospective chart review of the abdominal implant by Siami and colleagues [12]; eligible patients from the original retrospective chart review as well as patients receiving implants since the last retrospective review were evaluated. The primary objective of this extension study is to assess the long-term efficacy and tolerability of abdominal histrelin implants that have been placed for more than two years. This study is important clinically because it will allow evidence guided abdominal insertion of the histrelin acetate implant for five years, allowing physicians and patients to utilize benefits of the abdominal insertion site.

2. Materials and Methods

2.1. Subjects and Treatment. Data were collected retrospectively, at a single center during June 2007 to August 2013, from charts of all patients who received the histrelin acetate implant abdominally. Out of 113 patients in this study, 64 were followed up from the original chart review [12] and 49 new patients were added to the study. Patients included in the analysis were aged ≥45 years, were diagnosed with prostate cancer, and were deemed appropriate candidates for ADT. Patients receiving a shorter duration implant with leuprolide acetate or goserelin acetate for less than a year were included in the study. Patients who received prior LHRH antagonist were excluded from the study.

Patients were administered histrelin acetate using a sterile, diffusion-controlled reservoir drug delivery system (VANTAS; Endo Pharmaceuticals, Chadds Ford, PA, USA). The implant contains a histrelin acetate (50 mg) drug core inside a nonbiodegradable cylindrical hydrogel reservoir and releases the drug at ~50 μg/day [11]. During an aseptic office-based surgical procedure, the histrelin acetate implant was inserted subcutaneously into the abdominal area, approximately two fingerbreadths below the costal margins in the midaxillary (nipple) line using the insertion device supplied with the implant.

2.2. Ethics. The study was reviewed and found to be compliant with the Deaconess Health System Research Oversight and Privacy Committee policy. Under the NIH HIPAA Privacy Rule, investigators of the study signed a Limited Data Set Use Agreement in order to perform a retrospective review of patients receiving an abdominal histrelin acetate implant. The investigators of this study abide by good clinical practice and regulations in the current revision of the Declaration of Helsinki.

2.3. Statistics. Qualitative data from patient characteristics were presented as the number of patients and the percentage of the total population. Quantitative data were summarized using descriptive statistics including mean and standard errors of the mean. Continuous data with testosterone and PSA were analyzed with a standard t-test in the statistical software SAS.

3. Results

3.1. Patient Characteristics. Out of 64 patients from the original chart review, 39 received a second implant, 28 received a third implant, 17 received a fourth implant, and 10 received a fifth implant. A total of 25 patients died after five years, 24 had explantation, five were lost to follow-up, and one stopped treatment due to financial reasons. Out of the 49 new patients, 30 received a second implant, 11 had explantation, seven were lost to follow-up, and one died. Of the individuals who had explantation, the majority of patients decided to switch to intermittent therapy after consulting with a urologist regarding similar efficacy of intermittent and continuous therapy; some had explantation due to decreased libido, and minimal explanted due to experiencing hot flashes/not feeling well. Patient deaths were judged to be unrelated to histrelin acetate implant use.

3.2. Demographics. Baseline characteristics of patients according to the chart review were recorded as age, ethnicity, and prior medications. The mean (± standard error of the mean (SEM)) age was 74.91 (±0.98) years. Out of the 100 patients for whom race was recorded, 90 (90.9%) were

Table 1: Summary of baseline demographics.

Demographics	Mean
Age	74.9
Testosterone (ng/dL)	106.6
PSA (μg/L)	12.1
Demographics	Percent
Caucasian	90.9
African American	8.1
Hispanic	1.0
Testosterone ≤ 30 ng/dL	48.5
PSA ≥ 5 μg/L	55.7
Previous LHRH agonist	44.9

Caucasians, eight (8.1%) were African Americans, and one (1.0%) was Hispanic. Almost half of the patients (52/114, 44.9%) had been treated with LHRH agonist therapy prior to administration of the histrelin acetate implant; the most common LHRH agonist was leuprolide acetate. Among patients with available serum prostate-specific antigen (PSA) levels prior to the administration of the histrelin acetate implant (97/113), the mean PSA level was 12.1 μg/L, and 55.7% (54/97) of patients had PSA levels ≥5 μg/L. Among patients with available serum testosterone levels prior to the administration of the histrelin acetate implant (33/113), the mean serum testosterone level was 106.6 ng/dL and 48.5% (16/33) of patients had testosterone levels ≤30 ng/dL. Patients in the chart review population who had received prior short acting LHRH agonist therapy received the histrelin acetate implant during the prescribed end period of their prior LHRH agonist administration, and the length of time ranged from 3 months to 1 year of treatment; continued LHRH agonist therapy was indicated for all of these patients. The demographic information is summarized in Table 1.

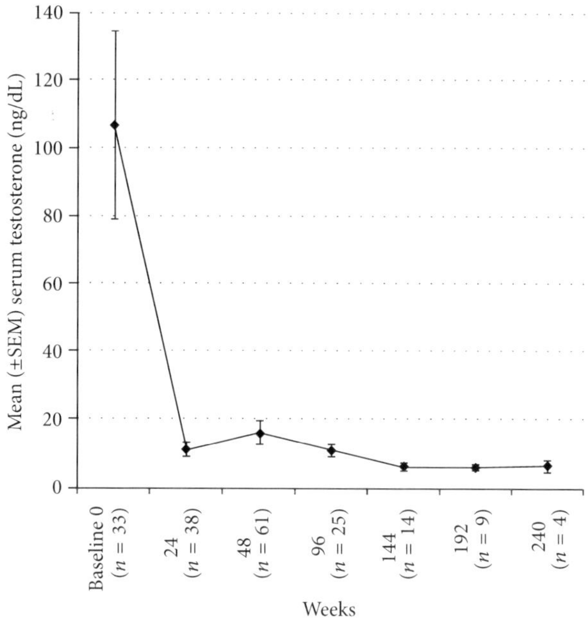

Figure 1: Mean serum testosterone levels (ng/dL) in patients after receiving once-yearly histrelin acetate implants for 240 weeks. The error bars represent the standard error of the mean (SEM).

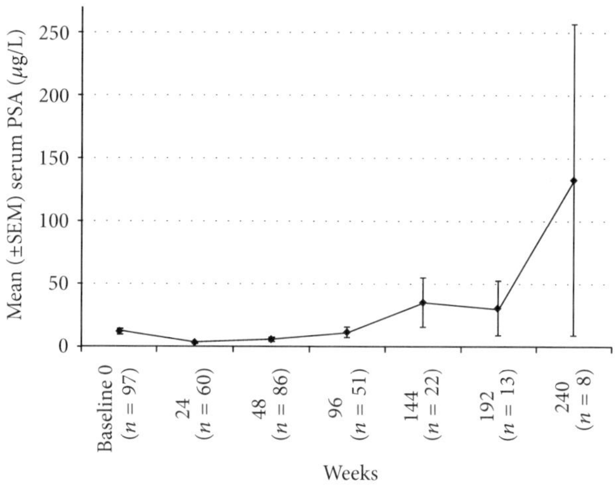

Figure 2: Mean serum prostate-specific antigen (PSA, μg/L) levels in patients after receiving once-yearly histrelin acetate implants for 240 weeks. The error bars represent the standard error of the mean (SEM).

3.3. Efficacy. Following abdominal insertion of the initial implant, the mean serum testosterone level was 11.1 ng/dL at 24 weeks ($n = 38$) and 16.0 ng/dL at 48 weeks ($n = 61$, Figure 1). The percentage of patients with a serum testosterone level ≤30 ng/dL was 92.1% (35/38 patients) at 24 weeks and 91.8% (56/61 patients) at 48 weeks. In addition, the mean serum PSA level decreased to 3.2 μg/L at 24 weeks ($n = 60$) and 5.6 μg/L at 48 weeks ($n = 86$, Figure 2). Both PSA and testosterone levels were significantly less than baseline ($P < 0.05$) at 24 and 48 weeks.

Continued long-term efficacy was seen in patients who had received second, third, and fourth implants at 5 years (Figure 1). The serum testosterone level remained <30 ng/dL for 96% (24/25) of patients at two years and 100% of patients at 3 years (14/14), 4 years (9/9), and 5 years (4/4). The mean testosterone levels for years 2–5 were 11.2 ng/dL, 6.2 ng/dL, 5.9 ng/dL, and 6.5 ng/dL, respectively (Figure 1). Testosterone levels remained significantly less than baseline during years 2–5 ($P < 0.05$). Six patients had androgen-independent progression of their disease at 144 weeks ($n = 2$), 192 weeks ($n = 3$), and 240 weeks ($n = 1$). The mean serum PSA level at 2, 3, 4, and 5 years was 11.3 μg/L ($n = 51$), 35.0 μg/L ($n = 22$), 30.7 μg/L ($n = 13$), and 132.9 μg/L ($n = 8$, Figure 2), respectively. The mean serum PSA level at 2 years was not significantly different compared to baseline ($P = 0.43$); however, the mean serum PSA was significantly greater than baseline at years 3, 4, and 5 ($P < 0.05$). The median serum PSA remained <1 μg/L for all 5 years.

3.4. Safety. Ten patients experienced difficulties with their implants during the retrospective chart review. At the time of reimplantation, the previous implant could not be located for removal in four patients. In another four patients, we clinically decided not to remove their previous implants. In one patient, the implant was reinserted after unintended expulsion less than one month after insertion. Subsequent clinical follow-up on this patient indicated maintenance of androgen suppression.

Eight patients experienced the following adverse events: redness and irritation around the implantation site (n = 1); pain at the implantation site 1 week after implantation, which is considered to be caused by muscle strain and is unrelated to the implant (n = 1); reactions to suture material (n = 2); and replacement of the implant due to erosion through the skin (n = 4). Drug related adverse effects were reported in 15% (17/113) of patients who experienced minor hot flashes, defined as tolerable/infrequent, and are consistent with patients undergoing ADT with an LHRH agonist. Twenty-six patients included in the chart review passed away after more than 5 years of evaluation; none of the deaths were related to histrelin acetate implant use.

4. Discussion

There is clinical interest in determining the long-term suitability of the abdomen as an insertion site for the VANTAS implant because of benefits to both the patient and the surgeon. From a surgeon's standpoint, the abdominal site is immobile, contains good anatomical landmarks, and is generally less vascular. Patients better tolerate the abdominal insertion site because it does not require strength/mobility of the shoulder joint to maintain the abducted and extended position; there is less positional risk as proximal arm insertion can cause irritation by deodorants/soaps/sweat and distal arm insertion can cause interferences from flexion/extension, and finally patients can easily visualize the abdominal site to evaluate for postprocedure wound changes. Our primary objective of this study was met because we were able to observe long-term efficacy and tolerability of the abdominal histrelin acetate subcutaneous implant used for prostate cancer management. The study's long-term data were consistent with the results from previous chart reviews regarding histrelin acetate abdominal implants and also the pivotal and extension study of the histrelin acetate arm implant [12–14].

The reviewed population in this study was similar to the population enrolled in a previous chart review, which was conducted to evaluate the abdominal implant, as well as the pivotal clinical trial and extension study, which evaluated the efficacy of histrelin acetate arm implants. In the current study, the mean patient age was 74.9 years and the percentage of Caucasian men was 90.9%. A major difference between the clinical trials of the arm implant and abdominal implant was that approximately 46% of patients in the current chart review received LHRH agonist. The clinical trials conducted by Schlegel et al. and Shore et al. to evaluate patients with arm implants excluded those who received previous ADT [13, 14].

In the current chart review, we demonstrated that the administration of the histrelin acetate implant subcutaneously into the abdomen reduced mean serum testosterone below castration levels (<50 ng/dL) for 24, 48, and 96 weeks. Data from the expanded chart review in the original abdominal implant study had mean serum testosterone values of 11.1, 16.0, and 11.2 ng/dL at 24, 48, and 96 weeks, respectively. These results are similar to the previously reported values by Siami and colleagues, who evaluated abdominal histrelin acetate subcutaneous implants. The mean serum testosterone value for 64 patients was 15.0 ng/dL at 24 weeks. In the study by Schlegel and colleagues, histrelin acetate implants were inserted for a similar duration of 52 weeks in the arm [13]. Schlegel et al. found that, in 134 patients, >99% of patients maintained chemical castration levels throughout the 52-week study duration [13].

In individuals with advanced prostate cancer, continuous long-term ADT may be clinically important. In this current chart review, we demonstrated that abdominal once-yearly histrelin acetate subcutaneous implants reduced mean serum testosterone below castration levels for 144, 192, and 240 weeks. Furthermore, the mean serum testosterone concentration remained <7 ng/dL with successive yearly cycles of insertion and removal of the abdominal implant during measurements (i.e., at 144, 192, and 240 weeks). These results are also similar to those of the study by Shore et al. In the study conducted by Shore et al., the mean serum testosterone concentration remained at <20 ng/dL for successive yearly cycles of insertion and removal for 234 weeks [14].

In our expanded chart review, a corresponding decrease in serum PSA level with testosterone level was observed in patients who had received the abdominal histrelin acetate implant during the first year. The mean serum PSA level was 3.2 and 5.6 during 24 and 48 weeks. Similar decreases were observed in both Siami et al. and Schlegel et al. [12, 13].

As expected, the natural progression of prostate cancer occurred with androgen-independent progression (AIP). AIP is defined as three consecutive increases in PSA levels after nadir. In the present study, six patients at 144 (n = 2), 192 (n = 3), and 240 weeks (n = 1) had AIP. Therefore, the mean serum PSA values increased above baseline to 35.0, 30.7, and 132.9 ng/dL during 144, 192, and 240 weeks, respectively. A similar progression in PSA levels was observed by Shore et al. Out of 104 patients, seven discontinued the study due to increasing PSA levels and <10% of the remaining patients experienced disease progression.

Abdominal administration of histrelin acetate was well tolerated by patients represented by the 5-year chart review and only minor adverse events were reported. Adverse events included insertion site reactions, hot flashes, and erosion of old implants through the skin. These adverse events were similar to those previously reported with the insertion of histrelin acetate implants [12–14].

The study encountered some limitations with the retrospective design. We were not able to evaluate patients' preference for the abdominal implant compared to the arm implant with a survey. Almost half of the patients (44.9%) received treatment with LHRH agonist prior to beginning the abdominal histrelin acetate yearly implant, which may confound mean testosterone levels, as patients do not recover testosterone levels immediately after stopping an agonist. Finally, the reason for patients being lost to follow-up could not be determined. Future prospective studies could help clarify some of these confounding factors in our study.

5. Conclusion

According to this retrospective chart review, abdominal histrelin acetate subcutaneous implants were effective on the long term at reducing serum testosterone levels below castration levels and reducing serum PSA levels. The subcutaneous abdominal insertion allows easier insertion of histrelin acetate implants for the surgeon, is well tolerated by patients, and thus is an indicated site to implant the histrelin acetate diffusion-controlled reservoir.

References

[1] American Cancer Society, "What are the key statistics for prostate cancer?" 2014, http://www.cancer.org/cancer/prostatecancer/detailedguide/prostate-cancer-key-statistics.

[2] National Cancer Institute, *SEER Stat Fact Sheets: Prostate Cancer*, 2014, http://seer.cancer.gov/statfacts/html/prost.html.

[3] T. J. Wilt, "Management of low risk and low PSA prostate cancer: long term results from the prostate cancer intervention versus observation trial," *Recent Results in Cancer Research*, vol. 202, pp. 149–169, 2014.

[4] F. Schröder, E. D. Crawford, K. Axcrona, H. Payne, and T. E. Keane, "Androgen deprivation therapy: past, present and future," *BJU International*, vol. 109, no. 6, pp. 1–12, 2012.

[5] M. E. Taplin and S.-M. Ho, "Clinical Review 134: the endocrinology of prostate cancer," *Journal of Clinical Endocrinology and Metabolism*, vol. 86, no. 8, pp. 3467–3477, 2001.

[6] National Comprehensive Cancer Network, NCCN Clinical Practice Guidelines in Oncology: Prostate Cancer, http://www.nccn.org/professionals/physician_gls/PDF/prostate.pdf.

[7] S. X. Bian and K. E. Hoffman, "Management of prostate cancer in elderly men," *Seminars in Radiation Oncology*, vol. 23, no. 3, pp. 198–205, 2013.

[8] J. Seidenfeld, D. J. Samson, V. Hasselblad et al., "Single-therapy androgen suppression in men with advanced prostate cancer: a systematic review and meta-analysis," *Annals of Internal Medicine*, vol. 132, no. 7, pp. 566–577, 2000.

[9] S. Chowdhury and R. Kirby, "Advances in the treatment of metastatic prostate cancer," *Practitioner*, vol. 257, pp. 15–18, 2013.

[10] I. M. Thompson, "Flare associated with LHRH-agonist therapy," *Reviews in Urology*, vol. 3, pp. 10–14, 2001.

[11] P. Schlegel, "A review of the pharmacokinetic and pharmacological properties of a once-yearly administered histrelin acetate implant in the treatment of prostate cancer," *BJU International*, vol. 103, no. 2, pp. 7–13, 2009.

[12] P. F. Siami, K. Beasley, S. Woolen, and J. Zahn, "A retrospective study evaluating the efficacy and tolerability of intra-abdominal, once-yearly histrelin acetate subcutaneous implants in patients with advanced prostate cancer," *UroToday International Journal*, vol. 5, no. 3, article 26, 2012.

[13] P. N. Schlegel and Histrelin Study Group, "Efficacy and safety of histrelin subdermal implant in patients with advanced prostate cancer," *The Journal of Urology*, vol. 175, no. 4, pp. 1353–1358, 2006.

[14] N. Shore, M. S. Cookson, and M. C. Gittelman, "Long-term efficacy and tolerability of once-yearly histrelin acetate subcutaneous implant in patients with advanced prostate cancer," *BJU International*, vol. 109, no. 2, pp. 226–232, 2012.

16

Obesity and the Odds of Weight Gain following Androgen Deprivation Therapy for Prostate Cancer

Lior Z. Braunstein,[1] Ming-Hui Chen,[2] Marian Loffredo,[3,4] Philip W. Kantoff,[3] and Anthony V. D'Amico[3,4]

[1] *Harvard Radiation Oncology Program, Brigham and Women's Hospital, ASB-I Radiation Oncology L2, 75 Francis Street, Boston, MA 02115, USA*
[2] *Department of Statistics, University of Connecticut, 215 Glenbrook Road, U-4120, Storrs, CT 06269-4120, USA*
[3] *Lank Center for Genitourinary Oncology, Dana-Farber Cancer Institute, Mailstop Dana 1230, 450 Brookline Avenue, Boston, MA 02215, USA*
[4] *Department of Radiation Oncology, Dana-Farber/Brigham and Women's Hospital, ASB-I Radiation Oncology L2, 75 Francis Street, Boston, MA 02115, USA*

Correspondence should be addressed to Lior Z. Braunstein; lbraunstein@partners.org

Academic Editor: Manfred Wirth

Background. Increasing body mass index (BMI) is associated with increased risk of mortality; however, quantifying weight gain in men undergoing androgen deprivation therapy (ADT) for prostate cancer (PC) remains unexplored. *Methods.* Between 1995 and 2001, 206 men were enrolled in a randomized trial evaluating the survival difference of adding 6 months of ADT to radiation therapy (RT). BMI measurements were available in 171 men comprising the study cohort. The primary endpoint was weight gain of ≥10 lbs by 6-month followup. Logistic regression analysis was performed to assess whether baseline BMI or treatment received was associated with this endpoint adjusting for known prognostic factors. *Results.* By the 6-month followup, 12 men gained ≥10 lbs, of which 10 (83%) received RT + ADT and, of these, 7 (70%) were obese at randomization. Men treated with RT as compared to RT + ADT were less likely to gain ≥10 lbs (adjusted odds ratio (AOR): 0.18 [95% CI: 0.04–0.89]; $P = 0.04$), whereas this risk increased with increasing BMI (AOR: 1.15 [95% CI: 1.01–1.31]; $P = 0.04$). *Conclusions.* Consideration should be given to avoid ADT in obese men with low- or favorable-intermediate risk PC where improved cancer control has not been observed, but shortened life expectancy from weight gain is expected.

1. Introduction

The addition of androgen deprivation therapy (ADT) to external beam radiation therapy (RT) has been shown to prolong overall survival in men with intermediate or high-risk prostate cancer (PC) enrolled on several randomized controlled trials [1–7]. Despite this well-established survival benefit, it is known that ADT has significant side effects that adversely affect quality of life [3, 5, 8]. These side effects include hot flashes, gynecomastia, decreased libido, nipple sensitivity, and decreased metabolism [9–14]. Moreover, ADT use in excess of 1 year has also been shown to increase the risk of osteoporosis [15, 16], diabetes [17–20], and cardiovascular disease [18, 21, 22].

With regard to decreased metabolism, several investigators have shown that ADT causes a decrease in lean body mass with a concomitant increase in total body fat of up to ~10% [14, 16]. Of note, the increase in fat mass appears to be distributed centrally about the abdominal compartment [23]. Based on these findings, men are commonly advised that weight gain is possible during ADT; however, the degree to which weight gain occurs and risk factors associated with weight gain are not well documented. Given the known association of an elevated BMI for men who are overweight

(BMI 25 to 29.9 kg/m^2) or obese (BMI $\geq$ 30 kg/m^2) and an increased risk of mortality [24], understanding weight changes during ADT use is important when counseling men about diet and exercise during ADT in order to minimize weight gain and thereby avoid increasing the risk of mortality.

Therefore, the purpose of this study was to use data from a prospective randomized trial in order to ascertain clinical factors at randomization associated with significant weight gain ($\geq$10 pounds) following the completion of RT and ADT [3]. In addition, we quantified weight gain across randomized treatment arms and within BMI categories as measured at baseline in order to quantify the effect of ADT on weight gain within each BMI category using the radiation-only arm as a control.

2. Methods

2.1. Patient Population and Treatment. Between December 1, 1995, and April 15, 2001, 206 men were enrolled in a prospective randomized trial evaluating the impact on the survival of adding 6 months of combined ADT to ~70 Gy RT [3]. Prior to randomization, patient age, prostate biopsy results, Gleason score, serum prostate-specific antigen level (PSA), digital rectal exam findings (DRE), and adult comorbidity evaluation 27 (ACE-27) scores were ascertained and recorded. Of 206 men, 11 did not have a body mass index (BMI) measured at randomization and 24 did not have BMI measured at the endpoint, leaving 171 patients who formed the current study cohort. Patients were randomized to RT alone consisting of 3-dimensional conformal RT to ~70 Gy or to the same RT regimen with 2 months of neoadjuvant, concurrent, and adjuvant combined ADT totaling 6 months and composed of a luteinizing hormone-releasing hormone (LHRH) agonist and the antiandrogen flutamide. This secondary analysis of the primary study was approved by the institutional review board of the Dana-Farber/Harvard Cancer Center; informed consent was obtained for the primary study. There is no funding for this secondary analysis.

2.2. Assessment of Weight Gain at End of Treatment. Following the completion of RT with or without 6 months of combined ADT, men were seen at approximately 6 months after randomization. At each followup, a digital rectal examination, serum PSA, and weight measurement were obtained. The scale used to measure patients at this 6-month followup was the same as at randomization and the difference in weight in pounds was ascertained and recorded between the two time-points.

2.3. Statistical Methods

2.3.1. Distribution and Comparison of Clinical Factors of the Study Cohort Stratified by Randomized Treatment Arm. Clinical characteristics at baseline were enumerated and compared across randomized treatment arms. For the continuous covariates of BMI, PSA, and age, the nonparametric Wilcoxon test [25, 26] was used to compare the distributions of these factors across randomized treatment arms. A Mantel-Haenszel chi-square metric [27, 28] was used to compare the distribution of categorical covariates including highest biopsy Gleason score, 2009 AJCC tumor (T) category [29], and ACE-27 comorbidity score across randomized treatment arms.

2.3.2. Logistic Regression Analysis. The primary endpoint of this study was whether the patient gained $\geq$10 lbs by the 6-month follow-up point after randomization. Univariable and multivariable logistic regression [30] analysis was performed to assess whether baseline BMI or treatment received was associated with this endpoint adjusting for comorbidity and known PC prognostic factors. Time zero was the date of randomization. BMI, PSA, and age were treated as continuous covariates, whereas treatment arm, Gleason score, tumor category, and ACE-27 score were considered as categorical covariates in the model. The baseline group for the categorical variables included the RT with ADT treatment arm, Gleason score $\leq$ 6, tumor category 1 (T1), and ACE-27 with no or minimal comorbidity, respectively. Adjusted odds ratios and their associated 95% confidence intervals and P values were calculated. Two-sided P values $\leq$ 0.05 were considered statistically significant. SAS version 9.3 was used for all statistical analyses.

2.3.3. Distribution of Weight Gain 6 Months following Randomization, Stratified by Treatment Received and BMI. The distribution of the 85 and 86 men, who underwent RT or RT and ADT, respectively, and experienced $\geq$10 lbs weight gain versus <10 lbs, 6 months following randomization, stratified by well-defined BMI cut-points for normal weight, overweight, and obese, was compared using Fisher's exact test [31].

3. Results

3.1. Distribution and Comparison of Clinical Factors of the Study Cohort Stratified by Randomized Treatment Arm. Table 1 illustrates the distribution of clinical factors stratified by randomized treatment arm (RT versus RT + ADT). As expected, given the randomization, all factors including BMI, PSA, patient age, Gleason score distribution, and ACE-27 comorbidity score were not significantly different between the two treatment arms (P value for each factor $\geq$ 0.11). Of note, the median BMI and its distribution were nearly equivalent between the two arms at baseline (27.44 kg/m^2 [IQR = 25.58, 30.23] versus 27.35 kg/m^2 [IQR = 24.68, 30.99]; P = 0.73).

3.2. Logistic Regression Analysis. By the 6-month followup, 12 men were observed to have gained $\geq$10 lbs of which 10 (83%) were treated with RT and ADT, and 7 (70%) were obese at the time of randomization. For these 7 men, the median increase in BMI was 5.21% (range: 3.60%–6.37%). As shown in Table 2, men treated with RT as compared to RT and ADT were significantly less likely to experience a weight gain of $\geq$10 lbs (AOR: 0.18 [95% CI 0.04–0.89]; P = 0.04), whereas this risk was increased with increasing BMI (AOR: 1.15 [95%

Table 1: Distribution and comparison of clinical factors at randomization of the study cohort stratified by randomized treatment arm.

Clinical factor	Treatment with RT $N = 85$	Treatment with RT and AST $N = 86$	P value
Median BMI (IQR)	27.44 kg/m^2 (25.58, 30.23)	27.35 kg/m^2 (24.68, 30.99)	0.73
Median PSA (IQR)	11.54 ng/mL (7.70, 16.40)	10.85 ng/mL (7.50, 15.51)	0.38
Median Age (IQR)	73.36 (70.82, 76.15)	72.12 (69.07, 74.71)	0.11
T1	37 (44%)	46 (53%)	0.19
T2	48 (56%)	40 (47%)	
Gleason score 6 or less	26 (31%)	25 (29%)	
7	45 (53%)	49 (57%)	0.92
8 to 10	14 (16%)	12 (14%)	
No or minimal cm	65 (76%)	65 (76%)	0.89
Moderate to severe cm	20 (24%)	21 (24%)	

RT indicates radiotherapy; ADT: androgen deprivation therapy; BMI: body mass index; IQR: interquartile range; PSA: prostate-specific antigen; cm: comorbidity.

Table 2: Univariate and multivariate odds ratios for the risk of ≥10 lbs weight gain 6 months after randomization for each clinical factor.

Clinical factor	Number of men	Number of men who gained ≥10 lbs by EOT	Univariable analysis OR (95% CI)	Univariable analysis P value	Multivariable analysis AOR (95% CI)	Multivariable analysis P value
RT	85	2	0.18 (0.04, 0.86)	0.03	0.18 (0.04, 0.89)	0.04
RT + AST	86	10	1 (Ref)	—	1 (Ref)	—
BMI increase per kg/m^2	171	12	1.18 (1.05, 1.33)	0.01	1.15 (1.01, 1.31)	0.04
PSA increase per ng/mL	171	12	0.98 (0.90, 1.06)	0.58	0.97 (0.87, 1.08)	0.57
Age	171	12	0.93 (0.85, 1.02)	0.14	0.95 (0.85, 1.06)	0.38
Gleason score 8 to 10	26	3	2.09 (0.39, 11.15)	0.39	1.17 (0.17, 7.93)	0.87
7	94	6	1.091 (0.26, 4.56)	0.90	0.55 (0.10, 3.06)	0.49
6 or less	51	3	1 (Ref)	—	1 (Ref)	—
T2	88	8	1.98 (0.57, 6.82)	0.28	1.99 (0.49, 7.99)	0.33
T1	83	4	1 (Ref)	—	1 (ref)	—
Mod to Sev cm	41	5	2.44 (0.73, 8.15)	0.15	2.11 (0.54, 8.26)	0.28
No or min cm	130	7	1 (Ref)	—	1 (Ref)	—

RT indicates radiotherapy; ADT: androgen deprivation therapy; BMI: body mass index; PSA: prostate-specific antigen; cm: comorbidity; OR: odds ratio; CI: confidence interval; AOR: adjusted odds ratio; EOT: end of treatment.

CI 1.01–1.31]; $P = 0.04$). No other clinical factors were found to be significantly associated with this endpoint.

3.3. Distribution of Men Observed to Experience at Least a 10 Pound Weight Gain 6 Months following Randomization, Stratified by Treatment Received and BMI Category. Table 3 illustrates the significant findings of the logistic regression multivariable analysis. Specifically, men treated with RT and ADT and who were obese at randomization were significantly more likely to gain ≥10 lbs as compared to <10 lbs by 6 months following randomization. These respective percentages were 70% versus 22%; $P = 0.006$. However, this significant trend was not noted for men who were obese at randomization and underwent RT alone where the respective values were 0% and 28%; $P = 0.45$. Of patients with a normal BMI

Table 3: Distribution of weight gain 6 months following randomization, stratified by treatment received and body mass index.

	RT only (N = 85)		RT + ADT (N = 86)	
	Weight change 6 months following randomization			
	<10 lbs (N = 83)	≥10 lbs (N = 2)	<10 lbs (N = 76)	≥10 lbs (N = 10)
BMI (range in kg/m^2)	(Range −13 to +9; median −1 lb)	(Range 10 to 13; median +11.5 lbs)	(Range −11 to +8; median +1 lb)	(Range 10 to 17 lbs; median +11.25 lbs)
Normal (18.5–24.9)	17 (20%)	1 (50%)	22 (29%)	2 (20%)
Overweight (25.0–29.9)	43 (52%)	1 (50%)	37 (49%)	1 (10%)
Obese (≥30.0)	23 (28%)	0 (0%)	17 (22%)	7 (70%)
	Fisher's exact test P value = 0.45		Fisher's exact test P value = 0.006	

RT indicates radiotherapy; ADT: androgen deprivation therapy; BMI: body mass index.

at the time of enrollment, only 1 out of 18 men (6%) who received RT alone and 2 out of 24 men (8%) who received RT and ADT gained ≥10 lbs (Fisher's exact test, P = 1.00), suggesting no significant risk to normal-weight men of becoming overweight from treatment with ADT.

4. Discussion

In this study, we observed that men at highest risk of ≥10 lbs weight gain following RT and 6 months of ADT were those who were obese at the outset of treatment. Specifically, for every 1 unit increase in BMI, there was a 15% increase in the odds of gaining at least 10 pounds by the 6-month follow-up visit and the median increase in BMI was 5.21%. Given the established association of increased mortality with additional weight gain in obese men [24], these findings suggest that some obese men may be at risk for a shortened survival with ADT use. Therefore, the clinical significance of this finding suggests taking a measured risk/benefit approach when deciding on ADT use in obese men. In particular, this consideration becomes extremely pertinent for obese men in whom ADT use may have little or no impact on reducing the risk of prostate cancer-specific mortality (PCSM) but can shorten life expectancy.

Several points require further clarification. First, weight gain in obese patients is known to reduce both quality of life (QoL) and longevity [24, 32, 33], in part due to increased risk of cardiovascular events [34–36] and the sequelae of diabetes [37, 38]. Yet, there is no proven benefit for the use of ADT in men with low risk PC despite its frequent use (up to 19%) documented within a large observational database between 1989 and 2002 (UCSF Cancer of the Prostate Strategic Urologic Research Endeavor—CaPSURE) [39].

Specifically, ADT has been used in men with benign prostatic hyperplasia and low risk PC who are not candidates for brachytherapy due to pubic arch interference as determined at the time of volume study [40, 41]. In such men, ADT has no proven benefit on reducing PCSM [5], but the results of the current study show that ADT use can lead to significant weight gain in men who are already obese, which places them at higher risk of earlier morbidity and mortality because of further increases in their BMI [13, 24, 33]. Second, recent literature suggests that men with favorable-intermediate risk prostate cancer [42] may not have a reduction in the risk of PCSM from the addition of ADT to high dose RT [43]. Moreover, randomized controlled trials that have established a survival benefit when ADT is added to RT in men with unfavorable-intermediate or high-risk prostate cancer did not have a prerandomization stratification by comorbidity, and a postrandomization analysis by comorbidity at randomization found no survival benefit for the addition of ADT to RT [44]. Therefore, by applying similar reasoning, obese men with favorable-intermediate risk PC may not benefit from ADT use and may also be at risk for shortened survival and declining quality of life, without reduction in PSA recurrence, metastasis, or death from PC from adding ADT to RT.

Therefore, ADT use should be discouraged in obese men with low- or favorable-intermediate risk PC. Moreover, future studies should employ a validated QoL metric [45] and a measurement of PC-specific and overall survival in obese men with unfavorable-intermediate and high-risk PC to ascertain the risk/benefit ratio of adding ADT to RT in obese men.

A limitation of the current analysis is the relatively small event rate (N = 12) of a ≥10 lbs weight gain following RT and 6 months of ADT. Therefore, validation of these results by other investigators is needed. However, while the overall event rate was small, the proportion of obese men who achieved this endpoint was substantial at 70%. Moreover, given that the proportion of men in the United States who are obese and over the age of 50 is increasing [32], and with the use of PSA screening, the proportion of men with low- or favorable-intermediate risk PC has also been increasing [46–48], and the potential negative impact of ADT use on life expectancy would be expected to also increase if ADT use is continued in these men. A strength of this study is that the data are from a prospective randomized trial. As a result, the radiation control arm is available for calculating the increased odds of weight gain from the multivariable logistic regression analysis for men who were randomized to receive RT and 6 months of ADT. Therefore, other reasons for weight gain besides ADT use are controlled for by the study design, lending additional support to both ADT and increasing BMI being the drivers of the weight gains observed.

In conclusion, obese men are at increased risk for ≥10 lbs weight gain by the end of 6 months of ADT, prompting serious consideration to limiting or avoiding the use of ADT in these men with low- or favorable-intermediate risk PC where improvement in cancer control has not been observed but a shortened life expectancy from further weight gain may be expected.

Disclosure

The material presented in this paper is original research, has not been previously published, and has not been submitted for publication elsewhere while under consideration.

References

[1] M. Bolla, G. Van Tienhoven, T. De Reijke, A. van den Bergh, A. van der Meijden, P. Poortmans et al., "Concomitant and adjuvant androgen deprivation (ADT) with external beam irradiation (RT) for locally advanced prostate cancer: 6 months versus 3 years ADT—results of the randomized EORTC phase III trial 22961," *Journal of Clinical Oncology*, vol. 25, supplement 18, 2007.

[2] M. Bolla, G. Van Tienhoven, P. Warde et al., "External irradiation with or without long-term androgen suppression for prostate cancer with high metastatic risk: 10-year results of an EORTC randomised study," *The Lancet Oncology*, vol. 11, no. 11, pp. 1066–1073, 2010.

[3] A. V. D'Amico, J. Manola, M. Loffredo, A. A. Renshaw, A. DellaCroce, and P. W. Kantoff, "6-Month androgen suppression plus radiation therapy vs radiation therapy alone for patients with clinically localized prostate cancer: a randomized controlled trial," *Journal of the American Medical Association*, vol. 292, no. 7, pp. 821–827, 2004.

[4] E. M. Horwitz, K. Bae, G. E. Hanks et al., "Ten-year follow-up of radiation therapy oncology group protocol 92-02: a phase III trial of the duration of elective androgen deprivation in locally advanced prostate cancer," *Journal of Clinical Oncology*, vol. 26, no. 15, pp. 2497–2504, 2008.

[5] C. U. Jones, D. Hunt, D. G. McGowan et al., "Radiotherapy and short-term androgen deprivation for localized prostate cancer," *The New England Journal of Medicine*, vol. 365, no. 2, pp. 107–118, 2011.

[6] M. V. Pilepich, K. Winter, M. J. John et al., "Phase III radiation therapy oncology group (RTOG) trial 86-10 of androgen deprivation adjuvant to definitive radiotherapy in locally advanced carcinoma of the prostate," *International Journal of Radiation Oncology Biology Physics*, vol. 50, no. 5, pp. 1243–1252, 2001.

[7] M. V. Pilepich, K. Winter, C. A. Lawton et al., "Androgen suppression adjuvant to definitive radiotherapy in prostate carcinoma—long-term results of phase III RTOG 85-31," *International Journal of Radiation Oncology Biology Physics*, vol. 61, no. 5, pp. 1285–1290, 2005.

[8] T. A. Guise, M. G. Oefelein, J. A. Eastham, M. S. Cookson, C. S. Higano, and M. R. Smith, "Estrogenic side effects of androgen deprivation therapy," *Reviews in Urology*, vol. 9, no. 4, pp. 163–180, 2007.

[9] J. M. Holzbeierlein, M. D. McLaughlin, and J. B. Thrasher, "Complications of androgen deprivation therapy for prostate cancer," *Current Opinion in Urology*, vol. 14, no. 3, pp. 177–183, 2004.

[10] C. S. Higano, "Side effects of androgen deprivation therapy: monitoring and minimizing toxicity," *Urology*, vol. 61, no. 2, pp. 32–38, 2003.

[11] J. A. Smith Jr., "A prospective comparison of treatments for symptomatic hot flushes following endocrine therapy for carcinoma of the prostate," *Journal of Urology*, vol. 152, no. 1, pp. 132–134, 1994.

[12] C. A. Thompson, T. D. Shanafelt, and C. L. Loprinzi, "Andropause: symptom management for prostate cancer patients treated with hormonal ablation," *Oncologist*, vol. 8, no. 5, pp. 474–487, 2003.

[13] A. C. Chen and D. P. Petrylak, "Complications of androgen deprivation therapy in men with prostate cancer," *Current Oncology Reports*, vol. 6, no. 3, pp. 209–215, 2004.

[14] M. R. Smith, J. S. Finkelstein, F. J. McGovern et al., "Changes in body composition during androgen deprivation therapy for prostate cancer," *Journal of Clinical Endocrinology and Metabolism*, vol. 87, no. 2, pp. 599–603, 2002.

[15] T. H. Diamond, C. S. Higano, M. R. Smith, T. A. Guise, and F. R. Singer, "Osteoporosis in men with prostate carcinoma receiving androgen, deprivation therapy," *Cancer*, vol. 100, no. 5, pp. 892–899, 2004.

[16] A. Berruti, L. Dogliotti, C. Terrone et al., "Changes in bone mineral density, lean body mass and fat content as measured by dual energy x-ray absorptiometry in patients with prostate cancer without apparent bone metastases given androgen deprivation therapy," *Journal of Urology*, vol. 167, no. 6, pp. 2361–2367, 2002.

[17] S. M. Haffner, J. Shaten, M. P. Stern, G. D. Smith, and L. Kuller, "Low levels of sex hormone-binding globulin and testosterone predict the development of non-insulin-dependent diabetes mellitus in men," *American Journal of Epidemiology*, vol. 143, no. 9, pp. 889–897, 1996.

[18] F. Dockery, C. J. Bulpitt, S. Agarwal, M. Donaldson, and C. Rajkumar, "Testosterone suppression in men with prostate cancer leads to an increase in arterial stiffness and hyperinsulinaemia," *Clinical Science*, vol. 104, no. 2, pp. 195–201, 2003.

[19] J.-Y. Oh, E. Barrett-Connor, N. M. Wedick, and D. L. Wingard, "Endogenous sex hormones and the development of type 2 diabetes in older men and women: the rancho bernardo study," *Diabetes Care*, vol. 25, no. 1, pp. 55–60, 2002.

[20] M. R. Smith, H. Lee, and D. M. Nathan, "Insulin sensitivity during combined androgen blockade for prostate cancer," *Journal of Clinical Endocrinology and Metabolism*, vol. 91, no. 4, pp. 1305–1308, 2006.

[21] J. C. Smith, S. Bennett, L. M. Evans et al., "The effects of induced hypogonadism on arterial stiffness, body composition, and metabolic parameters in males with prostate cancer," *Journal of Clinical Endocrinology and Metabolism*, vol. 86, no. 9, pp. 4261–4267, 2001.

[22] C. S. Higano, W. Ellis, K. Russell, and P. H. Lange, "Intermittent androgen suppression with leuprolide and flutamide for prostate cancer: a pilot study," *Urology*, vol. 48, no. 5, pp. 800–804, 1996.

[23] M. Braga-Basaria, A. S. Dobs, D. C. Muller et al., "Metabolic syndrome in men with prostate cancer undergoing long-term androgen-deprivation therapy," *Journal of Clinical Oncology*, vol. 24, no. 24, pp. 3979–3983, 2006.

[24] A. B. De Gonzalez, P. Hartge, J. R. Cerhan et al., "Body-mass index and mortality among 1.46 million white adults," *The New England Journal of Medicine*, vol. 363, no. 23, pp. 2211–2219, 2010.

[25] F. Wilcoxon, "Individual comparisons by ranking methods," *Biometrics Bulletin*, vol. 1, no. 6, pp. 80–83, 1945.

[26] H. B. Mann and D. R. Whitney, "On a test of whether one of two random variables is stochastically larger than the other," *The Annals of Mathematical Statistics*, vol. 18, no. 1, pp. 50–60, 1947.

[27] N. Mantel and W. Haenszel, "Statistical aspects of the analysis of data from retrospective studies of disease," *The Challenge of Epidemiology: Issues and Selected Readings*, vol. 1, no. 1, pp. 533–553, 2004.

[28] W. G. Cochran, "Some methods for strengthening the common χ^2 tests," *Biometrics*, vol. 10, no. 4, pp. 417–451, 1954.

[29] S. B. Edge and C. C. Compton, "The american joint committee on cancer: the 7th edition of the AJCC cancer staging manual and the future of TNM," *Annals of Surgical Oncology*, vol. 17, no. 6, pp. 1471–1474, 2010.

[30] J. M. Hilbe, *Logistic Regression Models*, CRC Press, Boca Raton, Fla, USA, 2009.

[31] R. A. Fisher, "On the interpretation of χ^2 from contingency tables, and the calculation of P," *Journal of the Royal Statistical Society*, vol. 85, no. 1, pp. 87–94, 1922.

[32] K. F. Adams, A. Schatzkin, T. B. Harris et al., "Overweight, obesity, and mortality in a large prospective cohort of persons 50 to 71 years old," *The New England Journal of Medicine*, vol. 355, no. 8, pp. 763–778, 2006.

[33] E. E. Calle, M. J. Thun, J. M. Petrelli, C. Rodriguez, and C. W. Heath Jr., "Body-mass index and mortality in a prospective cohort of U.S. adults," *The New England Journal of Medicine*, vol. 341, no. 15, pp. 1097–1105, 1999.

[34] P. W. Wilson, R. B. D'Agostino, L. Sullivan, H. Parise, and W. B. Kannel, "Overweight and obesity as determinants of cardiovascular risk: the Framingham experience," *Archives of Internal Medicine*, vol. 162, no. 16, pp. 1867–1872, 2002.

[35] L. F. Van Gaal, I. L. Mertens, and C. E. De Block, "Mechanisms linking obesity with cardiovascular disease," *Nature*, vol. 444, no. 7121, pp. 875–880, 2006.

[36] A. Rosengren, H. Wedel, and L. Wilhelmsen, "Body weight and weight gain during adult life in men in relation to coronary heart disease and mortality," *European Heart Journal*, vol. 20, no. 4, pp. 269–277, 1999.

[37] J. M. Chan, E. B. Rimm, G. A. Colditz, M. J. Stampfer, and W. C. Willett, "Obesity, fat distribution, and weight gain as risk factors for clinical diabetes in men," *Diabetes Care*, vol. 17, no. 9, pp. 961–969, 1994.

[38] M. A. Lazar, "How obesity causes diabetes: not a tall tale," *Science*, vol. 307, no. 5708, pp. 373–375, 2005.

[39] M. V. Meng, E. P. Elkin, D. M. Latini, J. DuChane, and P. R. Carroll, "Treatment of patients with high risk localized prostate cancer: results from cancer of the prostate strategic urological research endeavor (CaPSURE)," *The Journal of Urology*, vol. 173, no. 5, pp. 1557–1561, 2005.

[40] R. Kucway, F. Vicini, R. Huang, J. Stromberg, J. Gonzalez, and A. Martinez, "Prostate volume reduction with androgen deprivation therapy before interstitial brachytherapy," *The Journal of Urology*, vol. 167, no. 6, pp. 2443–2447, 2002.

[41] L. Potters, T. Torre, R. Ashley, and S. Leibel, "Examining the role of neoadjuvant androgen deprivation in patients undergoing prostate brachytherapy," *Journal of Clinical Oncology*, vol. 18, no. 6, pp. 1187–1192, 2000.

[42] J. L. Mohler, "NCCN clinical practice guidelines in oncology on prostate cancer," *Journal of the National Comprehensive Cancer Network*, vol. 8, no. 2, p. 145, 2010.

[43] Z. S. Zumsteg, D. E. Spratt, I. Pei, Z. Zhang, Y. Yamada, M. Kollmeier et al., "A new risk classification system for therapeutic decision making with intermediate-risk prostate cancer patients undergoing dose-escalated external-beam radiation therapy," *European Urology*, vol. 64, no. 6, pp. 895–902, 2013.

[44] A. V. D'Amico, M.-H. Chen, A. A. Renshaw, M. Loffredo, and P. W. Kantoff, "Androgen suppression and radiation vs radiation alone for prostate cancer: a randomized trial," *Journal of the American Medical Association*, vol. 299, no. 3, pp. 289–295, 2008.

[45] M. G. Sanda, R. L. Dunn, J. Michalski et al., "Quality of life and satisfaction with outcome among prostate-cancer survivors," *The New England Journal of Medicine*, vol. 358, no. 12, pp. 1250–1261, 2008.

[46] C. D. Berg, G. L. Andriole, E. D. Crawford et al., "Mortality results from a randomized prostate-cancer screening trial," *The New England Journal of Medicine*, vol. 360, no. 13, pp. 1310–1319, 2009.

[47] F. H. Schröder, J. Hugosson, M. J. Roobol et al., "Screening and prostate-cancer mortality in a randomized european study," *The New England Journal of Medicine*, vol. 360, no. 13, pp. 1320–1328, 2009.

[48] J. Hugosson, S. Carlsson, G. Aus et al., "Mortality results from the Göteborg randomised population-based prostate-cancer screening trial," *The Lancet Oncology*, vol. 11, no. 8, pp. 725–732, 2010.

17

Thioredoxin 1 in Prostate Tissue Is Associated with Gleason Score, Erythrocyte Antioxidant Enzyme Activity, and Dietary Antioxidants

Terrence M. Vance,[1] Gissou Azabdaftari,[2] Elena A. Pop,[2] Sang Gil Lee,[1] L. Joseph Su,[3] Elizabeth T. H. Fontham,[4] Jeannette T. Bensen,[5] Susan E. Steck,[6] Lenore Arab,[7] James L. Mohler,[2,5] Ming-Hui Chen,[8] Sung I. Koo,[1] and Ock K. Chun[1]

[1] *Department of Nutritional Sciences, University of Connecticut, Storrs, CT 06269, USA*
[2] *Roswell Park Cancer Institute, Buffalo, NY 14263, USA*
[3] *Epidemiology and Genomics Research Program, Division of Cancer Control and Population Sciences, National Cancer Institute, Bethesda, MD 20892, USA*
[4] *School of Public Health, Louisiana State University Health Sciences Center, New Orleans, LA 70112, USA*
[5] *School of Public Health, University of North Carolina at Chapel Hill, Chapel Hill, NC 27599, USA*
[6] *Department of Epidemiology and Biostatistics, Cancer Prevention and Control Program, University of South Carolina, Columbia, SC 29208, USA*
[7] *David Geffen School of Medicine, University of California, Los Angeles, CA 90095, USA*
[8] *Department of Statistics, University of Connecticut, Storrs, CT 06269, USA*

Correspondence should be addressed to Ock K. Chun; ock.chun@uconn.edu

Academic Editor: Craig Robson

Background. Prostate cancer is the most common noncutaneous cancer and second leading cause of cancer-related mortality in men in the US. Growing evidence suggests that oxidative stress is involved in prostate cancer. *Methods.* In this study, thioredoxin 1 (Trx 1), an enzyme and subcellular indicator of redox status, was measured in prostate biopsy tissue from 55 men from the North Carolina-Louisiana Prostate Cancer Project. A pathologist blindly scored levels of Trx 1. The association between Trx 1 and the Gleason score, erythrocyte antioxidant enzyme activity, and dietary antioxidant intake was determined using Fisher's exact test. *Results.* Trx 1 levels in benign prostate tissue in men with incident prostate cancer were positively associated with the Gleason score ($P = 0.01$) and inversely associated with dietary antioxidant intake ($P = 0.03$). In prostate cancer tissue, Trx 1 levels were associated with erythrocyte glutathione peroxidase activity ($P = 0.01$). No association was found for other erythrocyte enzymes. Greater Gleason score of malignant tissue corresponds to a greater difference in Trx 1 levels between malignant and benign tissue ($P = 0.04$). *Conclusion.* These results suggest that the redox status of prostate tissue is associated with prostate cancer grade and both endogenous and exogenous antioxidants.

1. Introduction

Prostate cancer is the most common noncutaneous cancer and second cause of cancer-related mortality in men in the US, with estimated 238,590 new cases and 29,720 deaths in 2013 [1]. The specific causes of prostate cancer have not yet been determined, but several risk factors have been identified for the disease, which include family history, age, and race [2, 3]. However, the mechanisms by which these and other risk factors, such as lifestyle, contribute to prostate cancer are not clear, and there is likely a great degree of heterogeneity in the causes of the disease.

At the cellular level, a growing body of evidence indicates that oxidative stress is involved in prostate carcinogenesis [4].

Reactive oxygen species can promote carcinogenesis by causing oxidative damage to DNA and macromolecules within cells, altering signal transduction pathways, and promoting a malignant phenotype. Furthermore, genetic polymorphisms in antioxidant enzymes have been associated with cancer risk [5], and prostate cancer risk may be modified by interactions between antioxidant enzyme genotype and dietary antioxidants [6, 7]. Men diagnosed with prostate cancer have been shown to have greater oxidative stress, lower antioxidant enzyme activity [8], and greater levels of urinary isoprostanes, a biomarker of oxidative stress and lipid peroxidation [9, 10]. Furthermore, *in vitro* experiments have implicated the production of reactive oxygen species in the aggressiveness of prostate cancer [11]. Thus, relatively consistent evidence suggests an association between oxidative stress and prostate cancer.

Oxidative stress is regulated in both benign and malignant cells via several nonenzymatic and enzymatic antioxidant mechanisms [4]. Malignant cells have relatively greater levels of reactive oxygen species and compensatory increases in antioxidant enzymes in order to tolerate increased oxidative stress [12]. The expression of several enzymes involved in oxidative stress and detoxification is repressed in prostate cancer, in particular glutathione S-transferase [13]. Furthermore, men with prostate cancer may be subject to greater oxidative stress and exhibit lower activity of erythrocyte glutathione peroxidase and superoxide dismutase, compared with controls [8]. These differences in activity and expression could indicate greater susceptibility to oxidative damage, potentially influencing the development or progression of cancer. Another antioxidant enzyme that is thought to be involved in prostate carcinogenesis is thioredoxin 1 (Trx 1). Thioredoxin reductase 1 (TrxR1) transfers electrons from NADPH to Trx 1, a process that occurs in most living cells and is essential for maintenance of cellular redox status [14]. Both Trx 1 and TrxR1 are increased in prostate cancer [15, 16], with a greater proportion of Trx 1 in an oxidized state, which may reflect redox imbalance and response to greater levels of oxidative stress. Reduced Trx 1 binds to apoptosis signal-regulating kinase 1 (ASK1) and regulates cell death [17]; thus, redox imbalance may promote cancer cell survival. TrxR1 is a selenoenzyme that can be modified by reaction with electrophilic compounds [14] and interact with several dietary phytochemicals that are considered antioxidants [18].

The role of TrxR1 in maintaining Trx 1 in a reduced state and the emerging role of both of these enzymes in carcinogenesis suggest a relationship between TrxR1 and dietary antioxidants. The evidence for a relationship between dietary antioxidants and prostate cancer is inconsistent in humans [19], which is partly due to the relatively small number of dietary antioxidants studied and their diversity in structure and possible mechanisms of action. However, dietary antioxidants, such as flavonoids, have been shown to reduce oxidative damage [20] and promote DNA repair [21] in prostate cancer cells *in vitro*. Dietary antioxidants could have some effect on prostate cancer, possibly by affecting oxidative stress.

The discrepant findings regarding prostate cancer and dietary antioxidants prompted a study of dietary antioxidant intake using total antioxidant capacity (TAC). TAC represents the cumulative antioxidant capacity of individual antioxidants present in diet and supplements [22]. Greater dietary TAC was recently found to be inversely associated with prostate cancer incidence [23]; however, the relationship between dietary antioxidants and redox status in prostate cancer remains unknown. Furthermore, the relationship between Trx 1 in prostate tissue and the activity of antioxidant enzymes in prostate cancer patients is relatively unknown.

The objectives of this study were to measure Trx 1 in benign and malignant prostate tissue of men diagnosed with incident prostate cancer and determine the association between prostate tissue Trx 1 and Gleason score, dietary antioxidant intake, and blood biomarkers of antioxidant enzyme activity. The hypotheses of the current study were as follows: (1) the level of Trx 1 in malignant prostate tissue would be positively associated with Gleason score, (2) high grade cancer would exhibit a greater difference between the Trx 1 level of benign and malignant tissue, and (3) measures of antioxidants and prostate tissue levels of Trx 1 would be inversely associated.

2. Materials and Methods

Data collected by the North Carolina-Louisiana Prostate Cancer Project (PCaP), a population based study of incident prostate cancer [24], was used for this study. Briefly, men between 40 and 79 years of age with a first diagnosis of histologically confirmed adenocarcinoma of the prostate on or after July 1, 2004, were eligible to participate in PCaP. Men had to be able to complete the study interview in English and could not live in an institution or nursing home, be cognitively impaired, be under the influence of alcohol, be severely medicated, or be apparently psychotic. Men must have self-identified as either African American or Black or Caucasian or White (European American), when responding to the question "What is your race?" This project was approved by the institutional review boards at the Department of Defense Prostate Cancer Research Program, the University of North Carolina, and Louisiana State University. The current study also was approved by the institutional review board at the University of Connecticut.

Dietary data were collected using a modified version of the National Cancer Institute Diet History Questionnaire (DHQ) [25]. Data for the flavonoid and proanthocyanidin content of foods were added to the DHQ database using Nutrition Data System for Research, version 2011 (Nutrition Coordinating Center, University of Minnesota, Minneapolis, MN). The ABTS (2,2′-azino-bis(3-ethylbenzothiazoline-6-sulfonic acid)) radical anion scavenging activity assay was used previously to measure the vitamin C equivalent antioxidant capacities of individual antioxidants [26] and values were applied to PCaP diet and supplement data. Total antioxidant capacity (TAC) was calculated from the vitamin C equivalent antioxidant capacity of 42 dietary antioxidants (carotenoids, vitamins C and E, flavonoids, proanthocyanidins, and isoflavones) and 5 antioxidants from dietary supplements (vitamin C, alpha-tocopherol, beta-carotene, lycopene, and lutein and zeaxanthin). The antioxidant capacity of an antioxidant was calculated as the product of its reported intake in grams and its vitamin C equivalent antioxidant capacity, and TAC was calculated as the sum of all individual antioxidant capacities.

Paraffin-embedded prostate tissue biopsy specimens were selected from PCaP research subjects who were untreated at the time of sample collection to provide an approximately equal distribution of subjects by site, race, and aggressiveness level to yield a subsample of 59 tissue sections (5 μm in thickness) for analysis. Sections were deparaffinized, rehydrated under an alcohol gradient, and antigen-retrieved using Reveal Decloaker (Biocare Medical, Concord, CA) for 15 minutes at 110°C in a decloaking chamber (Biocare Medical). Sections were blocked for endogenous peroxidase activity using 3% H_2O_2, rinsed with deionized, distilled water for 10 minutes at room temperature, blocked with normal goat serum for 1 hour, and incubated overnight at 4°C with rabbit anti-Trx 1 (1 : 1000; Cell Signaling, Danvers, MA). The next day, sections were incubated for 30 minutes at room temperature with Rabbit SignalStain Boost IHC Reagent; the enzymatic activity was revealed using diaminobenzidine (Sigma-Aldrich, St. Louis, MO), counterstained with hematoxylin (Vector Laboratories, Burlingame, CA), and mounted using a permanent mounting medium. Images of stained sections were collected using a Leica DFC0425C camera mounted on a Leica DMRA2 microscope equipped with automated stage. The optimal titer of the Trx 1 primary antibody was determined by assessing immunostain quality after using different dilutions on prostate cancer tissue control sections acquired from a deidentified research subject. Two sections from the deidentified research subject served as positive control, immunostained with Trx 1 or a negative control, immunostained with Trx 1 blocking peptide (Cell Signaling, Danvers, MA).

Prostate cancer Gleason score of biopsy sections was determined by a genitourinary pathologist (GA). Levels of Trx 1 in benign and malignant tissue were visually scored by a genitourinary pathologist (GA) in a blinded fashion. Slides were scored from 0 to 3, with 0 indicating absence of staining and 1 through 3 indicating greater intensity of staining. The difference in Trx 1 between benign and malignant tissue was determined by subtracting the score in benign tissue from that in malignant tissue.

Peripheral blood samples collected from PCaP research subjects were centrifuged and packed erythrocytes were aliquoted and stored at −80°C until analysis. The activities of erythrocyte glutathione peroxidase, glutathione S-transferase, glutathione reductase, and superoxide dismutase were measured in erythrocyte lysates using commercial kits following manufacturer instructions (Cayman Chemical Company, Ann Arbor, MI). Tertiles for dietary TAC and antioxidant enzyme activity were created using SAS PROC RANK. Associations between Trx 1 levels in prostate cancer tissue and Gleason score, erythrocyte antioxidant enzyme activity, and dietary TAC were determined using Fisher's exact test ($\alpha = 0.05$). All P values reported are two sided.

A total of 59 prostate biopsy specimens were randomly selected for analyses. Samples were excluded from analyses for the following reasons: (1) sections that contained malignant tissue were not available for four biopsies, (2) four sections fell off the slides during processing, and (3) blood samples were not available for 11 research subjects. The final number used in analyses was 51 for Gleason score, 45 for erythrocyte antioxidant enzymes, and 55 for dietary TAC. All statistical analyses were performed using SAS software, version 9.3 (SAS Institute Inc., Cary, NC).

Table 1: Descriptive statistics of research subjects.

Characteristic	Median	IQR
Age (years)	66	(61, 71)
PSA (ng/dL)	6.00	(4.7, 11.4)
TAC (mg VCE/d)	576.8	(312.9, 926.4)
GPx (nmol/min/mL)	815	(455.9, 1044.2)
GR (nmol/min/mL)	205.8	(151.8, 305.6)
GST (nmol/min/mL)	49.7	(32.6, 65.4)
SOD (units/mL)[1]	75.5	(68.1, 80)
Gleason score	N	%
3 + 3	12	20.3
3 + 4	24	40.7
4 + 3	12	20.3
4 + 4	2	3.4
4 + 5	1	1.7
Family history[2]	12	25.5
BMI[3]		
Underweight	1	1.8
Normal	10	18.2
Overweight	19	34.6
Obese	21	38.2
Morbidly obese	4	7.3
Race		
African American	28	50.9
European American	27	49.1

IQR: interquartile range; BMI: body mass index; PSA: prostate specific antigen; TAC: total antioxidant capacity; VCE/d: vitamin C equivalents per day; GPx: glutathione peroxidase; GR: glutathione reductase; GST: glutathione S-transferase; SOD: superoxide dismutase.

[1]One unit of SOD is the amount of enzyme needed to dismutate 50% of superoxide radicals.

[2]Family history defined as at least one first-degree relative diagnosed with prostate cancer.

[3]BMI categories defined as underweight (<18.5 kg/m^2), normal (18.5 to 24.9 kg/m^2), overweight (25.0 to 29.9 kg/m^2), obese (30.0 to 34.9 kg/m^2), and morbidly obese (>35.0 kg/m^2).

3. Results

Descriptive statistics for research subjects are presented in Table 1. The median age of research subjects was 66 years, the median level of prostate-specific antigen was 6.0 ng/dL, and the most common Gleason score was 3 + 4. Images of Trx 1 stained prostate biopsy specimens are shown in Figure 1 for benign tissue and malignant tissue with Gleason scores 3 + 3, 3 + 4, 4 + 3, and 4 + 4.

The associations between Gleason score and Trx 1 are displayed in Table 2. Prostate tissue Trx 1 levels in benign

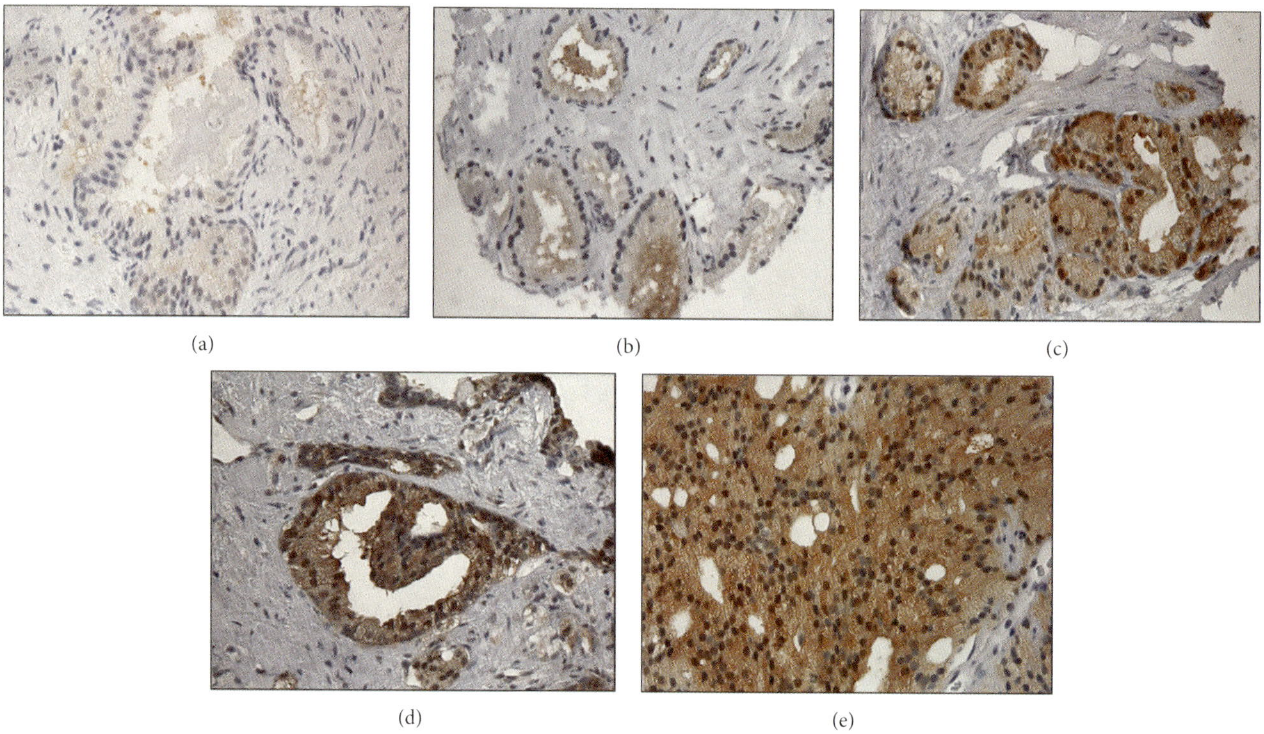

FIGURE 1: Images of immunohistochemical staining of Trx 1 diagnostic prostate cancer biopsy sections. Sections: (a) benign tissue, (b) Gleason score 3 + 3, (c) Gleason score 3 + 4, (d) Gleason score 4 + 3, and (e) Gleason score 4 + 4.

TABLE 2: Association between prostate tissue Trx 1 and Gleason score.

	Gleason score								Total
	3 + 3		3 + 4		4 + 3		4 + 4 or 5 + 4		
	n	%	*n*	%	*n*	%	*n*	%	
Malignant Trx 1									
1	4	(50)	3	(37)	0	(0)	1	(12)	8
2	6	(25)	13	(54)	4	(16)	1	(4)	24
3	2	(10)	8	(42)	8	(42)	1	(5)	19
Fisher's exact test, $P = 0.09$									
Benign Trx 1									
0	0	(0)	0	(0)	2	(66)	1	(33)	3
1	7	(23)	19	(63)	3	(10)	1	(3)	30
2	5	(33)	4	(26)	5	(33)	1	(6)	15
3	0	(0)	1	(33)	2	(66)	0	(0)	3
Fisher's exact test, $P = 0.01$									
ΔTrx 1									
−1	1	(33)	1	(33)	1	(33)	0	(0)	3
0	5	(31)	5	(31)	4	(25)	2	(12)	16
1	6	(30)	12	(60)	2	(10)	0	(0)	20
2	0	(0)	6	(66)	3	(33)	0	(0)	9
3	0	(0)	0	(0)	2	(66)	1	(33)	3
Total	**12**		**24**		**12**		**3**		**51**
Fisher's exact test, $P = 0.04$									

ΔTrx 1: difference in Trx 1 level between malignant and benign prostate cells.

TABLE 3: Association between prostate tissue Trx 1 and erythrocyte glutathione peroxidase activity.

	Erythrocyte glutathione peroxidase (GPx)						
	T1		T2		T3		Total
	n	%	n	%	n	%	
Malignant Trx 1							
0	2	(50)	0	(0)	2	(50)	4
1	1	(14)	5	(71)	1	(14)	7
2	7	(35)	3	(15)	10	(50)	20
3	6	(42)	7	(50)	1	(7)	14
Fisher's exact test, $P = 0.01$							
Benign Trx 1							
0	0	(0)	1	(100)	0	(0)	1
1	11	(39)	9	(32)	8	(28)	28
2	3	(23)	4	(30)	6	(46)	13
3	2	(66)	1	(33)	0	(0)	3
Fisher's exact test, $P = 0.55$							
ΔTrx 1							
−2	1	(50)	0	(0)	1	(50)	2
−1	1	(25)	2	(50)	1	(25)	4
0	4	(28)	4	(28)	6	(42)	14
1	7	(41)	5	(29)	5	(29)	17
2	3	(42)	3	(42)	1	(14)	7
3	0	(0)	1	(100)	0	(0)	1
Total	**16**		**15**		**14**		**45**
Fisher's exact test, $P = 0.93$							

ΔTrx 1: difference in Trx 1 level between malignant and benign prostate cells. Median values of tertiles of GPx activity are as follows: T1: 356.6 mol/min/mL; T2: 815.0 nmol/min/mL; T3: 1258.2 nmol/min/mL.

TABLE 4: Association between prostate tissue Trx 1 and erythrocyte glutathione reductase (GR) activity.

	Erythrocyte glutathione reductase (GR)						
	T1		T2		T3		Total
	n	%	n	%	n	%	
Malignant Trx 1							
0	2	(50)	1	(25)	1	(25)	4
1	0	(0)	3	(42)	4	(57)	7
2	9	(45)	6	(30)	5	(25)	20
3	3	(21)	6	(42)	5	(35)	14
Fisher's exact test, $P = 0.33$							
Benign Trx 1							
0	0	(0)	0	(0)	1	(100)	1
1	7	(25)	13	(46)	8	(28)	28
2	5	(38)	2	(14)	6	(46)	13
3	2	(66)	1	(33)	0	(0)	3
Fisher's exact test, $P = 0.17$							
ΔTrx 1							
−2	1	(50)	0	(0)	1	(50)	2
−1	1	(25)	2	(50)	1	(25)	4
0	6	(42)	4	(28)	4	(28)	14
1	5	(29)	5	(29)	7	(41)	17
2	1	(14)	5	(71)	1	(14)	7
3	0	(0)	0	(0)	1	(100)	1
Total	**14**		**16**		**15**		**45**
Fisher's exact test, $P = 0.62$							

ΔTrx 1: difference in Trx 1 level between malignant and benign prostate cells. Median values of tertiles of GR activity are as follows: T1: 137.8 mol/min/mL; T2: 205.8 nmol/min/mL; T3: 383.8 nmol/min/mL.

tissue appeared to increase significantly with the Gleason score of malignant tissue. Furthermore, the difference in Trx 1 between benign and malignant tissue was associated significantly with the Gleason score of malignant tissue ($P = 0.04$).

The relationship between prostate tissue Trx 1 and erythrocyte glutathione peroxidase, glutathione reductase, glutathione S-transferase, and superoxide dismutase is shown in Tables 3, 4, 5, and 6, respectively. No association was found between Trx 1 in prostate tissue and activity of erythrocyte glutathione reductase, glutathione S-transferase, or superoxide dismutase. However, Trx 1 levels were lower among research subjects with greater erythrocyte glutathione peroxidase activity ($P = 0.01$).

Dietary TAC, representing a combined dietary antioxidant index, was associated significantly with Trx 1 levels in benign tissue ($P = 0.03$), and greater levels of Trx 1 corresponded to lower dietary TAC (Table 7). There was no significant association between dietary TAC and Trx 1 levels in malignant tissue or the difference in Trx 1 levels between malignant and benign tissue. Table 8 provides a summary of the associations between Trx 1 and grade, antioxidant enzyme activity, and dietary antioxidant capacity.

4. Discussion

Levels of Trx 1 in prostate tissue were found to be associated with Gleason score, antioxidant enzyme activity, and dietary antioxidants. While no association was found between Gleason score and Trx 1 in malignant tissue, a positive association was found with Trx 1 in benign tissue and the difference in Trx 1 level between malignant and benign tissue, indicating that malignant cells have more Trx 1 compared with benign cells and that this difference increases with the Gleason score of malignant tissue (Table 2). While the clinical implications of these findings regarding prostate cancer is not clear, these results may reflect a compensatory response to redox imbalance, since the thioredoxin system is upregulated in prostate cancer [15, 16]. This suggests that more advanced cancer exhibits greater imbalance in redox status.

Glutathione peroxidase activity was associated significantly with Trx 1 level in malignant cells; levels of Trx 1 appeared lower in men with greater glutathione peroxidase activity (Table 3). Since no association was found between Trx 1 and the activity of other erythrocyte antioxidant enzymes, the observed association between Trx 1 and glutathione peroxidase could be due to chance. However, there are several explanations for an absence of effect. Arsova-Sarafinovska et al. [8]

Table 5: Association between prostate tissue Trx 1 and erythrocyte glutathione S-transferase activity.

	Erythrocyte glutathione S-transferase (GST)						
	T1		T2		T3		Total
	n	%	n	%	n	%	
Malignant Trx 1							
0	2	(50)	1	(25)	1	(25)	4
1	4	(57)	0	(0)	3	(42)	7
2	4	(20)	10	(50)	6	(30)	20
3	6	(42)	5	(35)	3	(21)	14
Fisher's exact test, $P = 0.21$							
Benign Trx 1							
0	0	(0)	1	(100)	0	(0)	1
1	8	(28)	11	(39)	9	(32)	28
2	7	(53)	3	(23)	3	(23)	13
3	1	(33)	1	(33)	1	(33)	3
Fisher's exact test, $P = 0.65$							
ΔTrx 1							
−2	1	(50)	1	(50)	0	(0)	2
−1	2	(50)	1	(25)	1	(25)	4
0	6	(42)	2	(14)	6	(42)	14
1	5	(29)	7	(41)	5	(29)	17
2	2	(28)	4	(57)	1	(14)	7
3	0	(0)	1	(100)	0	(0)	1
Total	**16**		**16**		**13**		**45**
Fisher's exact test, $P = 0.65$							

ΔTrx 1: difference in Trx 1 level between malignant and benign prostate cells. Median values of tertiles of GST activity are as follows: T1: 19.9 nmol/min/mL; T2: 49.7 nmol/min/mL; T3: 84.4 nmol/min/mL.

Table 6: Association between prostate tissue Trx 1 and erythrocyte superoxide dismutase activity.

	Erythrocyte superoxide dismutase (SOD)						
	T1		T2		T3		Total
	n	%	n	%	n	%	
Malignant Trx 1							
0	2	(50)	1	(25)	1	(25)	4
1	1	(14)	3	(42)	3	(42)	7
2	5	(25)	7	(35)	8	(40)	20
3	7	(50)	5	(35)	2	(14)	14
Fisher's exact test, $P = 0.53$							
Benign Trx 1							
0	0	(0)	1	(100)	0	(0)	1
1	11	(39)	8	(28)	9	(32)	28
2	2	(15)	6	(46)	5	(38)	13
3	2	(66)	1	(33)	0	(0)	3
Fisher's exact test, $P = 0.36$							
ΔTrx 1							
−2	1	(50)	0	(0)	1	(50)	2
−1	1	(25)	2	(50)	1	(25)	4
0	3	(21)	6	(42)	5	(35)	14
1	6	(35)	6	(35)	5	(29)	17
2	4	(57)	1	(14)	2	(28)	7
3	0	(0)	1	(100)	0	(0)	1
Total	**16**		**15**		**14**		**45**
Fisher's exact test, $P = 0.85$							

ΔTrx 1: difference in Trx 1 level between malignant and benign prostate cells. Median values of tertiles of SOD activity are as follows: T1: 66.3 units/mL; T2: 75.9 units/mL; T3: 80.8 units/mL.

found that erythrocyte antioxidant enzyme activity was decreased in prostate cancer patients compared to controls. Since the present study included only men diagnosed with prostate cancer, differences between healthy men and those with prostate cancer may be greater than differences among men with prostate cancer. Other studies have demonstrated that polymorphisms in antioxidant enzymes are related to prostate cancer [5, 6]; antioxidant enzyme activity, as assessed in this study, may not be sensitive enough to capture functional differences in antioxidant enzymes that result from differences in amino acid sequences. Furthermore, erythrocyte antioxidant activity may not reflect prostate tissue antioxidant activity.

Dietary TAC was used to represent antioxidant intake in the diet and was found to be associated significantly with the level of Trx 1 in benign prostate tissue ($P = 0.03$). Benign prostate tissue Trx 1 appears to be inversely associated with dietary TAC, with greater Trx 1 levels associated with lower dietary TAC (Table 7). Much of the evidence regarding dietary antioxidants and prostate cancer is inconsistent, but some dietary antioxidants may be beneficial for the chemoprevention of prostate cancer [19], although little evidence supports an effect of diet on prostate cancer progression. A summary of the associations observed in this study is presented in Table 8.

The primary strength of this study was use of Trx 1 to assess prostate tissue redox status. Trx 1 may indicate redox imbalance in prostate cancer [16]. Expression of TrxR1, the enzyme responsible for maintaining Trx 1 in a reduced form, is increased in castration-resistant prostate cancer [15]. Relatively few studies have been conducted on the thioredoxin system and prostate cancer, and while this system appears to play an important role in prostate cancer, the extent to which this system affects prostate cancer development and progression in humans remains uncertain. To the authors' knowledge, this is the first paper to demonstrate that the redox status of prostate tissue is associated with enzymatic and dietary antioxidants.

This study also has several limitations. The cross-sectional design of the study prohibits establishing a cause and effect relationship between prostate tissue Trx 1 and dietary and erythrocyte antioxidants. Dietary data were collected after diagnosis and knowledge of disease may have biased responses by research subjects, though this would likely have been nondifferential. The number of research subjects included in

TABLE 7: Association between prostate tissue Trx 1 level and dietary total antioxidant capacity.

	Dietary total antioxidant capacity (TAC)						
	T1		T2		T3		Total
	n	%	*n*	%	*n*	%	
Malignant Trx 1							
0	0	(0)	2	(50)	2	(50)	4
1	4	(50)	3	(38)	1	(13)	8
2	9	(38)	7	(29)	8	(33)	24
3	5	(26)	7	(37)	7	(37)	19
Fisher's exact test, $P = 0.64$							
Benign Trx 1							
0	0	(0)	3	(100)	0	(0)	3
1	12	(38)	11	(34)	9	(28)	32
2	3	(18)	5	(29)	9	(53)	17
3	3	(100)	0	(0)	0	(0)	3
Fisher's exact test, $P = 0.03$							
ΔTrx 1							
−2	0	(0)	1	(50)	1	(0)	2
−1	1	(20)	2	(40)	2	(40)	5
0	7	(44)	4	(25)	5	(32)	16
1	9	(45)	6	(30)	5	(25)	20
2	1	(11)	3	(33)	5	(56)	9
3	0	(0)	3	(100)	0	(0)	3
Total	**18**		**19**		**18**		**55**
Fisher's exact test, $P = 0.34$							

ΔTrx 1: difference in Trx 1 level between malignant and benign prostate cells. Median values of tertiles of dietary TAC are as follows: T1: 251.2 mg VCE/d; T2: 576.8 mg VCE/d; T3: 1181.0 mg VCE/d.

TABLE 8: Summary of associations between prostate cancer Gleason score, antioxidant enzymes, and dietary total antioxidant capacity and Trx 1 levels in prostate tissue based on results of the present study: (+) indicates a positive association and (−) a negative association; empty cells indicate no evidence of an association.

	Trx 1	
	Malignant tissue	Benign tissue
Gleason score	+	+
GPx	−	
GR		
GST		
SOD		
TAC		−

GPx: erythrocyte glutathione peroxidase activity; GR: erythrocyte glutathione reductase activity; GST: erythrocyte glutathione S-transferase activity; SOD: erythrocyte superoxide dismutase activity; TAC: dietary total antioxidant capacity.
*While the association between Gleason score and Trx 1 in malignant tissue was not statistically significant ($P = 0.09$), the data in Table 2 displays evidence of a positive association.

the study is relatively few, especially those with high Gleason score and Trx 1 levels, which may have contributed to some of the null results.

5. Conclusions

This study suggests that the redox status within the prostate is associated with endogenous and exogenous antioxidants. The results of this study and others warrant additional research in humans on the mechanisms underlying the relationship between prostate tissue redox status and carcinogenesis and determining whether the redox status within prostate tissue may influence prostate cancer aggressiveness.

Acknowledgments

The authors thank the staff, advisory committees, and research subjects participating in the PCaP study for their important contributions. The authors thank John Stocking and Sarah McEvoy for technical assistance with immunostaining. They would like to acknowledge the RPCI Department of Urology Tissue Microarray and Immuno-Analysis Core for their tissue processing, storage, and sample disbursement and to acknowledge the UNC BioSpecimen Facility and the LSUHSC Pathology Lab for their blood processing, storage, and sample disbursement (https://genome.unc.edu/bsp/). This study is supported by the NIH Cancer Epidemiology Small Grant no. 1R03CA159421-01A1 and Department of Defense contract DAMD 17-03-2-0052.

References

[1] R. Siegel, J. Ma, Z. Zou, and A. Jemal, "Cancer statistics, 2014," *CA Cancer Journal for Clinicians*, vol. 64, no. 1, pp. 9–29, 2014.

[2] O. W. Brawley, "Prostate cancer epidemiology in the United States," *World Journal of Urology*, vol. 30, no. 2, pp. 195–200, 2012.

[3] A. R. Patel and E. A. Klein, "Risk factors for prostate cancer," *Nature Clinical Practice Urology*, vol. 6, no. 2, pp. 87–95, 2009.

[4] A. Paschos, R. Pandya, W. C. M. Duivenvoorden, and J. H. Pinthus, "Oxidative stress in prostate cancer: changing research concepts towards a novel paradigm for prevention and therapeutics," *Prostate Cancer and Prostatic Diseases*, vol. 16, no. 3, pp. 217–225, 2013.

[5] J. E. Klaunig, L. M. Kamendulis, and B. A. Hocevar, "Oxidative stress and oxidative damage in carcinogenesis," *Toxicologic Pathology*, vol. 38, no. 1, pp. 96–109, 2010.

[6] H. Li, P. W. Kantoff, E. Giovannucci et al., "Manganese superoxide dismutase polymorphism, prediagnostic antioxidant status, and risk of clinical significant prostate cancer," *Cancer Research*, vol. 65, no. 6, pp. 2498–2504, 2005.

[7] M. Goodman, R. M. Bostick, K. C. Ward et al., "Lycopene intake and prostate cancer risk: effect modification by plasma antioxidants and the XRCC1 genotype," *Nutrition and Cancer*, vol. 55, no. 1, pp. 13–20, 2006.

[8] Z. Arsova-Sarafinovska, A. Eken, N. Matevska et al., "Increased oxidative/nitrosative stress and decreased antioxidant enzyme activities in prostate cancer," *Clinical Biochemistry*, vol. 42, no. 12, pp. 1228–1235, 2009.

[9] M. Brys, A. Morel, E. Forma et al., "Relationship of urinary isoprostanes to prostate cancer occurence," *Molecular and Cellular Biochemistry*, vol. 372, no. 1-2, pp. 149–153, 2013.

[10] D. A. Barocas, S. Motley, M. S. Cookson et al., "Oxidative stress measured by urine F2-isoprostane level is associated with prostate cancer," *Journal of Urology*, vol. 185, no. 6, pp. 2102–2107, 2011.

[11] B. Kumar, S. Koul, L. Khandrika, R. B. Meacham, and H. K. Koul, "Oxidative stress is inherent in prostate cancer cells and is required for aggressive phenotype," *Cancer Research*, vol. 68, no. 6, pp. 1777–1785, 2008.

[12] R. A. Cairns, I. S. Harris, and T. W. Mak, "Regulation of cancer cell metabolism," *Nature Reviews Cancer*, vol. 11, no. 2, pp. 85–95, 2011.

[13] R. Singal, J. van Wert, and M. Bashambu, "Cytosine methylation represses glutathione S-transferase P1 (GSTP1) gene expression in human prostate cancer cells," *Cancer Research*, vol. 61, no. 12, pp. 4820–4826, 2001.

[14] E. S. J. Arnér and A. Holmgren, "The thioredoxin system in cancer," *Seminars in Cancer Biology*, vol. 16, no. 6, pp. 420–426, 2006.

[15] S. S. Singh, Y. Li, O. H. Ford III et al., "Thioredoxin reductase 1 expression and castration-recurrent growth of prostate cancer," *Translational Oncology*, vol. 1, no. 3, pp. 153–157, 2008.

[16] W. Shan, W. Zhong, R. Zhao, and T. D. Oberley, "Thioredoxin 1 as a subcellular biomarker of redox imbalance in human prostate cancer progression," *Free Radical Biology & Medicine*, vol. 49, no. 12, pp. 2078–2087, 2010.

[17] A. Holmgren and J. Lu, "Thioredoxin and thioredoxin reductase: current research with special reference to human disease," *Biochemical and Biophysical Research Communications*, vol. 396, no. 1, pp. 120–124, 2010.

[18] E. S. J. Arnér, "Focus on mammalian thioredoxin reductases—important selenoproteins with versatile functions," *Biochimica et Biophysica Acta*, vol. 1790, no. 6, pp. 495–526, 2009.

[19] T. M. Vance, J. Su, E. T. H. Fontham, S. I. Koo, and O. K. Chun, "Dietary antioxidants and prostate cancer: a review," *Nutrition and Cancer*, vol. 65, no. 6, pp. 793–801, 2013.

[20] H. Sharma, R. Kanwal, N. Bhaskaran, and S. Gupta, "Plant flavone apigenin binds to nucleic acid bases and reduces oxidative DNA damage in prostate epithelial cells," *PLoS ONE*, vol. 9, no. 3, Article ID e91588, 2014.

[21] K. Gao, S. M. Henning, Y. Niu et al., "The citrus flavonoid naringenin stimulates DNA repair in prostate cancer cells," *Journal of Nutritional Biochemistry*, vol. 17, no. 2, pp. 89–95, 2006.

[22] M. Serafini and D. Del Rio, "Understanding the association between dietary antioxidants, redox status and disease: is the Total Antioxidant Capacity the right tool?" *Redox Report*, vol. 9, no. 3, pp. 145–152, 2004.

[23] K. M. Russnes, K. M. Wilson, M. M. Epstein et al., "Total antioxidant intake in relation to prostate cancer incidence in the health professionals follow-up study," *International Journal of Cancer*, vol. 134, no. 5, pp. 1156–1165, 2014.

[24] J. C. Schroeder, J. T. Bensen, L. J. Su et al., "The North Carolina-Louisiana Prostate Cancer Project (PCaP): methods and design of a multidisciplinary population-based cohort study of racial differences in prostate cancer outcomes," *Prostate*, vol. 66, no. 11, pp. 1162–1176, 2006.

[25] National Institutes of Health ARP and National Cancer Institute, *Diet History Questionnaire, Version 1.0*, 2007.

[26] A. Floegel, D.-O. Kim, S.-J. Chung et al., "Development and validation of an algorithm to establish a total antioxidant capacity database of the US diet," *International Journal of Food Sciences and Nutrition*, vol. 61, no. 6, pp. 600–623, 2010.

18

Biomarkers of Prostatic Cancer: An Attempt to Categorize Patients into Prostatic Carcinoma, Benign Prostatic Hyperplasia, or Prostatitis Based on Serum Prostate Specific Antigen, Prostatic Acid Phosphatase, Calcium, and Phosphorus

Shahana Sarwar,[1] Mohammed Abdul Majid Adil,[2] Parveen Nyamath,[3] and Mohammed Ishaq[3]

[1] *Department of Biochemistry, Owaisi Group of Hospitals, DCMS, Hyderabad, Telangana, India*
[2] *Department of Urology, Owaisi Group of Hospitals, DCMS, Hyderabad, Telangana, India*
[3] *Salar-e-Millat Research Centre, PEH, DCMS, Hyderabad, Telangana, India*

Correspondence should be addressed to Mohammed Abdul Majid Adil; drmamadil@yahoo.co.in

Academic Editor: Weide Zhong

Prostatitis, BPH, and P.Ca are the most frequent pathologies of the prostate gland that are responsible for morbidity in men. Raised levels of PSA are seen in different pathological conditions involving the prostate. PAP levels are altered in inflammatory or infectious or abnormal growth of the prostate tissue. Serum calcium and phosphorus levels were also found to be altered in prostate cancer and BPH. The present study was carried out to study the levels of PSA, PAP, calcium, and phosphorus in serum of patients with Prostatitis, BPH, or P.Ca and also to evaluate the relationship between them. Males in the age group of 50–85 years with LUTS disease symptoms and with PSA levels more than 4 ng/mL were included. A total of 114 patients were analyzed including 30 controls. Prostatitis in 35.7% of cases, BPH in 35.7% of the cases, and P.Ca in 28.57% of the cases were observed. Thus, the nonmalignant cases constitute a majority. PSA, a marker specific for prostatic conditions, was significantly high in all the diseases compared to controls. A rise in serum PSA and PAP indicates prostatitis or, in combination with these two tests, decreased serum calcium shows advanced disease.

1. Introduction

The diseases associated with prostate are prostatitis, benign prostatic hyperplasia (BPH), and prostate cancer (P.Ca) which leads to several metabolic disturbances. P.Ca is the second dreadful cancer in the world, common among men in US. Annually more than 2,30,000 men are diagnosed and approximately 30,000 die from it. African American men have high incidence of P.Ca and 60% more likely to develop when compared to Caucasian. It affects the young men with positive family history of P.Ca when compared to individuals without history. Men above 45 years are prone to BPH, a universal phenomenon which increases with age. Various factors are responsible for the prostate diseases in men especially elders [1, 2]. Screenings for P.Ca include serum PSA and digital rectal examination (DRE); a biopsy is required to diagnose P.Ca. The histopathological diagnosis of prostate cancer will only confirm the final diagnosis in 67% of cases whereas 33% are diagnosed with the other modalities [3].

Early detection and treatment in asymptomatic men may improve the mortality rate and the quality of life. Screening for markers such as prostate specific antigen (PSA) and prostate acid phosphatase (PAP) resulted in detection and treatment of the disease at an earlier stage.

Men of 50 years of age or above without any family history of cancer and those at 40 years of age with family history must undergo digital rectal examination (DRE) and PSA levels should be checked annually as recommended by of American Urological Association (AUA) and Food and Drug Administration (FDA).

The screening of PSA is not a common practice in India. The patients visiting department of urology of a hospital with complaints of lower urinary tract symptoms (LUTS) are checked for their PSA levels. Various studies reported that men with LUTS have the same risk of having P.Ca as asymptomatic men of the same age and have an increased risk of unnecessary biopsy if the threshold is taken as the same as that in case of the symptomatic men [4–6].

Several studies reported that markers such as PSA and PAP were used for confirming and monitoring P.Ca. PSA is one of the organ specific tumor markers produced by prostatic tissue [7]. In patients with BPH, PSA levels can increase 2-3 times the normal. The major limitation for using PSA, as a screening prostate cancer biomarker, is that majority of the men suffer from BPH and prostatitis as they become old, which increases their serum PSA levels. Therefore, PSA alone cannot be used as a biomarker for cancer detection. The elevated levels of PSA do not indicate cancer but the higher the PSA level, the more the chance of having cancer.

PAP is a tumor marker produced by the lysosomes of the prostate's epithelial cells [8]. The levels of PAP are high in 60% of men with P.Ca with metastases. However, the level of PAP in the serum is normal or slightly high when the carcinoma remains localized in the prostate gland and is elevated in some benign condition such as BPH and osteoporosis.

The association between high levels of serum calcium and risk of P.Ca has been demonstrated by various investigators [9]. The high level of calcium in serum is due to decrease in apoptosis and an increase in proliferation of P.Ca cells responsible for growth and metastasis. The increase in serum calcium or any factor that leads to it would increase the possibility for terminal P.Ca as has been reported by several researchers. Thus, analysis of calcium in serum may be used as a promising prospective biomarker for screening for P.Ca.

Several studies have reported a positive association between phosphorus intake and P.Ca [10, 11]. A recent study by Wilson et al. showed that calcium and phosphorus have independent effects at different time periods between exposure and diagnosis of P.Ca [12].

There is a need to use combination of markers and tests which can save the patient from unnecessary biopsies.

The present study was carried out to categorize the patients into prostatic carcinoma, benign prostatic hyperplasia, or prostatitis based on serum prostate specific antigen, prostatic acid phosphatase, calcium and phosphorus levels, and DRE and to evaluate the discriminating power of these in distinguishing controls and cases to reduce the risk of unnecessary biopsy. The diagnostic efficiency (DE) of these markers was confirmed by analyzing their sensitivity and specificity using receptor operative curves (ROC).

2. Methods

The study was approved by Institutional Ethical Committee. The informed consent was obtained from the patients. The patients with LUTS visiting the Department of Urology at Owaisi group of hospitals and research centre were enrolled in the study. A total of 114 subjects were included in the study. 84 patients served as cases whereas age and sex matched 30 individuals were selected from ENT, dental, and gastroenterology departments of the same hospital with complaints of disease other than LUTS and served as controls. From each department, 10 subjects were included.

2.1. Inclusion Criteria. Male patients in the age group of 50–85 years with LUTS and with PSA levels more than normal value (i.e. >4 ng/mL) were included. Age and sex matched persons without LUTS served as controls.

2.2. Exclusion Criteria. Patients with acute LUTS with fever and other symptoms, documented UTI, established cases of P.Ca, BPH and prostatitis, or history of previous biopsy or urological procedure were excluded.

The clinical diagnosis of prostatic disease was based on LUTS, elevated levels of PSA, DRE, TRUS, and TRUS guided biopsy, and histopathological examination of the biopsied tissue. The blood was collected at initial presentation in order to avoid any stimulation of the prostatic gland, which may increase PSA levels. Then, the patients were categorized into prostatitis, BPH, and P.Ca.

2.3. Sample Collection. 10 mL of venous blood (fasting) was collected under aseptic conditions in the plain tubes. Serum was used for the analysis of PSA, PAP, calcium, and phosphorus.

2.4. Procedure. Serum PSA was measured using commercially available kits based on enzyme immunoassay for the quantitative determination by Pathozyme ELISA [13]. The estimation of PAP was done by Kinetic method [14], calcium by O-cresolphthalein complexone method and End Point Assay [15], and the level of phosphorus was done by UV-End point method [16]. The ROC was plotted by Youden Index, to calculate the best cutoff value.

3. Results

The age of the subjects were given in the age range of 50–85 years (Table 1).

The mean values for PSA, PAP, and calcium are significantly higher in cases than controls (Table 2). The comparison of PSA and PAP levels in between the groups revealed that the levels are significantly higher in prostatitis as compared to BPH and controls. The level of PAP was significantly higher in prostatic carcinoma as compared to prostatitis. The serum calcium level was higher in BPH group when compared to prostate carcinoma. The phosphorus level was significantly more in BPH than controls.

In order to assess the maximum sensitivity, specificity, and DE of various parameters in identifying abnormality, the best cutoff values (BCV) were calculated using ROC analysis (Figures 1 and 2, Tables 3 and 4). The analysis of prostate gland in patients of various groups based on digital rectal examination (DRE) was given in Table 5. The PSA levels and

Table 1: The number of patients in each group along with their age.

Group	Age (years)				
	50–59	60–69	70–79	80+	Total
Controls	7	9	12	2	30
Prostatitis	13	11	5	1	30
BPH	8	11	6	5	30
P.Ca	3	8	9	4	24

This table shows the age range of patients and controls included in the study. A total of 114 patients were included in the study. The individuals were grouped into 4 groups based on the age range which was from 50 to 85 years.

Table 2: The table shows the mean levels of various biomarkers in different groups.

Group	PSA (ng/mL)	PAP (IU/L)	Calcium (mg/dL)	Phosphorus (mg/dL)
Control	2.27 ± 1.06	2.5 ± 1.12	8.94 ± 0.74	3.41 ± 0.91
Prostatitis	52 ± 6.45	11.4 ± 2.34	9.08 ± 0.93	3.77 ± 1.1
BPH	11.15 ± 2.23	3.9 ± 1.34	9.23 ± 0.78	4.85 ± 1.8
Prostate Carcinoma	70.64 ± 6.54	25.1 ± 3.4	8.45 ± 0.85	3.5 ± 1.98

The table showed the levels of biochemical parameters in different groups. The levels of PSA and PAP were higher in P.Ca group as compared to the others.

Table 3: The sensitivity and specificity of various biomarkers in different groups are given in the table.

Parameter		Control versus total	Prostatitis versus BPH	BPH versus P.Ca	Prostatitis versus P.Ca
PSA (ng/mL)	Best cutoff	4.75	16.75	22.5	36.3
	Sensitivity	100	70	99.2	70.8
	Specificity	100	83.3	96.2	50
PAP (IU/L)	Best cutoff	4.05	6.35	10.5	19.5
	Sensitivity	76.2	90	87.5	79.2
	Specificity	96.7	90	100	93
Calcium (mg/dL)	Best cutoff	8.95	10.6	5.8	5.8
	Sensitivity	47.6	6.7	100	100
	Specificity	63.3	100	0	0
Phosphorus (mg/dL)	Best cutoff	4.35	6.65	5.55	3.1
	Sensitivity	42.9	99.9	4.25	70.8
	Specificity	93.3	96.3	86.7	40

The table shows the sensitivity and specificity pattern of PSA and PAP in different groups. At BCV 4.75 ng/mL, the PSA showed 100% sensitivity and specificity whereas at BCV 4.05 IU/L PAP showed 76.2% sensitivity and 96.7% specificity. BCV at 5.8 mg/dL calcium showed 100% sensitivity in BPH versus P.Ca and prostatitis versus P.Ca.

staging of prostate carcinoma patients in different age groups were given in Table 6.

In cases and controls,

> PSA, at bcv 4.75 ng/mL, showed 100% sensitivity and specificity,
>
> PAP, at bcv 4.05 IU/L, showed 76% sensitivity and 96% specificity,
>
> serum phosphorus 4.35 mg/dL showed specificity of 93%.

In prostatitis and BPH,

> PSA, at bcv 16.75 ng/mL, showed 70% sensitivity and 83.3% specificity,
>
> PAP, at bcv 6.35 IU/L, showed 90% sensitivity and specificity,
>
> serum calcium 10.6 mg/dL showed 100% specificity,
>
> phosphorus 6.65 mg/dL showed 99.9% sensitivity and 96.7% specificity.

In BPH and P.Ca,

> PSA, at bcv 22.5 ng/mL, showed 99.27% sensitivity and 96.7% specificity,
>
> PAP, at bcv 10.5 IU/L, showed 87.5% sensitivity and 100% specificity,
>
> serum calcium, 5.8 mg/dL, showed 100% sensitivity.

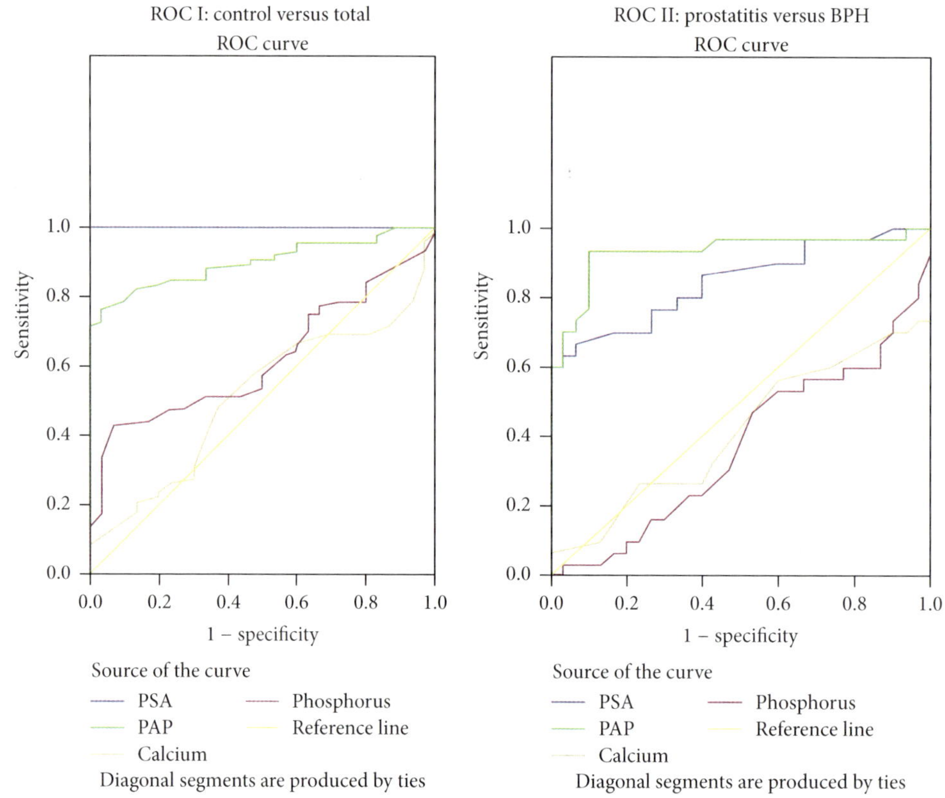

FIGURE 1: Receptor operative curves.

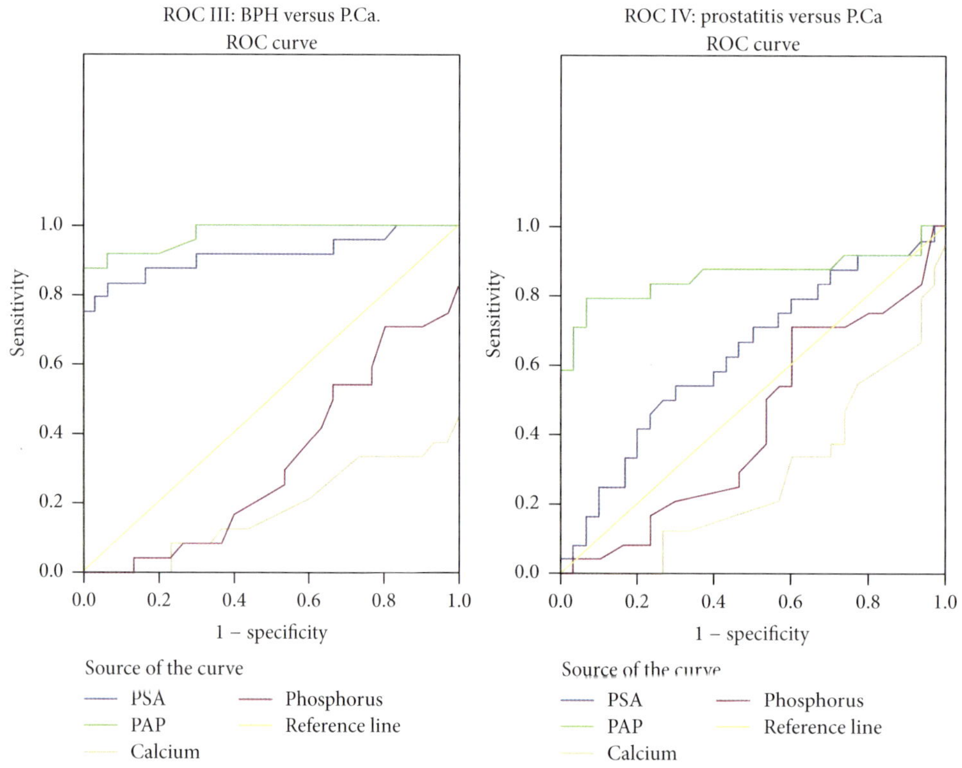

FIGURE 2: Receptor operative curves.

TABLE 4: The percentage of diagnostic efficiency (DE).

Parameter	Control versus total	Prostatitis versus BPH	BPH versus P.Ca
PSA	100%	76.6%	59.2%
PAP	82.4%	90%	83.35

The table showed the percentage of diagnostic efficiency of PSA and PAP in cases and controls. Serum PSA showed 100% DE in total cases and control whereas PAP showed only 82.4%. PSA showed DE of 76.6% and 59.2% in prostatitis versus BPH and BPH versus P.Ca, respectively, whereas DE of PAP was 90% and 83.3% in the above groups.

In prostatitis and P.Ca,

PSA, at bcv 36.3 ng/mL, showed 70.8% sensitivity and 50% specificity,

PAP, at bcv 19.5 IU/L, showed 79.2% sensitivity and 93% specificity,

serum calcium 5.8 mg/dL showed 100% sensitivity and no specificity.

4. Discussion

Prostate cancer, prostatitis, and BPH are the most frequent pathologies of the prostate gland, whose management strategies are diametrically different. P.Ca is the most frequently diagnosed malignancy in men and the second leading cause of cancer deaths especially in Western countries [1]. There is lack of epidemiological data on the exact prevalence of this disease in India due to lack of proper screening and underrecorded incidence of P.Ca. On the other hand, BPH and prostatitis are the other two most frequent pathologies of prostate gland that clinically/symptomatically mimic prostate cancer. P.Ca is notoriously difficult to treat, which makes its early detection a priority. There is an urgent need for appropriate diagnostic and prognostic markers to detect P.Ca and to differentiate it from other pathologies of prostate gland. The present study was undertaken to assess the levels of PSA, PAP, calcium, and phosphorus in different pathologies of prostate gland, in an attempt to use a combination of markers to differentiate the above conditions to avoid the use of unnecessary biopsies. Our observations revealed that PSA was significantly high in cases than controls ($p < 0.001$). These findings correlated with the studies by Jung et al. and Anim et al. confirming the increased levels of PSA in different pathologies of prostate gland [17, 18].

The discovery of PSA as a biomarker and demonstration of its utility in early diagnosis and monitoring of P.Ca date back to the early 1980s. However, the use of only PSA as an initial diagnostic tool has become controversial over the past decade due to its increased levels in other pathologies of prostate. This view is supported by our findings of significantly higher increase in PSA in prostatitis and prostate cancer compared to controls and BPH. The above marker, though it remains an early signal for the pathologies of prostate, may lead to overdiagnosis which in turn would result in over and aggressive treatment strategies. PAP was significantly increased in cases compared to controls ($p < 0.001$).

TABLE 5: The analysis of prostate gland in patients of various groups based on digital rectal examination (DRE).

Group	Number of patients	DRE details
Control ($n = 30$)	15	Normal, firm, nontender prostate with maintained landmarks
	13	Grade I-II, nontenderness and maintained land marks
	2	Grade III-IV, prostatomegaly
Prostatitis ($n = 30$)	16	Grade I-II prostatic enlargement with mild to moderate tenderness with maintained land marks
	7	Grade I-II with no tenderness with maintained landmarks
	4	Grade III-IV with mild to moderate tenderness and normal landmarks, firm consistency
	3	Grade III-IV with severe tenderness and soft prostate consistency
BPH ($n = 30$)	12	Grade I-II
	9	Grade III
	9	Grade IV, firm, nontender with maintained landmarks (median groove, etc.), no induration

Our findings were in agreement with the earlier studies by Taira et al. [19] and Nguyen et al. [20] thereby confirming the increased levels of PAP in different pathologies of prostate gland.

PAP emerged as the world's first clinically useful tumor marker in the 1940s and 1950s. With the introduction of the PSA test in the 1980s, which performed significantly better than PAP in terms of screening and monitoring response to treatment, PAP fell into disfavor. The recent studies have identified PAP as a significant prognostic factor for patients with intermediate and high-risk prostate cancer. PAP was known to have a low sensitivity for diagnosing new disease. In a study it was found that PAP has low sensitivity compared to PSA [21]. Since the goal of P.Ca screening is to identify early-stage treatable disease, PAP was rightly dropped as a screening tool. Several studies suggest that PAP could play a role in determining which early-stage patients are likely to benefit from more aggressive adjuvant therapy [21]. This view is supported by our findings of significantly higher increase in PAP in prostatitis and P.Ca compared to controls and BPH; in addition, we also observed significant increase in serum PAP in prostate cancer compared to prostatitis.

Moreover, it was observed that, at cutoff value of 4.75 ng/mL, PSA is indicative of prostate gland pathology at a sensitivity and specificity of 100% and DE of 100% which may lead to differentiating any pathology. However, the DE in discriminating prostatitis from BPH is 76.6%, between P.Ca and BPH is 90.7%, and between prostatitis and P.Ca is only 59.2%. Thus, the discriminating or diagnosing power of PSA into the type of pathology is limited. Our findings were in accordance with those of Yaman et al. and Simardi et al. who related the PSA elevation to pathologies of prostate

Table 6: The PSA levels and staging of prostate carcinoma patients.

Age (years)	Number of patients	PSA (ng/mL)	TNM staging	Stage	Gleason score
50–59	3	66.75	$T_1N_0M_0$	I-II	3 + 3 = 6
60–69	8	68.82	$T_1N_1M_0$	II-III	4 + 4 = 8
70–79	4	78.45	$T_3N_1M_1$	III-IV	5 + 4 = 9
	5	76.62	$T_3N_XM_1$	III-IV	3 + 4 = 7
80+	4	70.46	$T_2N_0M_1$	I-II	3 + 4 = 7

The table showed the TNM (tumor, lymph nodes, and metastases) staging and Gleason score in patients of various age groups. The level of PSA was also included.

tissues [22, 23]. It was also observed that, at a cutoff value of 4.05 IU/L, PAP is indicative of prostate gland pathology at a sensitivity of 76.2% and specificity of 96.7% in discriminating cases from controls and a DE of 82.4%. Thus, PAP was found to have a better discriminating power into the type of pathology. Its DE to differentiate between prostatitis and BPH is 90%, between BPH and P.Ca is 94.4%, and prostatitis from P.Ca is 85.5%.

A rise in PSA and PAP, in combination, indicates either prostatitis or P.Ca and rules out BPH. In combination to these two, a decrease in serum calcium is indicative of advanced disease in prostate cancer. This is in accordance with the findings of Kukreja et al. which show a significant decrease in P.Ca [9]. According to them, in patients with solid tumors like prostate, breast, or lung cancer, hypocalcaemia develops due to extensive osteoblastic metastases. Raskin et al. performed a retrospective analysis of serum calcium levels in patients with metastatic bone disease and reported a 33% prevalence of hypocalcaemia in patients with prostate cancer [24]. This is also in accordance with study by Szentirmai et al. which revealed that few patients with prostate cancer and bone metastases have a low serum calcium concentration, and some have severe hypocalcaemia [25]. Avid calcium uptake by osteoblastic bone metastases was postulated more than 30 years ago by Ludwig [26]. The hypocalcaemia in these patients may be most likely on the basis of extensive accretion of calcium into bones. Serum total calcium was significantly lower in patients with bone metastasis than those without. In this case, hypocalcaemia can be explained on the basis of hypoalbuminemia or renal failure. Therefore, apparent hypocalcaemia based on total calcium measurement is common in patients with P.Ca [9]. Men whose blood calcium levels fall at the high end of the normal range are more likely to develop 2.5 times fatal P.Ca when compared to men with lower levels, according to a recent study. If confirmed by other studies, the findings could have important implications for the prevention and treatment of P.Ca [27].

It has been known for many years that hypocalcaemia can occur in patients with osteoblastic metastases from prostate cancer. Ludwig postulated the following sequence: osteoblastic metastases cause increased deposition of calcium and phosphate in bone, tending to decrease serum concentrations of both ions [27]. P.Ca, BPH, and prostatitis are common prostatic clinical conditions whose management strategies are diametrically different. The final areas in differentiating these conditions are biopsy. Biopsies (8–10 needle core) have its own complications and side effects.

Though PSA has emerged as marker for prostatic conditions like P.Ca and BPH in the past decade, there has been an increasing realization by both biochemists and urologists, to have a better single marker or a combination of biochemical tests to differentiate the above conditions, to avoid frequency and unnecessary biopsies in nonmalignant conditions.

PSA is a marker specific for prostatic conditions and shown to be significant in all disease compared to controls. So, a rise in serum PSA and PAP indicates prostatitis or, in combination with these two tests, decreased serum calcium shows advanced disease.

Competing Interests

None of the contributing authors have any conflict of interests, including specific financial interests or relationships and affiliations relevant to the subject matter or materials discussed in the manuscript.

References

[1] P. Christudoss, R. Selvakumar, J. J. Fleming, and G. Gopalakrishnan, "Zinc status of patients with benign prostatic hyperplasia and prostate carcinoma," *Indian Journal of Urology*, vol. 27, no. 1, pp. 14–18, 2011.

[2] S. Bracarda, O. De Cobelli, C. Greco et al., "Cancer of the prostate," *Critical Reviews in Oncology/Hematology*, vol. 56, no. 3, pp. 379–396, 2005.

[3] J. E. McNeal, "Regional morphology and pathology of the prostate," *American Journal of Clinical Pathology*, vol. 49, no. 3, pp. 347–357, 1968.

[4] W. J. Catalona, A. W. Partin, K. M. Slawin et al., "Use of the percentage of free prostate-specific antigen to enhance differentiation of prostate cancer from benign prostatic disease: a prospective multicenter clinical trial," *The Journal of the American Medical Association*, vol. 279, no. 19, pp. 1542–1547, 1998.

[5] J. M. Young, D. J. Muscatello, and J. E. Ward, "Are men with lower urinary tract symptoms at increased risk of prostate cancer? A systematic review and critique of the available evidence," *BJU International*, vol. 85, no. 9, pp. 1037–1048, 2000.

[6] C. T. Brown, E. O'Flynn, J. Van Der Meulen, S. Newman, A. R. Mundy, and M. Emberton, "The fear of prostate cancer in men with lower urinary tract symptoms: should symptomatic men be screened?" *BJU International*, vol. 91, no. 1, pp. 30–32, 2003.

[7] D. F. Gleason and G. T. Mellinger, "Prediction of prognosis for prostatic adenocarcinoma by combined histological grading

and clinical staging," *The Journal of Urology*, vol. 111, no. 1, pp. 58–64, 1974.

[8] N. A. Romas, "Prostatic acid phosphatase: current concepts," *Seminars in urology*, vol. 1, no. 3, pp. 177–185, 1983.

[9] S. C. Kukreja, A. Shanmugam, and T. E. Lad, "Hypocalcemia in patients with prostate cancer," *Calcified Tissue International*, vol. 43, no. 6, pp. 340–345, 1988.

[10] S. Kapur, "Phosphorus balance and prostate cancer," *Indian Journal of Experimental Biology*, vol. 37, no. 7, pp. 623–626, 1999.

[11] E. Kesse, S. Bertrais, P. Astorg et al., "Dairy products, calcium and phosphorus intake, and the risk of prostate cancer: results of the French prospective SU.VI.MAX (Supplémentation en Vitamines et Minéraux Antioxydants) study," *British Journal of Nutrition*, vol. 95, no. 3, pp. 539–545, 2006.

[12] K. M. Wilson, I. M. Shui, L. A. Mucci, and E. Giovannucci, "Calcium and phosphorus intake and prostate cancer risk: a 24-y follow-up study," *American Journal of Clinical Nutrition*, vol. 101, no. 1, pp. 173–183, 2014.

[13] L. I. Stowell, L. E. Sharman, and K. Hamel, "An enzyme-linked immunosorbent assay (ELISA) for prostate-specific antigen," *Forensic Science International*, vol. 50, no. 1, pp. 125–138, 1991.

[14] A. B. Gutman and E. B. Gutman, "An 'ACID' phosphatase occurring in the serum of patients with metastasizing carcinoma of the prostate gland," *Journal of Clinical Investigation*, vol. 17, no. 4, pp. 473–478, 1938.

[15] H. J. Gitelman, "An improved automated procedure for the determination of calcium in biological specimens," *Analytical Biochemistry*, vol. 18, no. 3, pp. 521–531, 1967.

[16] N. W. Teitz, *Fundamentals of Clinical Chemistry*, W.B. Saunders, Philadelphia, Pa, USA, 2nd edition, 1976.

[17] K. Jung, J. Reiche, A. Boehme et al., "Analysis of subforms of free prostate-specific antigen in serum by two-dimensional gel electrophoresis: potential to improve diagnosis of prostate cancer," *Clinical Chemistry*, vol. 50, no. 12, pp. 2292–2301, 2004.

[18] J. Anim, E. Kehinde, M. Sheikh et al., "Serum prostate-specific antigen levels in middle eastern men with subclinical prostatitis," *Medical Principles and Practice*, vol. 16, no. 1, pp. 53–58, 2006.

[19] A. Taira, G. Merrick, K. Wallner, and M. Dattoli, "Reviving the acid phosphatase test for prostate cancer," *Oncology*, vol. 21, no. 8, pp. 1003–1010, 2007.

[20] L. Nguyen, A. Chapdelaine, and S. Chevalier, "Prostatic acid phosphatase in serum of patients with prostatic cancer is a specific phosphotyrosine acid phosphatase," *Clinical Chemistry*, vol. 36, no. 8, pp. 1450–1455, 1990.

[21] T. A. Stamey, N. Yang, and A. R. Hay, "Prostate-specific antigen as a serum marker for adenocarcinoma of the prostate," *New England Journal of Medicine*, vol. 317, no. 15, pp. 909–916, 1987.

[22] Ö. Yaman, Ç. Göğüş, Ö. Tulunay, Z. Tokatli, and E. Özden, "Increased prostate-specific antigen in subclinical prostatitis: the role of aggressiveness and extension of inflammation," *Urologia Internationalis*, vol. 71, no. 2, pp. 160–164, 2003.

[23] L. H. Simardi, M. Tobias-Machado, G. T. Kappaz, P. Taschner Goldenstein, J. M. Potts, and E. R. Wroclawski, "Influence of asymptomatic histologic prostatitis on serum prostate-specific antigen: a prospective study," *Urology*, vol. 64, no. 6, pp. 1098–1101, 2004.

[24] P. Raskin, C. J. McClain, and T. A. Medsger Jr., "Hypocalcemia associated with metastatic bone disease. A retrospective study," *Archives of Internal Medicine*, vol. 132, no. 4, pp. 539–543, 1973.

[25] M. Szentirmai, C. Constantinou, J. M. Rainey, and J. E. Loewenstein, "Hypocalcemia due to avid calcium uptake by osteoblastic metastases of prostate cancer," *Western Journal of Medicine*, vol. 163, no. 6, pp. 577–578, 1995.

[26] G. D. Ludwig, "Hypocalcemia and hypophosphatemia accompanying osteoblastic osseous metastases: studies of calcium and phosphate metabolism and parathyroid function," *Annals of Internal Medicine*, vol. 56, no. 4, pp. 676–677, 1962.

[27] H. G. Skinner and G. G. Schwartz, "Serum calcium and incident and fatal prostate cancer in the national health and nutrition examination survey," *Cancer Epidemiology, Biomarkers & Prevention*, vol. 17, no. 9, pp. 2302–2305, 2008.

19

Dissecting Major Signaling Pathways throughout the Development of Prostate Cancer

Henrique B. da Silva,[1] Eduardo P. Amaral,[1] Eduardo L. Nolasco,[2] Nathalia C. de Victo,[1] Rodrigo Atique,[3] Carina C. Jank,[1,4] Valesca Anschau,[3] Luiz F. Zerbini,[5] and Ricardo G. Correa[6]

[1] *Departamento de Imunologia, Instituto de Ciências Biomédicas, Universidade de São Paulo, Avenida Prof. Lineu Prestes 1730, 05508-900 São Paulo, SP, Brazil*
[2] *Departamento de Análises Clínicas e Toxicológicas, Faculdade de Ciências Farmacêuticas, Universidade de São Paulo, Avenida Prof. Lineu Prestes 580, 05508-000 São Paulo, SP, Brazil*
[3] *Departamento de Genética e Biologia Evolutiva, Instituto de Biociências, Universidade de São Paulo, Rua do Matão 277, 05508-900 São Paulo, SP, Brazil*
[4] *Instituto Israelita de Ensino e Pesquisa Albert Einstein, Avenida Albert Einstein 627/701, 05652-000 São Paulo, SP, Brazil*
[5] *International Center for Genetic Engineering & Biotechnology (ICGEB), Cancer Genomics Group and Division of Medical Biochemistry, University of Cape Town, Cape Town 7925, South Africa*
[6] *Sanford-Burnham Medical Research Institute, 10901 North Torrey Pines Road, La Jolla, CA 92037, USA*

Correspondence should be addressed to Ricardo G. Correa; rcorrea@burnham.org

Academic Editor: Craig Robson

Prostate cancer (PCa) is one of the most common malignancies found in males. The development of PCa involves several mutations in prostate epithelial cells, usually linked to developmental changes, such as enhanced resistance to apoptotic death, constitutive proliferation, and, in some cases, to differentiation into an androgen deprivation-resistant phenotype, leading to the appearance of castration-resistant PCa (CRPCa), which leads to a poor prognosis in patients. In this review, we summarize recent findings concerning the main deregulations into signaling pathways that will lead to the development of PCa and/or CRPCa. Key mutations in some pathway molecules are often linked to a higher prevalence of PCa, by directly affecting the respective cascade and, in some cases, by deregulating a cross-talk node or junction along the pathways. We also discuss the possible environmental and nonenvironmental inducers for these mutations, as well as the potential therapeutic strategies targeting these signaling pathways. A better understanding of how some risk factors induce deregulation of these signaling pathways, as well as how these deregulated pathways affect the development of PCa and CRPCa, will further help in the development of new treatments and prevention strategies for this disease.

1. Introduction

The long-term ineffectiveness of current treatments for prostate cancer (PCa) has spurred an increasing interest in understanding the molecular mechanisms that underlie PCa tumorigenesis [1]. Currently, PCa is considered the most common nonmelanoma neoplasia among men [2–4]. According to the current trends in population growth, the incidence of PCa will exceed 1.7 million new cases by 2030 [5]. In the United States, nearly 2.8 million men are potentially living with this condition, and approximately 240,000 new cases were diagnosed in 2012 [3]. PCa predominately affects elderly men with higher incidence [6], and it is more prevalent in Western countries [7], where the average life expectation is over 75 years old. In developing countries like Brazil, PCa has recently surpassed the population incidence of breast cancer, and it has become the most common tumor malignancy, with approximately 50,000 new cases occurring per year [4, 5]. Yet, there is a considerable heterogeneity in the mortality rates and incidence among different countries, probably due to the variable penetrance of some risk factors such as age, race, genetics (family history), diet and environmental factors [8], and also behavioral factors, like frequent consumption of dairy products and meat [9], smoking, and sexual behavior [10].

Several agents such as diet, life habits, and exposure to chemical agents have been correlated with risk of PCa development [8]. For instance, a broad study performed by a PCa prevention trial group (Seattle, USA) has found high correlations between the intake of polyunsaturated fat and the development of aggressive PCa [11]. Corroborating this study, a strong correlation has been found (over 50%) between obesity and aggressive PCa development in both African and Caucasian men [12]. In Brazil, for instance, PCa is more frequently related to higher socioeconomic classes [13]. The increase in animal fat consumption and reduction in fiber consumption, along with sedentarism, have been suggested to be related to higher risks of PCa progression, along other types for cancers [14]. Thus, fat consumption appears to be a major risk factor for PCa. The association between pesticide exposure and hormone-related cancers, such as PCa, has been extensively debated since the late 1990s [15]. On the other hand, several studies have inversely correlated mild exposure to sunlight to higher mortality or PCa incidence [16]. However, the exact factors responsible for a potential induction of PCa are still not fully understood.

The development of prostatic tumor in men is generally slow, taking up to 4 to 10 years to develop a 0.4 inch-size tumor [17]. PCa begins when the semen-secreting prostate gland cells mutate into tumor cells, proliferating at higher mitotic levels. Initially, the prostate cells begin to proliferate leading to tumor formation in the peripheral zone of the prostate gland. Over time these cancer cells eventually multiply to further invade nearby organs, such as the seminal vesicles, rectum, bladder and urethra [18]. During the initial metastatic stages, malignant cells from the primary tumor detach from their original site and migrate through blood and lymphatic vessels [19]. In the later stages, cancer cells eventually spread to more distal organs, including bones, liver, and lung [18].

PCa treatment has been conducted primarily by surgery and/or radiotherapy due to the intimate organ localization [4, 20]. A prostatectomy usually leads to an excellent prognosis with low risk of death from PCa after surgery [21]. However, deregulated production and secretion of growth factors by stromal cells within the PCa microenvironment, as well as mutations in androgen signaling pathway components and further physiological modifications, including angiogenesis, local migration, invasion, intravasation, circulation, and extravasation of the tumor, potentially lead to systemic recurrence of the cancer, including the appearance of focal tumor in advanced stage [22–26]. In this case, the preferred treatment is based on androgen-deprivation therapy (ADT), mostly including a luteinizing-hormone-releasing hormone (LHRH) [20]. In advanced PCa, ADT still remains the most effective therapy in initial stages, despite its temporary effectiveness (in general, between 18 and 24 months) [20, 27].

In order to study PCa, a variety of cell lines mimicking androgen-dependent and androgen-independent carcinogenic formations have been extensively used [28]. These cell lines have enabled researchers to directly test a series of antitumor drug candidates, such as tumor apoptosis inducers [29] or enhancers of antitumor immune response [30], as well as to evaluate the genomic foundations of PCa [31] and to further decipher the biological characteristics within cancer development [32, 33]. Alongside the *in vitro* studies, several animal models have been developed in order to confirm *in vitro* results by using a more clinically relevant approach [34, 35]. Mouse models for PCa can be obtained by systemic induction of gene mutations [36], xenografts [37], or by doxycycline-based inducible systems to overexpress certain target genes like in the case of AKT, which in turn induces tumorigenesis [38].

Many genetic alterations may be accountable for PCa induction, whereas mutations in genes responsible for the expression of proteins that participate in a variety of cell signaling processes can affect the decision of cell death or survival [39]. In this review, we will discuss the role of major cellular signaling pathways in the progression of PCa and some potential strategies to prevent this malignant outcome.

2. The Androgen Receptor Signaling Pathway in Prostate Cancer

2.1. Pathway Description. The androgen receptor (AR) signaling pathway promotes the differentiation of epithelial cells into male urogenital structures and encodes proteins that are necessary for the normal function of the prostate and for the initiation and maintenance of spermatogenesis [20, 40]. AR is a nuclear receptor that acts as a transcription factor [20], which is formed by four distinct functional domains like many other steroid-hormone receptors (Figure 1). The first region is composed of an N-terminal domain (NTD) that is constitutively active and has a transcriptional activation function (AF-1), executed by two transcriptional activation units (TAU-1 and TAU-2). The second region is a highly conserved DNA-binding domain (DBD), responsible for DNA binding specificity and for facilitating the dimerization and stabilization of the AR-DNA complex [20, 27]. The COOH-terminal ligand-binding domain (LBD) is another receptor site that is moderately conserved and equally important to mediate the binding to steroid hormones, which is the primary feature of the AR signaling pathway [20]. This site is also responsible for the direct binding between AR and the chaperone complex (Hsp90), which keeps the receptor in an inactive state but in a spatial conformation that allows affinity for androgens [41]. Upon binding to androgens, Hsp dissociates and releases AR from this complex, which further dimerizes and then translocates to the nucleus [27]. A fourth AR region contains the hinge region, a short amino-acid sequence that separates LBD from DBD and possesses a nuclear localization signal (NLS). This region is also important for the AR translocation to the nucleus through the interaction with the cytoskeletal protein Filamin-A (FlnA) [20], whose cytoplasmic localization is correlated with metastatic and hormone-refractory phenotype [20, 42].

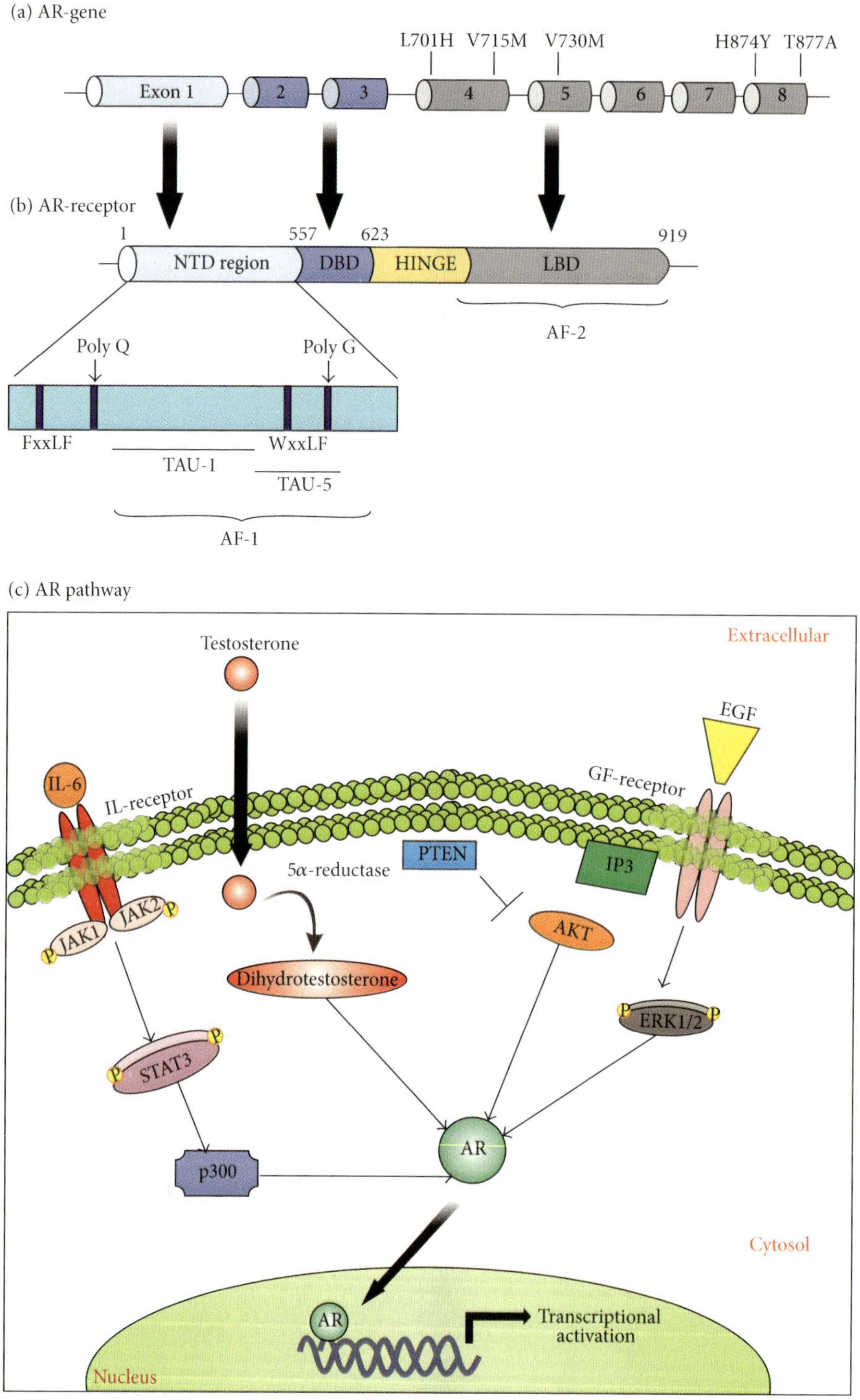

Figure 1: Androgen receptor (AR) signaling in prostate cancer. (a) Schematic representation of the AR gene, highlighting some major AR mutations and their exon localization. (b) Schematic representation of AR protein structure with indication of its functional domains. (c) AR-mediated signaling pathway. The androgen-receptor (AR) signaling pathway begins with the translocation of the testosterone to the cytoplasm, where it can be converted to dihydrotestosterone (DHT) and then promote the receptor dimerization and its further migration to the nucleus. A variety of signals, including PTEN-dependent downregulation, can also merge to AR stabilization and further activation (as indicated).

2.2. Pathway Disruptions Associated with PCa and Therapeutic Targets. One of the major causes of CRPCa is AR overexpression, which can be related to gene amplification or transcriptional and/or translational upregulation and decreased degradation. AR gene amplification is observed in approximately 80% of the CRPCa cases, being the most common genetic alteration in this type of cancer [43]. However, gene amplification can only partially explain AR overexpression, and other mechanisms that promote this enhancement have been investigated [27]. AR regulates many genes through the binding of the AR-ligand complex to the DNA, specifically to androgen receptor binding sites (ARBSs) or androgen-responsive elements (AREs). These binding sites might be close to the target genes or acting as distal enhancers. During PCa progression, many androgen-regulated genes including UBE2C, CND1, p21, and p27 are up-regulated [43, 44]. In most of CRPCa conditions, where AR overexpression is found, prostate cells show more sensitivity to lower concentrations of the ligand [45].

AR mutations are rare in the initial phases of PCa, but they are very common in CRPCa [43]. These mutations might broaden AR specificity towards nonandrogenic molecules, or they can bypass the necessity of a ligand for proper transcriptional activity [27]. A considerable number of AR mutations have been characterized, showing that the promiscuous behavior of the receptor culminates in activation by adrenal androgens and other steroids hormones, including dehydroepiandrosterone (DHEA), progesterone, estrogens, and cortisol [27]. This phenomenon allows the prostatic epithelial cells to grow in an androgen-refractory way [40, 43, 46]. For this, there are three particular AR regions where mutations appear to give specific properties (Figure 1). The first region is between residues 701 and 730, and it enables resistance to adrenal androgens, glucorticoids and progesterone [27, 43], and mutations like L701H, V715M, and V730M are responsible for affecting these properties [27, 43]. In the second region, between residues 874–910, a T877A mutation has been described as the most frequent in CRPCa [43]. This alteration appears to affect the AR ligand specificity by changing the stereochemistry of the binding pocket, which expands the spectrum of ligands able to bind AR. This allows other hormones like DHEA, estrogen, progesterone, cortisone, and cortisol to activate AR [27, 40, 43]. Another mutation (H874Y) is also responsible for enhancing the transcription sensitivity of AR towards steroids like adrenal androgens or antiandrogens [43]. The third mutational site occurs between residues 670–678, located at the boundary of the hinge and LBD regions, that enhances the transactivation activity of AR in response to dihydrotestosterone (DHT). Other mutations in the amino terminus also occur but at a low frequency [27].

Transcription factors play a key role in AR expression and act positively or negatively in gene regulation. For instance, cAMP response element-binding proteins (CREB) have been reported to significantly increase during PCa progression, which ultimately enhances AR transcriptional levels [46]. The proto-oncogene Myc is well known to be involved in cancer formation [46] and it also participates in AR transcription, acting as a predictor of biochemical recurrence after radical prostatectomy (RP) [46, 47]. The member of the activator protein-1 (AP-1) c-Jun is known to suppress AR expression, but it also acts as a coactivator of this receptor [46, 47]. Another transcription factor that positively regulates AR transcription is FOXO3a, which binds to the Foxo-response element in the AR promoter region. The Lymphoid enhancer-binding factor 1 (LEF1) is a nuclear transducer that indicates a link between Wnt signaling and PCa, as Wnt1 leads to activation of LEF1 and it increases AR transcription [46]. Other transcription factors, like NF-κB and Twist-1, have a positive correlation with AR expression, suggesting a key role in the progression and in the CRPCa state [46].

Another mechanism to bypass the requirement of ligands for AR activity is the presence of splice variants of AR transcripts. Alternative splicing events occur in approximately 90% of human genes and such events are evident in PCa [27, 43] where, in fact, it is an important mechanism of PCa resistance to AR-targeted therapy and further progression to CRPCa. Recent studies have identified several AR splice variants, and, despite having slightly different structures, a common characteristic is the absence of the LBD and the AF-2 domain in these isoforms [41]. The absence of LBD leads to loss of repression activity of this domain in the receptor, and potential hormone-independent AR activity [41]. It has been suggested that some AR variants may have an exclusive cytoplasmic function, although it has been demonstrated that truncated AR variants still show a nuclear localization that is enough to support transcriptional activity [41]. It has also been demonstrated that these AR variants can access the nucleus independently of the Hsp90 chaperone complex [41]. The clinical relevance of these variants is currently under investigation, and, due to the frequent identification of these splice variants in PCa metastases and CRPCa [27], these molecules could be envisioned as potential therapeutic targets.

Alterations of AR transcriptional activation induce deregulated proliferation and survival of prostate cells. For instance, it has been reported that androgens enhance the transcription of SENP1, a member of SUMO-specific protease family, showing that the regulation of AR signaling through this protease is based on a positive feedback mechanism [48]. Similarly, the regulation of the cell cycle regulator cyclin D1 by SENP1 contributes to cancer progression [49]. Therefore, SENP1 has emerged as an important prognostic marker and also a therapeutic target [38, 49]. Moreover, considering that the AR receptor is a phosphoprotein, changes to its phosphorylation profile would clearly have an impact on its function [20, 27, 40]. The use of pharmacological agents that modulate the AR posttranslational portfolio could be considered as an alternative approach for further interventions.

3. The NF-κB Pathway in Prostate Cancer

3.1. Pathway Description. The nuclear factor kappa B (NF-κB) signaling pathway is involved in a variety of physiopathological conditions, including inflammation, autoimmune disorders, and cancer. In humans, the NF-κB family is composed of five members: p65 (RelA), p100/p52, p105/p50, c-Rel and RelB (Figure 2(a)). NF-κB proteins form homo- or heterodimeric

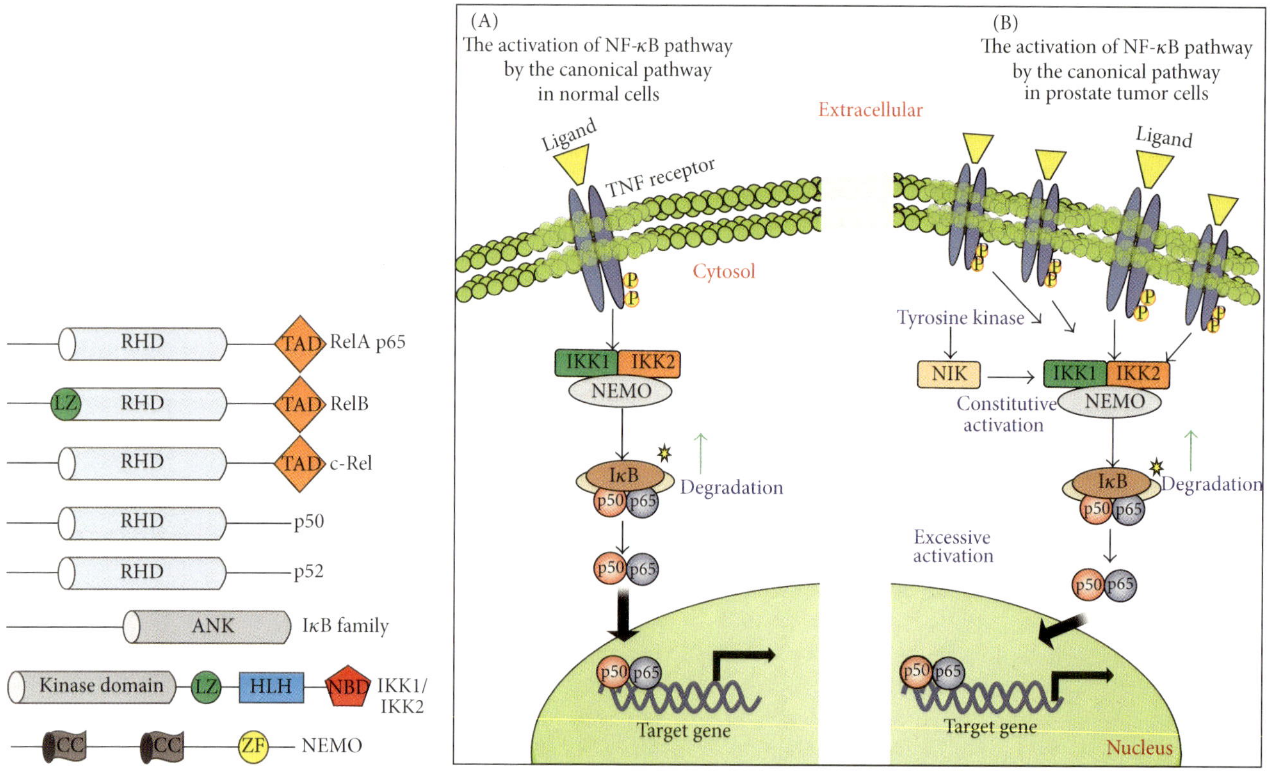

(a) (b)

Figure 2: The NF-κB signaling and prostate cancer. (a) Domain structure of NF-κB family members and its direct modulators IκB and IKK. The last two NF-κB members p50 and p52 are derived from the C-terminal processing of p105 and p100, respectively. All NF-κB family members contain an N-terminal Rel-homology domain (RHD) that governs the DNA binding, protein dimerization, and interaction to IκB. The Rel subfamily, RelA, RelB, and c-Rel, also contain a C-terminal transcriptional activation domain (TAD) and the subunit RelB has an additional leucine zipper (LZ) domain at the N-terminus. The IκB family mainly consists of IκBα, IκBβ, IκBγ, IκBε, and BCL-3 proteins (p100 also operates as an IκB-like protein in the non-canonical pathway). The IκB proteins contain ankyrin-repeat motifs (ANK) in their C-terminal region that interact with the RHD of NF-κB proteins and then prevent their nuclear translocation and DNA binding. The IκB kinase (IKK) complex is primarily composed of the two catalytic subunits IKK1 (or IKKα) and IKK2 (or IKKβ) and the scaffolding protein NEMO (or IKKγ). IKK1 and IKK2 are structurally related and both contain an LZ domain and a helix-loop-helix region (HLH), with a C-terminal portion containing a NEMO binding domain (NBD). NEMO has an alpha helical region along with two coiled-coil (CC) regions and a putative zinc finger (ZF) domain. (b) The TNF-dependent NF-κB signaling pathway. The canonical pathway in normal cells is used as an example for the signaling through TNF receptor. The activated IKK complex phosphorylates IκB that is then degraded by the proteasome. Upon degradation of IκB, the subunits of NF-κB are released and the complex is free to migrate to the nucleus. The canonical NF-κB pathway in prostate tumor cells is often constitutively activated, potentially due to increased levels of specific receptors like TNF receptors (TNFRs), which dramatically increase IκB degradation and the translocation of NF-κB dimers to the nucleus to activate κB-responsive genes involved in the development and progression of the tumor. Additionally, undetermined tyrosine kinase subpathways lead to NIK activation, which induces constitutive IKK activity and then constitutive NF-κB activation in androgen receptor-negative prostate cancer cell lines.

structures that, after activation, function as transcriptional factors through binding to κB enhancer sites along the DNA. The canonical NF-κB pathway involves the phosphorylation of the inhibitory IκB proteins by the IκB kinase complex (IKK) (composed of the catalytic subunits IKKα and IKKβ, and the regulatory scaffolding protein NEMO), which results in the ubiquitination and further degradation of IκB by the proteasome, thus releasing the NF-κB dimers to translocate to the nucleus and activate κB-responsive target genes. In contrast, a non-canonical NF-κB pathway is detected in a more cell-specific fashion (including lymphoid tissue and immune-related cells), and it involves an IKKα-dependent p100 processing instead of the typical IκB degradation. The non-canonical pathway is activated by specific stimuli that include Lymphotoxin-β (LTβ) and B cell-activating factor (BAFF), whereas the canonical pathway is activated by a broader spectrum of stimuli, such as tumor necrosis factor α (TNF-α) and interleukin 1 (IL-1) and is often related to tumorigenesis, including leukemias, lymphomas, and some solid tumors [50–54]. Some NF-κB target genes have important antiproliferative and apoptotic roles and may contribute to the development, progression, and resistance of certain tumor cells.

3.2. Pathway Disruptions Associated with PCa and Therapeutic Targets. Molecular strategies that target NF-κB have been shown to suppress prostate cancer, in terms of both prevention and further therapy [55–58]. For instance, the effect of specific IKK inhibitors in the growth and survival of androgen-dependent and independent PCa cell lines has been determined. The results indicate that, regardless of the AR status and androgen dependency, cell growth is remarkably affected [59]. Thus, the identification of NF-κB responsive genes linked to PCa progression represents a critical step toward a better understanding and treatment of this disease. Some genetic alterations have been identified by the differential mRNA expression between tumor tissues versus normal tissues. For example, during androgen-independent tumorigenesis in the prostate, NF-κB expression is elevated at both mRNA and protein level [60]. These studies indicate that the NF-κB pathway can be constitutively activated in PCa, since an increased expression of interleukin 6 (IL-6) in androgen-independent PCa cell lines (PC-3 and DU145) was consistently observed. This deregulation of IL-6 expression in prostate cancer cells is in fact mostly mediated by the constitutive NF-κB activation [61], and this activation occurs through signal transduction involving the upstream effectors NF-κB inducing kinase (NIK) and IKK. Therefore, NF-κB also targets a transcription regulatory element of the prostate-specific antigen PSA, which is an important marker for development and progression of PCa [62, 63].

The proinflammatory cytokine TNF-α, a prototypical NF-κB inducer and also a downstream target gene, is highly expressed in PCa, and the TNF receptors TNFR1 and TNFR2 are also expressed at higher levels in the tumor epithelium when compared to normal prostate epithelium (Figure 2(b)) [64]. The levels of TNF-α in the serum are associated with the pathological data and the prognosis of PCa patients [65]. High expression of TNF-α has been correlated with increased survival and proliferation of PCa cells, angiogenesis, metastasis, and changes in the response to chemotherapeutic agents [66]. Experiments using PC-3 and DU145 cell lines treated with psoralidin (TNF-α inhibitor) indicate that this cytokine could be one potential therapeutic target. TNF-α inhibition by psoralidin inhibits NF-κB via p65 and other upstream molecules, including the survival protein families IAPs (inhibitor of apoptosis proteins) [67]. The IAP proteins inhibit two major pathways that normally initiate the activation of the cysteine protease caspases, the mitochondrial (intrinsic) and the death receptor (extrinsic) pathways. The combined inhibition of IAPs and TNF-α could be attractive for PCa therapy, since IAPs modulate apoptotic events and TNF-α affects cell survival and proliferation via NF-κB [68].

Recent clinical data and *in vitro* studies have suggested that NF-κB directly interferes with AR signaling. NF-κB is associated with increased AR expression and higher binding activity in androgen-independent xenografts [69]. In fact, AR has been described as a NF-κB target gene, whereas p65/RelA activity causes an increase of AR at both mRNA and protein levels [70]. Moreover, endogenous AR expression can be induced by p65 in human prostate cancer cells, and this induction is associated with increased expression of downstream AR targets and enhanced growth and/or survival of prostate cancer cells [70]. Complex formation including the non-canonical p52 and AR has also been described, where it causes an increase in nuclear localization and binding of AR to DNA even in the absence of its ligand. This ligand-independent AR activation has similarities to the non-canonical NF-κB signaling, since both pathways depend on IKK1 activity to phosphorylate the p100 precursor and by STAT3 phosphorylation [71]. NF-κB and STAT3 share a subset of target genes during tumorigenesis, including PAI-1, Bcl-3, Bcl-2, and GADD45β. For this, the cooperation between STAT3 and NF-κB pathways is required [72], in such a way that NF-κB members physically interact with STAT3. This interaction can result in a synergy of specific gene transcription or repression regulated by NF-κB/STAT3. It has been suggested that nonphosphorylated STAT3 can bind to the NF-κB complex, thus facilitating its activation independently of IKK activity, supporting the idea that STAT3 may prolong the presence of active NF-κB dimers in the nucleus. Thus, STAT3 may represent an important mechanism that ensures continuous NF-κB activation in cancer cells [72].

The regulation of NF-κB by the tumor suppressor gene p53 has also been observed in many types of hematopoietic and solid tumors [73]. The interaction between p53 and NF-κB reveals that, despite its role as a tumor suppressor, NF-κB becomes activated after reactivation of p53 even when the p53-induced apoptosis requires the participation of NF-κB. Thus, activation of NF-κB in apoptosis is additionally related to a hyperactivation of p53 [73]. Because NF-κB and p53 can be eventually activated by the same stimuli, the balance of their activities is crucial for cell fate decision. An important mechanism of communication between these two pathways is the binding competition for CBP and p300, which are necessary for the selective activation of these factors [74].

4. The PI3K/AKT Pathway in Prostate Cancer

4.1. Pathway Description. The Phosphoinositide 3-kinase/AKT (PI3K/AKT) pathway is a key signal transduction pathway that links multiple classes of membrane receptors to many essential cellular functions, such as cell survival, proliferation, and differentiation [75–77]. PI3K molecules are divided into three major classes: class I (IA and IB) molecules, which have one catalytic and one regulatory subunit and can bind to receptor tyrosine kinases, G-protein coupled receptors and oncogenic proteins, such as small G protein RAS, to transduce their signals, and class II and III molecules which have a single catalytic subunit and can bind to several receptors, such as RTKs or cytokine receptors (class III molecules have been shown as important mediators of signaling through the mammalian target of rapamycin, mTOR). After activation of PI3K, these molecules can induce recruitment and activation of the serine/threonine-specific protein kinase AKT (also called protein kinase B, PKB) through phosphorylation-induced activation of transmembrane phosphatidylinositol (4,5) bisphosphate (PIP2) into phosphatidylinositol (3,4,5) trisphosphate (PIP3). PIP3 can recruit AKT through its pleckstrin homology domain [78, 79], a conserved protein module identified in many proteins involved in cell signaling or as cytoskeleton constituents. Activated AKT can subsequently phosphorylate and activate several other proteins, such as mTOR, glycogen synthase kinase 3, and FOXO members (the forkhead box family of transcription factors). Ultimately, AKT's action induces and regulates a large array of cellular processes [80, 81]. Considering that PI3K/AKT signaling is related to cell survival and proliferation, it is reasonable to link PI3K/AKT to cancer development.

4.2. Pathway Disruptions Associated with PCa and Therapeutic Targets. PI3K/AKT pathway is deregulated in the majority of solid tumors [82]. In PCa, it has been estimated that PI3K/AKT/mTOR signaling is up-regulated in 30%–50% of the cases, often due to the loss of PTEN function [83, 84], which leads to AKT hyperactivation. PTEN (phosphatase and tensin homolog) is responsible for the dephosphorylation of PIP3 to PIP2 and, in this way, negatively controls the activity of PI3K/AKT signaling. Interestingly, it is not clear whether or how direct mutations in AKT can lead to PCa [85]. PTEN is haploinsufficient in PCa, and its genetic dose is linked to PCa progression, in which total loss of function can be correlated with more advanced PCa, as seen in artificially created mouse models [86]. Complete PTEN inactivation in the prostate leads to a noninvasive PCa phenotype in mouse models, suggesting that other mutations might drive the appearance of more invasive tumors [87]. In fact, mutations in p53 or in the cyclin-dependent kinase inhibitor p27KIP1, when combined with loss of PTEN, have been linked to more aggressive PCa *in vivo* [87, 88]. Besides *PTEN* gene deletion, other mechanisms seem to contribute to loss of PTEN function. For instance, the action of microRNAs (miRNAs)—small, single-stranded RNA sequences which function as posttranscriptional regulators of gene expression—on PTEN inactivation has been recently described, with the characterization of miR-22 and miR-106b~25 as *PTEN*-targeting miRNAs aberrantly expressed in PCa [89]. It is also known that nuclear exclusion of PTEN is important for the development of tumors, including PCa [90]. In fact, it has been described that nuclear PTEN interacts with the anaphase-promoting complex (APC/C) and induces its association with CDH1 (APC/C activator protein), thereby enhancing the suppressive capacity of the APC-CDH1 complex to advance cell division [91], thus indicating a role for nuclear PTEN in PCa suppression.

The AKT hyperactivation induces high proliferative levels and resistance to apoptosis, an example of which is TRAIL resistance. TRAIL is a member of the tumor necrosis factor superfamily that specifically promotes apoptosis in cancer cells [92]. Indeed, treatment of PCa cells with the PI3K inhibitor LY294002 induces sensitization of these cells to TRAIL-induced apoptosis [93]. The excessive PI3K/AKT activation observed in PCa cells is accompanied by the presence of certain PI3K subunits that are not usually expressed in non-hematopoietic cells, such as p110δ. Augmented p110δ expression is correlated with inhibition of PTEN activity and further AKT activation [94]. Besides p110δ, transgenic mice with constitutive expression of p110β indicate that this molecule can be also linked to neoplasia formation [95].

PI3K/AKT pathway seems to act in conjunction with other proteins implicated in PCa cell growth. For example, AKT interacts with MST1, a hippo-like serine-threonine kinase [96]. Mst1 plays a critical role in the regulation of programmed cell death and it has been implicated in PCa development [96]. Interestingly, MST1 has been detected in AR-chromatin complexes, and forced expression of MST1 reduces AR binding to androgen-responsive elements along the PSA promoter [97]. MST1 also suppresses PCa cell growth *in vitro* and tumor growth *in vivo* [97]. AKT is able to phosphorylate a highly conserved residue Thr^{120} of MST1, which leads to inhibition of its kinase activity and nuclear translocation, as well as the autophosphorylation of Thr^{183} [98], having a positive role in PCa progression. Another example relates to a non-membrane tyrosine kinase called Acetate Kinase (Ack1) that is recruited by the upstream receptors and activates AKT through Tyr-176 phosphorylation, favoring the development of PCa [99]. Also, the polycomb group silencing protein Bmi1 can be phosphorylated by AKT, which enhances its oncogenic potential in PCa. Overexpression of Bmi1 can act in combination with PTEN haploinsufficiency to induce invasive carcinogenic formation in the prostate [100]. Recently, it was described that the deficiency of the Sprouty protein 2 (SPRY2) acts with the epidermal growth factor receptor (EGFR) system (RTK) and loss of PTEN to drive hyperactivation of PI3K/AKT via enhanced RTK trafficking in PCa [101]. It is also important to note that insulin-like growth factor (IGF) is an upstream effector on AKT signaling, and IGF up-regulation (which activates AKT) could promote the development of PCa *in vivo* [102, 103], suggesting an interrelationship between IGF and AKT signaling in PCa. Finally, the Myc oncogene, a downstream target of PI3K/AKT pathway, commonly upregulated in many types of cancer [104], appears to act synergistically with AKT in the development of prostate tumorigenesis by altering, for instance, its sensitivity to mTOR inhibitors [105]. The implications of PI3K/AKT signaling in PCa are detailed in Figure 3.

In the context of PCa, a variety of new drugs targeting deregulation of the PI3K/AKT pathway have been developed. Natural products such as Ethanolic Neem Leaf Extract (ENLE) [106], β-Caryophyllene Oxide [107], and Dietary flavonoid fisetin [108] have been described as having anti-PI3K/AKT activity in PCa cells. Other drugs, such as curcumin, can inhibit several signaling pathways including AKT [109–112]. Synthetic drugs, such as KN-93, can inhibit PCa cell growth in an androgen-independent manner, by activation and production of reactive oxygen species (ROS), which prevent AKT activation [113]. Other drugs, like GDC-0980, can inhibit PCa cell proliferation through direct inhibition of class I PI3K and mTORC1/2 [114]. HIF-1 proteins are regulators of transcriptional responses against hypoxia and equally important in angiogenesis and tumor growth. An HIF-1α inhibitor has been described to inhibit the PI3K/AKT pathway in PCa cell lines [115]. Another example is Gambogic Acid, which limits PCa development through inhibition of both PI3K/AKT and NF-κB pathways [116]. Several mTOR inhibitors have been tested to control the development of androgen-independent PCa [117]. It should be noted that there are currently several AKT inhibitors in clinical trials [118]. For instance, Celecoxib, an inhibitor of cyclooxygenase 2 (COX-2), is described to prevent AKT phosphorylation by inactivating its upstream kinase PDK1 [119]. Perifosine, a phospholipid analogue, can also arrest PCa cell cycle in G1/S

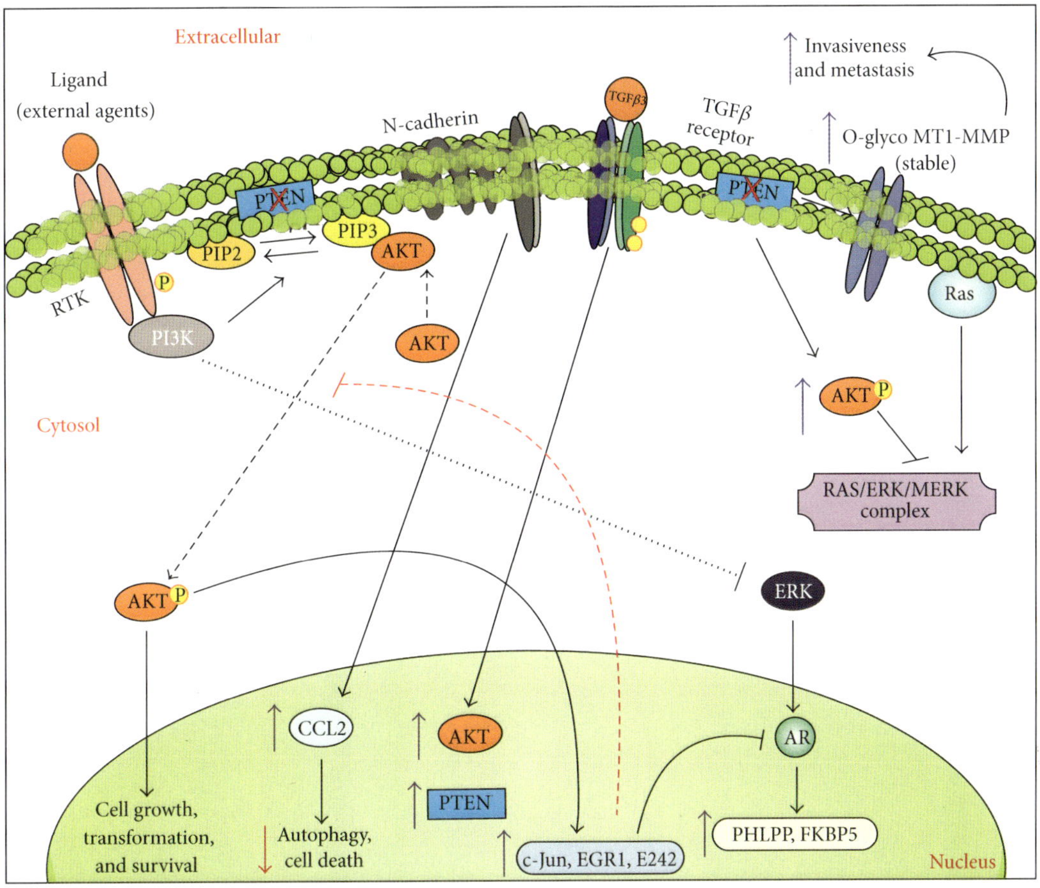

Figure 3: The PI3K/AKT signaling in prostate cancer. PI3K/AKT can induce enhanced activation of cancer cells by direct downstream effects. At the same time, this pathway (and downstream target genes) might affect the action of ERKs, which could lead to inhibition of AR-dependent activation, thus favoring an AR-independent growth. Conversely, AR pathway target genes can limit the PI3K/AKT pathway, favoring an AR-dependent tumor growth. A deregulated PI3K pathway (usually due to mutated or null PTEN) can also inhibit the Ras/MEK/ERK pathway, through enhanced activation of AKT. PI3K/AKT can also enhance the presence of stable metalloproteinase receptors (MT1-MMP), which favors invasive and metastatic phenotypes for these tumor cells. TGFβ signaling (through TGFβ3 ligation) can have a dual role in PI3K/AKT in PCa cells; for instance, benign cell lines enhance the expression of AKT and subsequent activation of this pathway following TGFβ3 engagement; malignant cell lines enhance PTEN expression in response to TGFβ3 engagement. Finally, N-cadherin enhanced expression in PCa cells leads to enhanced production of CCL2, which avoids autophagy in part through PI3K/AKT pathway.

or G2/M through AKT inhibition, although the mechanism of inactivation is still not fully understood (but possibly in a PDK1-independent manner) [120]. Genistein, a natural soy-based isoflavone, can inhibit AKT directly, subsequently inhibiting NF-κB activation and inducing apoptosis of PCa cells [121]. On the other hand, the deregulated PI3K/AKT pathway during PCa progression appears to be a reason for the resistance against some anticancer drugs; an example is the resistance to sunitinib in CRPCa, which is correlated with the loss of PTEN expression [122].

5. The JAK/STAT Pathway in Prostate Cancer

5.1. Pathway Description. Janus Kinase/signal transducers and activators of transcription (JAK/STAT) pathway is recognized as an important membrane-to-nucleus cascade, which may be activated by a wide variety of stimuli such as reactive oxygen species, cytokines, and growth factors [123–127]. JAK/STAT is one of the main cascades required for normal development and cell homeostasis, as well as in the control of cell proliferation, differentiation, cell migration, and apoptosis [124]. Specifically, this pathway is essential to regulate many physiopathological processes including hematopoiesis, gland development, immune response, adipogenesis, and sexually dimorphic growth [128, 129]. Briefly, the signaling activation occurs when specific inducers (e.g., IL-6) binds to and induces the oligomerization of respective receptor subunits (e.g., cytokine receptors), leading to signal propagation by phosphorylation of the receptor-associated tyrosine kinases, known as JAK1-3 and Tyk2 [130, 131]. Particularly, JAK activation occurs when the receptor subunit comes into close proximity (after ligand recognition) and allows the cross-phosphorylation of these tyrosine kinases. Subsequently, activated JAKs induce the phosphorylation of the receptor that now serves as a docking site for additional JAK targets including their major substrates known as signal transducer and activator transcription factors (STATs). STAT proteins have a dual function of signal transduction and transcription activation downstream of phosphorylation events. Indeed, STAT phosphorylation permits the dimerization of other STATs, culminating with the translocation to the nucleus mediated by importin α-5 and the Ran nuclear import system. Inside the nucleus, the dimerized STATs bind to specific regulatory sequences along the DNA, leading to activation or repression of target genes [132–135].

5.2. Pathway Disruptions Associated with PCa and Therapeutic Targets. The family of STAT transcription factors is constitutively activated in many human tumors. In this sense, these proteins control various cellular events such as proliferation, differentiation, and cell survival. Extensive studies have indicated that this pathway is upregulated in a broad range of cancers [136–140]. A particular member, STAT3, has been shown to be constitutively active in a number of human tumor cell lines as well as primary tumors, including haematological malignancies [141]. For instance, constitutive activation of STAT3 has been related to breast cancer susceptibility cancer 1 (BRCA1) expression in certain tumor cell lines [142]. Additionally, mutations in BRCA genes have been shown to increase predisposition to breast, ovarian, and prostate cancers [139, 143–145]. Both BRCA1 and BRCA2 are related to biological processes including DNA repair, control of cell-cycle checkpoint, and transcriptional regulation. Specifically, BRCA1 performs distinct but more general functions, working as a sensor/signal transducer and as an effector component in response to DNA damage by homologous recombination, while BRCA2 function is more restricted to DNA repair, modulating the activation of RAD51 recombinase, which is also required for homologous recombination [139, 146, 147]. It has been demonstrated that in PCa cells, BRCA1 interacts with JAK1/2, leading to STAT3 phosphorylation and culminating in the induction of cell proliferation and inhibition of apoptotic cell death [142].

STAT3 also targets other genes associated with cell cycle regulation [141, 148]. Upregulation of antiapoptotic STAT3 induces a subset of Bcl-related genes, including Bcl-2, Bcl-XL, Survivin, and Mcl-1, which have been described in PCa and many other tumors [141]. Another STAT3 target gene is the proangiogenic vascular endothelial growth factor (VEGF), involved in tumor invasion and spreading, which directly regulates several matrix metalloproteinases enzymes implicated in tumor cell invasion [141, 149–152]. Moreover, high levels of STAT3 in both malignant and normal tissues adjacent to the tumor have been detected, suggesting that STAT3 activation may occur before any detectable histological changes in the prostate [153]. Additionally, the inhibition of JAK/STAT3 signaling suppresses PCa cell growth and induces apoptosis [154]. In fact, STAT3 inhibition has been suggested as a good strategy to promote the control of cell proliferation and, consequently, tumor growth and metastasis formation [155].

IL-6 is another factor that has been found to be upregulated in the serum of PCa patients. IL-6 signaling is important to modulate cell growth and differentiation and immune-mediated resistance against infections. Unbalanced IL-6 production has a role in several diseases, such as osteoporosis, atherosclerosis, autoimmune disorders, rheumatoid arthritis, psoriasis, diabetes, and cancer [156, 157]. Several studies have indicated an important role of IL-6 in promoting PCa progression. PCa cells have upregulated expression of both IL-6 and its receptor IL-6R [158], as well as elevated circulating levels of IL-6 in patients with metastatic PCa and CRPCa [159–161], correlating IL-6 production to cancer morbidity [162–164] and differential autocrine and paracrine modulation of PCa cell lines [141, 164–166]. It has been shown that silencing of IL-6 expression by small-interfering RNA in PCa cell lines dramatically decreases cell growth, and this event is accompanied by downregulation of Bcl-2, Bcl-xL, and phosphorylation of AKT, MAPK, and STAT3 both *in vivo* and *in vitro* [167]. Upon IL-6 stimulation, androgen-responsive PCa cell lines also activate STAT3, which further binds to the C/EBPδ promoter region, inducing its expression. C/EBPδ is a member of the CCAAT/enhancer binding protein (C/EBP) family of transcription factors and plays a crucial role in the regulation of cell growth and fate [168–170]. In fact, C/EBPδ overexpression leads to inhibition of tumor growth in PCa [171]. On the other hand, after treatment with IL-6, androgen-independent PCa cells do not exhibit increased C/EBPδ gene expression or growth inhibition [171]. However, in PCa patients, the expression of C/EBPδ is significantly reduced in metastases when compared to primary PCa [172]. Altogether, the induction of C/EBPδ overexpression may function as an alternative of prevention and/or treatment of PCa. The implications of JAK/STAT pathway in PCa are detailed in Figure 4.

6. The MAPK Pathway in Prostate Cancer

6.1. Pathway Description. Mitogen activated protein kinases (MAPKs) comprise a family of kinases that have a major role in tumor growth and metastasis [173–175]. MAPKs can be divided into three subfamilies: the extracellular-signal-regulated kinases (ERKs), the c-Jun N-terminal kinases (JNKs), and p38 MAPKs that, together with the JNKs, compose the stress-activated protein kinase pathways [175]. All MAPKs have been linked to the regulation of intracellular metabolism, gene expression, cell growth and differentiation, apoptosis, and stress response [176–182]. There is a great body of evidence indicating that alterations in the regulation of MAPKs are extremely important in cancer development [183].

A plethora of extracellular signals initiate MAPK signaling by the binding and activation of receptor tyrosine kinases (RTKs) or G-protein coupled receptors (GPCRs) (Figure 5). In the case of ERK, the activation through these receptors leads to the recruitment of downstream effectors including growth factor receptor-bound protein 2 (Grb2) and protein tyrosine phosphatase non-receptor type 11 (PTPN11/Shp2), leading to the recruitment of Gab1 (GRB2-associated binding protein 1) and SOS (Son of Sevenless). Then, SOS protein exchanges the GDP in the Ras G-protein for a GTP. The Ras-GTP complex is able to activate the RAF kinase, a MAP-kinase-kinase-kinase (MAP3K) that is an upstream component of the ERK pathway, which in turn phosphorylates the MEK kinase (MAP2K) and, subsequently, phosphorylates and activates the next pathway component MAPK/ERK

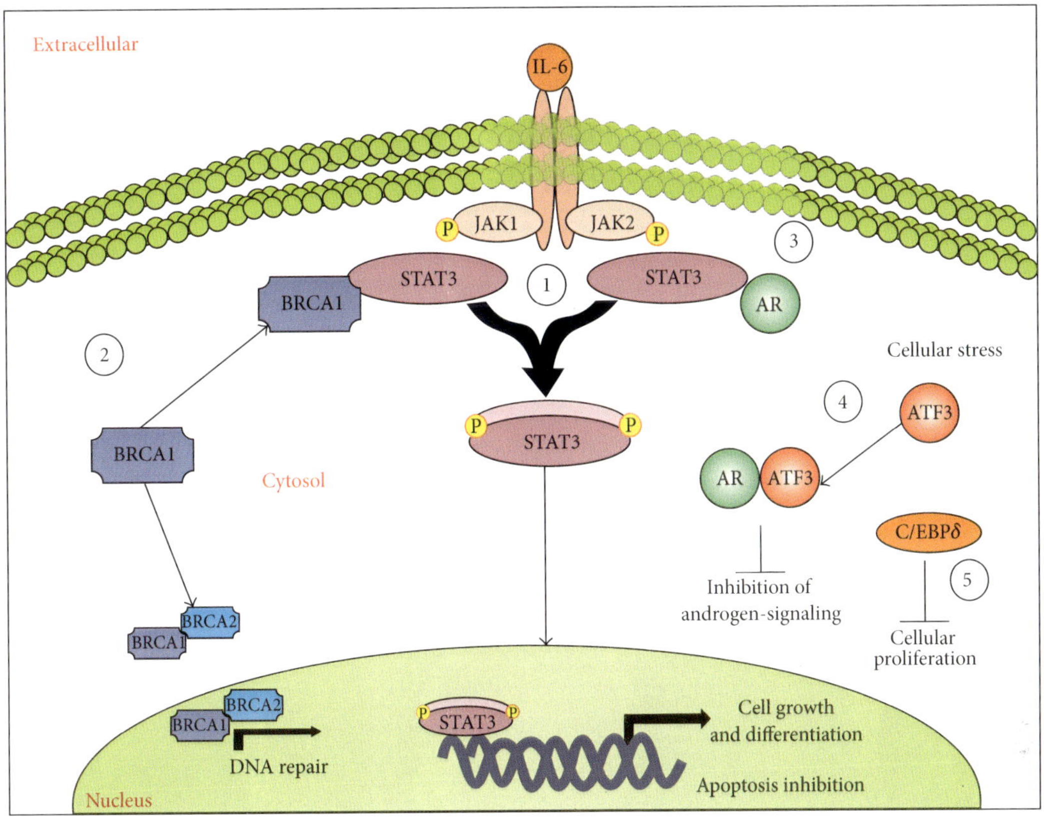

Figure 4: The JAK/STAT signaling in prostate cancer. (1) The JAK/STAT pathway has been found constitutively activated in PCa cells, leading to induction of tumor cell proliferation and apoptosis inhibition mediated by STAT3 activation. (2) BRCA1/2 is required for DNA repair in normal cells. However, in PCa, BRCA1 can bind STAT3 to promote JAK/STAT3 activation. (3) AR is a well-characterized cross-talk pathway in PCa. When activated, AR can bind to STAT3 leading to the activation of JAK/STAT cascade, being important in the induction of cell proliferation and apoptosis inhibition. (4) Under stress conditions, ATF3 is activated and plays a crucial role in the maintenance of cell integrity and homeostasis. ATF3 does so by interacting with AR, leading to inhibition of androgen signaling and, consequently, the inhibition of cell proliferation. However, ATF3 is downregulated in PCa cells, suggesting that this pathway provides an important mechanism of defense against cancer. (5) Similarly, C/EBPδ is required to inhibit cell proliferation by binding to STAT3. Nevertheless, C/EBPδ is typically downregulated in PCa, and, therefore, it could be used as an strategy in the development of therapeutic drugs against PCa growth.

[184]. The RTKs that interact with Ras, or other members of its superfamily, are diverse and include the epidermal growth factor receptor (EGFR), c-Kit, platelet-derived growth factor receptor (PDGFR), vascular endothelial growth factor receptor (VEGFR), fibroblast growth factor receptor (FGFR), and fms-related tyrosine kinase-3 (FLT-3) [185]. JNKs can be activated by the upstream MKK4 and MKK7 kinases [186, 187]. Although there are many JNK substrates, it is still challenging to identify the molecular networks regulated by the individual JNK family members. It has been found that JNK signaling can alternatively lead to apoptosis or cell survival [187–189]. Downstream targets of the MAPKs include c-Jun, c-Fos, and p53 [184]. c-Jun and c-Fos form a complex called AP-1 (activator protein 1) that acts as a transcription factor. MAPKs are able to translocate to the nucleus and then phosphorylate AP-1 transcription factors (c-Fos, c-Jun, ATF, and JDP family members) to mediate expression of target genes containing a TPA DNA response element (TRE) [190, 191].

6.2. Pathway Disruptions Associated with PCa and Therapeutic Targets. MAPK/ERK pathway is shown to be activated in PCa, especially in later stages of the disease, and is often deregulated with AKT signaling [192–194]. The upstream events that lead to activation of MAPK signaling are not well defined but are possibly related to aberrant growth factor signaling [195]. Although members of the Ras family are rarely mutated in PCa [22], Ras and the MEK/ERK pathway are stimulated by EGF, IGF-1, KGF, and FGFs, which are often overexpressed in PCa [196–198]. The expression of Ras or its effector-loop mutants reduces the androgen-dependent requirement of LNCaP cells for growth and increases their PSA expression and tumorigenicity, whereas dominant negative N17-Ras can restore androgen sensitivity to the CRPCa C4-2 cell line [22, 199]. Notably, expression of activated forms of Ras or Raf in the mouse prostate epithelium results in PCa formation [200, 201]. Interestingly, a small percentage of aggressive PCa contains chromosome translocations involving b- or c-Raf, which results in a constitutively activated hybrid protein due to the loss of the N-terminal RAS binding domain [202], which suggests that perturbations of Ras or Raf signaling may occur in PCa through mechanisms other than activating mutations. Also, p38 signals play an important role

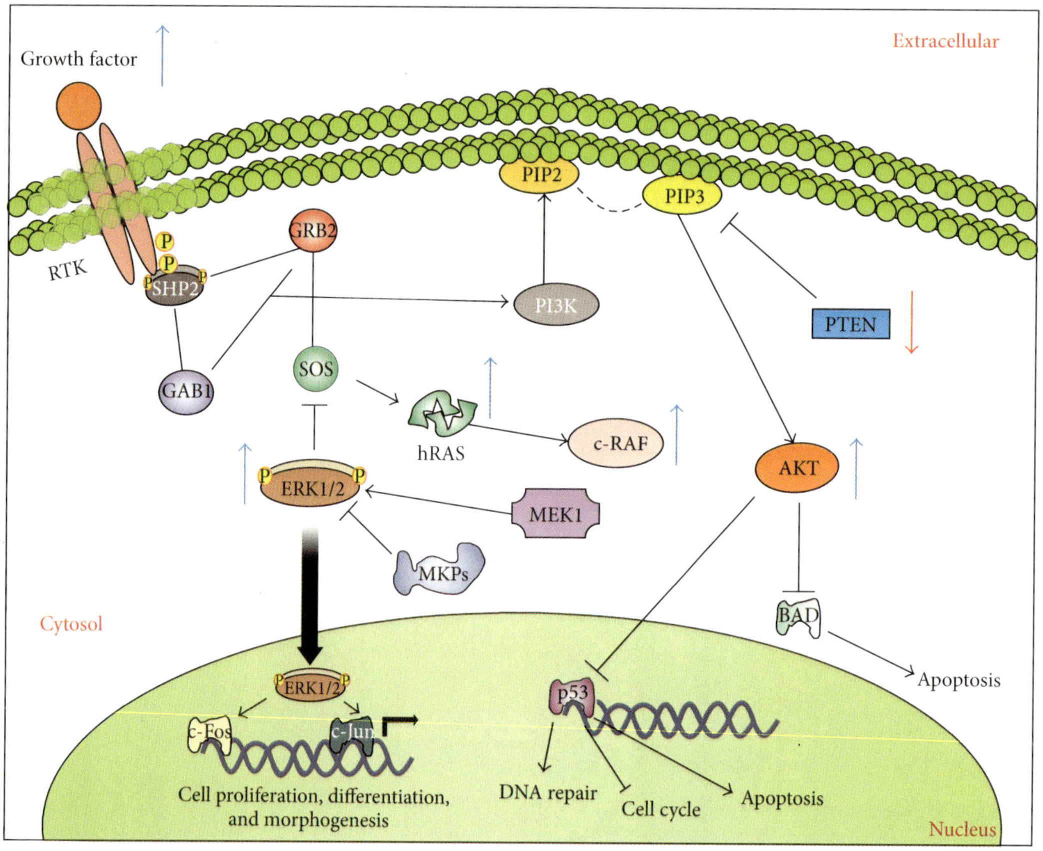

Figure 5: Overview of ERK and PI3K activation and their crosstalk. The binding of the ligand to RTK dimerizes and activates the receptor, leading to the recruitment of multiple Grb2 and Shp2 molecules, which further leads to the binding of a second anchoring protein Gab1 to the complex and to the activation of Son of Sevenless (SOS). This event leads to the activation of Raf/Ras/MEK/ERK pathway. Once phosphorylated, ERKs also phosphorylate a great number of substrates present in both nucleus and cytoplasm. In the nucleus, ERK phosphorylates a series of transcription factors including Elk1, c-Fos, p53, Ets1/2, and c-Jun, each one acting as regulators of cell proliferation, differentiation, and morphogenesis. The recruitment and activation of Grb2 and Shp2 also leads to the recruitment of another docking protein, Gab1. Once phosphorylated, Gab1 recruits PI3K to the membrane, where it phosphorylates the inositol ring of PIP-2 into PIP-3. PIP-3 facilitates the phosphorylation of AKT, which in turn regulates the activity of p53 and BAD. Blue and red arrows indicate up- and downregulated proteins in PCa, respectively.

in the adaptation of malignant cells to hypoxia by increasing the expression of the pore-forming proteins Aquaporins [203] and also by the increased resistance to apoptosis by overexpression of COX-2 [204].

MAPK and its upstream signals seem to be involved not only in PCa but also in the correct development of the prostate. For instance, FGFR2 is an RTK capable of recruiting Grb2 and Shp2 when activated, which acts as an upstream activator of the MAPK signaling pathway [205]. It has been demonstrated that FGFR2 is necessary for the embryological formation of the prostate [205]. Null mutants for *Fgf10* mostly lack prostate budding [206], while conditional deletion of *FGFR2* or *Frs2α*, a downstream signaling component in prostate epithelium, results in defects in branching morphogenesis [207, 208] It has been also demonstrated that ERK 1/2 is rapidly activated in the urogenital sinus (UGS) when induced by FGF10, and the inhibition of FGFR activity mostly inactivates phosphorylated ERK 1/2 in the UGS, suggesting that FGF10 may signal through MAPK pathway [209].

Simultaneous activation of the ERK and AKT signaling pathways has been shown to promote PCa and CRPCa both *in vitro* and *in vivo*, while combined inhibition of these pathways blocks cell proliferation and leads to Bcl-2 and Bim upregulation [192, 210] (Figure 5). Therefore, the MAPK signaling pathway may be a target for PCa therapy, especially if its modulation could be achieved concomitant with other pathways, including PI3K/AKT signaling. The aim of future studies in this area might be directed toward the factors and mechanisms that account for differential function of JNK, p38, and ERK MAPKs as pro- or anti-tumoral factors. In addition, it has been shown that the AKT/mTOR and MAPK pathways participate in the development of PCa. A therapeutic strategy using both rapamycin (mTOR inhibitor) and PD0325901 (MEK1 inhibitor) is shown to inhibit cell growth in a series of PCa cell lines and also to affect tumor growth in mouse models [192]. These results have been further confirmed [211] using inhibitors of both PI3K/AKT/mTOR and RAS/MEK/ERK pathways. These observations may lead to the development of therapeutic approaches to effectively target the pro-tumoral effects of the MAPK pathways.

7. The TGF-β/SMAD Signaling Pathway in Prostate Cancer

7.1. Pathway Description. The TGF-β/SMAD signaling pathway is involved in the regulation of many cellular functions including cell growth, adhesion, migration, cell differentiation, embryonic development, and apoptosis [212]. Accordingly, alterations in the TGF-β/SMAD signaling pathway are implicated in many human diseases such as cancer, fibrosis, and several hereditary conditions [213–215]. The pathway initiates when activated ligands (e.g., TGF-β) bind to respective receptors, composed of a very diverse cysteine-rich domain, a single-pass transmembrane domain, and a significantly conserved intracellular serine-threonine kinase domain. There are two types of functional receptors that bind to the TGF-β ligands, nominated as type I and type II receptors. Type II receptors are constitutively active receptors, and, upon ligand binding, they further activate type I receptors in a phosphorylation-dependent manner. The activated receptors then tetramerize and are able to recruit and activate SMAD proteins, the main effector proteins of this pathway [214–216]. SMADs are intracellular proteins that transduce signals from the TGF-β superfamily of ligands to the nucleus, where they activate or suppress the transcription of target genes. There are eight known types of SMADs, which can be divided into three different classes: receptor-regulated SMADs (R-SMADs), common-mediated SMAD (Co-SMAD), and inhibitory SMADs (I-SMADs). Once the receptors are activated, they recruit R-SMADs and phosphorylate them. Phosphorylated R-SMADs can then form complexes with the Co-SMAD SMAD4. This complex is translocated to the nucleus and acts as a transcription factor for many target genes (Figure 6). The I-SMADs, SMAD6 and SMAD7, inhibit SMAD transcriptional activity and the activation of the TGF-β/SMAD signaling pathway [214, 216].

7.2. Pathway Disruptions Associated with PCa and Therapeutic Targets. Despite the fact that enhanced TGF-β levels have been positively associated with prostate cancer progression (Figure 6), TGF-β-mediated suppression of growth and motility is also increased in metastatic CRPCa cells, and these events appear to be partially mediated by Smad2/3 signaling [217]. For instance, there is an increased sensitivity to TGF-β1-mediated growth inhibition and downregulation of cyclin D in prostate-derived metastatic cell lines C4-2 and C4-2B, when compared to the nonmetastatic cell line (LNCaP cells) and robust phosphorylation and nuclear translocation of Smad2 and Smad3 in metastatic cell lines [217]. The interactions of the stromal environment and epithelial tumor cells apparently dictate PCa progression, and it is likely that TGF-β pro-metastatic effects indirectly affects PCa cells through stromal cells, in contrast to its antiproliferative effect on the epithelium [217].

Using a *Cre/flox*-based system in mouse models, it has been observed that, in the absence of TGF-β1 produced by activated $CD4^+$ T cells and regulatory T cells, there is inhibition of tumor growth and protection from spontaneous PCa [218]. These findings have suggested that TGF-β1, produced by activated $CD4^+$ T cells, is necessary for tumor evasion from immune surveillance [218]. Furthermore, it is reported that LY2109761, a selective inhibitor of the TGF-β type I receptor, provides anti-tumoral effects against PCa cells after growth in bone tissue [219]. In addition, increased volume in normal bone and increased osteoblast and osteoclast numbers are observed after inhibition of the TGF-β type I receptor [219]. Thus, TGF-β1 has been detected at higher levels in the sera of PCa patients, is associated with bone metastasis, and correlates to a poor clinical outcome [220–222]. Many other studies have also linked changes in the levels of TGF-β and of pathway components to cancer progression and to further cellular responses [215, 223, 224].

Evidence for SMAD2 as a critical mediator of TGF-β-induced apoptosis has been reported [225]. Silencing of Smad2 expression in NRP-152, a nontumorigenic rat prostate basal epithelial cell line, inhibits TGF-β-induced apoptosis. Furthermore, rats injected with small hairpin RNA (shRNA) constructs targeting SMAD2 show palpable PCa tumors in over 80% of the injected sites by day 41 following injection [225].

The activation of the TGF-β signaling pathway in an SMAD-independent manner has also been described [226]. BMP-10 (bone morphogenetic protein 10) seems to inhibit growth of PCa cells, mainly by inducing caspase-3 mediated apoptosis and preventing PCa cell migration and invasiveness through SMAD-independent signaling (Figure 6) [226]. BMP-10 overexpression in PCa cells decreases tumor cell growth, cell matrix adhesion, invasion, and migration. These effects seem to be mediated through activation of TAK1 and ERK1/2 [226]. Nodal, another TGF-β ligand, has also been found to be overexpressed in some PCa cells and it can be involved in the inhibition of proliferation and induction of migration in these cells [227]. Furthermore, activin A, also known to inhibit growth of PCa cells and promote apoptosis, has been identified as a promoter of bone metastasis in PCa, possibly through SMAD signaling and concomitant elevation of the androgen receptor (AR) gene transcription [228]. Interestingly, the expression of activin A correlates with increased PSA expression, and, therefore, it might be considered as a novel biomarker or potential therapeutic target for the treatment of patients with metastatic PCa [228].

8. The Wnt Signaling Pathway in Prostate Cancer

8.1. Pathway Description. The Wnt family is composed of a large set of soluble proteins that play important roles in the embryonic developmental processes including cell proliferation, differentiation, and epithelial-mesenchymal interactions [229, 230]. Deregulations in the Wnt pathway have been implicated in cancer development in a variety of tissues including lung, skin, liver, and prostate [229, 231, 232]. Wnt proteins exert their biological effects through two signaling pathways (canonical and non-canonical), which

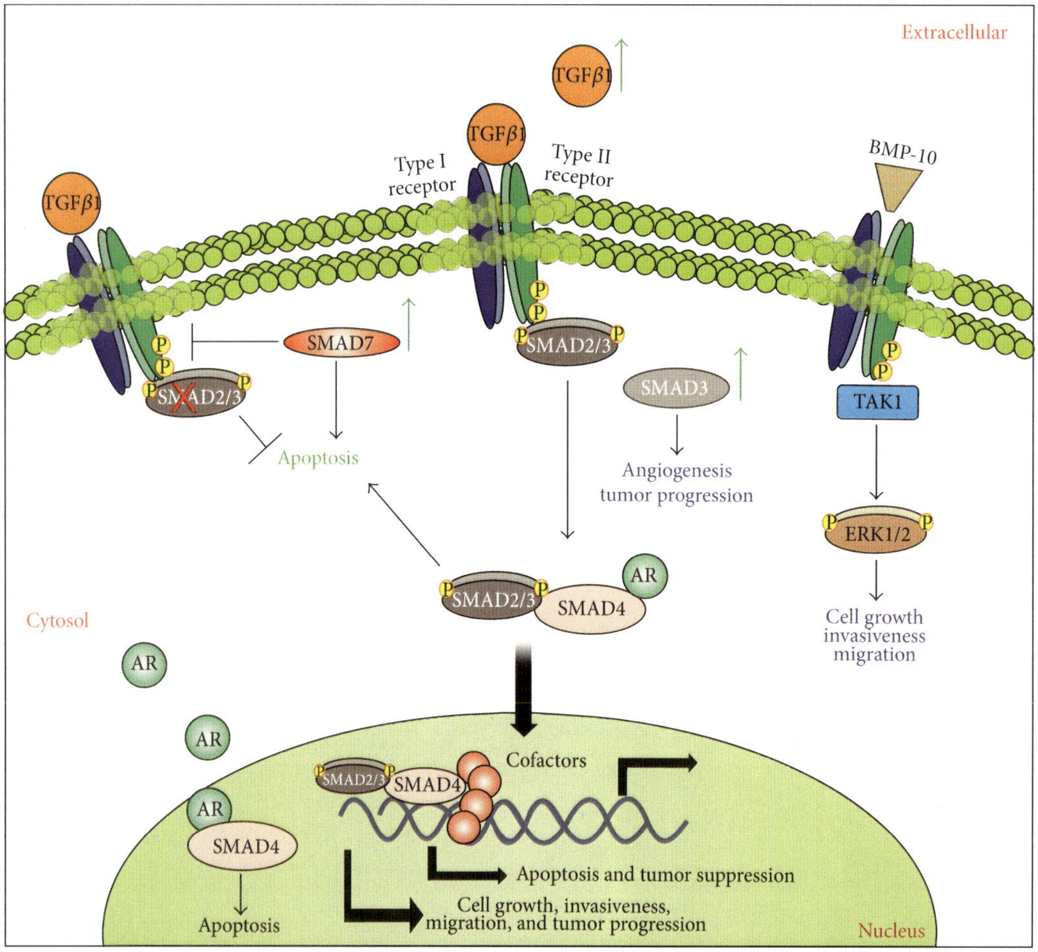

Figure 6: The TGF-β/SMAD signaling pathway and its implication in prostate cancer. When a TGF-β ligand binds to the constitutively active type II receptor, this complex associates with the type I receptor, forming a tetrameric receptor. The type II receptor phosphorylates and activates the type I receptor, which allows the recruitment of R-SMADs. The activated type I receptor then phosphorylates the MH2 domain of R-SMAD, activating it. Activated R-SMADs form complexes with SMAD4, which is then translocated to the nucleus. In the nucleus, SMAD complexes interact with nuclear proteins to activate or repress the transcription of target genes. Furthermore, BMP-10 can signal through SMAD-independent pathways and inhibit cell growth, invasiveness, and migration. TGF-β can also promote androgen receptor (AR) translocation into the nucleus and AR-dependent gene transcription. AR can combine with SMAD4 and regulate TGF-β-mediated apoptosis. According to the TGF-β central dogma, in normal epithelium or early-stage cancer cells, TGF-β acts as a tumor suppressor, by inhibiting cell growth, invasiveness, and motility and promoting apoptosis. In more advanced cancer cells, TGF-β has tumor-promoting functions; it promotes proliferation, invasion, and motility of cells and inhibits apoptosis. Green arrows indicate potentially up-regulated proteins in PCa.

are separated by their ability to stabilize β-catenin [233]. The β-catenin is a multirole protein that promotes cell proliferation by inducing gene transcription through the activation of transcription factors like T cell factor (TCF) and lymphoid enhancer factor (LEF) family of transcription factors [234]. β-Catenin exists in a cytoplasmic complex with Axin, APC (adenomatous polyposis coli gene), and glycogen synthase kinase 3β (GSK3β), which constitute the "β-catenin destruction complex." In the absence of Wnt, β-catenin is phosphorylated by casein kinase I (CKIα) at Ser45; this, in turn, enables GSK3β to phosphorylate serine/threonine residues 41, 37, and 33 [235]. Phosphorylation of these last two residues triggers ubiquitination of β-catenin and further degradation by the proteasome ([233, 236, 237], Figure 7(a)). The binding of Wnt proteins to transmembrane Frizzled receptors (FZD) activates the Disheveled protein (DVL), leading to the dephosphorylation of Axin which then reduces the formation of cytoplasmic β-catenin complexes. As a result, free β-catenin accumulates in the cytosol and it is further translocated to the nucleus, where it activates TCF/LEF transcriptional factors ([238], Figure 7(b)). The β-catenin/LEF/TCF complexes have been shown to interact with a variety of other nuclear factors to control specific transcriptional targets which include c-Myc, p300, CBP, Hrpt2, Foxo, Bcl9-2, reptin, pontin, c-Jun, Grouchos, Prmt2, CtBP, and cyclin D1 [239–241].

8.2. Pathway Disruptions Associated with PCa and Therapeutic Targets. The Wnt family members have been widely studied in PCa progression [241]. It has been hypothesized that PCa

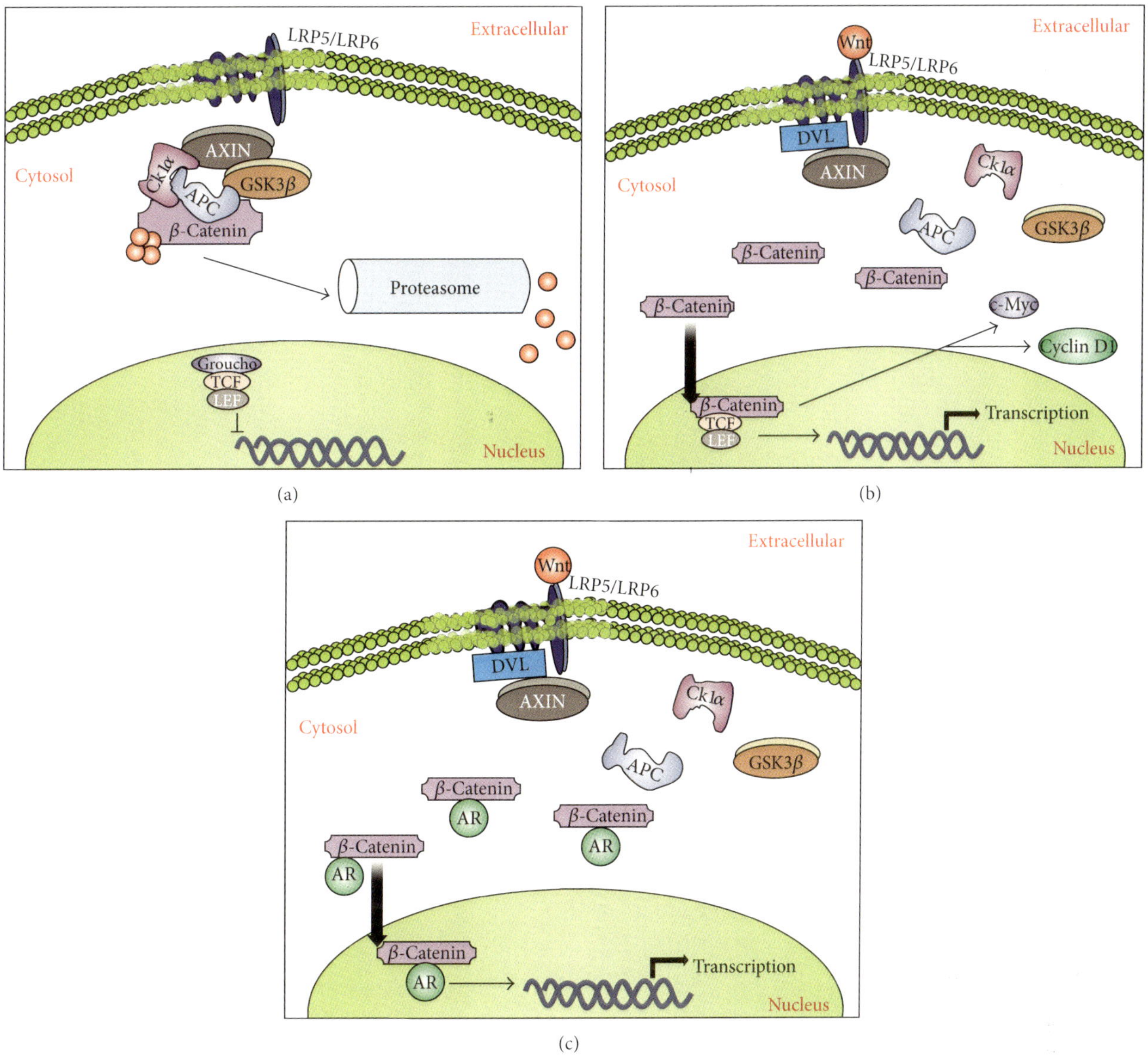

FIGURE 7: The Wnt signaling and its implications in the development of prostate cancer. (a) In an inactive state, the protein β-catenin is sequestered in a complex in the presence of Axin, GSK3β, CK1α, and APC. This complex allows ubiquitination of β-catenin and its subsequent degradation in a proteasome-dependent manner, maintaining this pathway inactive in the absence of Wnt. (b) After binding of Wnt to Frizzled receptor complex (which includes the adaptor molecules LRP5/LRP6), this allows the recruitment of Dishevelled (DVL) and Axin; the recruitment of Axin disrupts the inactivation complex and releases β-catenin, which translocates to the nucleus and functions as a transcription factor, inducing expression of several genes related to proliferation, such as *c-myc* and *cyclin D1*. (c) In the PCa environment, β-catenin can combine with AR proteins, whose levels are typically increased in PCa, enhancing their function as transcription factors and leading to increased gene expression of pro-survival and proliferative factors.

cells adopt embryonic signaling pathways that are generally silent in differentiated cells [242]. The role of β-catenin in tumorigenesis was first established in colon carcinoma, due to its complex formation with the adenomatous polyposis coli (APC) gene product [243]. APC is a well-known tumor suppressor, which plays a central role in the Wnt signaling pathway by targeting β-catenin for degradation. It has been shown that the APC gene is downregulated due to promoter hypermethylation [244], while β-catenin is frequently mutated to an active form [245] and it is typically found in early stages of prostate tumor formation. Indeed, APC exerts a variety of growth regulatory functions that, if disrupted, might lead to tumor formation [235]. A mouse model in which the APC gene has been inactivated results in PCa and adenocarcinoma [246]. Alterations in the APC gene are rare, although loss of heterozygosity and mutation have been detected in some PCa samples [243, 247]. As indicated, some studies have identified the genes *c-Myc* and *cyclin D1* as transcriptional targets activated by the β-catenin signaling pathway [248, 249]. The overexpression of *c-Myc* and *cyclin D1* increase cell growth and tumorigenicity in PCa cells, and these genes are apparently activated at the earliest phases of PCa progression [248, 249]. Noticeably, Wnt ligands are upregulated in PCa, and their expression often correlates with aggressiveness and metastasis [250]. It has been determined that 15 out of the 19 Wnt proteins are expressed in PCa cell lines [251]. Several Wnt ligands, such as Wnt-5a and Wnt-11, can induce the β-catenin-independent (non-canonical) pathway [252]. In particular, Wnt-11 is a secreted protein that modulates cell growth, differentiation, and morphogenesis during development; however, the prevalence of increased expression of Wnt-11 in tumours and the functions of Wnt-11 in PCa cells are not fully understood [253]. Recent data have shown an upregulation of Wnt-11 expression in a significant proportion of PCa tumors, and it has been positively correlated to higher Gleason scores as well as increased PSA levels [254]. Another Wnt ligand, Wnt-4, is highly expressed during embryonic development but is significantly less abundant in the adult prostate [251], suggesting that Wnt signaling might be temporally regulated during prostate development and that it can induce changes in cell fate for prostate progenitors.

Overexpression of Wnt ligands and high levels of β-catenin gene expression have been associated with advanced PCa *in vitro* [255]. Moreover, detection of mutant forms of β-catenin has been discovered in PCa [256, 257]. A series of studies have demonstrated that mutant forms of β-catenin that affect GSK3β-dependent phosphorylation site (which prevents its degradation and then allows its accumulation in the cytosol) are found in 5%–7% of radical prostatectomy specimens ([250, 258, 259], Figure 7(c)). Another mechanism for increased β-catenin expression in PCa may be loss of PTEN, which is common in advanced PCa and results in activation of the PI3K and downstream AKT signaling pathways [260]. AKT can phosphorylate and inactivate GSK3β, leading to stabilization and increased levels of β-catenin. Indeed, GSK3β suppression and subsequent β-catenin stabilization have been directly demonstrated in PTEN-deficient PCa cell lines [261]. Consistently, other members of the Wnt pathway are also deregulated in PCa [262]. For instance, Frizzled-4 (FZD4, a Wnt receptor) is co-expressed in human PCa samples with the ETS-related gene (ERG). Gene fusions involving ETS transcription factors (mostly ERG) are found in roughly 50% of all PCas [254]. Further experiments have shown that FZD4 overexpression in ERG-positive PCa leads to an epithelial-to-mesenchymal transition, which is a crucial step in metastasis initiation [254].

In summary, there are several ways that the Wnt pathway can be abnormally activated in cancer, due to the large number of proteins involved in this pathway [257]. For this reason, there is a great potential for the development of a wide array of Wnt antagonists. Several pharmaceutical and biotechnology companies have substantial programs designed to target this pathway [260], and a variety of drugs targeting Wnt pathway are currently on the market or under development [263, 264]. Some categories of drugs include non-steroidal anti-inflammatory drugs (NSAIDs) [265], vitamin D derivatives [266], antibody-based treatments [259], and other small molecule inhibitors [266, 267].

9. Conclusions

In the past several decades, an abundance of data related to the signaling events that trigger and maintain PCa have been collected. An increasing knowledge of the interconnections (crosstalks) of different signaling cascades, that ultimately promote the advance of PCa, is of seminal importance for the development of specific drugs which might promote the blockage and/or induction of specific molecules that could lead to the control of tumor progression. In fact, several drugs are currently in clinical trials or being tested in animal models, most of them acting as specific inhibitors of deregulated signaling pathways, such as those described in this review. Nevertheless, a more detailed and interactive panel of the external factors capable of inducing the deregulation(s) observed in the PCa microenvironment is still missing. Thus, it is crucial to pursue a more complete understanding of the cascade-dependent signals that lie behind PCa induction, to consequently lead to the development of fully functional strategies against PCa. This will also advance our knowledge towards more efficient screenings of PCa predisposition, which will certainly lead to increased prevention schemes and early treatments against this malady.

Authors' Contribution

H. B. da Silva and E. P. Amaral contributed equally to this paper.

Acknowledgments

The authors thank the Department of Genetics and Evolutionary Biology from the Institute of Biosciences (IB) of the University of Sao Paulo (USP, Sao Paulo, Brazil) and, particularly, Drs. Luis Eduardo Soares Netto and Regina Célia Mingroni Netto (IB-USP) for the academic support and opportunity to write this review. R. G. Correa is supported by grants from NIH.

References

[1] M. Verras and Z. Sun, "Roles and regulation of Wnt signaling and β-catenin in prostate cancer," *Cancer Letters*, vol. 237, no. 1, pp. 22–32, 2006.

[2] J. K. Mullins and S. Loeb, "Environmental exposures and prostate cancer," *Urologic Oncology*, vol. 30, pp. 216–219, 2012.

[3] R. Siegel, C. DeSantis, K. Virgo et al., "Cancer treatment and survivorship statistics, 2012," *CA: A Cancer Journal for Clinicians*, vol. 62, pp. 220–241, 2012.

[4] F. C. Maluf, O. Smaletz, and D. Herchenhorn, "Castration-resistant prostate cancer: systemic therapy in 2012," *Clinics*, vol. 67, pp. 389–394, 2012.

[5] M. M. Center, A. Jemal, J. Lortet-Tieulent et al., "International variation in prostate cancer incidence and mortality rates," *European Urology*, vol. 61, pp. 1079–1092, 2012.

[6] G. Arcangeli, B. Saracino, S. Gomellini et al., "A Prospective phase III randomized trial of hypofractionation versus conventional fractionation in patients with high-risk prostate cancer," *International Journal of Radiation Oncology Biology Physics*, vol. 78, no. 1, pp. 11–18, 2010.

[7] H. G. Sim and C. W. S. Cheng, "Changing demography of prostate cancer in Asia," *European Journal of Cancer*, vol. 41, no. 6, pp. 834–845, 2005.

[8] S. H. Reuben, "Reducing environmental cancer risk: what we can do now," *The President's Cancer Panel*, pp. 1–240, 2010.

[9] M. F. Leitzmann and S. Rohrmann, "Risk factors for the onset of prostatic cancer: age, location, and behavioral correlates," *Clinical Epidemiology*, vol. 4, pp. 1–11, 2012.

[10] B. G. Timms, "Prostate development: a historical perspective," *Differentiation*, vol. 76, no. 6, pp. 565–577, 2008.

[11] A. R. Kristal, K. B. Arnold, M. L. Neuhouser et al., "Diet, supplement use, and prostate cancer risk: results from the prostate cancer prevention trial," *American Journal of Epidemiology*, vol. 172, no. 5, pp. 566–577, 2010.

[12] L. J. Su, L. Arab, S. E. Steck et al., "Obesity and prostate cancer aggressiveness among African and Caucasian Americans in a population-based study," *Cancer Epidemiology Biomarkers and Prevention*, vol. 20, no. 5, pp. 844–853, 2011.

[13] S. Koifman and R. J. Koifman, "Environment and cancer in Brazil: an overview from a public health perspective," *Mutation Research*, vol. 544, no. 2-3, pp. 305–311, 2003.

[14] R. Sichieri, J. E. Everhart, and G. A. Mendonca, "Diet and mortality from common cancers in Brazil: an ecological study," *Cadernos de Saúde Pública*, vol. 12, pp. 53–59, 1996.

[15] P. Cocco, "On the rumors about the silent spring. Review of the scientific evidence linking occupational and environmental pesticide exposure to endocrine disruption health effects," *Cadernos de Saúde Pública*, vol. 18, no. 2, pp. 379–402, 2002.

[16] H. J. van der Rhee, E. de Vries, and J. W. W. Coebergh, "Does sunlight prevent cancer? A systematic review," *European Journal of Cancer*, vol. 42, no. 14, pp. 2222–2232, 2006.

[17] S. J. Freedland, W. B. Isaacs, E. A. Platz et al., "Prostate size and risk of high-grade, advanced prostate cancer and biochemical progression after radical prostatectomy: a search database study," *Journal of Clinical Oncology*, vol. 23, no. 30, pp. 7546–7554, 2005.

[18] H. T. Lynch and J. F. Lynch, "The Lynch syndrome: melding natural history and molecular genetics to genetic counseling and cancer control," *Cancer Control*, vol. 3, no. 1, pp. 13–19, 1996.

[19] J. K. Jin, F. Dayyani, and G. E. Gallick, "Steps in prostate cancer progression that lead to bone metastasis," *International Journal of Cancer*, vol. 128, no. 11, pp. 2545–2561, 2011.

[20] P. E. Lonergan and D. J. Tindall, "Androgen receptor signaling in prostate cancer development and progression," *Journal of Carcinogenesis*, vol. 10, article 20, 2011.

[21] S. A. Boorjian, J. A. Eastham, M. Graefen et al., "A critical analysis of the long-term impact of radical prostatectomy on cancer control and function outcomes," *European Urology*, vol. 61, pp. 664–675, 2012.

[22] Z. Culig, A. Hobisch, M. V. Cronauer et al., "Androgen receptor activation in prostatic tumor cell lines by insulin- like growth factor-I, keratinocyte growth factor, and epidermal growth factor," *Cancer Research*, vol. 54, no. 20, pp. 5474–5478, 1994.

[23] A. Wolk, C. S. Mantzoros, S. O. Andersson et al., "Insulin-like growth factor 1 and prostate cancer risk: a population-based, case-control study," *Journal of the National Cancer Institute*, vol. 90, no. 12, pp. 911–915, 1998.

[24] D. Gioeli, S. B. Ficarro, J. J. Kwiek et al., "Androgen receptor phosphorylation. Regulation and identification of the phosphorylation sites," *Journal of Biological Chemistry*, vol. 277, no. 32, pp. 29304–29314, 2002.

[25] Z. Guo, B. Dai, T. Jiang et al., "Regulation of androgen receptor activity by tyrosine phosphorylation," *Cancer Cell*, vol. 10, no. 4, pp. 309–319, 2006.

[26] E. Hernes, Fosså, A. Berner, B. Otnes, and J. M. Nesland, "Expression of the epidermal growth factor receptor family in prostate carcinoma before and during androgen-independence," *British Journal of Cancer*, vol. 90, no. 2, pp. 449–454, 2004.

[27] S. M. Green, E. A. Mostaghel, and P. S. Nelson, "Androgen action and metabolism in prostate cancer," *Molecular and Cellular Endocrinology*, vol. 360, pp. 3–13, 2012.

[28] S. Q. Yu, K. P. Lai, S. J. Xia, H. C. Chang, C. Chang, and S. Yeh, "The diverse and contrasting effects of using human prostate cancer cell lines to study androgen receptor roles in prostate cancer," *Asian Journal of Andrology*, vol. 11, no. 1, pp. 39–48, 2009.

[29] C. GIampietri, S. Petrungaro, F. Padula et al., "Autophagy modulators sensitize prostate epithelial cancer cell lines to TNF-alpha-dependent apoptosis," *Apoptosis*, vol. 17, no. 11, pp. 1210–1222, 2012.

[30] X. Huang, F. Yuan, M. Liang et al., "M-HIFU inhibits tumor growth, suppresses STAT3 activity and enhances tumor specific immunity in a transplant tumor model of prostate cancer," *PLoS ONE*, vol. 7, Article ID e41632, 2012.

[31] A. Vajda, L. Marignol, C. Barrett et al., "Gene expression analysis in prostate cancer: the importance of the endogenous control," *Prostate*, vol. 73, pp. 382–390, 2012.

[32] C. E. Lin, S. U. Chen, C. C. Lin et al., "Lysophosphatidic acid enhances vascular endothelial growth factor-C expression in human prostate cancer PC-3 cells," *PLoS ONE*, vol. 7, Article ID e41096, 2012.

[33] P. Saraon, N. Musrap, D. Cretu et al., "Proteomic profiling of androgen-independent prostate cancer cell lines reveals a role for protein S during the development of high grade and castration-resistant prostate cancer," *Journal of Biological Chemistry*, vol. 287, pp. 34019–34031, 2012.

[34] B. S. Carver, C. Chapinski, J. Wongvipat et al., "Reciprocal feedback regulation of PI3K and androgen receptor signaling in PTEN-deficient prostate cancer," *Cancer Cell*, vol. 19, no. 5, pp. 575–586, 2011.

[35] J. A. Ewald, J. A. Desotelle, D. R. Church et al., "Androgen deprivation induces senescence characteristics in prostate cancer cells in vitro and in vivo," *Prostate*, vol. 73, pp. 337–345, 2012.

[36] P. J. Maxwell, J. Coulter, S. M. Walker et al., "Potentiation of inflammatory CXCL8 signalling sustains cell survival in PTEN-deficient prostate carcinoma," *European Urology*, 2012.

[37] R. S. Jackson II, W. Placzek, A. Fernandez et al., "Sabutoclax, a Mcl-1 antagonist, inhibits tumorigenesis in transgenic mouse and human xenograft models of prostate cancer," *Neoplasia*, vol. 14, pp. 656–665, 2012.

[38] H. Wang, Y. Xu, Z. Fang, S. Chen, S. P. Balk, and X. Yuan, "Doxycycline regulated induction of AKT in murine prostate drives proliferation independently of p27 cyclin dependent kinase inhibitor downregulation," *PLoS ONE*, vol. 7, Article ID e41330, 2012.

[39] M. A. Reynolds, "Molecular alterations in prostate cancer," *Cancer Letters*, vol. 271, no. 1, pp. 13–24, 2008.

[40] M. E. Grossmann, H. Huang, and D. J. Tindall, "Androgen receptor signaling in androgen-refractory prostate cancer," *Journal of the National Cancer Institute*, vol. 93, no. 22, pp. 1687–1697, 2001.

[41] S. C. Chan, Y. Li, and S. M. Dehm, "Androgen receptor splice variants activate androgen receptor target genes and support aberrant prostate cancer cell growth independent of canonical

androgen receptor nuclear localization signal," *Journal of Biological Chemistry*, vol. 287, pp. 19736–19749, 2012.

[42] G. Castoria, L. D'Amato, A. Ciociola et al., "Androgen-induced cell migration: role of androgen receptor/filamin A association," *PLoS ONE*, vol. 6, Article ID e17218, 2012.

[43] K. K. Waltering, A. Urbanucci, and T. Visakorpi, "Androgen receptor (AR) aberrations in castration-resistant prostate cancer," *Molecular and Cellular Endocrinology*, vol. 360, pp. 38–43, 2012.

[44] H. Wang, C. Zhang, A. Rorick et al., "CCI-779 inhibits cell-cycle G2-M progression and invasion of castration-resistant prostate cancer via attenuation of UBE2C transcription and mRNA stability," *Cancer Research*, vol. 71, no. 14, pp. 4866–4876, 2011.

[45] A. Urbanucci, B. Sahu, J. Seppala et al., "Overexpression of androgen receptor enhances the binding of the receptor to the chromatin in prostate cancer," *Oncogene*, vol. 31, pp. 2153–2163, 2012.

[46] M. Shiota, A. Yokomizo, and S. Naito, "Increased androgen receptor transcription: a cause of castration-resistant prostate cancer and a possible therapeutic target," *Journal of Molecular Endocrinology*, vol. 47, no. 1, pp. R25–R41, 2011.

[47] M. Shiota, A. Yokomizo, and S. Naito, "Oxidative stress and androgen receptor signaling in the development and progression of castration-resistant prostate cancer," *Free Radical Biology and Medicine*, vol. 51, pp. 1320–1328, 2011.

[48] Y. Zuo and J. K. Cheng, "Small ubiquitin-like modifier protein-specific protease 1 and prostate cancer," *Asian Journal of Andrology*, vol. 11, no. 1, pp. 36–38, 2009.

[49] T. Bawa-Khalfe, J. Cheng, Z. Wang, and E. T. H. Yeh, "Induction of the SUMO-specific protease 1 transcription by the androgen receptor in prostate cancer cells," *Journal of Biological Chemistry*, vol. 282, no. 52, pp. 37341–37349, 2007.

[50] N. D. Perkins, "Integrating cell-signalling pathways with NF-kappaB and IKK function," *Nature Reviews Molecular Cell Biology*, vol. 8, pp. 49–62, 2007.

[51] C. Cai, F. N. Jiang, Y. X. Liang et al., "Classical and alternative nuclear factor-kappaB pathways: a comparison among normal prostate, benign prostate hyperplasia and prostate cancer," *Pathology and Oncology Research*, vol. 17, pp. 873–878, 2011.

[52] V. Tergaonkar, "NFκB pathway: a good signaling paradigm and therapeutic target," *International Journal of Biochemistry and Cell Biology*, vol. 38, no. 10, pp. 1647–1653, 2006.

[53] B. Razani, A. D. Reichardt, and G. Cheng, "Non-canonical NF-kappaB signaling activation and regulation: principles and perspectives," *Immunological Reviews*, vol. 244, pp. 44–54, 2011.

[54] R. C. Rickert, J. Jellusova, and A. V. Miletic, "Signaling by the tumor necrosis factor receptor superfamily in B-cell biology and disease," *Immunological Reviews*, vol. 244, pp. 115–133, 2011.

[55] L. Gu, A. Dagvadorj, J. Lutz et al., "Transcription factor Stat3 stimulates metastatic behavior of human prostate cancer cells in vivo, whereas Stat5b has a preferential role in the promotion of prostate cancer cell viability and tumor growth," *American Journal of Pathology*, vol. 176, no. 4, pp. 1959–1972, 2010.

[56] J. Chen, K. V. Giridhar, L. Zhang, S. Xu, and Q. Jane Wang, "A protein kinase C/protein kinase D pathway protects LNCaP prostate cancer cells from phorbol ester-induced apoptosis by promoting ERK1/2 and NF-κB activities," *Carcinogenesis*, vol. 32, no. 8, pp. 1198–1206, 2011.

[57] A. Hsu, R. S. Bruno, C. V. Löhr et al., "Dietary soy and tea mitigate chronic inflammation and prostate cancer via NFκB pathway in the Noble rat model," *Journal of Nutritional Biochemistry*, vol. 22, no. 5, pp. 502–510, 2011.

[58] R. Benelli, R. Vene, M. Ciarlo, S. Carlone, O. Barbieri, and N. Ferrari, "The AKT/NF-kappaB inhibitor xanthohumol is a potent anti-lymphocytic leukemia drug overcoming chemoresistance and cell infiltration," *Biochemical Pharmacology*, vol. 83, pp. 1634–1642, 2012.

[59] G. Jain, C. Voogdt, A. Tobias et al., "IkappaB kinases modulate the activity of the androgen receptor in prostate carcinoma cell lines," *Neoplasia*, vol. 14, pp. 178–189, 2012.

[60] Y. Fang, H. Sun, J. Zhai et al., "Antitumor activity of NF-kB decoy oligodeoxynucleotides in a prostate cancer cell line," *Asian Pacific Journal of Cancer Prevention*, vol. 12, pp. 2721–2726, 2012.

[61] W. Xiao, D. R. Hodge, L. Wang, X. Yang, X. Zhang, and W. L. Farrar, "Co-operative functions between nuclear factors NFκB and CCAT/enhancer-binding protein-β (C/EBP-β) regulate the IL-6 promoter in autocrine human prostate cancer cells," *Prostate*, vol. 61, no. 4, pp. 354–370, 2004.

[62] S. Shukla, G. T. MacLennan, P. Fu et al., "Nuclear factor-κB/p65 (Rel A) is constitutively activated in human prostate adenocarcinoma and correlates with disease progression," *Neoplasia*, vol. 6, no. 4, pp. 390–400, 2004.

[63] C. D. Chen and C. L. Sawyers, "NF-κB activates prostate-specific antigen expression and is upregulated in androgen-independent prostate cancer," *Molecular and Cellular Biology*, vol. 22, no. 8, pp. 2862–2870, 2002.

[64] M. Paz De Miguel, M. Royuela, F. R. Bethencourt, L. Santamaría, B. Fraile, and R. Paniagua, "Immunoexpression of tumour necrosis factor-α and its receptors 1 and 2 correlates with proliferation/apoptosis equilibrium in normal, hyperplasic and carcinomatous human prostrate," *Cytokine*, vol. 12, no. 5, pp. 535–538, 2000.

[65] G. Rodriguez-Berriguete, B. Fraile, R. Paniagua, P. Aller, and M. Royuela, "Expression of NF-kappaB-related proteins and their modulation during TNF-alpha-provoked apoptosis in prostate cancer cells," *Prostate*, vol. 72, pp. 40–50, 2012.

[66] Y. Bouraoui, M. Ricote, I. García-Tuñón et al., "Pro-inflammatory cytokines and prostate-specific antigen in hyperplasia and human prostate cancer," *Cancer Detection and Prevention*, vol. 32, no. 1, pp. 23–32, 2008.

[67] S. Srinivasan, R. Kumar, S. Koduru, A. Chandramouli, and C. Damodaran, "Inhibiting TNF-mediated signaling: a novel therapeutic paradigm for androgen independent prostate cancer," *Apoptosis*, vol. 15, no. 2, pp. 153–161, 2010.

[68] G. Rodríguez-Berriguete, B. Fraile, F. R. de Bethencourt et al., "Role of IAPs in prostate cancer progression: immunohistochemical study in normal and pathological (benign hyperplastic, prostatic intraepithelial neoplasia and cancer) human prostate," *BMC Cancer*, vol. 10, article 18, 2010.

[69] C. D. Chen, D. S. Welsbie, C. Tran et al., "Molecular determinants of resistance to antiandrogen therapy," *Nature Medicine*, vol. 10, no. 1, pp. 33–39, 2004.

[70] L. Zhang, S. Altuwaijri, F. Deng et al., "NF-κB regulates androgen receptor expression and prostate cancer growth," *American Journal of Pathology*, vol. 175, no. 2, pp. 489–499, 2009.

[71] G. Jain, M. V. Cronauer, M. Schrader, P. Moller, and R. B. Marienfeld, "NF-kappaB signaling in prostate cancer: a promising therapeutic target?" *World Journal of Urology*, vol. 30, pp. 303–310, 2012.

[72] S. I. Grivennikov and M. Karin, "Dangerous liaisons: STAT3 and NF-κB collaboration and crosstalk in cancer," *Cytokine and Growth Factor Reviews*, vol. 21, no. 1, pp. 11–19, 2010.

[73] G. Schneider and O. H. Kramer, "NFkappaB/p53 crosstalk-a promising new therapeutic target," *Biochimica et Biophysica Acta*, vol. 1815, pp. 90–103, 2011.

[74] A. Oeckinghaus, M. S. Hayden, and S. Ghosh, "Crosstalk in NF-kappaB signaling pathways," *Nature Immunology*, vol. 12, pp. 695–708, 2011.

[75] I. Vivanco and C. L. Sawyers, "The phosphatidylinositol 3-kinase-AKT pathway in human cancer," *Nature Reviews Cancer*, vol. 2, no. 7, pp. 489–501, 2002.

[76] A. G. Bader, S. Kang, L. Zhao, and P. K. Vogt, "Oncogenic PI3K deregulates transcription and translation," *Nature Reviews Cancer*, vol. 5, no. 12, pp. 921–929, 2005.

[77] J. A. Engelman, J. Luo, and L. C. Cantley, "The evolution of phosphatidylinositol 3-kinases as regulators of growth and metabolism," *Nature Reviews Genetics*, vol. 7, no. 8, pp. 606–619, 2006.

[78] D. A. Guertin and D. M. Sabatini, "Defining the role of mTOR in cancer," *Cancer Cell*, vol. 12, no. 1, pp. 9–22, 2007.

[79] L. Bozulic and B. A. Hemmings, "PIKKing on PKB: regulation of PKB activity by phosphorylation," *Current Opinion in Cell Biology*, vol. 21, no. 2, pp. 256–261, 2009.

[80] M. P. Scheid and J. R. Woodgett, "PKB/AKT: functional insights from genetic models," *Nature Reviews Molecular Cell Biology*, vol. 2, no. 10, pp. 760–768, 2001.

[81] B. D. Manning and L. C. Cantley, "AKT/PKB signaling: navigating downstream," *Cell*, vol. 129, no. 7, pp. 1261–1274, 2007.

[82] L. C. Cantley, "The phosphoinositide 3-kinase pathway," *Science*, vol. 296, no. 5573, pp. 1655–1657, 2002.

[83] T. M. Morgan, T. D. Koreckij, and E. Corey, "Targeted therapy for advanced prostate cancer: inhibition of the PI3K/Akt/mTOR pathway," *Current Cancer Drug Targets*, vol. 9, no. 2, pp. 237–249, 2009.

[84] A. Di Cristofano, B. Pesce, C. Cordon-Cardo, and P. P. Pandolfi, "Pten is essential for embryonic development and tumour suppression," *Nature Genetics*, vol. 19, no. 4, pp. 348–355, 1998.

[85] J. L. Boormans, H. Korsten, A. C. J. Ziel-Van Der Made, G. J. L. H. Van Leenders, P. C. M. S. Verhagen, and J. Trapman, "E17K substitution in AKT1 in prostate cancer," *British Journal of Cancer*, vol. 102, no. 10, pp. 1491–1494, 2010.

[86] L. C. Trotman, M. Niki, Z. A. Dotan et al., "Pten dose dictates cancer progression in the prostate," *PLoS Biology*, vol. 1, no. 3, article E59, 2003.

[87] Z. Chen, L. C. Trotman, D. Shaffer et al., "Crucial role of p53-dependent cellular senescence in suppression of Pten-deficient tumorigenesis," *Nature*, vol. 436, no. 7051, pp. 725–730, 2005.

[88] A. Di Cristofano, M. De Acetis, A. Koff, C. Cordon-Cardo, and P. P Pandolfi, "Pten and p27KIP1 cooperate in prostate cancer tumor suppression in the mouse," *Nature Genetics*, vol. 27, no. 2, pp. 222–224, 2001.

[89] L. Poliseno, L. Salmena, L. Riccardi et al., "Identification of the miR-106b~25 microRNA cluster as a proto-oncogenic PTEN-targeting intron that cooperates with its host gene MCM7 in transformation," *Science Signaling*, vol. 3, no. 117, article ra29, 2010.

[90] M. S. Song, L. Salmena, A. Carracedo et al., "The deubiquitinylation and localization of PTEN are regulated by a HAUSP-PML network," *Nature*, vol. 455, no. 7214, pp. 813–817, 2008.

[91] M. S. Song, L. Salmena, and P. P. Pandolfi, "The functions and regulation of the PTEN tumour suppressor," *Nature Reviews Molecular Cell Biology*, vol. 13, pp. 283–296, 2012.

[92] A. Almasan and A. Ashkenazi, "Apo2L/TRAIL: apoptosis signaling, biology, and potential for cancer therapy," *Cytokine and Growth Factor Reviews*, vol. 14, no. 3-4, pp. 337–348, 2003.

[93] J. Xu, J. Y. Zhou, W. Z. Wei, and G. S. Wu, "Activation of the Akt survival pathway contributes to TRAIL resistance in cancer cells," *PLoS ONE*, vol. 5, no. 4, Article ID e10226, 2010.

[94] N. Tzenaki, M. Andreou, K. Stratigi et al., "High levels of p110delta PI3K expression in solid tumor cells suppress PTEN activity, generating cellular sensitivity to p110delta inhibitors through PTEN activation," *FASEB Journal*, vol. 26, pp. 2498–2508, 2012.

[95] S. H. Lee, G. Poulogiannis, S. Pyne et al., "A constitutively activated form of the p110β isoform of PI3-kinase induces prostatic intraepithelial neoplasia in mice," *Proceedings of the National Academy of Sciences of the United States of America*, vol. 107, no. 24, pp. 11002–11007, 2010.

[96] B. Cinar, P. K. Fang, M. Lutchman et al., "The pro-apoptotic kinase Mst1 and its caspase cleavage products are direct inhibitors of Akt1," *EMBO Journal*, vol. 26, no. 21, pp. 4523–4534, 2007.

[97] B. Cinar, F. K. Collak, D. Lopez et al., "MST1 is a multifunctional caspase-independent inhibitor of androgenic signaling," *Cancer Research*, vol. 71, no. 12, pp. 4303–4313, 2011.

[98] Z. Yuan, D. Kim, S. Shu et al., "Phosphoinositide 3-kinase/Akt inhibits MST1-mediated pro-apoptotic signaling through phosphorylation of threonine 120," *Journal of Biological Chemistry*, vol. 285, no. 6, pp. 3815–3824, 2010.

[99] K. Mahajan, D. Coppola, S. Challa et al., "Ack1 mediated AKT/PKB tyrosine 176 phosphorylation regulates its activation," *PloS ONE*, vol. 5, no. 3, article e9646, 2010.

[100] K. Nacerddine, J. B. Beaudry, V. Ginjala et al., "Akt-mediated phosphorylation of Bmi1 modulates its oncogenic potential, E3 ligase activity, and DNA damage repair activity in mouse prostate cancer," *Journal of Clinical Investigation*, vol. 122, pp. 1920–1932, 2012.

[101] M. Gao, R. Patel, I. Ahmad et al., "SPRY2 loss enhances ErbB trafficking and PI3K/AKT signalling to drive human and mouse prostate carcinogenesis," *EMBO Molecular Medicine*, vol. 4, pp. 776–790, 2012.

[102] V. M. Adhami, I. A. Siddiqui, S. Sarfaraz et al., "Effective prostate cancer chemopreventive intervention with green tea polyphenols in the TRAMP model depends on Thestage of the disease," *Clinical Cancer Research*, vol. 15, no. 6, pp. 1947–1953, 2009.

[103] V. M. Adhami, I. A. Siddiqui, N. Ahmad, S. Gupta, and H. Mukhtar, "Oral consumption of green tea polyphenols inhibits insulin-like growth factor-I-induced signaling in an autochthonous mouse model of prostate cancer," *Cancer Research*, vol. 64, no. 23, pp. 8715–8722, 2004.

[104] H. J. Kung and C. P. Evans, "Oncogenic activation of androgen receptor," *Urologic Oncology*, vol. 27, no. 1, pp. 48–52, 2009.

[105] N. J. Clegg, S. S. Couto, J. Wongvipat et al., "MYC cooperates with AKT in prostate tumorigenesis and alters sensitivity to mTOR inhibitors," *PLoS ONE*, vol. 6, no. 3, Article ID e17449, 2011.

[106] D. N. Gunadharini, P. Elumalai, R. Arunkumar, K. Senthilkumar, and J. Arunakaran, "Induction of apoptosis and inhibition of PI3K/Akt pathway in PC-3 and LNCaP prostate cancer cells

by ethanolic neem leaf extract," *Journal of Ethnopharmacology*, vol. 134, no. 3, pp. 644–650, 2011.

[107] K. R. Park, D. Nam, H. M. Yun et al., "beta-Caryophyllene oxide inhibits growth and induces apoptosis through the suppression of PI3K/AKT/mTOR/S6K1 pathways and ROS-mediated MAPKs activation," *Cancer Letters*, vol. 312, pp. 178–188, 2011.

[108] V. M. Adhami, D. N. Syed, N. Khan, and H. Mukhtar, "Dietary flavonoid fisetin: a novel dual inhibitor of PI3K/Akt and mTOR for prostate cancer management," *Biochemical Pharmacology*, vol. 84, pp. 1277–1281, 2012.

[109] Z. Wang, Y. Zhang, S. Banerjee, Y. Li, and F. H. Sarkar, "Notch-1 down-regulation by curcumin is associated with the inhibition of cell growth and the induction of apoptosis in pancreatic cancer cells," *Cancer*, vol. 106, no. 11, pp. 2503–2513, 2006.

[110] M. J. Ryu, M. Cho, J. Y. Song et al., "Natural derivatives of curcumin attenuate the Wnt/β-catenin pathway through down-regulation of the transcriptional coactivator p300," *Biochemical and Biophysical Research Communications*, vol. 377, no. 4, pp. 1304–1308, 2008.

[111] S. Yu, G. Shen, O. K. Tin, J. H. Kim, and A. N. T. Kong, "Curcumin inhibits Akt/mammalian target of rapamycin signaling through protein phosphatase-dependent mechanism," *Molecular Cancer Therapeutics*, vol. 7, no. 9, pp. 2609–2620, 2008.

[112] A. Ślusarz, N. S. Shenouda, M. S. Sakla et al., "Common botanical compounds inhibit the hedgehog signaling pathway in prostate cancer," *Cancer Research*, vol. 70, no. 8, pp. 3382–3390, 2010.

[113] O. W. Rokhlin, N. V. Guseva, A. F. Taghiyev, R. A. Glover, and M. B. Cohen, "KN-93 inhibits androgen receptor activity and induces cell death irrespective of p53 and Akt status in prostate cancer," *Cancer Biology and Therapy*, vol. 9, no. 3, pp. 224–235, 2010.

[114] J. J. Wallin, K. A. Edgar, J. Guan et al., "GDC-0980 is a novel class I PI3K/mTOR kinase inhibitor with robust activity in cancer models driven by the PI3K pathway," *Molecular Cancer Therapeutics*, vol. 10, pp. 2426–2436, 2011.

[115] S. M. Manohar, A. A. Padgaonkar, A. J. Badhwar et al., "A novel inhibitor of hypoxia-inducible factor-1alpha P3155 also modulates PI3K pathway and inhibits growth of prostate cancer cells," *BMC Cancer*, vol. 11, article 338, 2011.

[116] L. Lu, D. Tang, L. Wang et al., "Gambogic acid inhibits TNF-alpha-induced invasion of human prostate cancer PC3 cells in vitro through PI3K/Akt and NF-kappaB signaling pathways," *Acta Pharmacologica Sinica*, vol. 33, pp. 531–541, 2012.

[117] S. L. Burgio, F. Fabbri, I. J. Seymour, W. Zoli, D. Amadori, and U. De Giorgi, "Perspectives on mTOR inhibitors for castration-refractory prostate cancer," *Current Cancer Drug Targets*, vol. 12, pp. 940–949, 2012.

[118] E. C. Nelson, C. P. Evans, P. C. Mack, R. W. Devere-White, and P. N. Lara Jr., "Inhibition of Akt pathways in the treatment of prostate cancer," *Prostate Cancer and Prostatic Diseases*, vol. 10, no. 4, pp. 331–339, 2007.

[119] C. A. Granville, R. M. Memmott, J. J. Gills, and P. A. Dennis, "Handicapping the race to develop inhibitors of the phosphoinositide 3-kinase/Akt/mammalian target of rapamycin pathway," *Clinical Cancer Research*, vol. 12, no. 3, pp. 679–689, 2006.

[120] S. B. Kondapaka, S. S. Singh, G. P. Dasmahapatra, E. A. Sausville, and K. K. Roy, "Perifosine, a novel alkylphospholipid, inhibits protein kinase B activation," *Molecular Cancer Therapeutics*, vol. 2, no. 11, pp. 1093–1103, 2003.

[121] C. G. Tepper, R. L. Vinall, C. B. Wee et al., "GCP-mediated growth inhibition and apoptosis of prostate cancer cells via androgen receptor-dependent and -independent mechanisms," *Prostate*, vol. 67, no. 5, pp. 521–535, 2007.

[122] P. B. Makhov, K. Golovine, A. Kutikov et al., "Modulation of Akt/mTOR signaling overcomes sunitinib resistance in renal and prostate cancer cells," *Molecular Cancer Therapeutics*, vol. 11, pp. 1510–1517, 2012.

[123] H. Kiu and S. E. Nicholson, "Biology and significance of the JAK/STAT signalling pathways," *Growth Factors*, vol. 30, pp. 88–106, 2012.

[124] D. A. Harrison, "The Jak/STAT pathway," *Cold Spring Harbor Perspectives in Biology*, vol. 4, 2012.

[125] W. X. Li, "Canonical and non-canonical JAK-STAT signaling," *Trends in Cell Biology*, vol. 18, no. 11, pp. 545–551, 2008.

[126] D. Hebenstreit, J. Horejs-Hoeck, and A. Duschl, "JAK/STAT-dependent gene regulation by cytokines," *Drug News and Perspectives*, vol. 18, no. 4, pp. 243–249, 2005.

[127] J. J. O'Shea, H. Park, M. Pesu, D. Borie, and P. Changelian, "New strategies for immunosuppression: interfering with cytokines by targeting the Jak/Stat pathway," *Current Opinion in Rheumatology*, vol. 17, no. 3, pp. 305–311, 2005.

[128] P. Igaz, S. Tóth, and A. Falus, "Biological and clinical significance of the JAK-STAT pathway; lessons from knockout mice," *Inflammation Research*, vol. 50, no. 9, pp. 435–441, 2001.

[129] J. J. O'Shea, M. Gadina, and R. D. Schreiber, "Cytokine signaling in 2002: new surprises in the Jak/Stat pathway," *Cell*, vol. 109, no. 2, pp. S121–S131, 2002.

[130] J. E. Darnell Jr., "STATs and gene regulation," *Science*, vol. 277, no. 5332, pp. 1630–1635, 1997.

[131] J. N. Ihle, W. Thierfelder, S. Teglund et al., "Signaling by the cytokine receptor superfamily," *Annals of the New York Academy of Sciences*, vol. 865, pp. 1–9, 1998.

[132] K. Shuai, C. M. Horvath, L. H. T. Huang, S. A. Qureshi, D. Cowburn, and J. E. Darnell Jr., "Interferon activation of the transcription factor Stat91 involves dimerization through SH2-phosphotyrosyl peptide interactions," *Cell*, vol. 76, no. 5, pp. 821–828, 1994.

[133] S. Gupta, T. Barrett, A. J. Whitmarsh et al., "Selective interaction of JNK protein kinase isoforms with transcription factors," *EMBO Journal*, vol. 15, no. 11, pp. 2760–2770, 1996.

[134] K. Mowen and M. David, "Role of the STAT1-SH2 domain and STAT2 in the activation and nuclear translocation of STAT1," *Journal of Biological Chemistry*, vol. 273, no. 46, pp. 30073–30076, 1998.

[135] J. S. Rawlings, K. M. Rosler, and D. A. Harrison, "The JAK/STAT signaling pathway," *Journal of Cell Science*, vol. 117, no. 8, pp. 1281–1283, 2004.

[136] J. Bromberg, "Stat proteins and oncogenesis," *Journal of Clinical Investigation*, vol. 109, no. 9, pp. 1139–1142, 2002.

[137] H. Yu and R. Jove, "The stats of cancer—new molecular targets come of age," *Nature Reviews Cancer*, vol. 4, no. 2, pp. 97–105, 2004.

[138] A. Tutt and A. Ashworth, "The relationship between the roles of BRCA genes in DNA repair and cancer predisposition," *Trends in Molecular Medicine*, vol. 8, no. 12, pp. 571–576, 2002.

[139] H. Wallerand, G. Robert, J. C. Bernhard, A. Ravaud, and J. J. Patard, "Tyrosine-kinase inhibitors in the treatment of muscle invasive bladder cancer and hormone refractory prostate cancer," *Archivos Espanoles de Urologia*, vol. 63, no. 9, pp. 773–787, 2010.

[140] E. M. Kwon, S. K. Holt, R. Fu et al., "Androgen metabolism and JAK/STAT pathway genes and prostate cancer risk," *Cancer Epidemiology*, vol. 36, pp. 347–353, 2012.

[141] D. A. Frank, "STAT3 as a central mediator of neoplastic cellular transformation," *Cancer Letters*, vol. 251, no. 2, pp. 199–210, 2007.

[142] B. Gao, X. Shen, G. Kunos et al., "Constitutive activation of JAK-STAT3 signaling by BRCA1 in human prostate cancer cells," *FEBS Letters*, vol. 488, no. 3, pp. 179–184, 2001.

[143] A. R. Venkitaraman, "Cancer susceptibility and the functions of BRCA1 and BRCA2," *Cell*, vol. 108, no. 2, pp. 171–182, 2002.

[144] E. A. Ostrander and M. S. Udler, "The role of the BRCA2 gene in susceptibility to prostate cancer revisited," *Cancer Epidemiology Biomarkers and Prevention*, vol. 17, no. 8, pp. 1843–1848, 2008.

[145] S. Panchal, O. Shachar, F. O'Malley et al., "Breast cancer in a BRCA2 mutation carrier with a history of prostate cancer," *Nature Reviews Clinical Oncology*, vol. 6, no. 10, pp. 604–607, 2009.

[146] N. Rahman and M. R. Stratton, "The genetics of breast cancer susceptibility," *Annual Review of Genetics*, vol. 32, pp. 95–121, 1998.

[147] P. Kerr and A. Ashworth, "New complexities for BRCA1 and BRCA2," *Current Biology*, vol. 11, no. 16, pp. R668–R676, 2001.

[148] M. Sakaguchi, M. Oka, T. Iwasaki, Y. Fukami, and C. Nishigori, "Role and regulation of STAT3 phosphorylation at Ser727 in melanocytes and melanoma cells," *Journal of Investigative Dermatology*, vol. 132, pp. 1877–1885, 2012.

[149] J. Cao, P. Kozarekar, M. Pavlaki, C. Chiarelli, W. F. Bahou, and S. Zucker, "Distinct roles for the catalytic and hemopexin domains of membrane type 1-matrix metalloproteinase in substrate degradation and cell migration," *Journal of Biological Chemistry*, vol. 279, no. 14, pp. 14129–14139, 2004.

[150] V. I. Romanov, T. Whyard, H. L. Adler, W. C. Waltzer, and S. Zucker, "Prostate cancer cell adhesion to bone marrow endothelium: the role of prostate-specific antigen," *Cancer Research*, vol. 64, no. 6, pp. 2083–2089, 2004.

[151] H. L. Nguyen, S. Zucker, K. Zarrabi, P. Kadam, C. Schmidt, and J. Cao, "Oxidative stress and prostate cancer progression are elicited by membrane-type 1 matrix metalloproteinase," *Molecular Cancer Research*, vol. 9, pp. 1305–1318, 2011.

[152] D. Kesanakurti, C. Chetty, D. H. Dinh, M. Gujrati, and J. S. Rao, "Role of MMP-2 in the regulation of IL-6/Stat3 survival signaling via interaction with alpha5beta1 integrin in glioma," *Oncogene*, vol. 32, pp. 327–340, 2012.

[153] R. Dhir, Z. Ni, W. Lou, F. DeMiguel, J. R. Grandis, and A. C. Gao, "Stat3 activation in prostatic carcinomas," *Prostate*, vol. 51, no. 4, pp. 241–246, 2002.

[154] X. Liu, Z. He, C. H. Li, G. Huang, C. Ding, and H. Liu, "Correlation analysis of JAK-STAT pathway components on prognosis of patients with prostate cancer," *Pathology and Oncology Research*, vol. 18, pp. 17–23, 2012.

[155] R. Aalinkeel, Z. Hu, B. B. Nair et al., "Genomic analysis highlights the role of the JAK-STAT signaling in the anti-proliferative effects of dietary—flavonoid "ashwagandha" in prostate cancer cells," *Evidence-Based Complementary and Alternative Medicine*, vol. 7, no. 2, pp. 177–187, 2010.

[156] K. Ishihara and T. Hirano, "IL-6 in autoimmune disease and chronic inflammatory proliferative disease," *Cytokine and Growth Factor Reviews*, vol. 13, no. 4-5, pp. 357–368, 2002.

[157] T. Kishimoto, "Interleukin-6: from basic science to medicine—40 years in immunology," *Annual Review of Immunology*, vol. 23, pp. 1–21, 2005.

[158] A. Hobisch, H. Rogatsch, A. Hittmair et al., "Immunohistochemical localization of interleukin-6 and its receptor in benign, premalignant and malignant prostate tissue," *Journal of Pathology*, vol. 191, pp. 239–244, 2000.

[159] P. C. Smith, A. Hobisch, D. L. Lin, Z. Culig, and E. T. Keller, "Interleukin-6 and prostate cancer progression," *Cytokine and Growth Factor Reviews*, vol. 12, no. 1, pp. 33–40, 2001.

[160] J. R. Stark, H. Li, P. Kraft et al., "Circulating prediagnostic interleukin-6 and C-reactive protein and prostate cancer incidence and mortality," *International Journal of Cancer*, vol. 124, no. 11, pp. 2683–2689, 2009.

[161] J. Karkera, H. Steiner, W. Li et al., "The anti-interleukin-6 antibody siltuximab down-regulates genes implicated in tumorigenesis in prostate cancer patients from a phase I study," *Prostate*, vol. 71, pp. 1455–1465, 2011.

[162] D. A. Twillie, M. A. Eisenberger, M. A. Carducci, W. S. Hseih, W. Y. Kim, and J. W. Simons, "Interleukin-6: a candidate mediator of human prostate cancer morbidity," *Urology*, vol. 45, no. 3, pp. 542–549, 1995.

[163] M. Okamoto, C. Lee, and R. Oyasu, "Interleukin-6 as a paracrine and autocrine growth factor in human prostatic carcinoma cells in vitro," *Cancer Research*, vol. 57, no. 1, pp. 141–146, 1997.

[164] I. T. Cavarretta, H. Neuwirt, G. Untergasser et al., "The antiapoptotic effect of IL-6 autocrine loop in a cellular model of advanced prostate cancer is mediated by Mcl-1," *Oncogene*, vol. 26, no. 20, pp. 2822–2832, 2007.

[165] T. D. Chung, J. J. Yu, M. T. Spiotto, M. Bartkowski, and J. W. Simons, "Characterization of the role of IL-6 in the progression of prostate cancer," *Prostate*, vol. 38, pp. 199–207, 1999.

[166] W. Lou, Z. Ni, K. Dyer, D. J. Tweardy, and A. C. Gao, "Interleukin-6 induces prostate cancer cell growth accompanied by activation of stat3 signaling pathway," *Prostate*, vol. 42, pp. 239–242, 2000.

[167] I. Sakai, H. Miyake, T. Terakawa, and M. Fujisawa, "Inhibition of tumor growth and sensitization to chemotherapy by RNA interference targeting interleukin-6 in the androgen-independent human prostate cancer PC3 model," *Cancer Science*, vol. 102, no. 4, pp. 769–775, 2011.

[168] L. R. Dearth and J. DeWille, "An AU-rich element in the 3′ untranslated region of the C/EBPδ mRNA is important for protein binding during G0 growth arrest," *Biochemical and Biophysical Research Communications*, vol. 304, no. 2, pp. 344–350, 2003.

[169] L. R. Dearth and J. DeWille, "Posttranscriptional and posttranslational regulation of C/EBPδ in Go growth-arrested mammary epithelial cells," *Journal of Biological Chemistry*, vol. 278, no. 13, pp. 11246–11255, 2003.

[170] D. P. Ramji and P. Foka, "CCAAT/enhancer-binding proteins: structure, function and regulation," *Biochemical Journal*, vol. 365, no. 3, pp. 561–575, 2002.

[171] D. C. Sanford and J. W. DeWille, "C/EBPδ is a downstream mediator of IL-6 induced growth inhibition of prostate cancer cells," *Prostate*, vol. 63, no. 2, pp. 143–154, 2005.

[172] E. LaTulippe, J. Satagopan, A. Smith et al., "Comprehensive gene expression analysis of prostate cancer reveals distinct transcriptional programs associated with metastatic disease," *Cancer Research*, vol. 62, no. 15, pp. 4499–4506, 2002.

[173] B. Binétruy, L. Heasley, F. Bost, L. Caron, and M. Aouadi, "Concise review: regulation of embryonic stem cell lineage commitment by mitogen-activated protein kinases," *Stem Cells*, vol. 25, no. 5, pp. 1090–1095, 2007.

[174] A. S. Dhillon, S. Hagan, O. Rath, and W. Kolch, "MAP kinase signalling pathways in cancer," *Oncogene*, vol. 26, no. 22, pp. 3279–3290, 2007.

[175] E. F. Wagner and A. R. Nebreda, "Signal integration by JNK and p38 MAPK pathways in cancer development," *Nature Reviews Cancer*, vol. 9, no. 8, pp. 537–549, 2009.

[176] Y. T. Ip and R. J. Davis, "Signal transduction by the c-Jun N-terminal kinase (JNK)—from inflammation to development," *Current Opinion in Cell Biology*, vol. 10, no. 2, pp. 205–219, 1998.

[177] T. H. Holmström, I. Schmitz, T. S. Söderström et al., "MAPK/ERK signaling in activated T cells inhibits CD95/Fas-mediated apoptosis downstream of DISC assembly," *EMBO Journal*, vol. 19, no. 20, pp. 5418–5428, 2000.

[178] K. Gupta, S. Kshirsagar, W. Li et al., "VEGF prevents apoptosis of human microvascular endothelial cells via opposing effects on MAPK/ERK and SAPK/JNK signaling," *Experimental Cell Research*, vol. 247, no. 2, pp. 495–504, 1999.

[179] A. Ogata, D. Chauhan, G. Teoh et al., "IL-6 triggers cell growth via the ras-dependent mitogen-activated protein kinase cascade," *Journal of Immunology*, vol. 159, no. 5, pp. 2212–2221, 1997.

[180] V. Flati, E. Pasini, G. D'Antona, S. Speca, E. Toniato, and S. Martinotti, "Intracellular mechanisms of metabolism regulation: the role of signaling via the mammalian target of rapamycin pathway and other routes," *American Journal of Cardiology*, vol. 101, no. 11, pp. S16–S21, 2008.

[181] S. Davis, P. Vanhoutte, C. Pagès, J. Caboche, and S. Laroche, "The MAPK/ERK cascade targets both Elk-1 and cAMP response element- binding protein to control long-term potentiation-dependent gene expression in the dentate gyrus in vivo," *Journal of Neuroscience*, vol. 20, no. 12, pp. 4563–4572, 2000.

[182] J. Guicheux, J. Lemonnier, C. Ghayor, A. Suzuki, G. Palmer, and J. Caverzasio, "Activation of p38 mitogen-activated protein kinase and c-Jun-NH2-terminal kinase by BMP-2 and their implication in the stimulation of osteoblastic cell differentiation," *Journal of Bone and Mineral Research*, vol. 18, no. 11, pp. 2060–2068, 2003.

[183] C. Huang, K. Jacobson, and M. D. Schaller, "MAP kinases and cell migration," *Journal of Cell Science*, vol. 117, no. 20, pp. 4619–4628, 2004.

[184] M. A. Lemmon and J. Schlessinger, "Cell signaling by receptor tyrosine kinases," *Cell*, vol. 141, no. 7, pp. 1117–1134, 2010.

[185] L. A. Fecher, R. K. Amaravadi, and K. T. Flaherty, "The MAPK pathway in melanoma," *Current Opinion in Oncology*, vol. 20, no. 2, pp. 183–189, 2008.

[186] Y. Fleming, C. G. Armstrong, N. Morrice, A. Paterson, M. Goedert, and P. Cohen, "Synergistic activation of stress-activated protein kinase 1/c-Jun N-terminal kinase (SAPK1/JNK) isoforms by mitogen-activated protein kinase kinase 4 (MKK4) and MKK7," *Biochemical Journal*, vol. 352, no. 1, pp. 145–154, 2000.

[187] W. Haeusgen, T. Herdegen, and V. Waetzig, "The bottleneck of JNK signaling: molecular and functional characteristics of MKK4 and MKK7," *European Journal of Cell Biology*, vol. 90, no. 6-7, pp. 536–544, 2011.

[188] W. Xin, K. J. Yun, F. Ricci et al., "MAP2K4/MKK4 expression in pancreatic cancer: genetic validation of immunohistochemistry and relationship to disease course," *Clinical Cancer Research*, vol. 10, no. 24, pp. 8516–8520, 2004.

[189] S. D. Yamada, J. A. Hickson, Y. Hrobowski et al., "Mitogen-activated protein kinase kinase 4 (MKK4) acts as a metastasis suppressor gene in human ovarian carcinoma," *Cancer Research*, vol. 62, no. 22, pp. 6717–6723, 2002.

[190] R. Chiu, W. J. Boyle, J. Meek, T. Smeal, T. Hunter, and M. Karin, "The c-Fos protein interacts with c-Jun/AP-1 to stimulate transcription of AP-1 responsive genes," *Cell*, vol. 54, no. 4, pp. 541–552, 1988.

[191] C. Jonat, H. J. Rahmsdorf, K. K. Park et al., "Antitumor promotion and antiinflammation: down-modulation of AP-1 (Fos/Jun) activity by glucocorticoid hormone," *Cell*, vol. 62, no. 6, pp. 1189–1204, 1990.

[192] C. W. Kinkade, M. Castillo-Martin, A. Puzio-Kuter et al., "Targeting AKT/mTOR and ERK MAPK signaling inhibits hormone-refractory prostate cancer in a preclinical mouse model," *Journal of Clinical Investigation*, vol. 118, no. 9, pp. 3051–3064, 2008.

[193] M. T. Abreu-Martin, A. Chari, A. A. Palladino, N. A. Craft, and C. L. Sawyers, "Mitogen-activated protein kinase kinase kinase 1 activates androgen receptor-dependent transcription and apoptosis in prostate cancer," *Molecular and Cellular Biology*, vol. 19, no. 7, pp. 5143–5154, 1999.

[194] D. Gioeli, J. W. Mandell, G. R. Petroni, H. F. Frierson, and M. J. Weber, "Activation of mitogen-activated protein kinase associated with prostate cancer progression," *Cancer Research*, vol. 59, no. 2, pp. 279–284, 1999.

[195] A. M. Carey, R. Pramanik, L. J. Nicholson et al., "Ras-MEK-ERK signaling cascade regulates androgen receptor element-inducible gene transcription and DNA synthesis in prostate cancer cells," *International Journal of Cancer*, vol. 121, no. 3, pp. 520–527, 2007.

[196] T. J. Dorkin, M. C. Robinson, C. Marsh, A. Bjartell, D. E. Neal, and H. Y. Leung, "FGF8 over-expression in prostate cancer is associated with decreased patient survival and persists in androgen independent disease," *Oncogene*, vol. 18, no. 17, pp. 2755–2761, 1999.

[197] H. Steiner, S. Godoy-Tundidor, H. Rogatsch et al., "Accelerated in vivo growth of prostate tumors that up-regulate interleukin-6 is associated with reduced retinoblastoma protein expression and activation of the mitogen-activated protein kinase pathway," *American Journal of Pathology*, vol. 162, no. 2, pp. 655–663, 2003.

[198] R. E. Bakin, D. Gioeli, E. A. Bissonette, and M. J. Weber, "Attenuation of Ras signaling restores androgen sensitivity to hormone-refractory C4-2 prostate cancer cells," *Cancer Research*, vol. 63, no. 8, pp. 1975–1980, 2003.

[199] J. H. Jeong, Z. Wang, A. S. Guimaraes et al., "BRAF activation initiates but does not maintain invasive prostate adenocarcinoma," *PLoS ONE*, vol. 3, no. 12, Article ID e3949, 2008.

[200] H. B. Pearson, T. J. Phesse, and A. R. Clarke, "K-ras and Wnt signaling synergize to accelerate prostate tumorigenesis in the mouse," *Cancer Research*, vol. 69, no. 1, pp. 94–101, 2009.

[201] N. Palanisamy, B. Ateeq, S. Kalyana-Sundaram et al., "Rearrangements of the RAF kinase pathway in prostate cancer, gastric cancer and melanoma," *Nature Medicine*, vol. 16, no. 7, pp. 793–798, 2010.

[202] L. Tie, N. Lu, X. Y. Pan et al., "Hypoxia-induced up-regulation of aquaporin-1 protein in prostate cancer cells in a p38-dependent manner," *Cellular Physiology and Biochemistry*, vol. 29, pp. 269–280, 2012.

[203] Y. Limami, A. Pinon, D. Y. Leger et al., "The P2Y2/Src/p38/COX-2 pathway is involved in the resistance to ursolic acid-induced apoptosis in colorectal and prostate cancer cells," *Biochimie*, vol. 94, pp. 1754–1763, 2012.

[204] M. Katoh, "FGFR2 abnormalities underlie a spectrum of bone, skin, and cancer pathologies," *Journal of Investigative Dermatology*, vol. 129, no. 8, pp. 1861–1867, 2009.

[205] P. C. Marker, A. A. Donjacour, R. Dahiya, and G. R. Cunha, "Hormonal, cellular, and molecular control of prostatic development," *Developmental Biology*, vol. 253, no. 2, pp. 165–174, 2003.

[206] A. A. Donjacour, A. A. Thomson, and G. R. Cunha, "FGF-10 plays an essential role in the growth of the fetal prostate," *Developmental Biology*, vol. 261, no. 1, pp. 39–54, 2003.

[207] Y. Lin, G. Liu, Y. Zhang et al., "Fibroblast growth factor receptor 2 tyrosine kinase is required for prostatic morphogenesis and the acquisition of strict androgen dependency for adult tissue homeostasis," *Development*, vol. 134, no. 4, pp. 723–734, 2007.

[208] Y. Zhang, J. Zhang, Y. Lin et al., "Role of epithelial cell fibroblast growth factor receptor substrate 2α in prostate development, regeneration and tumorigenesis," *Development*, vol. 135, no. 4, pp. 775–784, 2008.

[209] S. L. Kuslak and P. C. Marker, "Fibroblast growth factor receptor signaling through MEK-ERK is required for prostate bud induction," *Differentiation*, vol. 75, no. 7, pp. 638–651, 2007.

[210] M. J. Hour, S. C. Tsai, H. C. Wu et al., "Antitumor effects of the novel quinazolinone MJ-33: inhibition of metastasis through the MAPK, AKT, NF-kappaB and AP-1 signaling pathways in DU145 human prostate cancer cells," *International Journal of Oncology*, 2012.

[211] T. Shimizu, A. W. Tolcher, K. P. Papadopoulos et al., "The clinical effect of the dual-targeting strategy involving PI3K/AKT/mTOR and RAS/MEK/ERK pathways in patients with advanced cancer," *Clinical Cancer Research*, vol. 18, pp. 2316–2325, 2012.

[212] G. C. Blobe, W. P. Schiemann, and H. F. Lodish, "Role of transforming growth factor β in human disease," *New England Journal of Medicine*, vol. 342, no. 18, pp. 1350–1358, 2000.

[213] J. Massagué, S. W. Blain, and R. S. Lo, "TGFβ signaling in growth control, cancer, and heritable disorders," *Cell*, vol. 103, no. 2, pp. 295–309, 2000.

[214] B. Schmierer and C. S. Hill, "TGFβ-SMAD signal transduction: molecular specificity and functional flexibility," *Nature Reviews Molecular Cell Biology*, vol. 8, no. 12, pp. 970–982, 2007.

[215] J. Massague, "TGFbeta in cancer," *Cell*, vol. 134, pp. 215–230, 2008.

[216] Y. Shi and J. Massagué, "Mechanisms of TGF-β signaling from cell membrane to the nucleus," *Cell*, vol. 113, no. 6, pp. 685–700, 2003.

[217] F. L. Miles, N. S. Tung, A. A. Aguiar, S. Kurtoglu, and R. A. Sikes, "Increased TGF-beta1-mediated suppression of growth and motility in castrate-resistant prostate cancer cells is consistent with Smad2/3 signaling," *Prostate*, vol. 72, pp. 1339–1350, 2012.

[218] M. K. Donkor, A. Sarkar, and M. O. Li, "Tgf-beta1 produced by activated $CD4^+$ T cells antagonizes T cell surveillance of tumor development," *Oncoimmunology*, vol. 1, pp. 162–171, 2012.

[219] X. Wan, Z. G. Li, J. M. Yingling et al., "Effect of transforming growth factor beta (TGF-beta) receptor I kinase inhibitor on prostate cancer bone growth," *Bone*, vol. 50, pp. 695–703, 2012.

[220] P. Wikstrom, P. Stattin, I. Franck-Lissbrant, J. E. Damber, and A. Bergh, "Transforming growth factor beta1 is associated with angiogenesis, metastasis, and poor clinical outcome in prostate cancer," *Prostate*, vol. 37, pp. 19–29, 1998.

[221] H. L. Adler, M. A. McCurdy, M. W. Kattan, T. L. Timme, P. T. Scardino, and T. C. Thompson, "Elevated levels of circulating interleukin-6 and transforming growth factor-β1 in patients with metastatic prostatic carcinoma," *Journal of Urology*, vol. 161, no. 1, pp. 182–187, 1999.

[222] S. F. Shariat, M. Shalev, A. Menesses-Diaz et al., "Preoperative plasma levels of transforming growth factor beta1 (TGF-β1 strongly predict progression in patients undergoing radical prostatectomy," *Journal of Clinical Oncology*, vol. 19, no. 11, pp. 2856–2864, 2001.

[223] R. Derynck, R. J. Akhurst, and A. Balmain, "TGF-β signaling in tumor suppression and cancer progression," *Nature Genetics*, vol. 29, no. 2, pp. 117–129, 2001.

[224] L. M. Wakefield and A. B. Roberts, "TGF-β signaling: positive and negative effects on tumorigenesis," *Current Opinion in Genetics and Development*, vol. 12, no. 1, pp. 22–29, 2002.

[225] J. Yang, R. Wahdan-Alaswad, and D. Danielpour, "Critical role of smad2 in tumor suppression and transforming growth factor-β-Lnduced apoptosis of prostate epithelial cells," *Cancer Research*, vol. 69, no. 6, pp. 2185–2190, 2009.

[226] L. Ye, H. Kynaston, and W. G. Jiang, "Bone morphogenetic protein-10 suppresses the growth and aggressiveness of prostate cancer cells through a Smad independent pathway," *Journal of Urology*, vol. 181, no. 6, pp. 2749–2759, 2009.

[227] B. T. Vo and S. A. Khan, "Expression of nodal and nodal receptors in prostate stem cells and prostate cancer cells: autocrine effects on cell proliferation and migration," *Prostate*, vol. 71, no. 10, pp. 1084–1096, 2011.

[228] H. Y. Kang, H. Y. Huang, C. Y. Hsieh et al., "Activin A enhances prostate cancer cell migration through activation of androgen receptor and is overexpressed in metastatic prostate cancer," *Journal of Bone and Mineral Research*, vol. 24, no. 7, pp. 1180–1193, 2009.

[229] J. L. Whyte, A. A. Smith, and J. A. Helms, "Wnt signaling and injury repair," *Cold Spring Harbor Perspectives in Biology*, vol. 4, Article ID a008078, 2012.

[230] S. Angers and R. T. Moon, "Proximal events in Wnt signal transduction," *Nature Reviews Molecular Cell Biology*, vol. 10, no. 7, pp. 468–477, 2009.

[231] S. Thiele, M. Rauner, C. Goettsch et al., "Expression profile of WNT molecules in prostate cancer and its regulation by aminobisphosphonates," *Journal of Cellular Biochemistry*, vol. 112, no. 6, pp. 1593–1600, 2011.

[232] W. Lu, H. N. Tinsley, A. Keeton, Z. Qu, G. A. Piazza, and Y. Li, "Suppression of Wnt/β-catenin signaling inhibits prostate cancer cell proliferation," *European Journal of Pharmacology*, vol. 602, no. 1, pp. 8–14, 2009.

[233] C. L. Hall, S. Kang, O. A. MacDougald, and E. T. Keller, "Role of Wnts in prostate cancer bone metastases," *Journal of Cellular Biochemistry*, vol. 97, no. 4, pp. 661–672, 2006.

[234] D. Kimelman and W. Xu, "β-Catenin destruction complex: insights and questions from a structural perspective," *Oncogene*, vol. 25, no. 57, pp. 7482–7491, 2006.

[235] J. Huelsken and J. Behrens, "The Wnt signalling pathway," *Journal of Cell Science*, vol. 115, no. 21, pp. 3977–3978, 2002.

[236] H. C. Whitaker, J. Girling, A. Y. Warren, H. Leung, I. G. Mills, and D. E. Neal, "Alterations in β-catenin expression and localization in prostate cancer," *Prostate*, vol. 68, no. 11, pp. 1196–1205, 2008.

[237] S. Majid, S. Saini, and R. Dahiya, "Wnt signaling pathways in urological cancers: past decades and still growing," *Molecular Cancer*, vol. 11, article 7, 2012.

[238] S. Barolo, "Transgenic Wnt/TCF pathway reporters: all you need is Lef?" *Oncogene*, vol. 25, no. 57, pp. 7505–7511, 2006.

[239] C. Mosimann, G. Hausmann, and K. Basler, "β-Catenin hits chromatin: regulation of Wnt target gene activation," *Nature Reviews Molecular Cell Biology*, vol. 10, no. 4, pp. 276–286, 2009.

[240] J. Zhao, W. Yue, M. J. Zhu, N. Sreejayan, and M. Du, "AMP-activated protein kinase (AMPK) cross-talks with canonical Wnt signaling via phosphorylation of beta-catenin at Ser 552," *Biochemical and Biophysical Research Communications*, vol. 395, no. 1, pp. 146–151, 2010.

[241] W. J. Gullick, "Prevalence of aberrant expression of the epidermal growth factor receptor in human cancers," *British Medical Bulletin*, vol. 47, no. 1, pp. 87–98, 1991.

[242] K. K. Guturi, T. Mandal, A. Chatterjee et al., "Mechanism of beta-catenin-mediated transcriptional regulation of epidermal growth factor receptor expression in glycogen synthase kinase 3 beta-inactivated prostate cancer cells," *Journal of Biological Chemistry*, vol. 287, pp. 18287–18296, 2012.

[243] P. C. Marker, "Does prostate cancer co-opt the developmental program?" *Differentiation*, vol. 76, no. 6, pp. 736–744, 2008.

[244] N. S. Fearnhead, M. P. Britton, and W. F. Bodmer, "The ABC of APC," *Human Molecular Genetics*, vol. 10, no. 7, pp. 721–733, 2001.

[245] D. R. Chesire, C. M. Ewing, J. Sauvageot, G. S. Bova, and W. B. Isaacs, "Detection and analysis of beta-catenin mutations in prostate cancer," *Prostate*, vol. 45, pp. 323–334, 2000.

[246] L. Richiardi, V. Fiano, L. Vizzini et al., "Promoter methylation in APC, RUNX3, and GSTP1 and mortality in prostate cancer patients," *Journal of Clinical Oncology*, vol. 27, no. 19, pp. 3161–3168, 2009.

[247] L. E. Pascal, R. Z. N. Vêncio, L. S. Page et al., "Gene expression relationship between prostate cancer cells of Gleason 3, 4 and normal epithelial cells as revealed by cell type-specific transcriptomes," *BMC Cancer*, vol. 9, article 452, 2009.

[248] C. M. Koh, C. J. Bieberich, C. V. Dang, W. G. Nelson, S. Yegnasubramanian, and A. M. De Marzo, "MYC and prostate cancer," *Genes and Cancer*, vol. 1, no. 6, pp. 617–628, 2010.

[249] J. P. Alao, "The regulation of cyclin D1 degradation: roles in cancer development and the potential for therapeutic invention," *Molecular Cancer*, vol. 6, article 24, 2007.

[250] T. Grigoryan, P. Wend, A. Klaus, and W. Birchmeier, "Deciphering the function of canonical Wnt signals in development and disease: conditional loss- and gain-of-function mutations of β-catenin in mice," *Genes and Development*, vol. 22, no. 17, pp. 2308–2341, 2008.

[251] C. L. Hall, A. Bafico, J. Dai, S. A. Aaronson, and E. T. Keller, "Prostate cancer cells promote osteoblastic bone metastases through Wnts," *Cancer Research*, vol. 65, no. 17, pp. 7554–7560, 2005.

[252] K. J. Bruxvoort, H. M. Charbonneau, T. A. Giambernardi et al., "Inactivation of Apc in the mouse prostate causes prostate carcinoma," *Cancer Research*, vol. 67, no. 6, pp. 2490–2496, 2007.

[253] P. Uysal-Onganer, Y. Kawano, M. Caro et al., "Wnt-11 promotes neuroendocrine-like differentiation, survival and migration of prostate cancer cells," *Molecular Cancer*, vol. 9, article 55, 2010.

[254] S. Gupta, K. Iljin, H. Sara et al., "FZD4 as a mediator of ERG oncogene-induced WNT signaling and epithelial-to-mesenchymal transition in human prostate cancer cells," *Cancer Research*, vol. 70, no. 17, pp. 6735–6745, 2010.

[255] M. A. Liss, M. Schlicht, A. Kahler et al., "Characterization of soy-based changes in Wnt-frizzled signaling in prostate cancer," *Cancer Genomics and Proteomics*, vol. 7, no. 5, pp. 245–252, 2010.

[256] D. R. Chesire and W. B. Isaacs, "β-Catenin signaling in prostate cancer: an early perspective," *Endocrine-Related Cancer*, vol. 10, no. 4, pp. 537–560, 2003.

[257] B. He, L. You, K. Uematsu et al., "A monoclonal antibody against Wnt-1 induces apoptosis in human cancer cells," *Neoplasia*, vol. 6, no. 1, pp. 7–14, 2004.

[258] G. W. Yardy and S. F. Brewster, "Wnt signalling and prostate cancer," *Prostate Cancer and Prostatic Diseases*, vol. 8, no. 2, pp. 119–126, 2005.

[259] S. Le Guellec, I. Soubeyran, P. Rochaix et al., "CTNNB1 mutation analysis is a useful tool for the diagnosis of desmoid tumors: a study of 260 desmoid tumors and 191 potential morphologic mimics," *Modern Pathology*, vol. 25, pp. 1551–1558, 2012.

[260] K. Willert, J. D. Brown, E. Danenberg et al., "Wnt proteins are lipid-modified and can act as stem cell growth factors," *Nature*, vol. 423, no. 6938, pp. 448–452, 2003.

[261] M. Sharma, W. W. Chuang, and Z. Sun, "Phosphatidylinositol 3-kinase/Akt stimulates androgen pathway through GSK3β inhibition and nuclear β-catenin accumulation," *Journal of Biological Chemistry*, vol. 277, no. 34, pp. 30935–30941, 2002.

[262] P. Polakis, "The many ways of Wnt in cancer," *Current Opinion in Genetics and Development*, vol. 17, no. 1, pp. 45–51, 2007.

[263] P. Wend, J. D. Holland, U. Ziebold, and W. Birchmeier, "Wnt signaling in stem and cancer stem cells," *Seminars in Cell and Developmental Biology*, vol. 21, no. 8, pp. 855–863, 2010.

[264] T. Reya, S. J. Morrison, M. F. Clarke, and I. L. Weissman, "Stem cells, cancer, and cancer stem cells," *Nature*, vol. 414, no. 6859, pp. 105–111, 2001.

[265] M. D. Castellone, H. Teramoto, B. O. Williams, K. M. Druey, and J. S. Gutkind, "Medicine: prostaglandin E2 promotes colon cancer cell growth through a Gs-axin-β-catenin signaling axis," *Science*, vol. 310, no. 5753, pp. 1504–1510, 2005.

[266] M. Lepourcelet, Y. N. P. Chen, D. S. France et al., "Small-molecule antagonists of the oncogenic Tcf/β-catenin protein complex," *Cancer Cell*, vol. 5, no. 1, pp. 91–102, 2004.

[267] J. P. Rey and D. L. Ellies, "Wnt modulators in the biotech pipeline," *Developmental Dynamics*, vol. 239, no. 1, pp. 102–114, 2010.

Assessment of the Performance of Magnetic Resonance Imaging/Ultrasound Fusion Guided Prostate Biopsy against a Combined Targeted Plus Systematic Biopsy Approach Using 24-Core Transperineal Template Saturation Mapping Prostate Biopsy

Francis Ting,[1,2] Pim J. Van Leeuwen,[1,2] James Thompson,[1,2,3] Ron Shnier,[4] Daniel Moses,[3,5] Warick Delprado,[6] and Phillip D. Stricker[1,2]

[1] *St. Vincent's Prostate Cancer Centre, Darlinghurst, NSW 2010, Australia*
[2] *Garvan Institute of Medical Research, The Kinghorn Cancer Centre, Darlinghurst, NSW 2010, Australia*
[3] *School of Medicine, University of New South Wales, Kensington, NSW 2052, Australia*
[4] *Southern Radiology, Randwick, NSW 2031, Australia*
[5] *Spectrum Radiology, Randwick, NSW 2031, Australia*
[6] *Douglas Hanly Moir Pathology, Macquarie Park, NSW 2113, Australia*

Correspondence should be addressed to Francis Ting; francisting@gmail.com

Academic Editor: Bruce J. Trock

Objective. To compare the performance of multiparametric resonance imaging/ultrasound fusion targeted biopsy (MRI/US-TBx) to a combined biopsy strategy (MRI/US-TBx plus 24-core transperineal template saturation mapping biopsy (TTMB)). *Methods.* Between May 2012 and October 2015, all patients undergoing MRI/US-TBx at our institution were included for analysis. Patients underwent MRI/US-TBx of suspicious lesions detected on multiparametric MRI +/− simultaneous TTMB. Subgroup analysis was performed on patients undergoing simultaneous MRI/US-TBx + TTMB. Primary outcome was PCa detection. Significant PCa was defined as ≥Gleason score (GS) 3 + 4 = 7 PCa. McNemar's test was used to compare detection rates between MRI/US-TBx and the combined biopsy strategy. *Results.* 148 patients underwent MRI/US-TBx and 80 patients underwent MRI/US-TBx + TTMB. In the MRI/US-TBx versus combined biopsy strategy subgroup analysis ($n = 80$), there were 55 PCa and 38 significant PCa. The detection rate for the combined biopsy strategy versus MRI/US-TBx for significant PCa was 49% versus 40% ($p = 0.02$) and for insignificant PCa was 20% versus 10% ($p = 0.04$), respectively. Eleven cases (14%) of significant PCa were detected exclusively on MRI/US-TBx and 7 cases (8.7%) of significant PCa were detected exclusively on TTMB. *Conclusions.* A combined biopsy approach (MRI/US-TBx + TTMB) detects more significant PCa than MRI/US-TBx alone; however, it will double the detection rate of insignificant PCa.

1. Introduction

The generally accepted diagnostic approach for prostate cancer (PCa) involves performing random biopsies based on abnormal digital rectal examination (DRE) and prostate specific antigen (PSA) levels. However, this approach is limited by the fact that a negative DRE does not necessarily exclude PCa [1, 2] and although the risk of high-grade PCa increases with PSA level, there is no serum PSA threshold that can completely exclude significant PCa [3]. The drawbacks of the random systematic, template-based sampling approach are the potential for missing significant PCa and over-sampling of insignificant PCa [4]. Furthermore, random biopsies underestimate tumour grade compared with radical prostatectomy (RP) 30–40% of the time [5, 6].

Targeted biopsy to suspicious lesions on multiparametric magnetic resonance imaging (mp-MRI) has emerged with the potential advantages of increased diagnostic accuracy and fewer cores. It allows the sensitivity and negative predictive value (NPV) of mp-MRI to be utilised with the real-time capabilities of transrectal ultrasound. There are a number of MRI-targeted biopsy methods, which include in-gantry/in-bore MRI guided biopsy, MRI/ultrasound fusion targeted biopsy (MRI/US-TBx), and cognitive guided biopsy. Much of the rapidly growing body of literature on MRI-targeted biopsy has compared MRI/US-TBx to 10–12 core transrectal ultrasound guided biopsy (TRUSGB) and systematic reviews and meta-analysis have concluded that MRI/US-TBx detects more significant PCa [7, 8] and less insignificant PCa [9] compared with TRUSGB.

In order to improve standardisation of the reporting and interpretation of this continually growing body of literature, the standards of reporting for MRI-targeted biopsy studies (START) of the prostate were published in 2013 [10], written by an international working group. In addition, the European Society of Urogenital Radiology (ESUR) published the PI-RADS scoring system [11] in order to standardise the interpretation and reporting of prostate mp-MRI, and subsequently this scoring system has been validated in both primary and repeat biopsy cohorts [12–15].

Recent studies have utilised transperineal template saturation mapping biopsy (TTMB) as a reference test [16–18] in evaluation of MRI/US-TBx given the limited sensitivity and concordance with prostatectomy specimens of standard 10–12 core TRUSGB [19]. The consensus has been that the gold standard for cancer detection in primary biopsy is a combination of systematic and targeted cores. Our study aims to build on the current body of evidence by comparing the performance of MRI/US-TBx to that of a combined biopsy strategy (TTMB + MRI/US-TBx) in a meaningful way by adhering to START and PI-RADS guidelines.

2. Methods

2.1. Patient Selection and Study Design. Between May 2012 and October 2015, all patients undergoing MRI/US-TBx aged >40 years, with abnormal PSA or DRE, were included for retrospective study analysis. Patients underwent mp-MRI to identify regions suspicious for PCa followed by MRI/US-TBx of suspicious lesions ± simultaneous 24-core TTMB. Indications for MRI/US-TBx included previous negative biopsy, region of interest (ROI) on mp-MRI <1.5 cm, or ROI located in an unusual location not included in a standard TTMB template. A subgroup analysis was performed on all patients undergoing simultaneous MRI/US-TBx and TTMB. Informed consent was obtained from all patients and data collection performed as part of an approval from our institutional Human Research Ethics Committee (SVH File Number 12/231).

2.2. Imaging Protocol. All mp-MRIs were performed at 2 centres. Centre 1 used a 1.5 Tesla magnet (b-value 0–800 s/mm^2) and Centre 2 used a 3 Tesla magnet (b-value 0–1500 s/mm^2). Mp-MRI was performed using a standard MRI protocol described in [13]. Previous analysis has shown that there is no significant difference in diagnostic performance between these two centres [13]. All mp-MRIs were supervised and reported by subspecialised uroradiologists with at least 12 years of experience in >3000 cases each (RS and DM) following the standardised 5-point Prostate Imaging Reporting and Data System (PI-RADS) scale. Regions of interest (ROIs) were assigned a score of 1 to 5 for each parameter (T2WI, DCEI, and DWI) and then based on these individual parameter scores an overall impression ROI score was given. MRI-derived ROIs were assigned to twenty-seven regions of each prostate according to the standardised prostate reporting scheme [20]. ROI size was measured as the maximal diameter as taken from axial slices on the mp-MRI.

2.3. Biopsy Methodology. TTMB and MRI/US-TBx were conducted by a single urologist (PS) who had full access to all mp-MRI data and was aware of the location of ROIs for both systematic and targeted biopsies. MRI/US-TBx was generally conducted first followed by TTMB.

2.3.1. TTMB. Transperineal, grid-directed template mapping biopsy was used as the reference test and was taken from 18 template locations using a modified Barzell technique [21]. A median of 24 cores were taken per patient and adjusted for volume with relative periurethral zone sparing.

2.3.2. MRI/US-TBx. MRI/transrectal ultrasound (TRUS) fusion biopsy was performed with a floor mounted, transperineal grid TRUS platform (BK Medical, Herlev, Denmark) combined with Biojet rigid MRI/TRUS fusion software (Meditron, Melbourne, Victoria, Australia). The biopsy operator had access to all mp-MRI data with radiologist marked ROIs in digital format. These ROIs were sampled under live MRI/TRUS fusion visualisation with at least 2 cores taken, adjusted for ROI size.

Targeted and systematic cores were labelled and reported separately by a single experienced uropathologist (WD).

2.4. Statistical Methods. Primary outcome was PCa detection (overall, significant, and insignificant). Significant PCa was defined as ≥Gleason score (GS) 3 + 4 = 7 PCa. Gleason scores were compared between MRI/US-TBx and TTMB. GS upgrading on MRI/US-TBx compared to TTMB was defined as significant when the change was from nil/insignificant PCa to significant PCa or from GS 3 + 4 = 7 to ≥GS 4 + 3 = 7.

McNemar's test was used to evaluate differences in detection rates of PCa between MRI/US-TBx, TTMB, and the combined biopsy strategy. Binary logistic multivariate regression analysis was used to assess the significance of ROI size in detection of significant PCa. Sensitivity, specificity, negative predictive value (NPV), and positive predictive value (PPV) of PI-RADS scoring system were calculated based on PI-RADS 1/2 being negative and PI-RADS 3–5 being positive, and the combined biopsy strategy was used as the gold standard. Statistical analyses were performed using SPSS® V21. A p value <0.05 was considered statistically significant.

TABLE 1: Baseline characteristics of MRI/US fusion targeted biopsy cohort.

	All patients (n = 148)	Patients with both MRI/US-TBx + TTMB (n = 80)
Age (median, IQR)	65 (60–70)	64 (59–69)
PSA (median, IQR)	5.0 (3.6–7.5)	5.2 (3.8–7.5)
Prostate volume (median, IQR)	44 (34–60)	42 (32–59)
Positive DRE, n (%)	23 (16%)	12 (15%)
Patients with previous biopsy, n (%)	55 (37%)	15 (19%)
Positive biopsy in the past, n (%)	24 (16%)	8 (10%)
Negative biopsy in the past, n (%)	34 (23%)	7 (9%)
ROI size in mm	7 (5–10)	7 (5–10)
Number of cores taken per location (Median, IQR)	4 (3–5)	4 (3-4)

IQR = interquartile range, n = number, mm = millimetres, MRI/US-TBx = MRI/transrectal ultrasound fusion targeted biopsy, and TTMB = transperineal template guided mapping biopsy.

TABLE 2: PI-RADS score and cancer detection rates (n = 148).

PI-RADS	Frequency	MRI-fusion biopsy	
		All PCa	Sig PCa
1/2*	28	4 (14%)	2 (7%)
3	80	30 (38%)	17 (21%)
4	55	38 (69%)	33 (60%)
5	22	20 (91%)	18 (82%)
Total	185	92	70

PCa = prostate cancer, Sig = significant.
*Due to clinical reasons these patients with PI-RADS 1/2 ROIs underwent targeted biopsy.

TABLE 3: Detection rate MRI/US fusion targeted biopsy by size of ROI (n = 148).

Lesion size	Freq.	Any PCa	Sign PCa
		MRI/US Fusion targeted biopsy	
<5 mm	22	11 (50%)	7 (32%)
5–9 mm	93	39 (42%)	26 (28%)
≥10 mm	45	28 (62%)	25 (56%)

Freq. = frequency, PCa = prostate cancer, Sign = significant, and ROI = region of interest.

3. Results

3.1. MRI/US-TBx Patient Cohort. Demographic and baseline characteristics of the 148 included patients can be found in Table 1. Of these 148 patients, 93 (63%) were undergoing primary biopsy and 55 (37%) were undergoing repeat biopsy with 24 (16%) patients having a previous positive biopsy. 185 ROIs were targeted in these 148 men. There were 28 (15%) lesions scored as PI-RADS 1 or 2, 80 (43%) as PI-RADS 3, 55 (30%) as PI-RADS 4 and 22 (12%) as PI-RADS 5 (Table 2). An increasing PI-RADS score correlated with an increasing PCa detection rate with the detection rate of significant PCa ranging from 7% for PI-RADS 1/2 ROIs up to 82% for PI-RADS 5 ROIs. Overall, there were 92 cancers detected with 22 (24%) of these being GS 3 + 3 = 6 and 70 (76%) of these being GS 3 + 4 = 7 or greater.

ROI size data is displayed in Table 3. For ROIs <10 mm, the detection rate of significant PCa on MRI/US-TBx was 29% versus 56% for ROIs 10 mm or greater. Overall detection rate of PCa on MRI/US-TBx was 43% versus 62% for ROIs <10 mm versus ROIs 10 mm or greater, respectively. On multivariate analysis including age, PSA, DRE, primary versus repeat biopsy, prostate volume and PI-RADS score, ROI size was not significant (p = 0.09) but increasing age (p = 0.001) and PI-RADS score ≥4 (p = 0.02) were predictive in detection of significant PCa.

3.2. Comparison of Cancer Detection Performance: MRI/US-TBx versus Combined Biopsy Strategy. Eighty patients underwent both MRI-TBx and TTMB simultaneously. In this subgroup analysis, 65 (81%) patients underwent primary biopsy and 15 (19%) underwent repeat biopsy. Baseline characteristics of this subgroup can be found in Table 1.

There were 55 (69%) patients diagnosed with PCa and 38 (45%) of these were significant PCa. The detection rate of significant PCa for MRI/US-TBx and combined biopsy strategy was 40% versus 49% (p = 0.02) and the detection rate of insignificant PCa for MRI/US-TBx and combined biopsy strategy was 10% versus 20% (p = 0.04), respectively (Table 4). The proportion of detected cancers being significant for each biopsy technique was 32/40 (80%) for MRI/US-TBx and 39/55 (71%) for combined biopsy strategy (Table 4). Gleason score distribution for different biopsy techniques is displayed in Table 5.

Sixteen (20%) patients had a GS upgrade on combined biopsy strategy compared to their MRI/US-TBx with seven (9%) being significant upgrades. These missed cases are described in Table 6. All cancers were Gleason 3 + 4 = 7 PCa with a maximum of 15% Gleason 4. In addition, the location of the significant cancers detected on TTMB but missed on MRI/US-TBx did not correlate to the location of the ROI on mp-MRI in five of these seven cases.

Sensitivity and negative predictive value (NPV) of PI-RADS (when considering PI-RADS 1-2 negative, PI-RADS 3–5 positive) for detection of significant PCa were 98% and 92%,

TABLE 4: Detection rates for significant and insignificant prostate cancer of MRI/ultrasound fusion targeted biopsy versus transperineal template saturation mapping biopsy (n = 80).

	MRI/US-TBx	TTMB	p value (MRI versus TTMB)	CBS	p value (MRI versus CBS)
Any prostate cancer, n (%)	40 (50%)	48 (60%)	0.13	55 (69%)	<0.01
Significant prostate cancer, n (%)	32 (40%)	28 (35%)	0.48	39 (49%)	0.02
Insignificant prostate cancer, n (%)	8 (10%)	20 (25%)	0.01	16 (20%)	0.04

MRI/US-TBx = MRI/transrectal ultrasound fusion targeted biopsy, TTMB = transperineal template guided mapping biopsy, CBS = combined biopsy strategy (MRI/US-TBx + TTMB), and n = number.

TABLE 5: Gleason score breakdown for MRI/US-TBx and TTMB (n = 80).

Gleason score	MRI/US-TBx	TTMB	CBS	p value (MRI/US-TBx versus CBS)
No cancer	40 (50%)	32 (40%)	25 (31%)	
3 + 3	8 (10%)	20 (25%)	16 (20%)	
3 + 4	18 (22.5%)	24 (30%)	25 (31%)	
4 + 3	7 (9%)	3 (4%)	7 (9%)	
4 + 4	4 (5%)	1 (1%)	4 (5%)	
4 + 5	2 (2.5%)	0	2 (2.5%)	
5 + 4	1 (1%)	0	1 (1.5%)	
Total	80	80	80	
Low risk	8 (10%)	20 (25%)	16 (20%)	0.04
Int. risk	25 (31%)	27 (34%)	32 (40%)	0.02
High risk	7 (9%)	1 (1%)	7 (9%)	Not sig

CBS = combined biopsy strategy, MRI/US-TBx = MRI/transrectal ultrasound fusion targeted biopsy, and TTMB = transperineal template guided mapping biopsy.
Low risk = GS 6, intermediate risk = GS 7, and high risk = GS 8 or greater.

respectively (Table 7). The PPV of PI-RADS for detection of significant PCa when considering PI-RADS ≥3, ≥4, and 5 as positive was 56%, 74%, and 100%, respectively.

3.3. Comparison of Cancer Detection Performance: MRI/US-TBx versus TTMB. Median number of cores taken per patient was 24 (IQR 21–29) for TTMB and 4 (IQR 3-4) for MRI/US-TBx. Sampling efficiency was in favour of MRI/US-TBx with 20% of MRI/US-TBx versus 8% of TTMB cores detecting significant PCa.

The detection rate of significant PCa for MRI/US-TBx and TTMB was 40% versus 35% (p = 0.48) and the detection rate of insignificant PCa for MRI/US-TBx and TTMB was 10% versus 25% (p = 0.01).

Twenty patients (25%) had a GS upgrade on MRI/US-TBx compared to their TTMB with 15 (19%) being significant upgrades. Eleven cases of significant PCa were detected exclusively on MRI/US-TBx and 7 cases of significant PCa (all Gleason 3 + 4 = 7 with ≤15% Gleason 4) were detected exclusively on TTMB.

4. Discussion

Our results show that a biopsy strategy combining TTMB with MRI/US-TBx can increase the detection rate of significant PCa when compared to MRI/US-TBx alone; however this combined biopsy strategy also doubled the detection of insignificant PCa when compared to MRI/US-TBx alone. This is in line with recent data from a direct prospective comparison between MRI/US-TBx and TTMB which has shown that MRI/US-TBx can detect as many GS 7 or greater tumours while simultaneously avoiding the detection of 44% of lower grade disease [17]. Another series (n = 50) comparing both cognitive and software based MRI registration to TTMB has shown slightly lower rates of significant disease detection (68% for software based fusion versus 76% for TTMB) [18], and similarly, in another series (n = 437) more significant PCa was found exclusively in TTMB than exclusively in MRI/US-TBx (52 versus 18 cases) [16]. Thus, if the aim is purely to maximise the detection of significant PCa the combination of TTMB with MRI/US-TBx still appears to be the most effective biopsy strategy at present. However, in the current series it should be noted that all additional significant cancers detected by the addition of TTMB to the MRI/US-TBx biopsy strategy were GS 3 + 4 = 7 with a maximum GS 4 component of 15%. Given the slow natural history and high 10-year PCa specific survival of GS 3+4 PCa [22], a delayed diagnosis in the course of careful follow-up is unlikely to have resulted in missing the window of curability.

TRUSGB can miss 20–30% of clinically significant cancers due to undersampling, particularly in the anteroapical region of the prostate [23]. MRI/US-TBx overcomes this deficiency by sampling the suspicious region and thus is likely to be more effective than TRUSB in the detection of significant PCa. Accordingly, observational trials have shown that MRI/US-TBx has a higher detection rate for clinically significant cancer [24–26], a higher detection rate for high-risk PCa [27], and a lower sensitivity for clinically

Table 6: Missed cancers (cancers detected on TTMB but missed on MRI targeted biopsy: significant upgrades only).

TTMB data		MRI/US fusion targeted biopsy data				
GS (% Gleason 4)	Location of cancer	GS	Location of ROI	MRI ROI location correlates to TTMB	ROI size (mm)	PI-RAD score
3 + 4 (15%)	L ant	0	L base post	No	7	2
3 + 4 (5%)	R mid post	0	L post apex	No	4	3
3 + 4 (10%)	L post apex	0	Midline post	No	11	3
3 + 4 (10%)	R base PL + R ant	0	R mid apex	No	5	3
3 + 4 (10%)	R base PL	3 + 3	R base peripheral zone	Partial	12	3
3 + 4 (2%)	L ant apex, R mid PL, L mid PL	3 + 3	L post apex	Partial	9	4
3 + 4 (5%)	R base PL	0	L base	No	2	5

MRI/US-TBx = MRI/transrectal ultrasound fusion targeted biopsy, TTMB = transperineal template guided mapping biopsy, ROI = region of interest, L = left, R = right, ant = anterior, post = posterior, and PL = posterolateral.

Table 7: Sensitivity, specificity, NPV, and PPV of PI-RADS scoring system for prostate cancer detection, derived from combined biopsy strategy (MRI/US-TBx + TTMB). For this analysis PI-RADS 1/2 is considered negative and PI-RADS 3–5 is considered positive. N = 80.

	All PCa	Sign PCa	Insig PCa
Sensitivity	96	98	91
Specificity	32	22	13
NPV	75	92	83
PPV	78	56	23

PCa = prostate cancer, Sign = significant, Insig = insignificant, NPV = negative predictive value, and PPV = positive predictive value.

insignificant cancer compared to TRUSGB (0.51 versus 0.81, resp.) [9]. In addition, MRI/US-TBx has been shown to be able to detect as many GS ≥7 PCa compared to TTMB [17]. In the current series, we demonstrated a detection rate of MRI/US-TBx for significant PCa of 40%. A number of significant cancers were missed by MRI/US-TBx but the majority of these were outside of the ROI targeted on mp-MRI, which indicates that MRI/US-TBx is still a procedurally valid technique in our centre.

4.1. Magnetic Resonance Imaging Targeted Biopsy Can Reduce PCa Overdiagnosis. The disadvantage of using TTMB alone is the increased detection of insignificant PCa, with rates of insignificant PCa detection for TTMB of up to 25% being reported [28–30], which is consistent with the 25% rate of insignificant PCa detection by TTMB in the current series. Compared to this, MRI/US-TBx alone in the current series had a 10% detection rate of insignificant PCa and thus a future biopsy approach that replaces TTMB with MRI/US-TBx will significantly reduce the overdiagnosis of insignificant PCa.

4.2. Validation of the PI-RADS Scoring System. A PI-RADS score of 1/2 appeared to be effective in ruling out most cases of significant PCa and a PI-RADS score of 4/5 was able to predict prostate cancer; the data we present further validates the current data on the predictive information that is provided by PI-RADS scoring in prostate mp-MRI [14, 15]. In patients with PI-RADS 3 “equivocal” ROIs there were a significant proportion (21%) of patients with significant PCas, and comparable rates of significant PCa (26–29%) [13, 14] in PI-RADS 3 ROIs have been reported which supports the rationale of performing MRI-TBx on all patients with PI-RADS 3–5 lesions on mp-MRI.

Centres of excellence have reported sensitivity of 86–96% [13, 14, 31–34], and NPV of 90–92% [14, 33, 35] for mp-MRI in detection of significant PCa. Our reported sensitivity and NPV of 98% and 92%, respectively, is similar to these results and suggests the possibility of avoiding random biopsy in patients with negative mp-MRI, provided that standards are established for accreditation, training, and reporting of mp-MRI. Lower sensitivities of 58–76% [36, 37] and NPV of 79–89% [36, 37] have been reported in smaller series and this interstudy variability can be part-attributed to the significant learning curve associated with interpretation of prostate mp-MRI of about 100 cases [38, 39]. However, interstudy variability of NPV is also influenced by the overall prevalence of cancer and needs to be taken into account when comparing studies.

4.3. Limitations. Firstly, the primary operator was not blinded to the ROI when performing random biopsies and therefore an accurate direct comparison between TTMB and MRI/US-TBx alone is not possible from this study given this confounding factor. However, we are still able to draw an accurate comparison between MRI/US-TBx versus the combined biopsy strategy, which gives this study clinical utility. Secondly, this study was retrospective in nature but as noted above we have strict, standardised mp-MRI and biopsy protocols in place. Thirdly, longer follow-up is required, particularly in the biopsy negative patients and our operator and radiologists were not blinded to radiological or clinical data as per routine clinical practice. Fourthly, there are inherent limitations in using biopsy as the reference test: MRI/US-TBx could have missed MRI targets despite software registration [40] and there is a percentage of upgrading that occurs on radical prostatectomy. However in this cohort using radical prostatectomy as the reference test was not feasible due to ethical issues and positive selection bias. Finally, the binary logistic regression analysis performed to assess significance of ROI size in detection of significant PCa was performed on a per-lesion rather than a per-patient basis. Some patients had multiple ROIs/lesions and the ensuing correlation effect was not accounted for with a mixed model analysis, which resulted in the p values being more significant than they should be. However, this does not change the interpretation of nonsignificance for ROI size in detection of significant PCa.

4.4. Strengths. One of the main strengths of this study was the use of TTMB as a reference test. TTMB was used as it has been demonstrated as a robust reference test [13, 41], localises the index lesion [42] in most men with clinically significant disease [25], and detects more clinically significant cancer than 12-core TRUSGB [28]. Furthermore, another series demonstrated that in a significant proportion of men initially diagnosed with apparently low-risk disease on TRUSGB, subsequent TTMB revealed clinically significant PCa requiring more aggressive therapy [43]. Radical prostatectomy (RP), although the pathology gold standard reference test, could not be utilised in this study due to ethical considerations and positive selection bias.

5. Conclusion

A combined biopsy approach (MRI/US-TBx + TTMB) detects more significant PCa than MRI/US-TBx alone; however it will double the detection rate of insignificant PCa. MRI/US-TBx is the likely future of PCa diagnosis and in centres of excellence is a robust and valid technique. It has the potential to increase the specificity of PCa detection and reduce overdiagnosis of insignificant PCa. However, further prospective trials with longer follow-up are required, particularly for biopsy negative cases.

Competing Interests

The authors declare that they have no competing interests.

Acknowledgments

Anne-Maree Haynes and Quoc Nguyen from Australian Prostate Cancer Research Centre-NSW (APCRC-NSW), IT Applications Group, and CANSTO Database are gratefully acknowledged. This research is supported by the Department of Health and Ageing for its funding of the Australian Prostate Cancer Research Centre-NSW, the National Health and Medical Research Council, St. Vincent's Prostate Cancer Centre, and the RT Hall Trust.

References

[1] C. Gosselaar, R. Kranse, M. J. Roobol, S. Roemeling, and F. H. Schröder, "The interobserver variability of digital rectal examination in a large randomized trial for the screening of prostate cancer," *Prostate*, vol. 68, no. 9, pp. 985–993, 2008.

[2] F. H. Schroder, P. van der Maas, P. Beemsterboer, A. B. Kruger, R. Hoedemaeker, J. Rietbergen et al., "Evaluation of the digital rectal examination as a screening test for prostate cancer. Rotterdam section of the European Randomized Study of Screening for Prostate Cancer," *Journal of the National Cancer Institute*, vol. 90, no. 23, pp. 1817–1823, 1998.

[3] I. M. Thompson, D. P. Ankerst, C. Chi et al., "Operating characteristics of prostate-specific antigen in men with an initial PSA level of 3.0 ng/mL or lower," *The Journal of the American Medical Association*, vol. 294, no. 1, pp. 66–70, 2005.

[4] O. Ukimura, J. A. Coleman, A. de la Taille et al., "Contemporary role of systematic prostate biopsies: Indications, techniques, and implications for patient care," *European Urology*, vol. 63, no. 2, pp. 214–230, 2013.

[5] A. V. D'Amico, A. A. Renshaw, L. Arsenault, D. Schultz, and J. P. Richie, "Clinical predictors of upgrading to gleason grade 4 or 5 disease at radical prostatectomy: potential implications for patient selection for radiation and androgen suppression therapy," *International Journal of Radiation Oncology, Biology, Physics*, vol. 45, no. 4, pp. 841–846, 1999.

[6] S. Scott, H. Samaratunga, C. Chabert, M. Breckenridge, and T. Gianduzzo, "Is transperineal prostate biopsy more accurate than transrectal biopsy in determining final Gleason score and clinical risk category? A comparative analysis," *BJU International*, vol. 116, supplement 3, pp. 26–30, 2015.

[7] M. Valerio, I. Donaldson, M. Emberton et al., "Detection of clinically significant prostate cancer using magnetic resonance imaging-ultrasound fusion targeted biopsy: a systematic review," *European Urology*, vol. 68, no. 1, pp. 8–19, 2015.

[8] J. Wu, A. Ji, B. Xie et al., "Is magnetic resonance/ultrasound fusion prostate biopsy better than systematic prostate biopsy? An updated meta- and trial sequential analysis," *Oncotarget*, vol. 6, no. 41, pp. 43571–43580, 2015.

[9] I. G. Schoots, M. J. Roobol, D. Nieboer, C. H. Bangma, E. W. Steyerberg, and M. G. M. Hunink, "Magnetic resonance imaging-targeted biopsy may enhance the diagnostic accuracy of significant prostate cancer detection compared to standard transrectal ultrasound-guided biopsy: a systematic review and meta-analysis," *European Urology*, vol. 68, no. 3, pp. 438–450, 2015.

[10] C. M. Moore, V. Kasivisvanathan, S. Eggener et al., "Standards of reporting for MRI-targeted biopsy studies (START) of the prostate: recommendations from an international working group," *European Urology*, vol. 64, no. 4, pp. 544–552, 2013.

[11] J. C. Weinreb, J. O. Barentsz, P. L. Choyke et al., "Pi-rads prostate imaging—reporting and data system: 2015, version 2," *European Urology*, vol. 69, no. 1, pp. 16–40, 2015.

[12] H. Cash, A. Maxeiner, C. Stephan et al., "The detection of significant prostate cancer is correlated with the Prostate Imaging Reporting and Data System (PI-RADS) in MRI/transrectal ultrasound fusion biopsy," *World Journal of Urology*, vol. 34, no. 4, pp. 525–532, 2016.

[13] J. E. Thompson, D. Moses, R. Shnier et al., "Multiparametric magnetic resonance imaging guided diagnostic biopsy detects significant prostate cancer and could reduce unnecessary biopsies and over detection: a prospective study," *The Journal of Urology*, vol. 192, no. 1, pp. 67–74, 2014.

[14] J. E. Thompson, P. J. van Leeuwen, D. Moses et al., "The diagnostic performance of multiparametric magnetic resonance imaging to detect significant prostate cancer," *The Journal of Urology*, 2015.

[15] D. Portalez, P. Mozer, F. Cornud et al., "Validation of the European Society of Urogenital Radiology scoring system for prostate cancer diagnosis on multiparametric magnetic resonance imaging in a cohort of repeat biopsy patients," *European Urology*, vol. 62, no. 6, pp. 986–996, 2012.

[16] F. Distler, J. P. Radtke, C. Kesch et al., "Value of MRI/ultrasound fusion in primary biopsy for the diagnosis of prostate cancer," *Der Urologe*, vol. 55, no. 2, pp. 146–155, 2016.

[17] J. P. Radtke, T. H. Kuru, S. Boxler et al., "Comparative Analysis of transperineal template saturation prostate biopsy versus magnetic resonance imaging targeted biopsy with magnetic resonance imaging-ultrasound fusion guidance," *The Journal of Urology*, vol. 193, no. 1, pp. 87–94, 2015.

[18] M. Valerio, N. McCartan, A. Freeman, S. Punwani, M. Emberton, and H. U. Ahmed, "Visually directed vs. software-based targeted biopsy compared to transperineal template mapping biopsy in the detection of clinically significant prostate cancer," *Urologic Oncology*, vol. 33, no. 10, pp. 424.e9–424.e16, 2015.

[19] M. A. Bjurlin, H. B. Carter, P. Schellhammer et al., "Optimization of initial prostate biopsy in clinical practice: sampling, labeling and specimen processing," *The Journal of Urology*, vol. 189, no. 6, pp. 2039–2046, 2013.

[20] L. Dickinson, H. U. Ahmed, C. Allen et al., "Magnetic resonance imaging for the detection, localisation, and characterisation of prostate cancer: recommendations from a European consensus meeting," *European Urology*, vol. 59, no. 4, pp. 477–494, 2011.

[21] W. Barzell WIW and G. Andriole, *Transperineal Template Guided Saturation Biopsy of the Prostate: Rationale, Indications and Technique. Urology Times*, vol. 31, Andriole G. Transperineal Template Guided Saturation Biopsy of the Prostate, Rationale, 2003.

[22] J. L. Wright, C. A. Salinas, D. W. Lin et al., "Prostate cancer specific mortality and gleason 7 disease differences in prostate cancer outcomes between cases with gleason 4 + 3 and gleason 3 + 4 tumors in a population based cohort," *The Journal of Urology*, vol. 182, no. 6, pp. 2702–2707, 2009.

[23] B. Gershman, A. L. Zietman, A. S. Feldman, and W. S. McDougal, "Transperineal template-guided prostate biopsy for patients with persistently elevated PSA and multiple prior negative biopsies," *Urologic Oncology: Seminars and Original Investigations*, vol. 31, no. 7, pp. 1093–1097, 2013.

[24] P. Mozer, M. Rouprêt, C. Le Cossec et al., "First round of targeted biopsies using magnetic resonance imaging/ultrasonography fusion compared with conventional transrectal ultrasonography-guided biopsies for the diagnosis of localised prostate cancer," *BJU International*, vol. 115, no. 1, pp. 50–57, 2014.

[25] A. R. Rastinehad, B. Turkbey, S. S. Salami et al., "Improving detection of clinically significant prostate cancer: magnetic resonance imaging/transrectal ultrasound fusion guided prostate biopsy," *The Journal of Urology*, vol. 191, no. 6, pp. 1749–1754, 2014.

[26] M. M. Siddiqui, S. Rais-Bahrami, H. Truong et al., "Magnetic resonance imaging/ultrasound-fusion biopsy significantly upgrades prostate cancer versus systematic 12-core transrectal ultrasound biopsy," *European Urology*, vol. 64, no. 5, pp. 713–719, 2013.

[27] M. M. Siddiqui, S. Rais-Bahrami, B. Turkbey et al., "Comparison of MR/ultrasound fusion-guided biopsy with ultrasound-guided biopsy for the diagnosis of prostate cancer," *The Journal of the American Medical Association*, vol. 313, no. 4, pp. 390–397, 2015.

[28] N. Bittner, G. S. Merrick, A. Bennett et al., "Diagnostic performance of initial transperineal template-guided mapping biopsy of the prostate gland," *American Journal of Clinical Oncology*, vol. 38, no. 3, pp. 300–303, 2015.

[29] T. Klatte, N. Swietek, G. Schatzl, and M. Waldert, "Transperineal template-guided biopsy for diagnosis of prostate cancer in patients with at least two prior negative biopsies," *Wiener Klinische Wochenschrift*, vol. 125, no. 21-22, pp. 669–673, 2013.

[30] N. Bittner, G. S. Merrick, W. M. Butler, A. Bennett, and R. W. Galbreath, "Incidence and pathological features of prostate cancer detected on transperineal template guided mapping biopsy after negative transrectal ultrasound guided biopsy," *The Journal of Urology*, vol. 190, no. 2, pp. 509–514, 2013.

[31] M. Abd-Alazeez, A. Kirkham, H. U. Ahmed et al., "Performance of multiparametric MRI in men at risk of prostate cancer before the first biopsy: a paired validating cohort study using template prostate mapping biopsies as the reference standard," *Prostate Cancer and Prostatic Diseases*, vol. 17, no. 1, pp. 40–46, 2014.

[32] K. Chamie, G. A. Sonn, D. S. Finley et al., "The role of magnetic resonance imaging in delineating clinically significant prostate cancer," *Urology*, vol. 83, no. 2, pp. 369–375, 2014.

[33] S. Rais-Bahrami, M. M. Siddiqui, B. Turkbey et al., "Utility of multiparametric magnetic resonance imaging suspicion levels for detecting prostate cancer," *The Journal of Urology*, vol. 190, no. 5, pp. 1721–1727, 2013.

[34] P. Rouse, G. Shaw, H. U. Ahmed, A. Freeman, C. Allen, and M. Emberton, "Multi-parametric magnetic resonance imaging to rule-in and rule-out clinically important prostate cancer in men at risk: a cohort study," *Urologia Internationalis*, vol. 87, no. 1, pp. 49–53, 2011.

[35] P. J. De Visschere, L. Naesens, L. Libbrecht et al., "What kind of prostate cancers do we miss on multiparametric magnetic resonance imaging?" *European Radiology*, vol. 26, no. 4, pp. 1098–1107, 2015.

[36] N. Arumainayagam, H. U. Ahmed, C. M. Moore et al., "Multiparametric MR imaging for detection of clinically significant prostate cancer: a validation cohort study with transperineal template prostate mapping as the reference standard," *Radiology*, vol. 268, no. 3, pp. 761–769, 2013.

[37] M. Abd-Alazeez, H. U. Ahmed, M. Arya et al., "The accuracy of multiparametric MRI in men with negative biopsy and elevated PSA level-can it rule out clinically significant prostate cancer?" *Urologic Oncology: Seminars and Original Investigations*, vol. 32, no. 1, pp. 45–e22, 2014.

[38] K. C. Latchamsetty, L. S. Borden Jr., C. R. Porter et al., "Experience improves staging accuracy of endorectal magnetic resonance imaging in prostate cancer: what is the learning curve?" *The Canadian Journal of Urology*, vol. 14, no. 1, pp. 3429–3434, 2007.

[39] O. Akin, C. C. Riedl, N. M. Ishill, C. S. Moskowitz, J. Zhang, and H. Hricak, "Interactive dedicated training curriculum improves accuracy in the interpretation of MR imaging of prostate cancer," *European Radiology*, vol. 20, no. 4, pp. 995–1002, 2010.

[40] H. Cash, K. Günzel, A. Maxeiner et al., "Prostate cancer detection on transrectal ultrasonography-guided random biopsy despite negative real-time magnetic resonance imaging/ultrasonography fusion-guided targeted biopsy: reasons for targeted biopsy failure," *BJU International*, 2015.

[41] G. Ploussard, N. Nicolaiew, C. Marchand et al., "Prospective evaluation of an extended 21-core biopsy scheme as initial prostate cancer diagnostic strategy," *European Urology*, vol. 65, no. 1, pp. 154–161, 2014.

[42] M. Valerio, C. Anele, A. Freeman et al., "Identifying the index lesion with template prostate mapping biopsies," *The Journal of Urology*, vol. 193, no. 4, pp. 1185–1190, 2015.

[43] A. B. Barqawi, K. O. Rove, S. Gholizadeh, C. I. O'Donnell, H. Koul, and E. D. Crawford, "The role of 3-dimensional mapping biopsy in decision making for treatment of apparent early stage prostate cancer," *The Journal of Urology*, vol. 186, no. 1, pp. 80–85, 2011.

21

Prostate Cancer: Epigenetic Alterations, Risk Factors, and Therapy

Mankgopo M. Kgatle,[1] Asgar A. Kalla,[2] Muhammed M. Islam,[3] Mike Sathekge,[4] and Razia Moorad[5]

[1]*Division of Hepatology and Liver Research, Department of Medicine, Faculty of Health Sciences, University of Cape Town and Groote Schuur Hospital, Observatory, Western Cape 7925, South Africa*
[2]*Division of Rheumatology, Department of Medicine, Faculty of Health Sciences, University of Cape Town and Groote Schuur Hospital, Observatory, Western Cape 7925, South Africa*
[3]*Department of Integrative Biomedical Sciences, Institute of Infectious Disease and Molecular Medicine, Faculty of Health Sciences, University of Cape Town, Observatory, Western Cape 7925, South Africa*
[4]*Department of Nuclear Medicine, University of Pretoria and Steve Biko Academic Hospital, Private Bag X169, Pretoria, Gauteng 0001, South Africa*
[5]*Department of Surgery, Faculty of Health Science, University of Cape Town and Groote Schuur Hospital, Observatory, Western Cape 7925, South Africa*

Correspondence should be addressed to Mankgopo M. Kgatle; mankgopo.kgatle@gmail.com

Academic Editor: Cristina Magi-Galluzzi

Prostate cancer (PCa) is the most prevalent urological cancer that affects aging men in South Africa, and mechanisms underlying prostate tumorigenesis remain elusive. Research advancements in the field of PCa and epigenetics have allowed for the identification of specific alterations that occur beyond genetics but are still critically important in the pathogenesis of tumorigenesis. Anomalous epigenetic changes associated with PCa include histone modifications, DNA methylation, and noncoding miRNA. These mechanisms regulate and silence hundreds of target genes including some which are key components of cellular signalling pathways that, when perturbed, promote tumorigenesis. Elucidation of mechanisms underlying epigenetic alterations and the manner in which these mechanisms interact in regulating gene transcription in PCa are an unmet necessity that may lead to novel chemotherapeutic approaches. This will, therefore, aid in developing combination therapies that will target multiple epigenetic pathways, which can be used in conjunction with the current conventional PCa treatment.

1. Introduction

According to the World Cancer Research Fund's list, South Africa is ranked 50th among countries with the highest cancer prevalence [1]. Recent article published in Lancet projected cancer to become a leading cause of deaths in South Africa, with an increase from 77 400 cases in 2008 to 112 921 new cases in 2030 [2]. Prostate cancer (PCa) is the most prevalent urological cancer and one of the four top cancers including Kaposi sarcoma and colorectal and lung cancers, which affect aging men in South Africa [2]. It is estimated that 1 in 8 South African aging men will develop PCa at some point in their lifetime. The most common type of PCa is acinar adenocarcinoma, representing 90% of the PCa cases [3].

Prostate is a walnut sized organ located just between the bladder and penis, and it slowly grows larger to an average weight of 40 grams in aging men. A prostate gland surrounds the urethra that empties urine from the bladder and also secretes prostate fluid that protects sperm. These physiological functions may be compromised during various prostate diseases including prostatitis, benign prostatic hyperplasia or hypertrophy, and cancer. PCa begins when aberrant semen-secreting prostate gland cells develop and proliferate uncontrollably. If left untreated, PCa may metastasise to other parts of the body, particularly to the lymph nodes and bones. Although most patients may remain asymptomatic in the early stages, advanced PCa may be accompanied by a variety of urinary symptoms including troublesome nocturia, dysuria, hematuria, hematospermia, pain and swelling in the legs and pelvic area, loss of bladder, and erection control. On the other hand, benign prostatic hyperplasia or hypertrophy may show similar symptoms but is rarely life-threatening. In this case, the use of total plasma prostate specific antigen (tPSA) level becomes important. According to ASC, a tPSA level of more than the cut-off value of 4 ng/mL may indicate the occurrence of PCa [4]. To overrule the possibility of an elevated tPSA level in a subset in nonmalignant conditions, transrectal biopsy guided by ultrasound can be used to validate the diagnosis [4, 5].

Owing to its slow growth, PCa may take up to 10 years to progress from precursor prostatic intraepithelial neoplasia (PIN) to an invasive carcinoma. Histologically, PIN can be classified into low and high grade, which are generally characterised by various molecular or cellular architecture [6]. The Gleason grading system developed by Dr. Donald F. Gleason between 1966 and 1974 and recently reviewed and improved by the 2014 International Society of Urological Pathology remains one of the most powerful predictors for the prognostic outcome of PCa. An alternative to the current Gleason score was recently proposed with the potential to lessen the overtreatment of low-grade PCa detected by PSA screening. The new simplified PCa grading incorporates five grades, and these include grade group 1 (Gleason score ≤ 6), grade group 2 (Gleason score $3 + 4 = 7$), grade group 3 (Gleason score $4 + 3 = 7$), grade group 4 (Gleason score 8), and finally grade group 5 (Gleason score 9-10) [7].

PCa is a heterogeneous disease, and its occurrence differs extremely from patient to patient even within the same tumour. The great disparity in the PCa architecture and incidence rates may be attributable to genomic instabilities and alterations associated with various PCa risk factors. Therefore, this review aims to provide a comprehensive understanding of the prostate carcinogenesis-related epigenetic signatures and their mediators. In addition, the associated PCa risk factors and recent treatment options are discussed.

2. Current Prostate Cancer Treatment

Depending on the severity of the disease, current therapies for PCa may include watchful waiting, hormone therapy, therapeutic vaccines, bone-directed treatment, cryotherapy, radiation therapy, and surgery. Although these treatment options may improve the quality of life of patients by significantly delaying or inhibiting the progression of the disease, chemotherapeutic resistance commonly develops often resulting in death [8, 9]. In addition, an estimated 30% of patients relapse following the initial treatment. The 5-year survival rate for the localised and regional PCa is nearly 100%; however, this percentage drops to 28% in cases where cancer has metastasised to distant organs [9, 10].

Two recently approved hormone therapy agents, the AR antagonist enzalutamide and the CYP17A1-inhibitor abiraterone, have proven to be well tolerated and effective in many metastasised castration-resistant PCa patients [11]. Nonetheless, these therapy agents remain noncurative, suggesting an urgent need of novel systemic treatment that can improve the overall survival of PCa patients. This encouraged the development of novel therapeutic approaches such as the prostate specific membrane antigen-targeted radioligand therapy (PSMA-RLT) [12]. PSMA-RLT allows the delivery of high dose of therapeutic radiation to cancer cells, while lessening the exposure of normal cells. PSMA, also known as folate hydrolase I or glutamate carboxypeptidase II, is a cell surface protein that is significantly overexpressed in refractory or metastasised castration-resistant PCa cells. The PSMA-RLT involves binding of a ligand PSMA to a radioactive isotope Lu-177, and this facilitates the detection of metastatic sites for treatment as illustrated in Figure 1. The widely used radiopharmaceutical is ^{177}Lu-PSMA. The radionuclide is transported directly to the tumour cells and radioactive decay of ^{177}Lu emits beta particles, which are absorbed by the disease targeted sites thereby damaging the surrounding PCa cells [13, 14]. PSMA-RLT with ^{177}Lu-PSMA holds a great promise to be a magic bullet for patients with metastasised castration-resistant PCa with appropriate selection and follow-up by ^{68}Ga-PSMA PET/CT as it follows a theranostic approach, which is the basis for successful radionuclide therapy [14–16].

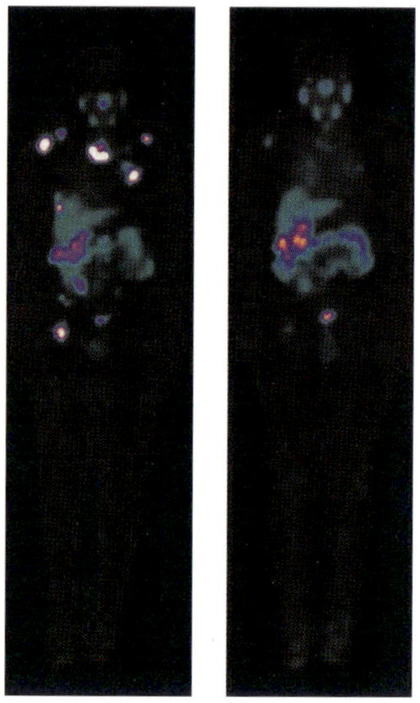

FIGURE 1: Anterior whole body ^{177}Lu-PSMA scan of a 72-year-old patient with metastasised castration-resistant prostate cancer. This demonstrates normal biodistribution in the nasal region, salivary glands, liver, and spleen gastrointestinal and urinary system, with multiple PSMA-avid metastases in the prostate bed, clavicle, sternum, clavicle, vertebrae, iliac bone, and femora. An excellent response to therapy was observed after 3 cycles of ^{177}Lu-PSMA-RLT with decrease in serum PSA level (from 63 to 4.25 ng/mL).

Radiomics is a high throughput approach used to extract a large number of qualitative and quantitative features from medical images, which could improve tumour phenotype characterisation and treatment outcome prediction [17]. Positive ^{68}Ga-prostate-specific membrane antigen for diagnostics with positron emission tomography/computed tomography (PET/CT) has the ability to capture intratumoural heterogeneity in a noninvasive way as well as to assess the response to PSMA-RLT. This imaging has brought radiomics closer to reality when it significantly reduced false-negative biopsies by guiding the needle to the highest Gleason score lesion in a comparative trial of biopsied PCa patients [18]. ^{68}Ga-PSMA PET/CT imaging and the use of PSMA-RLT with ^{177}Lu-PSMA may provide better risk stratification of PCa patients, if the findings are complemented with the knowledge of somatic mutations and epimutations. Recent data on a mouse model have shown that combining epigenetic drugs with immunomodulatory antibodies that target cytotoxic T-lymphocyte antigen 4 (CTLA-4) and programmed cell death 1 (PD-1) improves antitumor activity compared to the case when they were used individually [19]. For instance, syngeneic mammary and colorectal carcinoma models demonstrated that combination of 5-azacytidine (DNA demethylating agent) plus entinostat (histone deacetylase inhibitor) and CTL-4 plus CD-1 significantly improved therapeutic outcomes. The same study have also shown that anti-CD40 plus anti-CD137 immunotherapy combined with panobinostat (another histone deacetylase inhibitor) delayed tumour growth in syngeneic mammary (i.e., 4T1.2), colon (i.e., CT26), and prostate carcinoma mouse models [20].

3. Epigenetic Signatures and Mediators in Prostate Cancer

The epigenetic regulation of gene expression has been substantially studied for over 19 years now and is embraced as the well-known hallmark of tumorigenesis. Perturbed key multiple and important cellular processes that are normally suppressed or activated to inhibit malignant transformation is the common phenotype of aberrant gene expression. Cancer-related epigenetics, also known as epimutations, involves anomalous epigenetic alterations of gene transcription in cancer cells that are not attributable to any change in the nucleotide sequence [21, 22]. Advanced research in this rapidly growing and evolving landscape of cancer epigenetics has revealed a large amount of data showing global and specific epigenetic alterations, which are characterised by suppressed cell apoptosis, sustained cell proliferation, and invasion. These cellular manifestations are associated with hijacked or disrupted physiological pathways mediated by inactivating mutations and silencing of the transcriptional activities of cell-cycle activators [23, 24]. Several lines of evidence show that histone modifications, DNA methylation, and noncoding microRNA (miRNA/miR) are the most common epigenetic signatures responsible for the aberrant suppression of gene transcription observed in many malignancies. PCa is also influenced by a combination of genetic and/or epigenetic alterations that are strongly linked to perturbed cellular processes and tumour initiation. However, how these aberrant epigenetic signatures are established still remains poorly understood.

4. DNA Methylation

DNA methylation can be categorised as hypermethylation (increased methylation) and hypomethylation (decreased methylation). It involves chemical attachment of a methyl group to the carbon 5 on the genome, thereby leading to an alteration in gene transcription and normal function [21]. This phenomenon is established and maintained by various active DNA methyltransferase (DNMTs) enzymes including DNMT1, DNMT3A, and DNMT3B [21, 22, 25]. Hypermethylation is one of the best dissected epigenetic alterations in PCa and involves well-known genes that are important in DNA damage repair (*GSTP1* and *MGMT*), apoptosis (*DAPK1*; *RASSF1*), hormonal response (*androgen receptor-AR*, *estrogen receptor-ER*, and *RARβ*), inflammatory responses (*prostaglandin endoperoxide synthase 2-PTGS2*), cell-cycle control (*CDKN2A*), and metastases (*Cadherins*, *CD44*, and *tissue inhibitor metallopeptidase* (*TIMP*)) [26]. Like in other malignancies, silence in gene expression is the most common trait associated with promoter hypermethylation in PCa. This is often highly detected in advanced pathologic grades or clinical stages and usually accompanied by cancer development, invasion, and metastasis. More recently, hypermethylation of genes such as *Ephrin-A5* (*Eph-A5*) and *transmembrane protease serine 2* (*TMPRSS2*) has been revealed in PCa. Aberrant hypermethylation of the *Eph5A* CpG promoter regions was observed in advanced PCa patients with a Gleason score of 8. *Eph5A* is one of the Eph family of receptors of tyrosine kinases that are implicated in several human malignancies including PCa and hepatocellular carcinoma [27, 28]. TMPRSS2, an AR signalling downstream gene, is a type II transmembrane protease abundantly expressed in the prostate gland that has been shown to induce tumorigenesis when altered. DNMT1-induced hypermethylation at the promoter region of *TMPRSS2* was observed in PCa cells. This was accompanied by a suppressed expression of *AR* and *TMPRSS2*, which was restored through treatment with demethylating agent 5-Aza-2′-deoxycytidine [28]. Overexpression of *ERα* is directly proportional to PCa disease progression and promotes oncogenic events such as fusion of *TMPRSS2* and *estrogen-regulated gene* (*ERG*) located on chromosome 21. It was discovered that *TMPRSS2* is fused to either *ERG* or *ETS variant 1* (*ETV1*) and this frequent event contributes to PCa tumour progression [29–31]. Global DNA hypomethylation was hypothesised to occur later in PCa than CpG island hypermethylation and therefore is more likely to contribute to PCa metastasis than initiation and progression. Genes that are hypomethylated in PCa cells are limited, and these include LINE1, X-inactive specific transcript, plasminogen activator urokinase, and heparanase [32].

Androgen receptors (ARs) play a fundamental role by interacting with testosterone or dihydrotestosterone, which are crucial for the development of the male reproductive system during embryogenesis and sexual development at puberty. In PCa, aberrant hypermethylation of the AR correlates with suppressed gene transcription and increased PCa cell growth and proliferation [33]. A significant difference in methylation profiles that affect genes including caspase 8,

CD14, multiple drug resistant 1, and glypican 3 was observed between the AR-resistant and AR-negative cancer cells [34]. Matthew Freedman and his colleagues from Dana-Farber Cancer Institute and Harvard Medical School have recently shown in the human PCa tissues that the AR cistrome undergoes extensive reprogramming, which is an erasure and remodelling of DNA methylation [35]. This phenomenon was accompanied by localisation of forkhead Box A1 (FOXA1) and homeobox B13 (HOXB13) at the programmed AR binding sites, suggesting the implication of transcription factors in establishing aberrant epigenetic reprogramming [35].

The transcription factor E twenty-six-related gene (ERG) mediates epigenetic alterations in the AR cistrome and prime prostate tumorigenesis in a mouse model [36]. Ten-eleven translocation methylcytosine dioxygenase (Tet) proteins 1, 2, and 3 were demonstrated to preserve the unmethylated CpG islands by converting 5-methylcytosine to hydroxymethylcytosine via oxidation induced through interaction and catalytic activities of iron and alpha-ketoglutarate. In PCa, androgen hormone induced global hydroxymethylation silences Tet 2 expression, leading to poor prognosis. This was detected largely among global *FOXA1*-binding sites and inhibited *FOXA1* binding at specific loci, suggesting that alterations in Tet 2-mediated pathway may have a significant implication for treating advanced PCa [37].

5. Interaction among Epigenetic Mechanisms in Prostate Cancer

Histones commonly undergo extensive covalent modifications that alter chromatin structure or function, and these include methylation, acetylation, ubiquitylation, and sumoylation. Histone methylation/demethylation and acetylation/deacetylation are extensively studied [38, 39]. Histone acetylation (or deacetylation) involves the addition (or removal) of an acetyl group on lysine (K) residues within the N-terminal tail protruding from the histone core of the nucleosome and is generally linked to gene activation. When methyl groups are added to (or removed from) histone protein amino acids and result in the transcriptional activation or silence, the process is known as histone methylation (or demethylation) [22]. Lysines can be mono-, di-, or trimethylated, and this can be associated with either silence or active in-gene transcription. For instance, methylation on H3K4 and H3K36 is associated with active gene transcription, whereas mono-, di-, and trimethylation on H3K9, H3K27, and H4K20 mark transcriptionally silent chromatin. Histone acetylation/deacetylation and methylation/demethylation are driven by histone acetyltransferases (HATs)/deacetylases (HDACs) and methyltransferases (HMTs)/demethylases [22, 25].

The polycomb group of proteins including polycomb repressive complex 1 (PRC1) and PRC2 are key transcriptional repressor complexes that induce histone methylation to repress *Hox* genes involved in early development and stem cell differentiation. The main complex, PRC2, is composed of four core subunits: embryonic ectoderm development, suppressor of zeste 12, retinoblastoma binding protein 4, and enhancer of zeste 1 (EZH1) or EZH2 [40, 41]. PRC2 silences gene expression through trimethylation of H3K27, which is catalysed by its enzymatic units EZH1 and EZH2 [42, 43]. Disrupted activity of EZH2 through aberrant histone methylation promotes transcriptional instability that favours tumorigenesis and drug resistance. In castration-resistant PCa, overexpression of EZH2 via H3K27me3 is associated with poor clinical outcome, prognosis, and metastasis [44]. The role of EZH2 in tumorigenesis was strengthened by its knockdown in both castrated xenograft mouse model and human PCa cells that led to androgen-independence growth arrest, significant reduction of tumour growth, and metastasis. The activity of EZH2 can also be regulated by other non-PRC2 independent pathways such as phosphatidylinositol-3-kinases (PI3K)/AKT signalling pathways. Dysregulation in PI3K/AKT signalling pathway is associated with perturbed cellular processes including apoptosis, cell growth, and survival, which in turn leads to tumour progression. PI3K/AKT signalling pathway switches the function of EZH2 from a PRC2 to a transcriptional coactivator of AR in PCa. Moreover, EZH2 may also methylate AR at lysines 630 and 632 and enhance its transcriptional activity without any synergistic relationship with polycomb repressors, suggesting that targeting more pathways including those that regulate the activity of EZH2 independent polycomb repressors would have therapeutic efficacy in suppressing PCa tumorigenesis and metastasis [44].

Other PRC2 binding partners that mediate aberrant epigenetic activities in PCa are bromodomain adjacent to zinc finger domain 2A (BAZ2A), JARID1A/B/D, and KDM4A. The BAZ2A, also known as TTF-1 interacting 5, represses numerous protein-coding genes that promote cell growth and proliferation. Overexpression of BAZ2A correlates with molecular subtype displaying a CpG island methylator phenotype that aberrantly alters gene expression, leading to PCa aggressiveness, metastasis, and recurrence [45]. BAZ2A harbours C-termini with tandem PHD finger/bromodomain that interacts with EZH2, which is a key mediator for heterochromatic histone signatures and *de novo* DNA methylation. Jumonji AT-rich interactive domain 1 protein (JARID1) is one of the JARID family proteins that partners with PRC2 to induce H3K4me2/3 through EZH2. JARID1 is also known to disrupt the activation of pathways such as Fe(II)/α-ketoglutarate-dependent oxygenase and regulates cell survival and metastasis. Overexpression of JARID1A/B/D has been observed in PCa and metastasis, and its deletion or knockdown is associated with poor prognosis [46]. The prognostic value of JARID1D in PCa was also observed when upregulated JARID1D repressed the transcription of *Snail family zinc finger 2* and *miR-21-targeted matrix metallopeptidase* (*MMP*) family genes, leading to reduced invasion and metastasis [47–49]. Regulation of AR-regulated and BTG2-targeted *miR-32* is associated with PCa chemoresistance [50]. Upregulation of JMJD2A, also known as lysine-specific demethylase 4A (KDM4A), has also been observed in both human and mice models with PCa. This significantly correlates with advanced PCa and metastasis. JMJD2A appears to interact with ETS transcription factor ETV1 as well as tumour suppressor genes phosphatase and tensin homolog

(*Pten*) and yes associated protein 1 (YAP1), which promotes PCa initiation and aggressiveness [51]. Additionally, KDM4A was demonstrated to cooperate with miRNAs in regulating gene transcription and cellular processes in PCa, supporting an interaction between epigenetic alterations and miRNAs profiles [52].

6. MicroRNA and Epigenetics Alterations in Prostate Cancer

Noncoding miRNAs are evolutionary conserved short regulatory endogenous RNA molecules (~24 nucleotides in length) that are not translated into protein even though they are transcribed from DNA. They disrupt the function of messenger RNA, leading to dysregulation in RNA silencing and gene expression at posttranscriptional and translational levels. The miRNAs may function as tumour suppressors or oncogenes and can be either downregulated or upregulated in PCa. The miRNA profiling studies demonstrate that mRNAs may act independently or in partnership with other transcription factors to regulate gene transcription, which ultimately leads to perturbed cellular processes in PCa. Several *miRs* in addition to those described and reviewed by Lo et al. 2013 are dysregulated in PCa [53]. The *miR-101/31* was found to be downregulated in metastatic PCa, affecting the expression of EZH2 and regulation of PRC1 and B lymphoma Mo-MLV insertion region 1 homolog (BMI1) [54, 55]. This promotes tumour progression by targeting AR, Stathmin 1, and cyclooxygenase-2, which were shown to be an independent prognostic indicator for recurrent PCa [55, 56]. The *miR-24* was demonstrated to target proapoptotic gene Fas associated factor 1 by binding to its open reading frame, thereby enhancing apoptosis in DU-145 PCa cells [57]. In other studies, suppression of p63-mediated *miR-205*, Frizzled7-mediated *miR-613*, and *Myc*-mediated *miR-26a* expression levels was observed in PCa tissues as compared to their normal counterparts [24, 58]. Moreover, stable *miR-26a* induced G1 phase arrest and epithelial mesenchymal transition (EMT), leading to significantly reduced proliferation and metastasis via activation of Wnt5a pathway [58]. Similar effects in relation to EMT regulation were observed with downregulation of the *miR-182/203* via suppression of SNAI2 and with the *miR-144/145* associated with bone, skeletal, and seminal vesicle metastases in PCa patients [59, 60]. Genistein downregulates *miR-205/31*, *miR-221/222*, *miR-574-36b*, and *miR-574-36b* and confers resistance to chemotherapy-induced apoptosis in PCa cells [61–63]. Demethylation of *miR-146a* promoter by 5-Aza-2′-deoxycytidine significantly enhanced *miR-146a* expression, leading to delayed progression of castration-resistant PCa. [64].

7. Risk Factors for Prostate Cancer and Associated Epigenetics Alterations

A significant amount of data has shown that certain risk factors including old age, familial hereditary, and ethnicity/race may induce PCa growth by influencing both genetic and epigenetic factors [65]. Advancing age and ethnicity are the greatest nonmodifiable risk factors and play a pivotal role in PCa development (Figure 2). The risk of developing PCa increases exponentially after the age of 50 years [66]. Seminal work published by Kwabi-Addu and his coauthors in the Clinical Cancer Research showed that methylation of *GSTPi*, *RARβ2*, *RASSF1A*, *NK2 homeobox 5* (*NKX-2-5*), and *estrogen receptor 1* (*ESR1*) tumours suppressor genes in prostate tissues is age-independent [67]. Methylation of these genes was shown to initiate in normal prostate tissues as old age strikes and markedly increases during the progression of PCa [67]. Age-related CpG island methylation is significantly enriched with DNA binding and transcriptional factors [68]. Jung et al. and his team in Van Andel Research Institute are currently investigating the epigenomic changes following environmental factors including aging. They developed the methylated CpG island recovery assay, which is a reliable method for comparing genome-wide DNA methylations in normal and cancer tissues [69]. More recently, the same group hypothesised that polycomb complex resulting from KDM2B interaction with PRC1/2 that recognize unmethylated CpG islands may degrade with age. This would, in turn, allow access of CpG islands to the DNMT3A and DNMT3B, leading to partial DNA methylation in aging men [70].

The risk of PCa is increased in black African and American men compared to Caucasian men, suggesting an important role of ethnicity/race in PCa development [71]. Several studies showed that black South African men present with higher PSA levels and more aggressive and metastatic PCa than black American men. The presence of these phenotypes correlates with socioeconomic status, poor PCa awareness, and screening facilities associated with developing countries [66, 71]. Racial/ethnic disparities in epigenetic alterations have been observed in PCa tissues and correlate with racial differences in cancer prognosis and survival [72]. Devaney et al. [73] revealed that genome-wide methylation profiles differ in the PCa tissues between African-American and Caucasian men. However, considerable research investigations are still required to elucidate the role of these methylation differences in PCa disparity.

Similar to most cancers, PCa is a genetic disease that can also be caused by both germline and somatic mutations. Family hereditary has been postulated to increase the risk of PCa development. Men older than 55 years who have a first-degree male relative (i.e., father, son, and brother) diagnosed with PCa are at higher risk of acquiring PCa [74]. Genetic susceptibility and aberrant epigenetics may predispose individuals to PCa [65]. For instance, mutations or abnormal gene expression associated with classic genes such as *p53*, *PTEN*, *BRCA1*, and *BRCA2* may contribute to PCa development and metastasis [75–77]. Epidemiological studies have also indicated that male carriers of *BRCA1 and BRCA2* mutations have the highest risk of developing PCa compared to noncarriers of these mutations. This coincides with more aggressive disease and low rates of survival [78, 79].

Diet and environmental and occupational factors are hypothesised to be modifiable PCa-related risk factors.

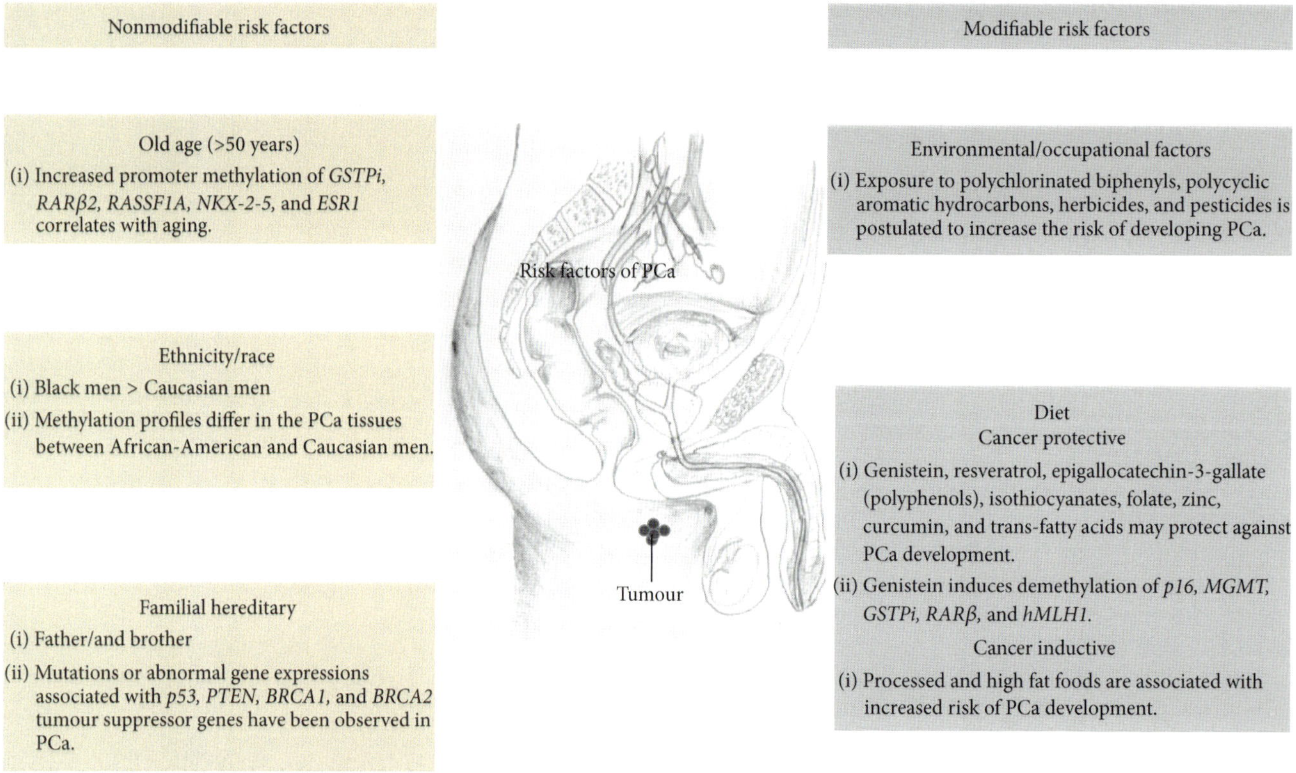

Figure 2: Risk factors associated with the development of prostate cancer. PCa risk factors can be categorised as nonmodifiable (e.g., old age, ethnicity/race, and familial hereditary) and modifiable (diet and environmental/occupational factors).

However, the mechanisms underlying the link of these factors and PCa development remain unclear [80, 81]. The α-methylacyl-CoA racemase is a peroxisomal enzyme required for the oxidation of branched-chain trans-fatty acids from red meat and dairy products. This enzyme was found to be aberrantly upregulated in PCa cells, supporting the hypothesis that a diet high in saturated or trans fats is associated with increased risk for PCa development [82, 83]. Certain diets containing antioxidant or anticancer properties such as genistein, resveratrol, epigallocatechin-3-gallate (polyphenols), isothiocyanates, folate, zinc, curcumin, and mono- or polyunsaturated fatty acids may serve as protective factors for PCa (Figure 2). Some of these anticancer agents were found to inhibit tumour proliferation and promote apoptosis by suppressing trimethylation of H3K27 through PRC2 arrest [84, 85]. Genistein is an important nutraceutical compound derived from soy products and has been shown to confer protection from developing cancer. Genistein suppresses multiple cellular processes such as proliferation and angiogenesis by demethylating tumour suppressor genes *p16*, *MGMT*, *GSTPi*, *RARβ*, and *hMLH1*. Rajvir Dahiya and his colleagues from University of Southern California at San Francisco have recently demonstrated that genistein regulates various miRs including *miR-1260b*, leading to the upregulation of *sFRP1* and *Smad4* in PCa cell lines via DNA demethylation and histone modifications, suggesting that diet may also prompt epigenetic alterations and contribute to PCa development [86].

8. Epigenetic Therapy in Prostate Cancer

Substantial knowledge on abnormal epigenetic alterations and cancer development is now being translated into novel anticancer therapeutic approaches [87, 88]. Unlike genetic mutations, aberrant epigenetic alterations are potentially pharmaceutically reversible making them attractive targets for chemotherapeutic approaches. DNMTs, HDACs, EZH2, DOT1-like histone H3K79 methyltransferase (DOT1L), and bromodomain and extraterminal (BET) are the current targets of epigenetic therapies (Figure 3). Inhibitors against these epigenetic mediators emerged as promising chemotherapeutic agents in several cancer models [87, 89].

Available demethylating agents that inhibit the action of DNMT include nucleoside (5-azacytidine, 5-azacytidine-2′-deoxycytidine/decitabine, and zebularine) and nonnucleoside (procaine, procainamide, disulfiram, and RG108) inhibitors [88]. These inhibitors have exhibited efficient antitumorigenic activities by suppressing an altered expression of tumour suppressor genes in haematological malignancies, breast, gastric, lung, ovarian, and hepatocellular carcinomas. Convincing clinical evidence of most DNMT inhibitors in PCa is still lacking and remains elusive. However, the epigenetic therapeutic potential of decitabine, procainamide, disulfiram, and RG108 was recently observed in human PCa cell lines and xenograft models, correlating with significant reduction in tumour growth and increased apoptosis [87–91].

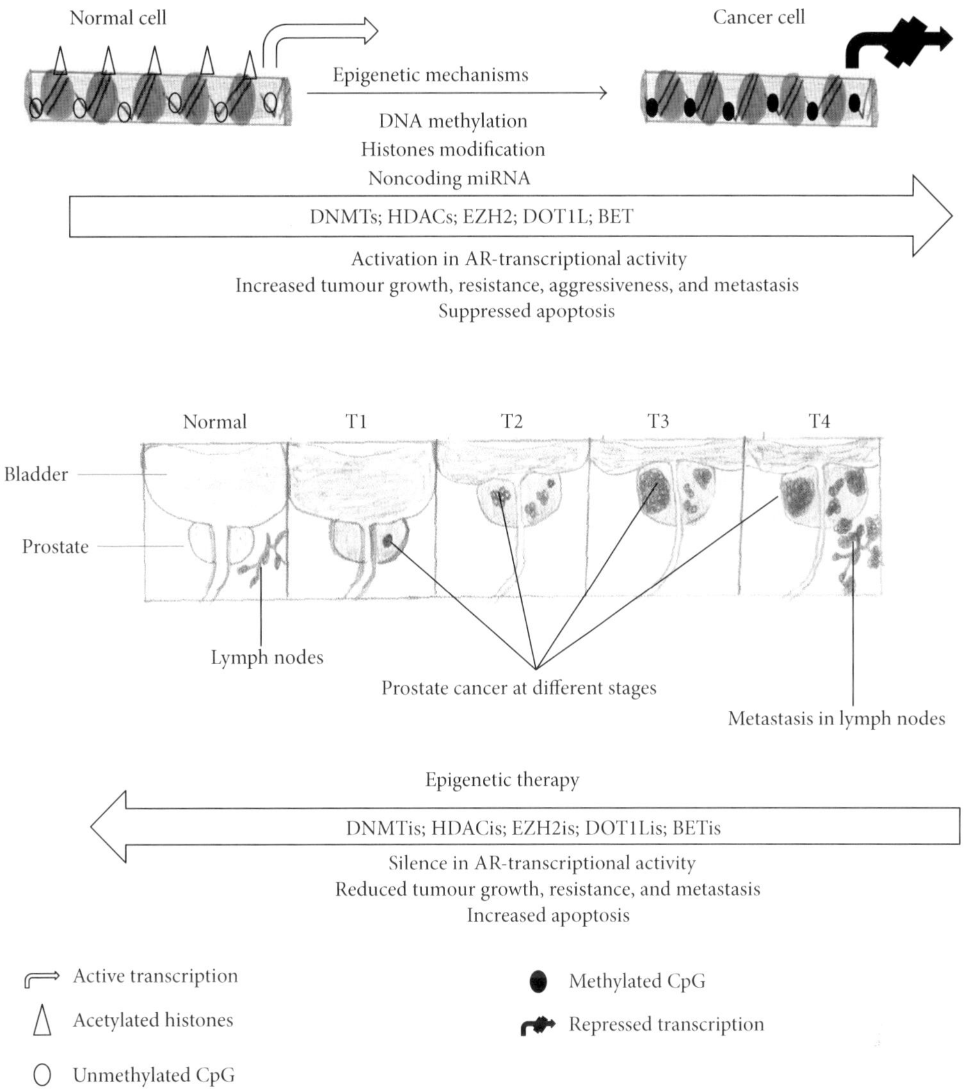

FIGURE 3: Epigenetic mechanisms and therapy in advanced prostate cancer. Prostate cancer follows aberrant epigenetic alterations that are associated with perturbed cellular processes that are critical in tumorigenesis. In normal cell, CpG islands are protected from DNA methylation and deacetylation whereas a prostate cancer cell is characterised by tumour growth, differentiation, resistance, and metastasis resulting from aberrant DNA methylation and deacetylation. AR: androgen receptor; BET: bromodomain and extraterminal; CpG: cytosine-phosphate-guanine island; DNMTs: DNA methyltransferases; DOT1L: DOT1-like histone H3K79 methyltransferase; EZH2: enhancer of zeste 1; HDACs: histone deacetylases; DNMTs: DNA methyltransferase inhibitors; HDACs: histone deacetylase inhibitors.

HDAC inhibitors (HDACis) are class of anticancer agents that reverse autonomous epigenetic alterations by disrupting the activity of HDACs, and their action coincides with sustained apoptosis resulting from impeded cell differentiation, angiogenesis, and metastasis. Vorinostat and romidepsin are the first FDA and EMEA approved HDACis and are currently used to treat uncontrolled cutaneous T cell lymphoma. Vorinostat has been investigated extensively in biologic, preclinical, and clinical studies involving several cancers and has emerged as a promising antitumor and antimetastatic agent with a favourable safety profile. Treatment with vorinostat represses PC-3 xenograft tumours and inhibits cell proliferation and metastasis in PC-3, LNCaP, and DU-145 human PCa cell lines [92]. Similar effects were observed in vorinostat-treated mice transplanted with CWR222 PCa tumours [93]. Romidepsin disrupts the interaction between Hsp90 and its binding partners, thereby inducing the *Hsp90* hyperacetylation and abrogation of AR signalling. In castration-resistant PCa clinical models, romidepsin correlates with minimal clinical activity. Other new HDACis that are currently undergoing investigation in PCa cell line models include panobinostat, MCL33(S)-2, and MHY219 [94, 95]. Combination therapy of vorinostat and romidepsin with other chemotherapeutic drugs including demethylating agents was shown to have more maximal activity than monotherapy and synergistically enhanced apoptosis in PCa cell lines ALVA-31,

LNCaP, and DU-154 [96, 97]. Recently, a new hybrid of vorinostat and a topoisomerase inhibitor WJ3543 exhibited potential antitumor activities, which overlapped with repressed cell growth, proliferation, and increased apoptosis in metastatic PCa [98].

While the efficacy of most lysine methyltransferases inhibitors in PCa remains obscure, there has been some advancement in preclinical development and phase 1 clinical studies with inhibitors targeting EZH2, DOT1L, and BET. BET inhibitor I-BET762 potentially suppressed cell growth and tumour aggressiveness *in vivo* by reducing *MYC* expression in PCa cancer cell lines, xenograft mouse model, and human tissues [99, 100]. EZH2 inhibitors GlaxoSmithKline-126 (GSK-126) and 3-deazaneplanocin-A reduced AR-transcriptional activity, leading to the inhibition of cancer cells self-renewal mechanisms, tumorigenesis, and metastasis mediated by aberrant EZH2 upregulation in PCa cells [101, 102]. Furthermore, combinations of nontoxic topoisomerase poisons VP-16 and GSK-126 significantly enhanced apoptosis in *in vitro* viability assays [102]. Other EZH2 inhibitors such as EPZ005667, GSK343, EP2-6436, Novartis, and EI1 also demonstrated their chemotherapeutic potential in treating several malignancies. Anti-DOT1L inhibitors such as EPZ004777, EPZ003696, EPZ5676, Yao CMP4, BrSAH, and SGC946 have been identified and tested in leukemic cells, where they were associated with suppression of H3K27 and tumour growth [103–107]. These inhibitors and other EZH2 inhibitors including EPZ005667, GSK343, EP2-6436, Novartis, and EI1 warrant clinical investigations in PCa.

9. Conclusion

Current evidence supports previous studies and demonstrates that epigenetic mechanisms play a critical role in PCa development. PCa-related epigenetic alterations may be triggered by induced genomic instabilities as well as various modifiable and nonmodifiable risk factors. Aberrant DNA methylation, histone modification, and noncoding RNA are tightly linked and synergistically alter gene transcription and normal gene function. These mechanisms lead to perturbed cellular pathways that are associated with abnormal or pathological phenotypes in prostate gland. Although several transcriptional factors have been demonstrated to interact with epigenetic regulators and modifiers, the underlying mechanisms are clearly complex and remain elusive. In terms of clinical application, epigenetic alterations in PCA are also potentially pharmacologically reversible. However, more preclinical and clinical studies are still needed to explore the chemotherapeutic potential of demethylation agents including EZH2, DOT1L, and BET. This may enable the development of more novel chemotherapeutic drugs that will be used in conjunction with current conventional treatments such as ^{77}Lu-PSMA-RLT to improve the management of refractory and metastasised PCa.

Competing Interests

The authors declare no conflict of interests.

Acknowledgments

This work was supported by grants from Oppenheimer Memorial Trust, Poliomyelitis Research Foundation, and National Research Foundation.

References

[1] S. J. Fourie, A. McMaster, R. Mothilal, and K. I. Maart, "A phase IV clinical trial of patients with solid tumors receiving lenog rastim as primary prophylaxis for chemotherapy-induced neutropenia, in a docetaxel-based regimen," *Journal of Cancer Research*, vol. 2014, Article ID 684936, 7 pages, 2014.

[2] G. Alleyne, A. Binagwaho, A. Haines et al., "Embedding non-communicable diseases in the post-2015 development agenda," *The Lancet*, vol. 381, no. 9866, pp. 566–574, 2013.

[3] R. Siegel, D. Naishadham, and A. Jemal, "Cancer statistics, 2013," *CA Cancer Journal for Clinicians*, vol. 63, no. 1, pp. 11–30, 2013.

[4] W. Catalona, J. Richie, F. Ahmann et al., "In reply: re comparison of prostate specific antigen concentration versus prostate specific antigen density in the early detection of prostate cancer receiver operating characteristic curves; re selection of optimal prostate specific antigen cutoffs for early detection of prostate cancer receiver operating characteristic curves," *The Journal of Urology*, vol. 154, pp. 1145–1146, 1995.

[5] M. J. Barry, "Screening for prostate cancer-the controversy that refuses to die," *New England Journal of Medicine*, vol. 360, no. 13, pp. 1351–1354, 2009.

[6] B. A. Lipski, R. L. Garcia, and M. K. Brawer, "Prostatic intraepithelial neoplasia: significance and management," *Seminars in Urologic Oncology*, vol. 14, no. 3, pp. 149–155, 1996.

[7] J. I. Epstein, M. J. Zelefsky, D. D. Sjoberg et al., "A contemporary prostate cancer grading system: a validated alternative to the gleason score," *European Urology*, vol. 69, pp. 428–435, 2016.

[8] A. O. Sartor, "Progression of metastatic castrate-resistant prostate cancer: impact of therapeutic intervention in the post-docetaxel space," *Journal of Hematology & Oncology*, vol. 4, article 18, 2011.

[9] T. A. Skolarus, A. M. D. Wolf, N. L. Erb et al., "American Cancer Society prostate cancer survivorship care guidelines," *CA: Cancer Journal for Clinicians*, vol. 64, no. 4, pp. 225–249, 2014.

[10] H. Hieronymus, N. Schultz, A. Gopalan et al., "Copy number alteration burden predicts prostate cancer relapse," *Proceedings of the National Academy of Sciences of the United States of America*, vol. 111, no. 30, pp. 11139–11144, 2014.

[11] E. D. Crawford, C. S. Higano, N. D. Shore, M. Hussain, and D. P. Petrylak, "Treating patients with metastatic castration resistant prostate cancer: a comprehensive review of available therapies," *The Journal of Urology*, vol. 194, no. 6, pp. 1537–1547, 2015.

[12] A. Afshar-Oromieh, E. Avtzi, F. L. Giesel et al., "The diagnostic value of PET/CT imaging with the ^{68}Ga-labelled PSMA ligand HBED-CC in the diagnosis of recurrent prostate cancer," *European Journal of Nuclear Medicine and Molecular Imaging*, vol. 42, no. 2, pp. 197–209, 2015.

[13] D. A. Silver, I. Pellicer, W. R. Fair, W. D. W. Heston, and C. Cordon-Cardo, "Prostate-specific membrane antigen expression in normal and malignant human tissues," *Clinical Cancer Research*, vol. 3, no. 1, pp. 81–85, 1997.

[14] C. Kratochwil, F. L. Giesel, M. Stefanova et al., "PSMA-targeted radionuclide therapy of metastatic castration-resistant prostate cancer with 177Lu-labeled PSMA-617," *Journal of Nuclear Medicine*, vol. 57, no. 8, pp. 1170–1176, 2016.

[15] R. P. Baum, H. R. Kulkarni, C. Schuchardt et al., "^{177}Lu-labeled prostate-specific membrane antigen radioligand therapy of metastatic castration-resistant prostate cancer: safety and efficacy," *Journal of Nuclear Medicine*, vol. 57, no. 7, pp. 1006–1013, 2016.

[16] G. J. Kelloff, P. Choyke, and D. S. Coffey, "Challenges in clinical prostate cancer: role of imaging," *American Journal of Roentgenology*, vol. 192, no. 6, pp. 1455–1470, 2009.

[17] P. Lambin, E. Rios-Velazquez, R. Leijenaar et al., "Radiomics: extracting more information from medical images using advanced feature analysis," *European Journal of Cancer*, vol. 48, no. 4, pp. 441–446, 2012.

[18] A. Rajinikanth, M. Manoharan, C. T. Soloway, F. J. Civantos, and M. S. Soloway, "Trends in Gleason score: concordance between biopsy and prostatectomy over 15 years," *Urology*, vol. 72, no. 1, pp. 177–182, 2008.

[19] M. Maio, A. Covre, E. Fratta et al., "Molecular pathways: at the crossroads of cancer epigenetics and immunotherapy," *Clinical Cancer Research*, vol. 21, no. 18, pp. 4040–4047, 2015.

[20] A. J. Christiansen, A. West, K.-M. Banks et al., "Eradication of solid tumors using histone deacetylase inhibitors combined with immune-stimulating antibodies," *Proceedings of the National Academy of Sciences of the United States of America*, vol. 108, no. 10, pp. 4141–4146, 2011.

[21] P. A. Jones and S. B. Baylin, "The fundamental role of epigenetic events in cancer," *Nature Reviews Genetics*, vol. 3, no. 6, pp. 415–428, 2002.

[22] G. Egger, G. Liang, A. Aparicio, and P. A. Jones, "Epigenetics in human disease and prospects for epigenetic therapy," *Nature*, vol. 429, no. 6990, pp. 457–463, 2004.

[23] Z. Kote-Jarai, C. Mikropoulos, D. A. Leongamornlert et al., "Prevalence of the HOXB13 G84E germline mutation in British men and correlation with prostate cancer risk, tumour characteristics and clinical outcomes," *Annals of Oncology*, vol. 26, no. 4, pp. 756–761, 2015.

[24] W. Ren, C. Li, W. Duan et al., "MicroRNA-613 represses prostate cancer cell proliferation and invasion through targeting Frizzled7," *Biochemical and Biophysical Research Communications*, vol. 469, no. 3, pp. 633–638, 2016.

[25] K. D. Robertson, "DNA methylation and chromatin—unraveling the tangled web," *Oncogene*, vol. 21, no. 35, pp. 5361–5379, 2002.

[26] L.-C. Li, P. R. Carroll, and R. Dahiya, "Epigenetic changes in prostate cancer: implication for diagnosis and treatment," *Journal of the National Cancer Institute*, vol. 97, no. 2, pp. 103–115, 2005.

[27] D. E. Linn, K. L. Penney, R. T. Bronson, L. A. Mucci, and Z. Li, "Deletion of interstitial genes between TMPRSS2 and ERG promotes prostate cancer progression," *Cancer Research*, vol. 76, no. 7, pp. 1869–1881, 2016.

[28] M. Chu, Y. Chang, N. Wang, W. Li, P. Li, and W.-Q. Gao, "Hypermethylation-mediated transcriptional repression of TMPRSS2 in androgen receptor-negative prostate cancer cells," *Experimental Biology and Medicine*, vol. 239, no. 7, pp. 823–828, 2014.

[29] B. G. Barwick, M. Abramovitz, M. Kodani et al., "Prostate cancer genes associated with *TMPRSS2-ERG* gene fusion and prognostic of biochemical recurrence in multiple cohorts," *British Journal of Cancer*, vol. 102, no. 3, pp. 570–576, 2010.

[30] S. A. Tomlins, B. Laxman, S. Varambally et al., "Role of the TMPRSS2-ERG gene fusion in prostate cancer," *Neoplasia*, vol. 10, no. 2, pp. 177–188, 2008.

[31] S. A. Tomlins, D. R. Rhodes, S. Perner et al., "Recurrent fusion of TMPRSS2 and ETS transcription factor genes in prostate cancer," *Science*, vol. 310, no. 5748, pp. 644–648, 2005.

[32] R. Zelic, V. Fiano, C. Grasso et al., "Global DNA hypomethylation in prostate cancer development and progression: a systematic review," *Prostate Cancer and Prostatic Diseases*, vol. 18, no. 1, pp. 1–12, 2015.

[33] H. Kinoshita, Y. Shi, C. Sandefur et al., "Methylation of the androgen receptor minimal promoter silences transcription in human prostate cancer," *Cancer Research*, vol. 60, no. 13, pp. 3623–3630, 2000.

[34] D. K. Mishra, Z. Chen, Y. Wu, M. Sarkissyan, H. P. Koeffler, and J. V. Vadgama, "Global methylation pattern of genes in androgen-sensitive and androgen-independent prostate cancer cells," *Molecular Cancer Therapeutics*, vol. 9, no. 1, pp. 33–45, 2010.

[35] M. M. Pomerantz, F. Li, D. Y. Takeda et al., "The androgen receptor cistrome is extensively reprogrammed in human prostate tumorigenesis," *Nature Genetics*, vol. 47, no. 11, pp. 1346–1351, 2015.

[36] Y. Chen, P. Chi, S. Rockowitz et al., "ETS factors reprogram the androgen receptor cistrome and prime prostate tumorigenesis in response to PTEN loss," *Nature Medicine*, vol. 19, no. 8, pp. 1023–1029, 2013.

[37] K.-I. Takayama, A. Misawa, T. Suzuki et al., "TET2 repression by androgen hormone regulates global hydroxymethylation status and prostate cancer progression," *Nature Communications*, vol. 6, article 8219, 2015.

[38] X.-J. Yang and E. Seto, "Lysine acetylation: codified crosstalk with other posttranslational modifications," *Molecular Cell*, vol. 31, no. 4, pp. 449–461, 2008.

[39] L. Ringrose and R. Paro, "Epigenetic regulation of cellular memory by the polycomb and trithorax group proteins," *Annual Review of Genetics*, vol. 38, pp. 413–443, 2004.

[40] S. Varambally, S. M. Dhanasekaran, M. Zhou et al., "The polycomb group protein EZH2 is involved in progression of prostate cancer," *Nature*, vol. 419, no. 6907, pp. 624–629, 2002.

[41] P. L. Clermont, D. Lin, F. Crea et al., "Polycomb-mediated silencing in neuroendocrine prostate cancer," *Clinical Epigenetics*, vol. 7, article 40, 2015.

[42] G. P. Souroullas, W. R. Jeck, J. S. Parker et al., "An oncogenic Ezh2 mutation induces tumors through global redistribution of histone 3 lysine 27 trimethylation," *Nature Medicine*, vol. 22, no. 6, pp. 632–640, 2016.

[43] L. Jiao and X. Liu, "Structural basis of histone H3K27 trimethylation by an active polycomb repressive complex 2," *Science*, vol. 350, no. 6258, article aac4383, 2015.

[44] K. Xu, Z. J. Wu, A. C. Groner et al., "EZH2 oncogenic activity in castration-resistant prostate cancer cells is polycomb-independent," *Science*, vol. 338, no. 6113, pp. 1465–1469, 2012.

[45] L. Gu, S. C. Frommel, C. C. Oakes et al., "BAZ2A (TIP5) is involved in epigenetic alterations in Prostate cancer and its overexpression predicts disease recurrence," *Nature Genetics*, vol. 47, no. 1, pp. 22–30, 2015.

[46] J. Qi, K. Nakayama, R. D. Cardiff et al., "Siah2-dependent concerted activity of HIF and FoxA2 regulates formation of neuroendocrine phenotype and neuroendocrine prostate tumors," *Cancer Cell*, vol. 18, no. 1, pp. 23–38, 2010.

[47] N. Li, S. S. Dhar, T. Y. Chen et al., "JARID1D is a suppressor and prognostic marker of prostate cancer invasion and metastasis," *Cancer Research*, vol. 76, no. 4, pp. 831–843, 2016.

[48] J. Sayegh, J. Cao, M. R. Zou et al., "Identification of small molecule inhibitors of Jumonji AT-rich interactive domain 1B (JARID1B) histone demethylase by a sensitive high throughput screen," *Journal of Biological Chemistry*, vol. 288, no. 13, pp. 9408–9417, 2013.

[49] S. T. Reis, J. Pontes-Junior, A. A. Antunes et al., "miR-21 may acts as an oncomir by targeting RECK, a matrix metalloproteinase regulator, in prostate cancer," *BMC Urology*, vol. 12, no. 1, article 14, 2012.

[50] S. E. Jalava, A. Urbanucci, L. Latonen et al., "Androgen-regulated miR-32 targets BTG2 and is overexpressed in castration-resistant prostate cancer," *Oncogene*, vol. 31, no. 41, pp. 4460–4471, 2012.

[51] S. Kaneko, R. Bonasio, R. Saldaña-Meyer et al., "Interactions between JARID2 and noncoding RNAs regulate PRC2 recruitment to chromatin," *Molecular Cell*, vol. 53, no. 2, pp. 290–300, 2014.

[52] S. N. Kamdar, L. T. Ho, K. J. Kron et al., "Dynamic interplay between locus-specific DNA methylation and hydroxymethylation regulates distinct biological pathways in prostate carcinogenesis," *Clinical Epigenetics*, vol. 8, article 32, 2016.

[53] U. Lo, D. Yang, and J. Hsieh, "The role of microRNAs in prostate cancer progression," *Translational Andrology and Urology*, vol. 2, no. 3, pp. 228–241, 2013.

[54] Q. Zhang, S. K. R. Padi, D. J. Tindall, and B. Guo, "Polycomb protein EZH2 suppresses apoptosis by silencing the proapoptotic miR-31," *Cell Death and Disease*, vol. 5, no. 10, article e1486, 2014.

[55] P. Cao, Z. Deng, M. Wan et al., "MicroRNA-101 negatively regulates Ezh2 and its expression is modulated by androgen receptor and HIF-1α/HIF-1β," *Molecular Cancer*, vol. 9, no. 1, article 108, 2010.

[56] M. R. M. Roduan, N. Mohtarrudin, C. P. Pei, M. Osman, and N. M. Dusa, "High expression of cyclooxygenase-2 in high grade human prostate adenocarcinoma," *Sains Malaysiana*, vol. 44, no. 5, pp. 727–733, 2015.

[57] W. Qin, Y. Shi, B. Zhao et al., "miR-24 regulates apoptosis by targeting the Open Reading Frame (ORF) region of FAF1 in cancer cells," *PLoS ONE*, vol. 5, no. 2, article e9429, 2010.

[58] S. Zhao, X. Ye, L. Xiao et al., "MiR-26a inhibits prostate cancer progression by repression of Wnt5a," *Tumor Biology*, vol. 35, no. 10, pp. 9725–9733, 2014.

[59] Y. Qu, W. Li, M. R. Hellem et al., "MiR–182 and miR–203 induce mesenchymal to epithelial transition and self–sufficiency of growth signals via repressing SNAI2 in prostate cells," *International Journal of Cancer*, vol. 133, no. 3, pp. 544–555, 2013.

[60] X. Peng, W. Guo, T. Liu et al., "Identification of miRs-143 and -145 that is associated with bone metastasis of prostate cancer and involved in the regulation of EMT," *PLoS ONE*, vol. 6, no. 5, article e20341, 2011.

[61] N. Bhatnagar, X. Li, S. K. R. Padi, Q. Zhang, M.-S. Tang, and B. Guo, "Downregulation of miR-205 and miR-31 confers resistance to chemotherapy-induced apoptosis in prostate cancer cells," *Cell Death & Disease*, vol. 1, no. 12, article e105, 2010.

[62] Y. Chen, M. S. Zaman, G. Deng et al., "MicroRNAs 221/222 and genistein-mediated regulation of ARHI tumor suppressor gene in prostate cancer," *Cancer Prevention Research*, vol. 4, no. 1, pp. 76–86, 2011.

[63] T. Chiyomaru, S. Yamamura, S. Fukuhara et al., "Genistein up-regulates tumor suppressor MicroRNA-574-3p in prostate cancer," *PLoS ONE*, vol. 8, no. 3, Article ID e58929, 2013.

[64] X. Wang, H. Gao, L. Ren, J. Gu, Y. Zhang, and Y. Zhang, "Demethylation of the miR-146a promoter by 5-Aza-2'-deoxycytidine correlates with delayed progression of castration-resistant prostate cancer," *BMC Cancer*, vol. 14, no. 1, article 308, 2014.

[65] D. Karan, J. Thrasher, and D. Lubaroff, "Prostate cancer: genes, environment, immunity and the use of immunotherapy," *Prostate Cancer and Prostatic Diseases*, vol. 11, no. 3, pp. 230–236, 2008.

[66] C. F. Heyns, M. Fisher, A. Lecuona, and A. van der Merwe, "Prostate cancer among different racial groups in the western cape: presenting features and management," *South African Medical Journal*, vol. 101, no. 4, pp. 267–270, 2011.

[67] B. Kwabi-Addo, W. Chung, L. Shen et al., "Age-related DNA methylation changes in normal human prostate tissues," *Clinical Cancer Research*, vol. 13, no. 13, pp. 3796–3802, 2007.

[68] T. Yuan, Y. Jiao, S. de Jong, R. A. Ophoff, S. Beck, and A. E. Teschendorff, "An integrative multi-scale analysis of the dynamic DNA methylation landscape in aging," *PLoS Genetics*, vol. 11, no. 2, Article ID e1004996, 2015.

[69] M. Jung, S. Kadam, W. Xiong, T. A. Rauch, S.-G. Jin, and G. P. Pfeifer, "MIRA-seq for DNA methylation analysis of CpG islands," *Epigenomics*, vol. 7, no. 5, pp. 695–706, 2015.

[70] M. Jung and G. P. Pfeifer, "Aging and DNA methylation," *BMC Biology*, vol. 13, no. 1, 2015.

[71] N. Mofolo, O. Betshu, O. Kenna et al., "Knowledge of prostate cancer among males attending a urology clinic, a South African study," *SpringerPlus*, vol. 4, article 67, 2015.

[72] Y.-Y. Xia, Y.-B. Ding, X.-Q. Liu et al., "Racial/ethnic disparities in human DNA methylation," *Biochimica et Biophysica Acta-Reviews on Cancer*, vol. 1846, no. 1, pp. 258–262, 2014.

[73] J. M. Devaney, S. Wang, P. Furbert-Harris et al., "Genome-wide differentially methylated genes in prostate cancer tissues from African-American and Caucasian men," *Epigenetics*, vol. 10, no. 4, pp. 319–328, 2015.

[74] A. Bjartell, "Genetic markers and the risk of developing prostate cancer," *European Urology*, vol. 60, no. 1, pp. 29–31, 2011.

[75] E. Castro and R. Eeles, "The role of BRCA1 and BRCA2 in prostate cancer," *Asian Journal of Andrology*, vol. 14, no. 3, pp. 409–414, 2012.

[76] N. Rivlin, R. Brosh, M. Oren, and V. Rotter, "Mutations in the p53 tumor suppressor gene: important milestones at the various steps of tumorigenesis," *Genes & Cancer*, vol. 2, no. 4, pp. 466–474, 2011.

[77] C. E. Barbieri, C. H. Bangma, A. Bjartell et al., "The mutational landscape of prostate cancer," *European Urology*, vol. 64, no. 4, pp. 567–576, 2013.

[78] H. Cavanagh and K. M. A. Rogers, "The role of *BRCA1* and *BRCA2* mutations in prostate, pancreatic and stomach cancers," *Hereditary Cancer in Clinical Practice*, vol. 13, no. 1, article 16, pp. 1–7, 2015.

[79] C. Rosty, M. D. Walsh, N. M. Lindor et al., "High prevalence of mismatch repair deficiency in prostate cancers diagnosed in mismatch repair gene mutation carriers from the colon cancer family registry," *Familial Cancer*, vol. 13, no. 4, pp. 573–582, 2014.

[80] J. Peto, "Cancer epidemiology in the last century and the next decade," *Nature*, vol. 411, no. 6835, pp. 390–395, 2001.

[81] H. Shimizu, R. K. Ross, L. Bernstein, R. Yatani, B. E. Henderson, and T. M. Mack, "Cancers of the prostate and breast among Japanese and white immigrants in Los Angeles County," *British Journal of Cancer*, vol. 63, no. 6, pp. 963–966, 1991.

[82] M. D. Lloyd, M. Yevglevskis, G. L. Lee, P. J. Wood, M. D. Threadgill, and T. J. Woodman, "α-methylacyl-CoA racemase (AMACR): metabolic enzyme, drug metabolizer and cancer marker P504S," *Progress in Lipid Research*, vol. 52, no. 2, pp. 220–230, 2013.

[83] Y. Liu, "Fatty acid oxidation is a dominant bioenergetic pathway in prostate cancer," *Prostate Cancer and Prostatic Diseases*, vol. 9, no. 3, pp. 230–234, 2006.

[84] L. J. Gudas and J. A. Wagner, "Retinoids regulate stem cell differentiation," *Journal of Cellular Physiology*, vol. 226, no. 2, pp. 322–330, 2011.

[85] A. P. Bracken and K. Helin, "Polycomb group proteins: navigators of lineage pathways led astray in cancer," *Nature Reviews Cancer*, vol. 9, no. 11, pp. 773–784, 2009.

[86] H. Hirata, K. Ueno, K. Nakajima et al., "Genistein downregulates onco-miR-1260b and inhibits Wnt-signalling in renal cancer cells," *British Journal of Cancer*, vol. 108, no. 10, pp. 2070–2078, 2013.

[87] I. Naldi, M. Taranta, L. Gherardini et al., "Novel epigenetic target therapy for prostate cancer: a preclinical study," *PLoS ONE*, vol. 9, no. 5, Article ID e98101, 2014.

[88] I. Graça, E. J. Sousa, T. Baptista et al., "Anti-tumoral effect of the non-nucleoside DNMT inhibitor RG108 in human prostate cancer cells," *Current Pharmaceutical Design*, vol. 20, no. 11, pp. 1803–1811, 2014.

[89] M. Karahoca and R. L. Momparler, "Pharmacokinetic and pharmacodynamic analysis of 5-aza-2′- deoxycytidine (decitabine) in the design of its dose-schedule for cancer therapy," *Clinical Epigenetics*, vol. 5, no. 1, article 3, 2013.

[90] A. Hagelgans, M. Menschikowski, S. Fuessel et al., "Deregulated expression of urokinase and its inhibitor type 1 in prostate cancer cells: role of epigenetic mechanisms," *Experimental and Molecular Pathology*, vol. 94, no. 3, pp. 458–465, 2013.

[91] B. Fialova, K. S. Trtkova, L. Paskova, K. Langova, and Z. Kolar, "Effect of histone deacetylase and DNA methyltransferase inhibitors on the expression of the androgen receptor gene in androgen-independent prostate cancer cell lines," *Oncology Reports*, vol. 29, no. 5, pp. 2039–2045, 2013.

[92] S. K. Kulp, C. S. Chen, D. S. Wang, C. Y. Chen, and C. S. Chen, "Antitumor effects of a novel phenylbutyrate-based histone deacetylase inhibitor, (S)-HDAC-42, in prostate cancer," *Clinical Cancer Research*, vol. 12, no. 17, pp. 5199–5206, 2006.

[93] L. M. Butler, D. B. Agus, H. I. Scher et al., "Suberoylanilide hydroxamic acid, an inhibitor of histone deacetylase, suppresses the growth of prostate cancer cells in vitro and in vivo," *Cancer Research*, vol. 60, no. 18, pp. 5165–5170, 2000.

[94] A. Laurenzana, M. Balliu, C. Cellai, M. N. Romanelli, and F. Paoletti, "Effectiveness of the histone deacetylase inhibitor (S)-2 against LNCaP and PC3 human prostate cancer cells," *PLoS ONE*, vol. 8, no. 3, Article ID e58267, 2013.

[95] N. Patra, U. De, T. H. Kim et al., "A novel histone deacetylase (HDAC) inhibitor MHY219 induces apoptosis via up-regulation of androgen receptor expression in human prostate cancer cells," *Biomedicine and Pharmacotherapy*, vol. 67, no. 5, pp. 407–415, 2013.

[96] V. Lakshmikanthan, I. Kaddour-Djebbar, R. W. Lewis, and M. V. Kumar, "SAHA-sensitized prostate cancer cells to TNFα-related apoptosis-inducing ligand (TRAIL): mechanisms leading to synergistic apoptosis," *International Journal of Cancer*, vol. 119, no. 1, pp. 221–228, 2006.

[97] R. L. VanOosten, J. K. Earel Jr., and T. S. Griffith, "Histone deacetylase inhibitors enhance Ad5-TRAIL killing of TRAIL-resistant prostate tumor cells through increased caspase-2 activity," *Apoptosis*, vol. 12, no. 3, pp. 561–571, 2007.

[98] C. Yu, S. Pan, S. Chao et al., "A novel small molecule hybrid of vorinostat and DACA displays anticancer activity against human hormone-refractory metastatic prostate cancer through dual inhibition of histone deacetylase and topoisomerase I," *Biochemical Pharmacology*, vol. 90, no. 3, pp. 320–330, 2014.

[99] I. A. Asangani, V. L. Dommeti, X. Wang et al., "Therapeutic targeting of BET bromodomain proteins in castration-resistant prostate cancer," *Nature*, vol. 510, no. 7504, pp. 278–282, 2014.

[100] A. Wyce, Y. Degenhardt, Y. Bai et al., "Inhibition of BET bromodomain proteins as a therapeutic approach in prostate cancer," *Oncotarget*, vol. 4, no. 12, pp. 2419–2429, 2013.

[101] F. Crea, E. M. Hurt, L. A. Mathews et al., "Pharmacologic disruption of Polycomb Repressive Complex 2 inhibits tumorigenicity and tumor progression in prostate cancer," *Molecular Cancer*, vol. 10, article 40, 2011.

[102] K. F. Schaarschuch, *Co-Regulators of Androgen Receptor Transcriptional Activity as a Novel Therapeutic Target for Advanced Prostate Cancer*, 2014.

[103] S. R. Daigle, E. J. Olhava, C. A. Therkelsen et al., "Potent inhibition of DOT1L as treatment of MLL-fusion leukemia," *Blood*, vol. 122, no. 6, pp. 1017–1025, 2013.

[104] E. Olhava, R. Chesworth, K. Kuntz, V. Richon, R. Pollock, and S. Daigle, "Preparation of substituted purine and 7-deazapurine compounds as modulators of epigenetic enzymes," PCT Int.Appl.WO, 2011.

[105] A. Basavapathruni, E. J. Olhava, S. R. Daigle et al., "Nonclinical pharmacokinetics and metabolism of EPZ-5676, a novel DOT1L histone methyltransferase inhibitor," *Biopharmaceutics and Drug Disposition*, vol. 35, no. 4, pp. 237–252, 2014.

[106] W. Yu, E. J. Chory, A. K. Wernimont et al., "Catalytic site remodelling of the DOT1L methyltransferase by selective inhibitors," *Nature Communications*, vol. 3, article 1288, 2012.

[107] Y. Yao, P. Chen, J. Diao et al., "Selective inhibitors of histone methyltransferase DOT1L: design, synthesis, and crystallographic studies," *Journal of the American Chemical Society*, vol. 133, no. 42, pp. 16746–16749, 2011.

22

Atypical Small Acinar Proliferation: Repeat Biopsy and Detection of High Grade Prostate Cancer

Andrew Leone,[1] Katherine Rotker,[1] Christi Butler,[2] Anthony Mega,[3] Jianhong Li,[4] Ali Amin,[4] Stephen F. Schiff,[1] Gyan Pareek,[5] Dragan Golijanin,[5] and Joseph F. Renzulli II[5]

[1]*Division of Urology, Rhode Island Hospital and The Warren Alpert Medical School of Brown University, Providence, RI 02905, USA*
[2]*The Warren Alpert Medical School of Brown University, Providence, RI 02905, USA*
[3]*Department of Hematology/Oncology, The Miriam Hospital, Providence, RI 02905, USA*
[4]*Pathology and Laboratory Medicine, Rhode Island Hospital, Providence, RI 02905, USA*
[5]*Section of Minimally Invasive Urology, The Warren Alpert Medical School of Brown University, Providence, RI 02905, USA*

Correspondence should be addressed to Joseph F. Renzulli II; jrenzulli@lifespan.org

Academic Editor: Michael Fröhner

Purpose. Atypical small acinar proliferation (ASAP) is diagnosed in 1-2% of prostate biopsies. 30–40% of patients with ASAP may be diagnosed with prostate cancer (PCa) on repeat biopsy. Our objective was to examine the association between ASAP and subsequent diagnosis of intermediate/high risk PCa. *Materials and Methods.* Ninety-six patients who underwent prostate biopsy from 2000 to 2013 and were diagnosed with ASAP were identified. Clinicopathologic features were analyzed. Comparison was made between those with subsequent PCa on repeat biopsy and those with benign repeat pathology. *Results.* 56/96 (58%) patients had a repeat biopsy. 22/56 (39%) were subsequently diagnosed with PCa. There was no significant difference in patients' characteristics. Presence of HGPIN on initial biopsy was associated with a benign repeat biopsy (68% versus 23%). 17/22 (77%) had Gleason grade (GG) 3+3 disease and only 5/22 (23%) had GG 3+4 disease. *Conclusions.* 22/56 patients (39%) of patients who underwent a subsequent prostate biopsy following a diagnosis of ASAP were found to have PCa. 77% of these men were diagnosed with GG 3+3 PCa. Only 23% were found to have intermediate risk PCa and no high risk PCa was identified. Immediate repeat prostate biopsy in patients diagnosed with ASAP may be safely delayed. A multi-institutional cohort is being analyzed.

1. Introduction

There are over one million prostate biopsies performed annually in the United States [1]. It has become clear that the potential risks, costs, and overdiagnosis of insignificant prostate cancer (PCa) have been underappreciated. Recent literature has demonstrated an increase in the incidence of significant postbiopsy infections and the consequences of overtreatment of indolent disease. Post-prostate biopsy hospitalization rates for infectious complications now approximate 1% [2].

Atypical small acinar proliferation (ASAP) is a diagnosis that occurs in about 1-2% of prostate biopsies [3]. The term ASAP, first defined by Bostwick, represents suspicious glands without adequate histologic atypia for a definitive diagnosis of prostate adenocarcinoma [4]. Previous studies have suggested that 17–70% of patients with ASAP have adenocarcinoma present on subsequent prostate biopsies [5, 6]. Current guidelines recommend immediate repeat biopsy within 3–6 months after the initial diagnosis of ASAP [7, 8]. However, up to 80% of the patients who are found to have adenocarcinoma on repeat biopsy have low risk GG 6 PCa [9]. With the recent trend toward adoption of active surveillance (AS) for low risk PCa defined by NCCN criteria, such patients are followed using serum PSA and digital rectal exam (DRE) every 4–6 months with a repeat biopsy in 1 year. However, there is concern with the potential for undersampling of intermediate risk PCa (GG 3+4). Recent evidence suggests that AS may be an acceptable treatment option in select patients with GG 3+4 PCa. Cooperberg et al. demonstrated that when patients do progress, the progression rate is slow and delayed intervention does not impact overall survival [10]. Also, recent research using MRI/TRUS targeted

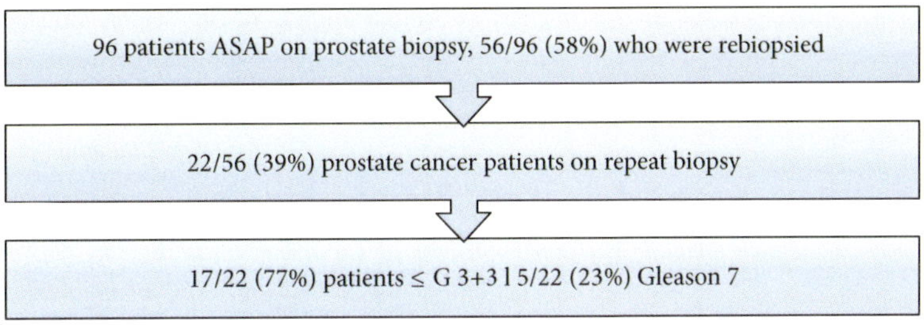

FIGURE 1: Flowchart of patients diagnosed with ASAP.

fusion biopsy has confirmed that patients diagnosed with subsequent PCa all had low risk disease [11]. We sought to explore the natural history of ASAP and the infrequent diagnosis of high risk PCa on repeat biopsy.

2. Materials and Methods

After obtaining appropriate institutional review board approval, a retrospective chart review of patients of an academic group practice from January of 2000 to December of 2013 was performed. Prostate biopsies were performed using transrectal ultrasound guided prostate biopsy for elevated PSA and/or abnormal DRE (standard 12-core template) and 96 patients were diagnosed with ASAP. Patient-specific data including age, prostate size on transrectal ultrasound, PSA, interval between repeat biopsies, GG on repeat biopsy, and subsequent treatment modality were recorded. Patients who had undergone previous prostate biopsy or those who had concomitant adenocarcinoma on biopsy or ASAP diagnosis prior to 2000 were excluded. Repeat prostate biopsy was performed with standard 12-core template with increased sampling performed at the previous site of ASAP at the discretion of the urologist. The diagnosis of ASAP was confirmed by a single genitourinary pathologist (AA). The pathologist reviewed all slides to confirm diagnosis of ASAP.

Clinicopathologic features recorded included age at biopsy, prebiopsy PSA, DRE findings, number of cores with ASAP, presence of high grade prostatic intraepithelial neoplasia (HGPIN), presence of cancer on repeat biopsy, Gleason score at repeat biopsy, and GG at radical prostatectomy (RP) for patients treated with RP. The primary outcome was detection of intermediate/high risk PCa, defined as GG ≥7 on repeat biopsy, in accordance with prior studies [12, 13]. Secondary outcome was diagnosis of any grade of PCa on repeat biopsy.

Continuous variables were compared using Student's t-test and Wilcoxon rank-sum test, and categorical variables were compared using chi-square and Fisher's Exact test, as appropriate. Separate logistic regression analyses were performed to evaluate the associations of clinicopathologic features with subsequent diagnosis of any grade and high risk cancer. Statistical analyses were performed using SPSS (version 21.0 (IBM, Chicago, IL, USA)). All tests were two-sided with p values < 0.05 considered statistically significant.

TABLE 1: (a) Demographic data. (b) Demographic data patients who underwent rebiopsy versus no rebiopsy.

(a)

Parameters	Data (IQR)
Number of patients ASAP on initial biopsy	96
Median number of cores positive ASAP	1.3 (1.0–1.7)
Median time to rebiopsy (months)	4.4 (1.2–5.6)
Percentage of patients repeat biopsy	58%
Median age (yrs.)	62 (56–67)
Median PSA (ng/mL)	6 (4.0–6.8)
DRE abnormal (%)	17%
Median follow-up (years)	2.8 (1.5–3.6)

(b)

	Underwent rebiopsy	No rebiopsy	p value
	$N = 56$	$N = 40$	
Age (yrs.) (IQR)	62 (55–67)	65 (57–68)	**0.05**
PSA (ng/mL) (IQR)	6.0 (3.3–6.3)	6 (3.5–6.1)	0.92

3. Results

Overall, 96 patients were diagnosed with ASAP. Median age was 62 years (IQR 56, 67), median PSA at presentation was 6.0 ng/mL (4.0, 6.8). 17% of patients had abnormal DRE demonstrating cT2a or cT2b disease. Median follow-up was 2.8 years (1.5, 3.6) and no deaths were recorded in the cohort (Table 1).

Of the 96 patients with ASAP on initial diagnosis, 56 (58%) had a repeat biopsy (Figure 1), with 45 patients undergoing repeat biopsy within 3–6 months of the initial ASAP diagnosis. The reasons for a lack of repeat biopsies were patients' preference and noncompliance. Table 1(b) depicts the comparative demographic data for patients who did undergo repeat biopsy to those who did not undergo repeat biopsy.

Age was statistically different, 62 versus 65 years (p = 0.051), but PSA did not differ between the two groups. The remaining 12 patients underwent repeat sampling within 2.5 years. Median time to repeat biopsy was 4.4 months (1.2, 5.6). 22/56 (39%) patients were diagnosed with PCa on repeat biopsy. Of those 22 patients, 17 (17%) patients had GG 3+3 disease and 5 had GG 3+4 disease (Table 2). Median number of cores positive was 1.8 (1.0, 1.7). None of the cases revealed

TABLE 2: Outcomes of rebiopsy on patients with CaP.

Gleason grade biopsy	Number of patients	RP	Upgraded (RP path)
3+3	17	8	1
3+4	5	1	0

higher grade prostate adenocarcinoma on repeat sampling. Median PSA prebiopsy was 6 ng/mL (4, 6.8).

Radical prostatectomy (RP) was performed in 9 patients, while 3 received external beam radiation. One patient was upgraded from GG 3+3 to 3+4 in radical prostatectomy. No biopsies revealed GG 4+3 or higher in this cohort. The remaining patients underwent active surveillance and remained on active surveillance at last follow-up.

To identify features associated with a subsequent diagnosis of any grade cancer, we examined bivariate associations of clinicopathologic characteristics among men with and without subsequent cancer diagnosis (Table 3). There was no significant statistical difference in the number of initial biopsy cores positive for ASAP between the two cohorts (those with cancer = 1.76 versus those without 1.33, $p < 0.21$). Concomitant HGPIN was identified in 23% of the patients that progressed to PCa compared to 67% of those not diagnosed with cancer on repeat biopsy ($p < 0.001$). Median age and PSA level at time of initial biopsy were not statistically different between the two cohorts.

4. Discussion

In this study, we examined the natural history of ASAP and the subsequent diagnosis of intermediate or high risk PCa on repeat biopsy. Notably, only 9% of men who underwent a repeat prostate biopsy were found to have intermediate risk PCa. No cases of high risk PCa were detected. Thus, for every thirteen repeat biopsies, one intermediate risk PCa was detected.

PCa is the leading noncutaneous cancer diagnosis among men and the second leading cause of cancer death in the United States [14]. Recently, the utility of PCa screening has come under scrutiny because of the suspected overdiagnosis and overtreatment of PCa.

ASAP generally encompasses marginally sampled adenocarcinomas or benign acini with reactive atypia or partial atrophy. ASAP differs histologically from PCa since it has a smaller size with fewer acini, more prominent nuclear hyperchromasia, and less prominent nuclear enlargement [15]. Current recommendations for ASAP diagnosis suggest repeating the biopsy within 3–6 months of the initial biopsy. This is based on the study by Iczkowski et al., which revealed that most PCas found in patients with ASAP are detected within the first 6 months after the initial biopsy [16]. Similarly, in the study by Epstein and Herawi, 90% of PCa following an ASAP were found on the first repeat biopsy [17]. This would most likely represent undersampling rather than disease progression. Dorin et al. reported that 51% of men subsequently diagnosed with cancer harbored clinically significant disease by the modified Epstein criteria [18], and Leone et al. noted that 43% of men treated with RP after a subsequent PCa harbored clinically significant disease [19]. Conversely, Warlick et al. observed that only 17.3% of men diagnosed with ASAP were subsequently found to have high grade (Gleason ≥7) cancer [20], and Raskolnikov et al. identified Gleason ≥7 disease in only 5% of patients with ASAP using MRI/TRUS-fusion guided biopsy [21]. While such findings appear to imply disparate conclusions, the differences in interpretation are largely related to choice of denominator. The prevalence of intermediate or high grade PCa is approximately 30–50% among men initially diagnosed with cancer. Also, the prevalence of significant or intermediate or high risk cancer among men with ASAP who undergo repeat biopsy is only 5–20%.

Other studies have suggested that concomitant HGPIN and ASAP increase the risk of PCa in repeat biopsy [22]. Conversely, our study suggests that a finding of concomitant HGPIN confers a statistically significant difference in the identification of PCa in ASAP patients undergoing repeat prostate biopsy (23% versus 67%, resp.) ($p < 0.001$).

Prostate biopsies can be associated with significant morbidity including pain, bleeding, and infectious complications. Also, a recent study has shown appreciable erectile dysfunction after transrectal prostate biopsy as early as three months after the biopsy [23]. Further, with increasing fluoroquinolone resistance and emergence of extended spectrum beta lactamase (ESBL) producing organisms, hospital admission rates following prostate biopsy are increasing and in some countries may be as high as 4% [24]. There are numerous studies demonstrating a relationship between ASAP diagnosis and low frequency of intermediate/high grade PCa [25]. Our study confirms this notion and suggests that, in appropriate patients, a 3–6 month repeat biopsy can be safely delayed.

In our opinion, patients with ASAP can be followed with parameters similar to AS for very low risk or low risk PCa [26]. In our series, the patients who were subsequently diagnosed with PCa after initial ASAP diagnosis were optimal AS candidates given the low volume (low number of cores and percentage of cores) as well as low prebiopsy PSA. We recommend placing newly diagnosed ASAP patients on an AS protocol abrogating the need for immediate repeat biopsy.

The limitations of our study include its retrospective nature and limited number of repeat biopsies. A substantial portion of patients were lost to follow-up. Variability in time to repeat biopsy for ASAP also demonstrates the lack of uniformity in practice patters within a group on academic urologists. There is significant interobserver variability in the diagnosis of ASAP. To address this issue, we utilized one fellowship trained genitourinary pathologist to review all cases and confirm the diagnosis of ASAP prior to their inclusion.

Over the last decade, there has been a trend to more aggressive grading of PCa known as the Will Rogers phenomenon [27]. Further, there has been a paradigm shift in the treatment of low risk PCa in recent years. Current advocacy is for very low and low risk PCa to be treated with AS. Long term follow-up (>10 years) is not available; however, some limited evidence suggests ASAP rarely progresses to intermediate PCa and does not progress to high grade PCa.

TABLE 3: Comparison of patients with and without PCa and high grade versus low grade PCa on repeat biopsy.

Feature	Any cancer on repeat biopsy ($N = 56$)		p value	GG ≥ 7 on repeat biopsy ($N = 5$)		p value
	Yes ($N = 22$)	No ($N = 34$)		Yes ($N = 5$)	No ($N = 17$)	
Mean age (years)	63	60	0.18	65 (59–69)	62 (57–66)	0.58
Abnormal DRE (%)	24	28	0.74	20	23	0.76
Mean PSA (ng/dL)	6	6	—	11 (5–15)	6 (4–7.3)	0.09
Mean # cores with ASAP	1.76	1.33	0.21	1	1.7 (1–3)	0.23
Presence of concomitant HGPIN	**22.7%**	**67.6%**	**0.001**	20%	9%	0.47

Our results demonstrate that a limited number of patients (39%) with an initial diagnosis of ASAP were subsequently diagnosed with PCa. However, only 9% of this patient population was diagnosed with intermediate risk PCa. No high risk PCa was detected. Prospective studies are needed to corroborate the natural history of men diagnosed with ASAP seen in our cohort.

Abbreviations

ASAP: Atypical small acinar proliferation
CaP: Prostate adenocarcinoma
DRE: Digital rectal exam
AS: Active surveillance
GG: Gleason grade
HGPIN: High grade prostatic intraepithelial neoplasia.

References

[1] S. Loeb, H. B. Carter, S. I. Berndt, W. Ricker, and E. M. Schaeffer, "Complications after prostate biopsy: data from SEER-Medicare," *The Journal of Urology*, vol. 186, no. 5, pp. 1830–1834, 2011.

[2] K.-J. Lundström, L. Drevin, S. Carlsson et al., "Nationwide population based study of infections after transrectal ultrasound guided prostate biopsy," *Journal of Urology*, vol. 192, no. 4, pp. 1116–1122, 2014.

[3] J. C. Cheville, M. J. Reznicek, J. R. Clark et al., "The focus of atypical glands suspicious for malignancy in prostate needle biopsy specimens: incidence, histologic features, and clinical follow-up of cases diagnosed in a community practice," *American Journal of Clinical Pathology*, vol. 108, pp. 633–640, 1997.

[4] R. Montironi, V. Scattoni, R. Mazzucchelli, A. Lopez-Beltran, D. G. Bostwick, and F. Montorsi, "Atypical foci suspicious but not diagnostic of malignancy in prostate needle biopsies (also referred to as 'atypical small acinar proliferation suspicious for but not diagnostic of malignancy')," *European Urology*, vol. 50, no. 4, pp. 666–674, 2006.

[5] V. Scattoni, M. Roscigno, M. Freschi et al., "Atypical small acinar proliferation (ASAP) on extended prostatic biopsies: predictive factors of cancer detection on repeat biopsies," *Archivio Italiano di Urologia e Andrologia*, vol. 77, no. 1, pp. 31–36, 2005.

[6] P. G. Borboroglu, R. L. Sur, J. L. Roberts, and C. L. Amling, "Repeat biopsy strategy in patients with atypical small acinar proliferation or high grade prostatic intraepithelial neoplasia on initial prostate needle biopsy," *The Journal of Urology*, vol. 166, no. 3, pp. 866–870, 2001.

[7] A. El-Hakim and S. Moussa, "CUA guidelines on prostate biopsy methodology," *Canadian Urological Association Journal*, vol. 4, pp. 89–94, 2010.

[8] A. Heidenreich, P. J. Bastian, J. Bellmunt et al., "EAU guidelines on prostate cancer. Part 1: screening, diagnosis, and local treatment with curative intent-Update 2013," *European Urology*, vol. 65, no. 1, pp. 124–137, 2014.

[9] D. G. Bostwick and I. Meiers, "Atypical small acinar proliferation in the prostate: clinical significance in 2006," *Archives of Pathology and Laboratory Medicine*, vol. 130, no. 7, pp. 952–957, 2006.

[10] M. R. Cooperberg, J. E. Cowan, J. F. Hilton et al., "Outcomes of active surveillance for men with intermediate-risk prostate cancer," *Journal of Clinical Oncology*, vol. 29, no. 2, pp. 228–234, 2011.

[11] D. Raskolnikov, S. Rais-Bahrami, A. K. George et al., "The role of image guided biopsy targeting in patients with atypical small acinar proliferation," *The Journal of Urology*, vol. 193, no. 2, pp. 473–478, 2015.

[12] H. A. van Vugt, M. J. Roobol, R. Kranse et al., "Prediction of prostate cancer in unscreened men: external validation of a risk calculator," *European Journal of Cancer*, vol. 47, no. 6, pp. 903–909, 2011.

[13] D. P. Ankerst, J. Hoefler, S. Bock et al., "Prostate Cancer Prevention Trial risk calculator 2.0 for the prediction of low-vs high-grade prostate cancer," *Urology*, vol. 83, no. 6, pp. 1362–1367, 2014.

[14] Surveillance, Epidemiology, and End Results (SEER) Program, Research Data (1973–2011), National Cancer Institute, DCCPS, Surveillance Research Program, Surveillance Systems Branch, April 2014.

[15] K. A. Iczkowski, "Current prostate biopsy interpretation: Criteria for cancer, atypical small acinar proliferation, high-grade prostatic intraepithelial neoplasia, and use of immunostains," *Archives of Pathology and Laboratory Medicine*, vol. 130, no. 6, pp. 835–843, 2006.

[16] K. A. Iczkowski, T. J. Bassler, V. S. Schwob et al., "Diagnosis of "suspicious for malignancy" in pros-tate biopsies: predictive value for cancer," *Urology*, vol. 51, no. 5, pp. 749–757, 1998.

[17] J. I. Epstein and M. Herawi, "Prostate needle biopsies containing prostatic intraepithelial neoplasia or atypical foci suspicious for carcinoma: implications for patient care," *Journal of Urology*, vol. 175, no. 3, pp. 820–834, 2006.

[18] R. P. Dorin, S. Wiener, C. D. Harris, and J. R. Wagner, "Prostate atypia: does repeat biopsy detect clinically significant prostate cancer?" *Prostate*, vol. 75, no. 7, pp. 673–678, 2015.

[19] L. Leone, V. Lacetera, R. Montironi et al., "Biopsy follow-up in patients with isolated atypical small acinar proliferation (ASAP) in prostate biopsy," *Archivio Italiano di Urologia e Andrologia*, vol. 86, no. 4, pp. 332–335, 2014.

[20] C. Warlick, K. Feia, J. Tomasini, C. Iwamoto, B. Lindgren, and M. Risk, "Rate of Gleason 7 or higher prostate cancer on repeat biopsy after a diagnosis of atypical small acinar proliferation," *Prostate Cancer and Prostatic Disease*, vol. 18, no. 3, pp. 255–259, 2015.

[21] D. Raskolnikov, S. Rais-Bahrami, A. K. George et al., "The role of image guided biopsy targeting in patients with atypical small acinar proliferation," *Journal of Urology*, vol. 193, no. 2, pp. 473–478, 2015.

[22] G. Ploussard, G. Plennevaux, Y. Allory et al., "High-grade prostatic intraepithelial neoplasia and atypical small acinar proliferation on initial 21-core extended biopsy scheme: incidence and implications for patient care and surveillance," *World Journal of Urology*, vol. 27, no. 5, pp. 587–592, 2009.

[23] K. S. Murray, J. Bailey, K. Zuk, E. Lopez-Corona, and J. B. Thrasher, "A prospective study of erectile function after transrectal ultrasonography-guided prostate biopsy," *BJU International*, vol. 116, no. 2, pp. 190–195, 2015.

[24] R. K. Nam, R. Saskin, Y. Lee et al., "Increasing hospital admission rates for urological complications after transrectal ultrasound guided prostate biopsy," *Journal of Urology*, vol. 183, no. 3, pp. 963–969, 2010.

[25] R. Postma, M. Roobol, F. H. Schröder, and T. H. van der Kwast, "Lesions predictive for prostate cancer in a screened population: first and second screening round findings," *Prostate*, vol. 61, no. 3, pp. 260–266, 2004.

[26] J. J. Tosoian, B. J. Trock, P. Landis et al., "Active surveillance program for prostate cancer: an update of the Johns Hopkins experience," *Journal of Clinical Oncology*, vol. 29, no. 16, pp. 2185–2190, 2011.

[27] P. C. Albertsen, J. A. H. Hanley, G. H. Barrows et al., "Prostate cancer and the Will Rogers phenomenon," *Journal of the National Cancer Institute*, vol. 97, no. 17, pp. 1248–1253, 2005.

23

The Prognostic PDE4D7 Score in a Diagnostic Biopsy Prostate Cancer Patient Cohort with Longitudinal Biological Outcomes

Dianne van Strijp,[1] Christiane de Witz,[1] Pieter C. Vos,[1] Eveline den Biezen-Timmermans,[1] Anne van Brussel,[1] Janneke Wrobel,[1] George S. Baillie,[2] Pierre Tennstedt,[3] Thorsten Schlomm,[4] Birthe Heitkötter,[5] Sebastian Huss,[5] Martin Bögemann,[6] Miles D. Houslay,[7,8] Chris Bangma,[9] Axel Semjonow,[6] and Ralf Hoffmann[1,2]

[1]*Philips Research Europe, High Tech Campus 34, 5656AE Eindhoven, Netherlands*
[2]*Institute of Cardiovascular and Medical Science, University of Glasgow, G12 8TA Glasgow, Scotland, UK*
[3]*Martini-Klinik Prostate Cancer Center, University Medical Center Hamburg-Eppendorf, 20246 Hamburg, Germany*
[4]*Klinik für Urologie, Charité–Universitätsmedizin Berlin, 10117 Berlin, Germany*
[5]*Gerhard-Domagk-Institute of Pathology, University Hospital Münster, 48149 Münster, Germany*
[6]*Prostate Center, University Hospital Münster, 48149 Münster, Germany*
[7]*Institute of Pharmaceutical Science, King's College London, WC2R 2LS London, UK*
[8]*Mironid Ltd, BioCity Scotland, ML1 5UH Newhouse, Scotland, UK*
[9]*Department of Urology, 3000CA Erasmus Medical Center, Rotterdam, Netherlands*

Correspondence should be addressed to Ralf Hoffmann; ralf.hoffmann@philips.com

Academic Editor: Craig Robson

Purpose. To further validate the prognostic power of the biomarker PDE4D7, we investigated the correlation of PDE4D7 scores adjusted for presurgical clinical variables with longitudinal postsurgical biological outcomes. *Methods.* RNA was extracted from biopsy punches of resected tumors (550 patients; RP cohort) and diagnostic needle biopsies (168 patients; DB cohort). Cox regression and survival were applied to correlate PDE4D7 scores with patient outcomes. Logistic regression was used to combine the clinical CAPRA score with PDE4D7. *Results.* In univariate analysis, the PDE4D7 score was significantly associated with PSA recurrence after prostatectomy in both studied patient cohorts' analysis (HR 0.53; 95% CI 0.41-0.67; p<1.0E-04 and HR 0.47; 95% CI 0.33-0.65; p<1.0E-04, respectively). After adjustment for the presurgical clinical variables preoperative PSA, PSA density, biopsy Gleason, clinical stage, percentage tumor in the biopsy (data only available for RP cohort), and percentage of positive biopsies, the HR was 0.49 (95% CI 0.38-0.64; p<1.0E-04) and 0.43 (95% CI 0.29-0.63; p<1.0E-04), respectively. The addition of the PDE4D7 to the clinical CAPRA score increased the AUC by 5% over the CAPRA score alone (0.82 versus 0.77; p=0.004). This combination model stratified 14.6% patients of the DB cohort to no risk of biochemical relapse (NPV 100%) over a follow-up period of up to 15 years. *Conclusions.* The PDE4D7 score provides independent risk information for pretreatment risk stratification. Combining CAPRA with PDE4D7 scores significantly improved the clinical risk stratification before surgery.

1. Introduction

Prostate cancer displays as a heterogeneous disease with varying potential to develop progressively to deadly forms of the disease [1]. Clinically, various schemes for pretreatment risk classification have been developed based upon longitudinal biological patient outcomes [2]. While active surveillance (AS) is recommended by the various guidelines for men with very low and low risk prostate cancer [3], there is a significant subgroup in this patient population with a risk of 10-25% cancer recurrence after primary treatment [4–6]. These patients suffer from the burden of follow-up treatments that are typically triggered by biochemical relapse. Likewise, in the intermediate risk group, there is a subpopulation with low risk of biochemical progression [7, 8]. Nevertheless, this group is heterogeneous, comprising patients with varied outcomes, including those with aggressive pathological characteristics [9, 10].

Clinical risk descriptors do not delineate effectively either the extent of the disease or its aggressiveness for all patients. Additional molecular information representing the biology of the disease offers the potential to achieve this.

Cyclic AMP is an ubiquitous second messenger that critically impacts on the functioning of all cell types in the body through its effectors, protein kinase A (PKA) and Exchange Protein Activated by cAMP (Epac) [11, 12]. It has the ability to regulate independently distinct processes within a single cell type due to compartmentalisation of signalling processes to spatially discrete loci (signalosomes) [13, 14]. This is achieved not only by the sequestration of effector molecules and their targets, but also by the formation and shaping of intracellular gradients of cyclic AMP by its targeted degradation through the action of cAMP degrading phosphodiesterases (PDEs) that are specifically sequestered to distinct signalosomes in discrete cell locales [14]. Playing a critical role in this are members of the cAMP specific PDE4 family. Indeed, this four-gene family (PDE4A/B/C/D), which encodes 20+ isoforms, appears to be designed specifically to underpin compartmentalisation as their isoform-specific N-terminal regions contain motifs that allow for their targeting to distinct signalling complexes [15]. Consistent with the importance of particular PDE4 isoforms, their selective knockdown leads to distinct phenotypic changes [16] and genetic lesions in particular PDE4 subfamilies have been shown to provide the underpinning molecular pathology [17]. PDE4D7 is the so-called long isoform as it contains both the UCR1 and UCR2 regulatory domains that allow for regulation by various protein kinases, including PKA and MK2 as well as determining the functional outcome of catalytic unit phosphorylation by ERK [14]. Functionally, then it contributes to the cellular desensitization system towards cAMP and enables cross-talk between signalling pathways that lead to the activation of ERK and AMPK.

Recently, we have demonstrated that PDE4D7 transcript levels correlate to the longitudinal outcome of prostate cancer and independently add to postsurgical risk stratification in a consecutively operated prostate cancer patient cohort [18, 19]. To further explore the prognostic power of PDE4D7 in pretreatment patient risk assessment, we have investigated here the correlation to disease recurrence in the context of presurgical risk variables and algorithms like the CAPRA (Cancer of the Prostate Risk Assessment) score. We have developed a combination model of CAPRA and PDE4D7 scores in a surgery cohort and validated this model in an independent patient cohort on diagnostic biopsy tissue. We conclude that PDE4D7 does not only provide value in postsurgical risk stratification as we have shown before but also increases the stratification power of the CAPRA score in a pretreatment setting.

2. Patients and Methods

2.1. Patient Cohorts and Samples. RP patient cohort (n=550): patients consecutively managed at a single, large-volume prostate cancer center were included into the study (Martini-Klinik, Hamburg, Germany). Two small biopsy punches (~1x2 mm) of a representative resected tumor area of patients operated on between 2000 and 2004 were collected from the tumors index lesion. Patients who underwent adjuvant hormone therapy were removed from the study cohort. RP∗ patient cohort (n=130): detailed characteristics of this cohort and analysis of the respective gene expression data were described previously [20]. DB patient cohort (n=168): from the tumor positive diagnostic biopsy with the highest Gleason grade per patient a single biopsy punch (~1x2 mm) was collected. Patients were diagnosed with prostate cancer and operated on between 1994 and 2011 at the Prostate Center (University Hospital Münster, Germany). After quality control of the study data based on predefined criteria [18] 503 and 151 patient samples were defined eligible for statistical analysis in the RP and the DB cohort, respectively. The local Institutional Review Boards approved the collection of patient tissue for clinical research with appropriate patient consent (for cohort design see Supplementary Figures 3A & 3B).

2.2. Laboratory Methods. To account for potential tumor heterogeneity, the two tissue punches of the RP cohort were combined before nucleic acid extraction. A potential difference in tumor cellularity of the tissue punches was addressed by normalization of the qPCR results of the PDE4D transcript to four reference genes which were selected based on stable gene expression across multiple tumor sample types [18]. All used molecular laboratory methods including oligonucleotide primers and probes for RT-qPCR (quantitative real-time PCR), RNA extraction, and quality control and procedures to include/discard samples from the statistical analysis were described before [18].

2.3. Data Analysis and Statistics. Generation of normalized PDE4D transcript expression was performed by subtracting the Cq of the respective PDE4D transcript from the averaged Cq of the reference genes. Normalized PDE4D7 expression was transformed to the PDE4D7 score [19] (Supplementary Figures 1A & 1B). In correlation analysis for various available biological and treatment related outcomes (Table 1), the PDE4D7 score was used either as a continuous or as a categorical variable defined as (a) PDE4D7 score (1≤2); (b) PDE4D7 score (>2 and ≤3); (c) PDE4D7 score (>3 and ≤4); (d) PDE4D7 score (>4 and ≤5). The CAPRA risk score and corresponding low (1), intermediate (2), and high risk (3) categories were calculated as described earlier [21]. Uni- and multivariate Cox regression and Kaplan-Meier analyses were applied to correlate biochemical recurrence (BCR) progression-free survival or secondary treatment (salvage radiation and/or androgen deprivation) free survival (STFS) to the PDE4D7 score in the RP cohorts (n=503 [18], and Taylor et al. [20] (n=130)) and the DB cohort (n=151; this study). Decision curve analyses were performed as described [22]. For statistical analysis, the software package MedCalc (MedCalc Software BVBA, Ostend, Belgium) was used. The data analysis strategy is outlined in Supplementary Figure 2.

Table 1: Aggregated summary of the characteristics of the studied patient cohorts. (**A**) Demographics of the radical prostatectomy (RP) patient cohort including the 503 patients eligible for statistical data analysis. For patient age, preoperative PSA, percentage of tumor in biopsy, prostate volume, and PSA density the min and max values in the cohort are shown; median and IQR are depicted in parentheses. Pre- and postsurgical pathology are given (note: extracapsular extension was derived from pathology stage information). The outcome category illustrates the cumulative 5- and 10-year biochemical recurrence (BCR) and clinical recurrence to metastases (CR) postsurgical primary treatment. The treatment category lists the cumulative 5- and 10-year start to SRT (salvage radiation therapy) or SADT (salvage androgen deprivation therapy) after surgery. Mortality is shown as prostate cancer specific survival (PCSS) as well as overall survival (OS). (**B**) Demographics of the diagnostic biopsy (DB) patient cohort. In total diagnostic needle biopsy tissues of 151 were eligible for statistical data analysis. The demographics and clinical data of this cohort are presented equivalent to the RP cohort (N/A=not available).

	Parameter	(A) RP cohort (n=503)	(B) DB cohort (n=151)
Demographic & Clinical Range (median; IQR)	Age range (at RP)	41.3-74.5 (62.6; 7.4)	47.4-77.4 (64.9; 8.5)
	Preoperative PSA range	0.18-73.16 (6.7; 5.5)	2.0-49.1 (8.1; 5.7)
	Percent tumor in biopsy range	0.2-79.7 (10.3; 16.0)	N/A
	Prostate Volume range	9-148 (42; 22.5)	13.6-148.0 (38.5; 19.2)
	PSA density range	0.01-2.03 (0.16; 0.14)	0.03-1.6 (0.2; 0.17)
CAPRA Risk Category—No. of patients (percentage)	Low Risk (NCCN)	211 (41.9%)	38 (25.2%)
	Intermediate Risk (NCCN)	248 (49.3%)	82(54.3%)
	High Risk (NCCN)	44 (8.7%)	31 (20.5%)
Pre-Surgery Pathology—Number of patients (percentage)	Biopsy Gleason 3+3 (GG1)	316 (62.8%)	77 (51.0%)
	Biopsy Gleason 3+4 (GG2)	149 (29.6%)	38 (25.2%)
	Biopsy Gleason 4+3 (GG3)	25 (5.0%)	20 (13.2%)
	Biopsy Gleason >=4+4 (>=GG4)	13 (2.6%)	16 (10.6%)
	cT1	342 (68%)	97 (64.2%)
	cT2	150 (29.8%)	
	cT3	11 (2.2%)	54 (35.8%)
Post-Surgery Pathology—No. of patients (percentage)	Pathology Gleason 3+3 (GG1)	201 (40%)	46 (30.5%)
	Pathology Gleason 3+4 (GG2)	257 (51.1%)	52 (34.4%)
	Pathology Gleason 4+3 (GG3)	41 (8.2%)	31 (20.5%)
	Pathology Gleason >=4+4 (>=GG4)	4 (0.8%)	22 (14.6%)
	pT2	331 (65.8%)	88 (58.3%)
	pT3	172 (34.2%)	63 (41.7%)
	pT4	0 (0%)	0 (0%)
	Positive Surgical Margins	120 (23.9%)	33 (21.9%)
	Capsular Status	113 (22.5%) (=T3a)	57/145 (39.3%) infiltrated; 75/145 (51.7%) penetrated
	Positive Seminal Vesicle Invasion	60 (11.9%)	20 (13.2%)
	Positive Lymph Node Invasion	5 (1%)	10 (6.6%)
Follow-up [months] (IQR median follow-up)	Mean	123.6	73.7
	Median	141.8	73.6
Outcome—No events / total patient number (percentage; median follow-up; IQR)	BCR within 5 years	92/446 (20.6%; 121.2; 87.5)	49/151 (32.5%; 73.7; 43.9)
	BCR within 10 years	134/347 (38.6%; 134.0; 95.6)	N/A
	CR within 5 years	5/441 (1.1%; 144.4; 37.8)	4/151 (2.6%; 73.7; 42.6)
	CR within 10 years	13/306 (4.2%; 154.7; 32.85)	N/A
Salvage Therapy—No events / total patient number (percentage; median follow-up; IQR)	SRT within 5 years	53/439 (12.1%; 120.4; 53.5)	12/151 (7.9%; N/A; N/A)
	SRT within 10 years	83/320 (25.9%; 132.3; 39.6)	N/A
	SADT within 5 years	27/441 (6.1%; 120.7; 46.6)	16/151 (10.6%; N/A; N/A)
	SADT within 10 years	54/312 (17.3%; 132.4; 24.2)	N/A
Survival—No events / total patient number (percentage; median follow-up; IQR)	PCSS within 5 years	17/453 (1.1%; 144.4; 37.7)	1/151 (0.7%; N/A; N/A)
	PCSS within 10 years	38/330 (2.6%; 154.8; 30.3)	0/151 (0%; N/A; N/A)
	OS within 5 years	5/441 (3.7%; 144.4; 45.1)	1/151 (0.7%; N/A; N/A)
	OS within 10 years	10/302 (11.2%; 146.0; 35.4)	5/151 (3.3%; N/A; N/A)

3. Results

3.1. Correlation of PDE4D7 Score to Longitudinal Clinical Outcomes. We recently described the association of the expression of the prostate cancer biomarker PDE4D7 to postsurgical biochemical relapse based on the quantitation of the PDE4D transcript in surgical resection tissues [18]. Here we set out to translate this earlier finding to a presurgical setting using three independent patient cohorts. Firstly, we evaluated a radical prostatectomy (RP) cohort comprising 550 patients (Supplementary Figure 3A) [18]. In this patient cohort, a logistic regression model of the PDE4D7 score together with the presurgical CAPRA risk score was developed to predict the risk of postsurgical BCR. Secondly, we tested this PDE4D7 & CAPRA risk model for BCR outcome in an independent surgery cohort (RP∗; n=130 [20]). It is well known that >30% of tumors with an initial biopsy Gleason 3+3 undergo grade migration to a pathology Gleason 3+4 after surgery; we could confirm this effect in the RP cohort used in this study while any other stage migration with initial biopsy Gleason scores >3+3 was much less frequent (<5%). However, we could not find a significant PDE4D7 expression difference in tumors that were upgraded postsurgically from a biopsy Gleason 3+3 to a pathology Gleason 3+4 versus those tumors that remained Gleason 3+3 after radical prostatectomy (data not shown). Therefore, we hypothesized that the association of PDE4D7 measured on resection tissue with presurgical clinical variables will translate into equivalent results on preoperatively prostate needle biopsy tissue. To test this hypothesis, we validated the PDE4D7 & CAPRA risk model to predict postoperative BCR which we developed using the RP cohort in a presurgical needle biopsy (DB) cohort. This cohort comprised 168 patients of which 151 were eligible for subsequent data analysis (Table 1; Supplementary Figure 3B).

Univariate Cox regression analysis demonstrated a very significant association of the continuous PDE4D7 score to time to BCR in the RP and DB patient cohorts with HR=0.53; 95% CI=0.41-0.67; p<0.0001, and HR=0.47; 95% CI=0.33-0.65, p=<0.0001, respectively. Adjusting the multivariate Cox regression analysis for the presurgical variables age, preoperative PSA, PSA density, biopsy Gleason grade group, percent tumor positive biopsy cores, clinical stage, or the prognostic CAPRA score [21] resulted in a significant independent contribution to the prediction of postsurgical BCR for the continuous PDE4D7 score (Tables 2(a), 2(b)).

3.2. Outcome Modeling of Combined CAPRA and PDE4D7 Scores. To explore this further we set out to test the benefit of a combination of the PDE4D7 score with clinical variables used to predict postsurgical risk of disease progression. Based on our multivariate Cox regression data we hypothesized that a combination of the CAPRA score, together with the PDE4D7 score, might provide a significant improvement in prognostic power over the CAPRA score alone. The CAPRA algorithm combines age, preoperative PSA, biopsy Gleason, and percent of tumor positive biopsy cores. The resulting score categorized patients into low risk (CAPRA scores 0-2), intermediate risk (CAPRA scores 3-5), and high risk (CAPRA scores 6-10). The CAPRA score has been shown to predict, significantly, postsurgical PSA relapse in several studies [23]. To evaluate our postulation we selected a subcohort of 449 patients (92 events; 20.5%) of the RP cohort with complete 5-year outcome histories and generated a logistic regression model to combine PDE4D7 with the CAPRA score so as to predict the 5-year risk of biochemical recurrence after surgery (odds ratio 0.46; 95% CI 0.3-0.69; p=0.0002; data not shown). Next, we tested this CAPRA & PDE4D7 score logistic regression model on 130 patients from the independent RP∗ cohort [20] as well as on the 151 patients of the DB cohort for Kaplan-Meier survival analysis and ROC curve analysis, as well as decision curve analysis (see Supplementary Figure 2 for data analysis strategy).

In Kaplan-Meier survival studies on the DB patient cohort, we observed a significant separation of patients into different risks to experience postoperative PSA relapse based on the presurgical measurement of the PDE4D7 score in a tissue punch of a diagnostic needle biopsy (Figure 1(a)). We then compared postsurgical progression-free survival curves of the three CAPRA score categories (low, intermediate, and high risk) with progression-free survival based on the CAPRA & PDE4D7 logistic regression combination model in the DB (n=151) patient cohort. Concerning the logistic regression model we categorized the model-calculated risk probability to experience the clinical endpoint into four groups (p<0.1; p=0.1 to <0.25; p=0.25 to <0.5; p=0.5 to 1.0) and compared the hazard ratio (HR) difference between the lowest versus highest recurrence risk groups between the tested models (Figures 1(b) and 1(c)). The addition of the PDE4D7 score to the clinical CAPRA categories proved to significantly increase in the hazard ratio difference from the lowest to the highest risk group in the DB cohort (HR=9.0 for the CAPRA score; HR for the CAPRA & PDE4D7 combination score could not be determined due to no event in the lowest risk group which is used as the reference; Figures 1(b) and 1(c)).

We then set out to test the clinically relevant endpoint of secondary treatment free survival (STFS). This endpoint comprises start of any salvage therapy (radiation, hormone ablation) after postsurgical PSA failure. As before, we noticed an improved risk separation between patients with lowest versus highest risk groups to receive postsurgical secondary treatment when combining the CAPRA with PDE4D7 scores versus CAPRA score categories alone (Figures 1(d)–1(f)). Finally, we confirmed the performance of the CAPRA & PDE4D7 combination model versus the CAPRA score categories on the RP∗ cohort (HR=11.8 for CAPRA score versus HR=16.4 for the CAPRA & PDE4D7 combination score, respectively (Supplementary Figures 4A & 4B)).

Next, we analysed the prediction of risk of 5-year PSA relapse after primary treatment using the CAPRA score alone versus the CAPRA & PDE4D7 score combination model, which was previously developed using the RP cohort. In ROC analysis, we calculated the 5-year BCR AUCs as 0.77 for the CAPRA score alone and 0.82 for the combination model of CAPRA & PDE4D7 score model (p=0.004; Figure 2(a)). Further, the CAPRA & PDE4D7 combination model showed equivalent performance in a subcohort analysis including only patients with biopsy Gleason ≥7 over CAPRA

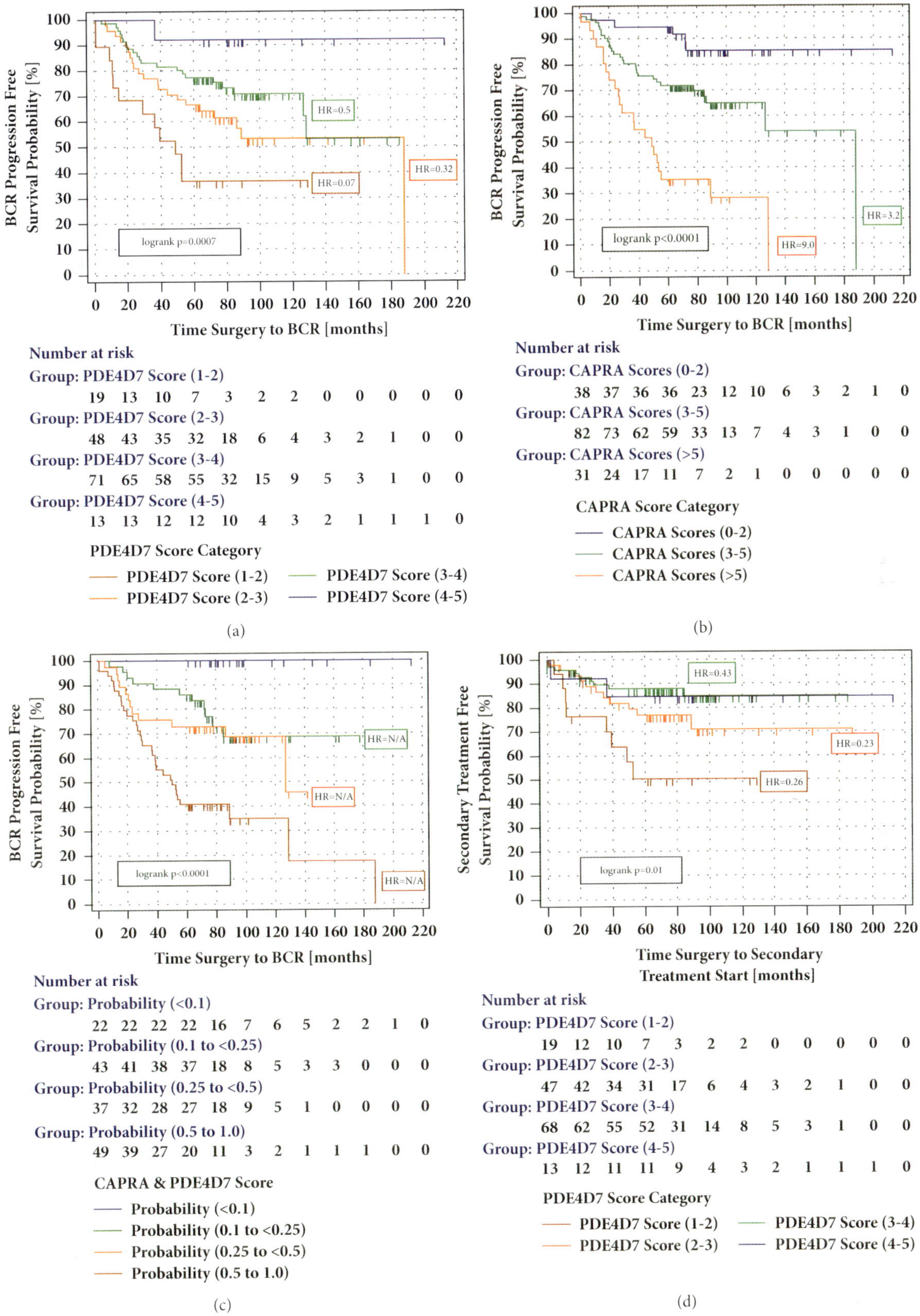

FIGURE 1: Continued.

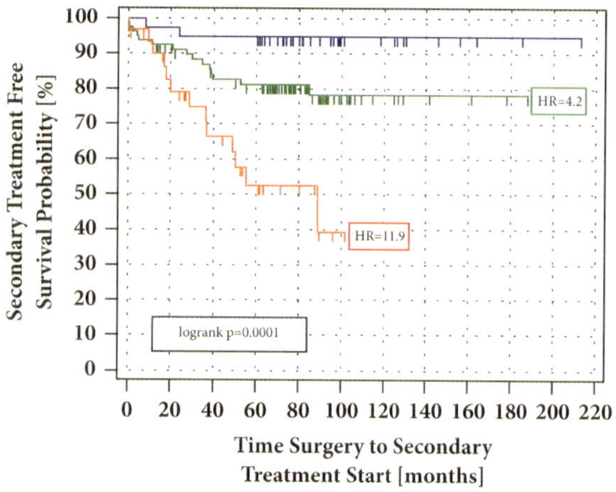

Number at risk

Group: CAPRA Scores (0-2)

38 37 36 36 23 12 10 6 3 2 1 0

Group: CAPRA Scores (3-5)

79 68 58 55 31 13 7 4 3 1 0 0

Group: CAPRA Scores (>5)

30 23 16 10 6 1 0 0 0 0 0 0

CAPRA Score Category

- CAPRA Scores (0-2)
- CAPRA Scores (3-5)
- CAPRA Scores (>5)

(e)

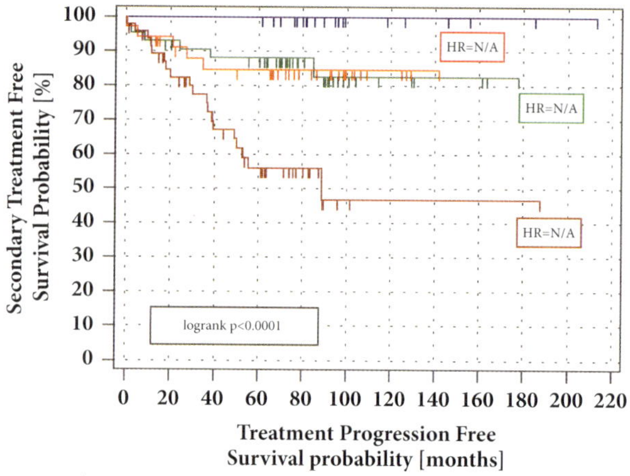

Number at risk

Group: Probability (<0.1)

22 22 22 22 16 7 6 5 2 2 1 0

Group: Probability (0.1 to <0.25)

42 39 36 35 17 8 5 3 3 0 0 0

Group: Probability (0.25 to <0.5)

35 30 26 25 17 9 5 1 0 0 0 0

Group: Probability (0.5 to 1.0)

48 37 26 19 10 2 1 1 1 1 0 0

CAPRA & PDE4D7 Score

- Probability (<0.1)
- Probability (0.1 to <0.25)
- Probability (0.25 to <0.5)
- Probability (0.5 to 1.0)

(f)

FIGURE 1: Kaplan-Meier survival analysis of the time to PSA relapse (endpoint: BCR) or start of any salvage therapy after radical prostatectomy (endpoint: STFS) in the DB patient cohort (n=151). **((a)-(c))** Kaplan-Meier analysis of the biochemical recurrence (BCR) free survival in the patient diagnostic biopsy (DB) cohort of the categorized PDE4D7 score, the CAPRA score categories, and the CAPRA & PDE4D7 score combination model. **((d)-(f))** Kaplan-Meier analysis of postsurgical secondary treatment free survival (STFS) in the patient diagnostic biopsy (DB) cohort of the categorized PDE4D7 score, the CAPRA score categories, and the CAPRA & PDE4D7 score combination model. The CAPRA & PDE4D7 combination model was developed by logistic regression in the RP patient cohort and used as such for testing in the DB patient cohort. Censored patients are indicated by vertical bars. PDE4D7 score categories were defined as PDE4D7 (1-2): PDE4D7 scores (1 to <2); PDE4D7 (2-3): PDE4D7 scores (2 to <3); PDE4D7 (3-4): PDE4D7 scores (3 to <4); PDE4D7 (4-5): PDE4D7 scores (4 to <=5). The CAPRA score categories were defined as CAPRA (1): CAPRA scores 0-2; CAPRA (2): CAPRA scores 3-5; CAPRA (3): CAPRA scores ≥6. The CAPRA & PDE4D7 score categories were defined according to the probability to experience PSA failure after surgery based on the logit(p) function of the logistic regression model. Four categories of probabilities were selected: p<0.1; p=0.1 to <0.25; p=0.25 to <0.5; p=0.5 to 1.0 to risk categorize the DB patients.

score alone (AUC=0.8 versus 0.73, respectively; Figure 2(b); p=0.026). This data may indicate an improved discrimination performance of the combination model in patients with higher risk characteristics.

Recently, the concept of decision curve analysis (DCA) was introduced to test the value of a biomarker or prediction model in clinical practice [24]. DCA is a net benefit analysis, which compares the true-positive to the weighted false-positive rates across different risk thresholds. We explored the net benefit of avoiding primary treatment based on the predicted risk of a PSA relapse after surgery for the CAPRA score, and the CAPRA & PDE4D7 combination model. The analysis demonstrated that the two models showed better net benefit compared to the "treat all" strategy while the combined CAPRA & PDE4D7 score revealed the best net benefit across all modeled decision thresholds (0-50%; Figure 3(a)). Similarly, the net reduction analysis in primary treatment based on the two tested decision models revealed a substantial difference in treatment reduction between the CARPA score and the CARPA & PDE4D7 combination model with decision thresholds ≤30% (Figure 3(b)). At higher decision thresholds above 30% the CAPRA score might perform equivalent to the CAPRA & PDE4D7 score. However, it seems questionable whether such thresholds of 30% and higher risk of disease recurrence and progression are of any practical relevance for a patient to avoid a primary treatment like surgery.

We have illustrated that a predictive model of the clinical risk algorithm CAPRA with the prostate cancer biomarker PDE4D7 in a diagnostic needle biopsy sample provides value

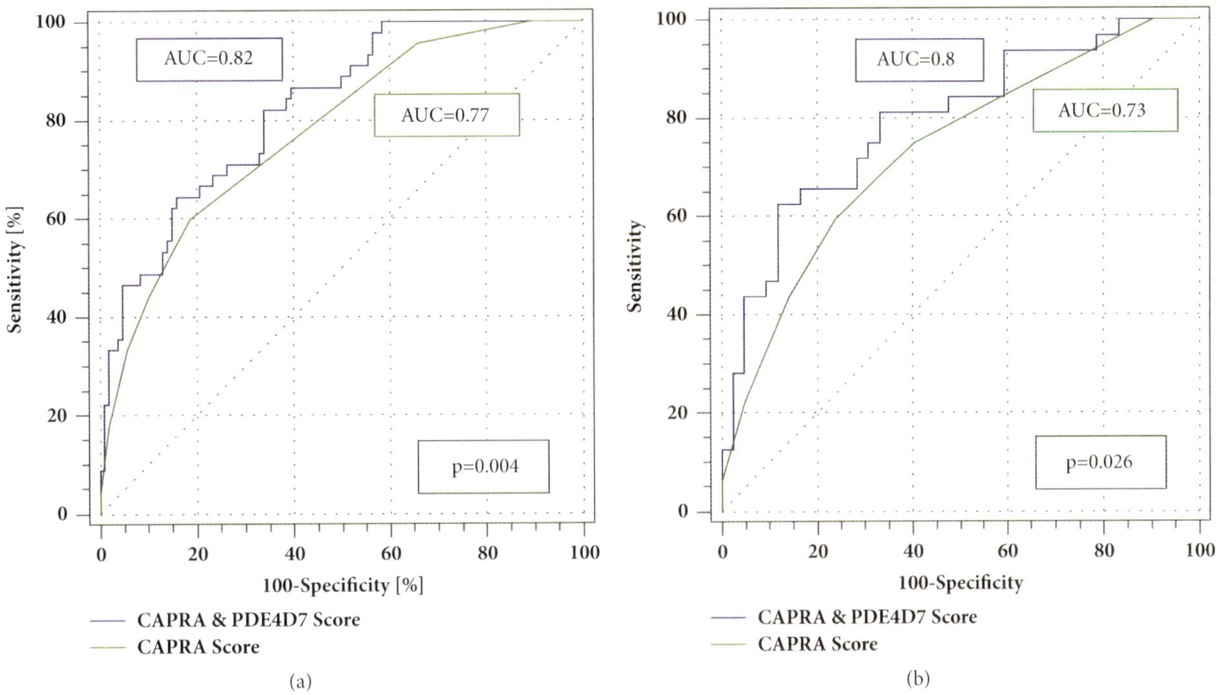

FIGURE 2: **(a)** ROC curve analysis of 5-year biochemical recurrence (BCR) in the DB cohort (n=151) of the CAPRAP score versus the CAPRA & PDE4D7 logistic regression model which was developed on the RP patient cohort with complete 5-year follow-up (n=449). **(b)** Subcohort ROC curve analysis of the 5-year biochemical recurrence (BCR) of CAPRA & PDE4D7 logistic regression model compared to the CAPRA model alone. In this analysis, only patients with a biopsy Gleason ≥7 were included (n=74).

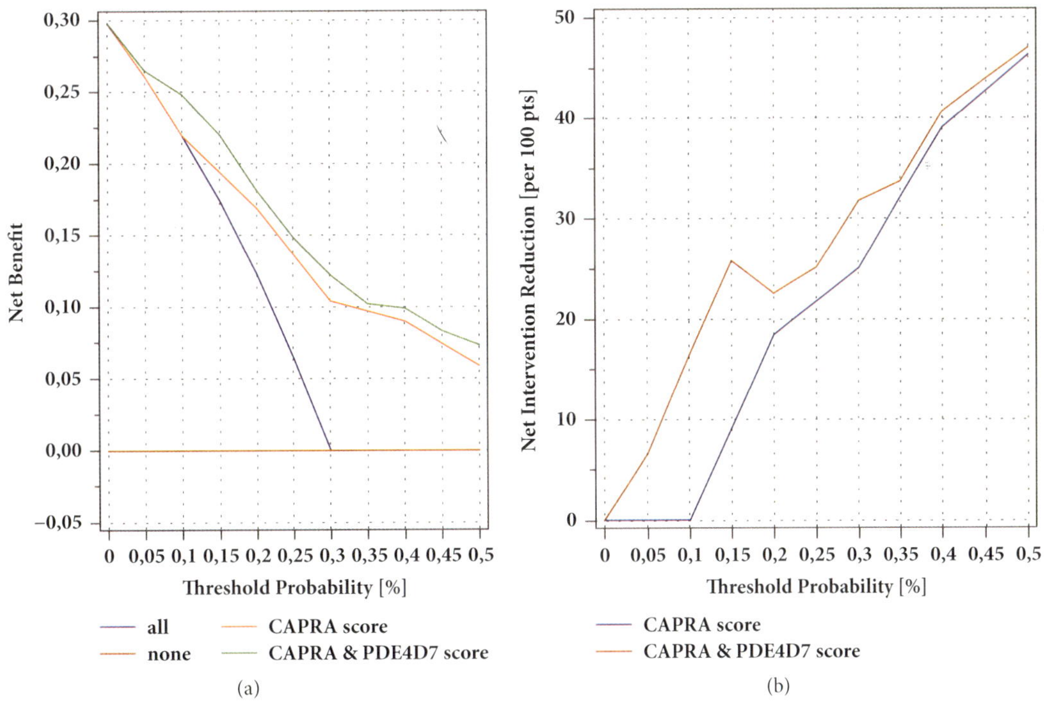

FIGURE 3: **(a)** Decision curve analysis in the diagnostic biopsy (DB) patient cohort of the net benefit of four different treatment decision strategies for men at risk of disease recurrence within 5 years after surgery. In total 45 of the 151 investigated patients failed the initial primary treatment of surgery by PSA recurrence (29.8%) within 5 years after intervention. Treatment strategies were tested for their net benefit across indicated threshold probabilities (0.05 step size) to trigger prostate surgery based on the probability of future disease recurrence. The CAPRA scores and the CAPRA & PDE4D7 scores were converted into 5-year BCR probabilities with logistic regression on the RP cohort (n=449 men with completed 5-year follow-up) before estimating net benefit. **(b)** Net reduction analyses demonstrating in how many patients a resection can be avoided based on the predicted risk of BCR derived from the CAPRA score and CAPRA & PDE4D7 score model, respectively.

to risk stratification. We have demonstrated in multiple analyses that this risk prediction model performs better in stratifying prostate cancer patients to treatment relevant risk categories compared to risk schemas solely based on clinical parameters.

4. Discussion

Recently, we have reported the association of the PDE4D7 score to postsurgical disease recurrence in a radical prostatectomy (RP) patient cohort. Here we aimed to demonstrate that a logistic regression model developed on the same RP cohort using the preclinical risk score CAPRA with the PDE4D7 score remains its prognostic power in diagnostic needle biopsy (DB) patients. Thus, we were able to confirm the associated hazard ratio (~0.5 per score unit change) in this DB cohort to predict biochemical failure after surgery in the same order of magnitude as shown on surgical tumor tissue. We conclude that the associated hazard of the PDE4D7 score is stable across independent patient cohorts as well as in different tissue collection settings (diagnostic biopsies versus surgical resections).

Treatment decisions in primary, localized prostate cancer are largely subject to a combination of the risk of future disease progression and life expectancy. The National Comprehensive Cancer Network (NCCN) has defined six risk categories based on pretreatment clinical variables [3]. Depending on the clinical risk various options of interventions are presented in the guidelines. Multiple tools of clinical risk prediction have been developed in the form of mathematical models, which combine the value of clinical variables into a single score [25]. One of the most extensively validated clinical risk algorithms for pretreatment decision support is the CAPRA score [21]. The score is a combination of clinically available information. Originally reported in 2005, this score has been validated in several studies since then [23]. Our data illustrate that the PDE4D7 score adds important prognostic value to clinical prediction models, such as the CAPRA score, for disease-specific outcomes to support treatment decision-making.

Recently, the long-term results of the active surveillance cohort within the Göteborg randomized prostate cancer screening trial were published [26]. This data indicated that men with clinically low risk disease may have a considerable risk to experience progressive disease under a deferred treatment regime. Therefore, the authors questioned whether men other than those with very low risk disease would be eligible for expectant management strategies. The recent publication of the 10-year outcomes of the ProtecT study indicates similar conclusions in the active monitoring arm of the trial [27]. Although there is some debate about the validity of these results to contemporary practice [28] they suggest that only patients with the very lowest risk are safe of any progression during deferred treatment management. While the use of clinical criteria like CAPRA allow the selection of such a low risk patient cohort the addition of molecular markers can be expected to enlarge this very low risk patient group or further reduce the risk within this cohort. In fact, our combined CAPRA & PDE4D7 regression model defines a very low risk cohort of 22 out of 151 patients (14.6%) in the DB patient cohort with a progression-free survival (PFS) of 100% over a follow-up period of more than 15 years compared to a PFS of 85.6% for the CAPRA score alone.

Active surveillance (AS) has been established as a safe treatment alternative for men with low risk prostate cancer over the last years [29]. However, the challenge associated with AS relates to the strict monitoring schedules that men are advised to follow in order not to miss signs of progressive disease. These include the identification of elevations in PSA and upgrading of biopsy Gleason scores, which are typically "protocol triggers" to switch from AS to active treatment. Longitudinal AS studies have published decreasing patient compliance to the monitoring protocols in AS over time in particular when it comes to additional biopsy procedures [30, 31]. This issue might be addressed with a selection algorithm such as that proposed here, i.e., the combination of the CAPRA score with the prognostic genomic biomarker PDE4D7, in order to define a patient cohort with virtually no risk of future disease progression. Although this finding has to be confirmed in an AS setting, this might provide a way forward to include men into active surveillance on the basis of very limited (or no) follow-up for a given time period after the initiation of AS.

4.1. Limitations. A potential limitation of this study might be the sample size of the diagnostic biopsy cohort used for the CAPRA & PDE4D7 model validation. However, the measured endpoints of BCR and of secondary treatment start provide a relevant number of events (36.4% and 19.9%, respectively) for validation testing. Nevertheless, we appreciate the fact that further validation of this model is required which is warranted by the so far presented results. Another limitation might be in the selection of BCR (biochemical recurrence) as a tested endpoint. The follow-up of the diagnostic biopsy cohort was too limited to enable the testing for clinical recurrence or prostate cancer death. However, to our opinion, BCR is still a treatment relevant endpoint and is used as a decision point to a start secondary treatment in a majority of the patients (e.g., in 73.2% of patients in the RP cohort who experienced BCR a secondary treatment was started). Furthermore, PSA progression is also a typical protocol-based trigger to stop active surveillance and initiate an active intervention. Ultimately, we believe that it is important to understand the risk to experience this endpoint for an optimal treatment decision.

5. Conclusions

With the data presented here we have further validated the prognostic power of the prostate cancer biomarker PDE4D7. We have demonstrated that the PDE4D7 score has equivalent performance to predict longitudinal prostate cancer outcomes when tested on tumor tissue of a diagnostic biopsy sample compared to a cancer sample that was collected after prostate resection during surgery. This study illustrates the potential of PDE4D7 for clinical use to improve presurgical risk stratification in conjunction with the routinely used prognostic clinical risk models.

TABLE 2: Uni- and multivariate Cox regression analysis of biochemical recurrence (BCR) free survival and overall survival (OS) of the continuous PDE4D7 scores. In multivariate analysis, the PDE4D7 scores were adjusted by presurgical clinical variables or the CAPRA score as indicated. Biopsy Gleason and pathology stage were modeled as categories. All other demographic and clinical variables as well as the PDE4D7 scores were modeled as continuous variables. All variables were entered into the multivariate modeling. **(a)** Uni- and multivariate Cox regression analysis of the biochemical recurrence (BCR) free survival of the PDE4D7 score in the RP study cohort (n=503; 148 (29.4%) events); multivariate analysis was adjusted for presurgical variables or CAPRA scores. **(b)** Uni- and multivariate Cox regression analysis of the biochemical recurrence (BCR) free survival of the PDE4D7 score in the DB study cohort (n=151; 55 (36.4%) events); multivariate analysis was adjusted for presurgical variables or CAPRA scores. PDE4D7 score categories were defined as PDE4D7 (1-2): PDE4D7 scores (1 to <2); PDE4D7 (2-3): PDE4D7 scores (2 to <3); PDE4D7 (3-4): PDE4D7 scores (3 to <4); PDE4D7 (4-5): PDE4D7 scores (4 to <=5).

(a)

Pre-Surgical Clinical Parameters		**univariate**			**multivariate**	
Endpoint BCR (#148/#503; 29.4%)	**p value**	**HR**	**95% CI of HR**	**p value**	**HR**	**95% CI of HR**
Age at surgery	0,88	1,0	0.97 -1.03	0,77	1,00	0.96 to 1.02
Preoperative PSA	0,0002	1,03	1.01-1.04	0,00	1,08	1.03 to 1.1
PSA density	0,0100	2,15	1.2 to 3.8	0,03	0,12	0.02 to 0.8
Biopsy Gleason Score 3+3 (N=316); reference						
Biopsy Gleason Score 3+4 (N=149)	0,0003	1,9	1.4-2.8	0,02	1,56	1.06 to 2.3
Biopsy Gleason Score >=4+3 (N=38)	<0.0001	6,2	3.9-9.7	<0.0001	4,82	2.9 to 7.9
Percentage Positive Biopsy Cores	<0.0001	4,2	2.3-7.7	0,08	2,29	0.91 to 5.7
Percentage Tumor in Biopsy	<0.0001	1,0	1.02-1.04	0,00	1,02	1.01 to 1.04
Clinical stage cT1c (N= 342); reference						
Clinical stages cT2 & cT3 (N=161)	<0.0001	2,1	1.5 to 2.9	0,20	1,27	0.88 to 1.8
PDE4D7 (continuous)	<0.0001	0,53	0.41 to 0.67	<0.0001	0,52	0.4 to 0.68
Pre-Surgical Clinical Parameters		**univariate**			**multivariate**	
Endpoint BCR (#148/#503; 29.4%)	**p value**	**HR**	**95% CI of HR**	**p value**	**HR**	**95% CI of HR**
CAPRA Score	<0.0001	1,5	1.3 to 1.6	<0.0001	1,7	1.5 to 1.9
PDE4D7 (continuous)	<0.0001	0,47	0.33 to 0.65	<0.0001	0,56	0.43 to 0.72

(b)

Pre-Surgical Clinical Parameters		**univariate**			**multivariate**	
Endpoint BCR (#55/#151; 36.4%)	**p value**	**HR**	**95% CI of HR**	**p value**	**HR**	**95% CI of HR**
Age at surgery	0,81	0,99	0.95 to 1.04	0,006	0,94	0.89 to 0.98
Preoperative PSA	0,0001	1,04	1.02 to 1.06	0,002	1,1	1.03 to 1.2
PSA Density	0,003	2,7	1.4 to 5.3	0,18	0,26	0.04 to 1.9
Biopsy Gleason GG1 (n=85); reference						
Biopsy Gleason GG2 (n=44)	0,07	1,9	0.95 to 3.8	0,10	1,9	0.89 to 3.9
Biopsy Gleason GG3 (n=20)	0,0001	4,3	2.04 to 9.2	0,02	2,6	1.2 to 5.7
Biopsy Gleason GG4 (n=7)	0,0007	5,7	2.1 to 15.8	0,01	4,1	1.4 to 11.6
Biopsy Gleason GG5 (n=11)	<0.0001	8,0	3.5 to 18.4	0,03	2,9	1.1 to 7.6
Percentage Positive Biopsy Cores	0,013	4,6	1.4 to 15.2	0,19	2,4	0.63 to 9.4
Clinical stage cT2 (n= 108); reference						
Clinical stage cT3 (n=60)	0,007	2,0	1.2 to 3.4	0,05	1,7	0.99 to 3.1
PDE4D7 (continuous)	<0.0001	0,47	0.33 to 0.65	<0.0001	0,43	0.29 to 0.63
Pre-Surgical Clinical Parameters		**univariate**			**multivariate**	
Endpoint BCR (#55/#151; 36.4%)	**p value**	**HR**	**95% CI of HR**	**p value**	**HR**	**95% CI of HR**
CAPRA Score	<0.0001	1,5	1.3 to 1.6	<0.0001	1,4	1.2 to 1.6
PDE4D7 (continuous)	<0.0001	0,47	0.33 to 0.65	0,0001	0,53	0.38 to 0.74

Abbreviations

AS:	Active surveillance
RP:	Radical prostatectomy
DB:	Diagnostic biopsy
BCR:	Biochemical recurrence
STFS:	Secondary treatment free survival
HR:	Hazard ratio
CI:	Confidence interval
NPV:	Negative predictive value
AUC:	Area under the curve
DCA:	Decision curve analysis
CAPRA score:	Cancer of the Prostate Risk Assessment score.

Acknowledgments

This project was supported by the framework of CTMM (The Center for Translational Molecular Medicine, The Netherlands), PCMM project (Grant 03O-203). The authors gratefully thank Dr. G. Sauter and Ms. C. Koop for providing the surgical biopsy punches.

References

[1] J. Ferlay, I. Soerjomataram, and M. Ervik, "GLOBOCAN 2012 v1.0, Cancer Incidence and Mortality Worldwide: IARC CancerBase. No. 11 [Internet]," Lyon. Fr. Int. Agency Res. Cancer 11: http://globocan.iarc.fr, 2013.

[2] G. Rodrigues, P. Warde, T. Pickles et al., "Pre-treatment risk stratification of prostate cancer patients: A critical review," *Canadian Urological Association Journal*, vol. 6, no. 2, pp. 121–127, 2012.

[3] J. L. Mohler, A. J. Armstrong, R. R. Bahnson et al., "NCCN clinical practice guidelines in oncology: Prostate cancer Version 1," *Journal of the National Comprehensive Cancer Network*, vol. 14, no. 1, pp. 19–30, 2016.

[4] D. J. Hernandez, M. E. Nielsen, M. Han, and A. W. Partin, "Contemporary Evaluation of the D'Amico Risk Classification of Prostate Cancer," *Urology*, vol. 70, no. 5, pp. 931–935, 2007.

[5] S. A. Boorjian, R. J. Karnes, L. J. Rangel, E. J. Bergstralh, and M. L. Blute, "Mayo Clinic Validation of the D'Amico Risk Group Classification for Predicting Survival Following Radical Prostatectomy," *The Journal of Urology*, vol. 179, no. 4, pp. 1354–1361, 2008.

[6] A. C. Reese, P. M. Pierorazio, M. Han et al., "Contemporary evaluation of the national comprehensive cancer network prostate cancer risk classification system," *Urology*, vol. 80, no. 5, pp. 1075–1079, 2012.

[7] G. Gandaglia, J. Schiffmann, T. Schlomm et al., "Identification of pathologically favorable disease in intermediate-risk prostate cancer patients: Implications for active surveillance candidates selection," *The Prostate*, vol. 75, no. 13, pp. 1484–1491, 2015.

[8] J.-W. Jung, J. K. Lee, S. K. Hong, S.-S. Byun, and S. E. Lee, "Stratification of patients with intermediate-risk prostate cancer," *BJU International*, vol. 115, no. 6, pp. 907–912, 2015.

[9] S. K. Hong, E. Vertosick, D. D. Sjoberg, P. T. Scardino, and J. A. Eastham, "Insignificant disease among men with intermediate-risk prostate cancer," *World Journal of Urology*, vol. 32, no. 6, pp. 1417–1421, 2014.

[10] M. R. Abern, W. J. Aronson, M. K. Terris et al., "Delayed radical prostatectomy for intermediate-risk prostate cancer is associated with biochemical recurrence: Possible implications for active surveillance from the SEARCH database," *The Prostate*, vol. 73, no. 4, pp. 409–417, 2013.

[11] K. Taskén and E. M. Aandahl, "Localized Effects of cAMP Mediated by Distinct Routes of Protein Kinase A," *Physiological Reviews*, vol. 84, no. 1, pp. 137–167, 2004.

[12] U. Banerjee and X. Cheng, "Exchange protein directly activated by cAMP encoded by the mammalian rapgef3 gene: Structure, function and therapeutics," *Gene*, vol. 570, no. 2, pp. 157–167, 2015.

[13] G. Pidoux and K. Tasken, "Specificity and spatial dynamics of PKA signaling organized by A kinase anchoring proteins," *Molecular Endocrinology*, vol. 44, no. 5, pp. 271–284, 2010.

[14] M. D. Houslay, "Underpinning compartmentalised cAMP signalling through targeted cAMP breakdown," *Trends in Biochemical Sciences*, vol. 35, no. 2, pp. 91–100, 2010.

[15] K. F. Houslay, F. Christian, R. MacLeod, D. R. Adams, M. D. Houslay, and G. S. Baillie, "Identification of a multifunctional docking site on the catalytic unit of phosphodiesterase-4 (PDE4) that is utilised by multiple interaction partners," *Biochemical Journal*, vol. 474, no. 4, pp. 597–609, 2017.

[16] E. Huston, M. J. Lynch, A. Mohamed et al., "EPAC and PKA allow cAMP dual control over DNA-PK nuclear translocation," *Proceedings of the National Acadamy of Sciences of the United States of America*, vol. 105, no. 35, pp. 12791–12796, 2008.

[17] T. Kaname, C.-S. Ki, N. Niikawa et al., "Heterozygous mutations in cyclic AMP phosphodiesterase-4D (PDE4D) and protein kinase A (PKA) provide new insights into the molecular pathology of acrodysostosis," *Cellular Signalling*, vol. 26, no. 11, pp. 2446–2459, 2014.

[18] M. Alves de Inda, D. van Strijp, E. den Biezen-Timmermans et al., "Validation of Cyclic Adenosine Monophosphate Phosphodiesterase-4D7 for its Independent Contribution to Risk Stratification in a Prostate Cancer Patient Cohort with Longitudinal Biological Outcomes," *European Urology Focus*, vol. 13, 2017.

[19] R. Böttcher, K. Dulla, D. Van Strijp et al., "Human PDE4D isoform composition is deregulated in primary prostate cancer and indicative for disease progression and development of distant metastases," *Oncotarget*, vol. 7, no. 43, pp. 70669–70684, 2016.

[20] B. S. Taylor, N. Schultz, H. Hieronymus et al., "Integrative genomic profiling of human prostate cancer," *Cancer Cell*, vol. 18, no. 1, pp. 11–22, 2010.

[21] M. R. Cooperberg, D. J. Pasta, E. P. Elkin et al., "The UCSF Cancer of the Prostate Risk Assessment (CAPRA) Score: a straightforward and reliable preoperative predictor of disease recurrence after radical prostatectomy," *The Journal of Urology*, vol. 173, pp. 1938–1942, 2005.

[22] A. J. Vickers, A. M. Cronin, E. B. Elkin, and M. Gonen, "Extensions to decision curve analysis, a novel method for evaluating diagnostic tests, prediction models and molecular markers," *BMC Medical Informatics and Decision Making*, vol. 8, pp. 1–17, 2008.

[23] J. S. Brajtbord, M. S. Leapman, and M. R. Cooperberg, "The CAPRA Score at 10 Years: Contemporary Perspectives and Analysis of Supporting Studies," *European Urology*, vol. 71, no. 5, pp. 705–709, 2017.

[24] A. J. Vickers, B. Van Calster, and E. W. Steyerberg, "Net benefit approaches to the evaluation of prediction models, molecular markers, and diagnostic tests," *BMJ*, vol. 25, p. 352, 2016.

[25] G. Lughezzani, A. Briganti, P. I. Karakiewicz et al., "Predictive and prognostic models in radical prostatectomy candidates: A critical analysis of the literature," *European Urology*, vol. 58, no. 5, pp. 687–700, 2010.

[26] R. A. Godtman, E. Holmberg, A. Khatami, C.-G. Pihl, J. Stranne, and J. Hugosson, "Long-term Results of Active Surveillance in the Göteborg Randomized, Population-based Prostate Cancer Screening Trial," *European Urology*, vol. 70, no. 5, pp. 760–766, 2016.

[27] F. C. Hamdy, J. L. Donovan, J. A. Lane et al., "10-Year outcomes after monitoring, surgery, or radiotherapy for localized prostate cancer," *The New England Journal of Medicine*, vol. 375, no. 15, pp. 1415–1424, 2016.

[28] R. C. N. van den Bergh, D. G. Murphy, and H. G. van der Poel, "Expectant Management for Prostate Cancer: Lessons from the Past, Challenges for the Future," *European Urology*, vol. 70, no. 5, pp. 767-768, 2016.

[29] L. Klotz, "Active surveillance for low-risk prostate cancer," *Current Opinion in Urology*, vol. 27, pp. 225–230, 2016.

[30] L. P. Bokhorst, A. R. Alberts, A. Rannikko et al., "Compliance rates with the Prostate Cancer Research International Active Surveillance (PRIAS) protocol and disease reclassification in noncompliers," *European Urology*, vol. 68, no. 5, pp. 814–821, 2015.

[31] M. S. Leapman and P. R. Carroll, "What is the best way not to treat prostate cancer?" *Urologic Oncology: Seminars and Original Investigations*, vol. 35, no. 2, pp. 42–50, 2017.

24

Systematic Review of Focal Prostate Brachytherapy and the Future Implementation of Image-Guided Prostate HDR Brachytherapy Using MR-Ultrasound Fusion

M. Sean Peach, Daniel M. Trifiletti, and Bruce Libby

Department of Radiation Oncology, University of Virginia School of Medicine, Charlottesville, VA 22908, USA

Correspondence should be addressed to Bruce Libby; bl8b@hscmail.mcc.virginia.edu

Academic Editor: Hendrik Van Poppel

Prostate cancer is the most common malignancy found in North American and European men and the second most common cause of cancer related death. Since the practice of PSA screening has become common the disease is most often found early and can have a long indolent course. Current definitive therapy treats the whole gland but has considerable long-term side effects. Focal therapies may be able to target the cancer while decreasing dose to organs at risk. Our objective was to determine if focal prostate brachytherapy could meet target objectives while permitting a decrease in dose to organs at risk in a way that would allow future salvage treatments. Further, we wanted to determine if focal treatment results in less toxicity. Utilizing the Medline repository, dosimetric papers comparing whole gland to partial gland brachytherapy and clinical papers that reported toxicity of focal brachytherapy were selected. A total of 9 dosimetric and 6 clinical papers met these inclusion criteria. Together, these manuscripts suggest that focal brachytherapy may be employed to decrease dose to organs at risk with decreased toxicity. Of current technology, image-guided HDR brachytherapy using MRI registered to transrectal ultrasound offers the flexibility and efficiency to achieve such focal treatments.

1. Introduction

Radiation therapy (RT) for prostate cancer came into common use in the United States utilizing an external beam approach during the 1920s. However, disease was often inadequately treated due to poor tissue penetration along with significant dermal morbidity produced by the treatment [1]. Combined with the development of androgen therapy there was lost interest in RT. Additionally, there was a decrease utilization of brachytherapy for all disease sites in the first half of the 20th century due to the significant radiation exposure to nurses and physicians. These shortcomings were overcome by the development of low activity radioactive iodine seeds that required minimal shielding during handling and, once placed in patients, released a negligible dose to the outside environment [2]. These seeds were first successfully employed for prostate cancer at Memorial Sloan Kettering in 1967, with hundreds of subsequent cases in the 1970s using the Whitmore open hand technique. Briefly, a laparotomy was performed and the prostate was mobilized from all but the posterior rectal facing wall. Evenly spaced empty catheters were then placed through the exposed prostate until felt by the physician rectally, followed by permanent seed placement. It was determined that doses greater than 100 Gy produced a five-year disease-free survival rate of 80%. However, there were considerable long-term issues with inadequate coverage and morbidity from the invasive nature of the procedure; thus the technique was abandoned by the mid 1980s.

At the time that the free hand technique was in decline there were several advancements made in diagnostic imaging that would have profound impact on prostate brachytherapy. Holm was able to combine the application of ultrasound (US) guided seed placement for pancreatic cancer with transrectal US (TRUS) to develop US guided low dose rate (LDR) prostate brachytherapy. In Europe this was combined with external beam radiation therapy (EBRT) on a series of patients. However the high dose (160 Gy LDR and 46 Gy EBRT) resulted in significant side effects [3]. In the early

1990s this technique was refined by utilizing lower doses, achieving outcomes similar to prostatectomy with less overall side effects [4]. By the mid 1990s high dose rate brachytherapy (HDR) was practiced at a handful of centers, which offered an additional degree of conformity by being able to shape the delivered dose based on computer optimization of source dwell times. As a result of these developments prostate brachytherapy either as monotherapy or as part of a combined EBRT regimen has become a mainstream therapeutic option for low risk and intermediate risk prostate cancer [5].

There are significant risks of side effects associated with either surgery or RT, including urinary toxicity, erectile dysfunction, and, in the case of RT, rectal toxicity. In the pre-PSA era, prostate disease was not detected until it was more advanced, requiring treatment of the entire gland and immediate periphery to control disease and impart increased survival. Thus such symptoms were viewed as an acceptable necessity. With the advent of PSA screening in the 1990s and a better understanding of the behavior of prostate cancer, disease in the modern PSA era is found significantly earlier and typically has a more indolent course [6]. In patients with low risk disease active surveillance is an acceptable option, as well as prostatectomy or brachytherapy +/− EBRT [5]. However, for younger patients with isolated lesions a more ideal treatment would be to treat the focus of disease without affecting the urethra or neurovascular bundles which cause the most detrimental side effects of traditional therapies, namely, genitourinary toxicity and erectile dysfunction (ED). These treatment related issues become increasingly significant as the average life span of the population increases, with future patients living increasingly longer with whatever side effects treatment imparts. With advances in imaging modalities partial prostate brachytherapy may be applied with limited toxicity to what is a large patient population who want a temporary measure, with low side effects, but still affords salvage RT or surgery in the future if needed.

In this paper, we perform a systematic review to explore the up-to-date dosimetric and clinical studies of focal and focused prostate brachytherapy. We postulate that focal brachytherapy may offer a salvageable therapy that provides lower side effects. Given the dosimetric advantages of HDR prostate brachytherapy [7, 8] and the expanded use of prostate/pelvic MRI in clinical workups, intraoperative planned HDR brachytherapy utilizing TRUS registered, MRI tumor delineation would provide a reliable and efficient strategy to implant focal prostate brachytherapy at most radiotherapy centers.

2. Methods

2.1. Selection of Studies. Two separate searches were performed with two slightly different search criteria. A PubMed database search for the terms "focal + brachytherapy + prostate" and for "partial + brachytherapy + prostate" with no limits placed on publication date was completed (10/16/2015). All non-English language manuscripts were then removed at which point the abstracts of the remaining manuscripts were read. Those manuscripts that did not concentrate on focal or focused prostate brachytherapy or were review papers were removed from this pool. Focused treatments where deemed as those in which the whole gland was treated with brachytherapy; however there was a focal boost in the plan in an attempt to deliver more dose to the gross tumor volume (GTV) and/or decrease toxicity to nearby organs at risk (OARs). Inclusion criteria for manuscripts in the final analysis included dosimetric studies that demonstrated treatment and organ at risk dosimetric data of whole gland (HG) compared to focal or focused treatments. Clinical study inclusion criteria included works involving focal or focused brachytherapy that reported treatment toxicity.

2.2. Data Extraction and Clinical Endpoints. Data extraction was conducted according to the Preferred Reporting Items for Systematic Reviews and Meta-Analyses (PRISMA) statement [9]. For each study, the following information was extracted: name of the first author, year of publication, number of participants included in analysis, brachytherapy type (HDR versus LDR), RT protocol (whether focal or focused and whether monotherapy or with EBRT), planning imaging modality, and treatment imaging modality. The primary measure of interest for the analysis of dosimetric studies was if OAR and GTV doses were reported for both partial and whole gland treatments which would provide evidence as to whether partial gland therapy is amenable to future definitive salvage therapy (what will be referred to as salvageability). The primary measure of interest for the analysis of clinical studies was toxicity, with secondary interests, if available, in treatment efficacy in regard to survival parameters and treatment dosimetry details. Preliminary analysis indicated that the data provided was insufficient for meta-analysis, thus this work was followed as a PRISMA style systematic review.

3. Results

3.1. Selection of Manuscripts. As outlined in Figure 1, the initial search yielded combined 154 results. Removal of duplicates and non-English language manuscripts reduced this number to 138. All review articles were removed which reduced the pool of papers to 99. The abstracts of these manuscripts were then read to determine if the work concentrated on focal or focused prostate brachytherapy. Resulting 32 papers met these eligibility criteria and were read in entirety for final inclusion. Criteria for dosimetric papers considered for final inclusion were those in which disease target prescription and dose to OARs were characterized between whole gland and focal/focused treatments. Clinical papers were required to demonstrate side effects of focal/focused brachytherapy treatments. In total, 9 dosimetric manuscripts (Table 1) and 6 clinical manuscripts (Table 2) met all eligibility requirements.

3.2. Patterns between Selected Dosimetric Manuscripts. The nine dosimetric studies included in this systematic review were published between 2009 and 2015 with a heavy weighting towards more recent publications. There were three different groups/collaborators that contributed more than

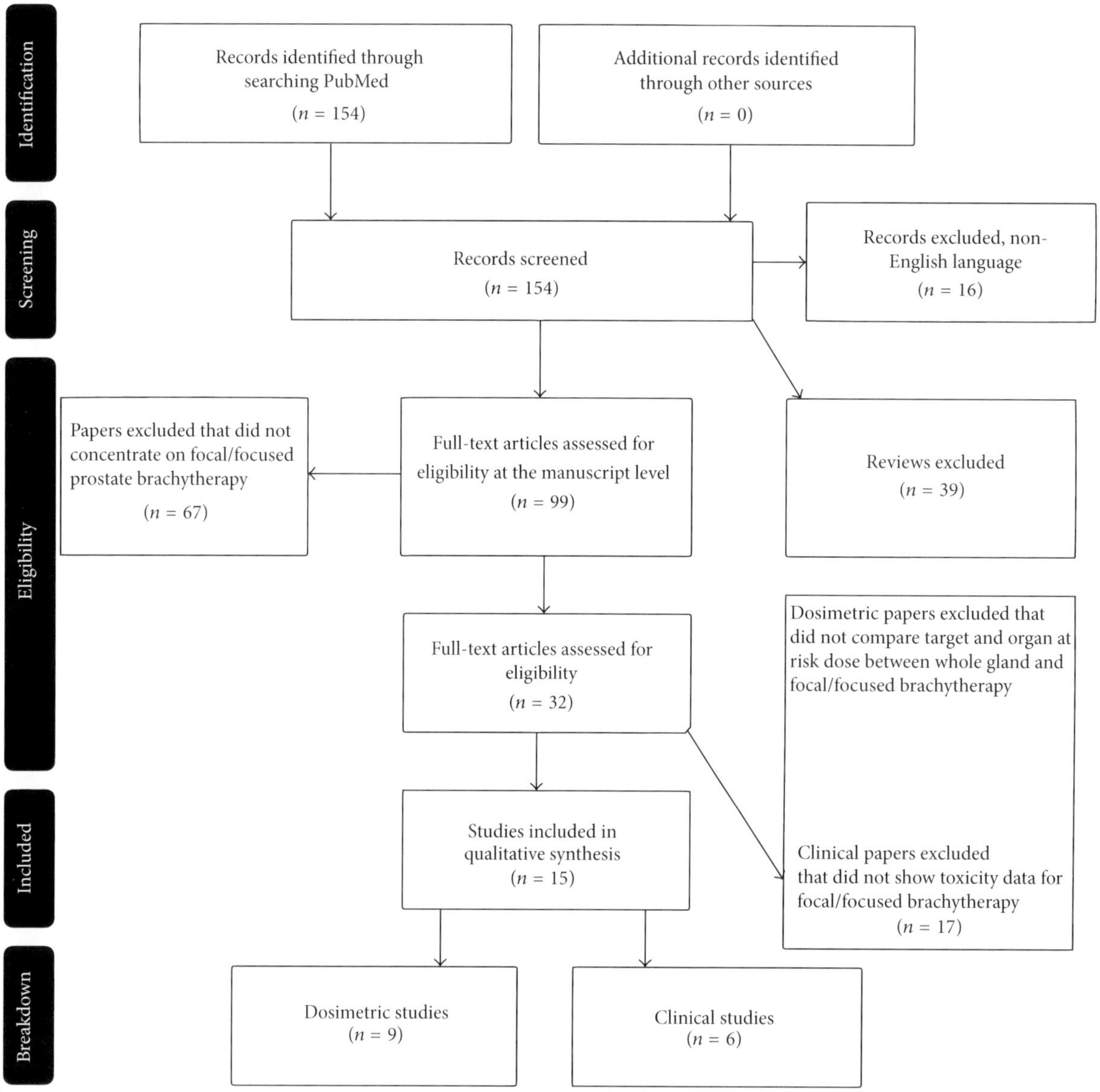

FIGURE 1: Literature selection process (PRISMA flow diagram).

one publication but looked at different aspects of focal and focused brachytherapy. These included significant work by Mason et al. and Al-Qaisieh et al. [10–13], Kamrava et al. and Banerjee et al. [14, 15], and Peters et al. and Moman et al. [16, 17]. Sample size ranged from 2 to 15 with an average of 9 subjects per study. Of the manuscripts, 3 involved focused treatments [11, 13, 18], one hemigland treatment [14], two focal treatments [17, 19], and three hemi/focal treatments [10, 12, 13], all of which were compared to whole gland therapy (Table 1). One work involved focal treatment as salvage therapy [17], while the rest were initial cancer treatment studies. In regard to planning imaging two manuscripts utilized CT to treat the whole prostate and an arbitrary focus [14, 15]. The remaining works used various MRI sequences alone [11–13, 19], MRI with MR spectroscopy (MRS) [18], or MRI combined with positional information from prostate biopsy [10, 17]. HDR was employed in 6 of the 9 studies [11–15, 17] with LDR seeds in the rest [10, 18, 19]. Two of the HDR studies were plans combined with EBRT [11, 13], while the rest were brachytherapy monotherapy. In regard to HDR monotherapy fractionation, two studies employed a single fraction [12] (one of which was a salvage treatment [17]), while the rest used 6 fractions [14, 15].

Comparison of the target/OAR doses of the partial gland plans to whole gland therapy demonstrated three patterns. Two works using partial gland therapy demonstrated a similar dose to tumor volume and less dose to OARs [14, 19]. Higher dose to the GTV was achieved by partial therapy while maintaining the same dose to the OARs as whole gland in two publications [11, 13]. The remaining 5 manuscripts were able to achieve superior tumor dose with less involvement of the OARs with partial therapy [10, 12, 15, 17, 18]. As previously

Table 1: Summary of dosimetric manuscripts.

Author/year	Focal/focused	Tumor imaging	Treatment imaging	Patient number/technique	Dosing data summary	Sal
Todor et al. 2011 [18]	Focused	MRI/MRS	MRI reg US	$n = 2$ LDR standard versus boost mix of I^{125}, Pd^{103}, and Cs^{131} seeds	Mixed seeds allowed 20%–66% increase in dose to tumor PTV while decreasing urethra dose by 10% compared to standard single type seed plans	No
Kamrava et al. 2013 [14]	Focal	CT	CT	$n = 10$ HDR 7.25 Gy × 6, WG versus HG plans	WG: D90 112%, V100 97.6%, V150 33.8%, $D2cc_{Rectum}$ 64.1%, $D2cc_{Bladder}$ 67.5%, $D2cc_{Urethra}$ 95.2% HG: D90 108%, V100 98.8%, V150 26.5%, $D2cc_{Rectum}$ 53.1%, $D2cc_{Bladder}$ 55.9%, $D2cc_{Urethra}$ 69.3%	Yes
Mason et al. 2014 [11]	Focused	MRI	MRI reg US	$n = 15$ HDR 15 Gy × 1 fx and then 37.5 Gy in 15 fx EBRT fG versus WG	WG: median D90 17.6 Gy, V150 27.3%, $D10cc_{Urethra}$ 17.2 Gy, $D2cc_{Rectum}$ 8 Gy fG: median D90 20.9 Gy, V150 75.9%, $D10cc_{Urethra}$ 17.4 Gy, $D2cc_{Rectum}$ 9 Gy	No
Mason et al. 2014 [12]	Focal	MRI	MRI reg US	$n = 9$ HDR 19 Gy × 1, WG versus HG versus FG	WG: D90 20.4 Gy, V100 97.9%, $D2cc_{Rectal}$ 20.3 Gy, $D10_{Urethra}$ 12.5 Gy HG: D90 22.2 Gy, V100 98.1%, $D2cc_{Rectal}$ 19.7 Gy, $D10_{Urethra}$ 9.8 Gy FG: D90 23.0 Gy, V100 98.2%, $D2cc_{Rectal}$ 9.2 Gy, $D10_{Urethra}$ 4.6 Gy	Yes
Polders et al. 2015 [19]	Focal	MRI	MRI reg US	$n = 15$ LDR I^{125} 145 Gy × 1 fx, WG versus FG	WG: $D90_{GTV}$ 198 ± 44 Gy, $V100_{GTV}$ 94% (89–100), $D2cc_{Rectal}$ 99 ± 19 Gy, $D10_{Urethra}$ 214 ± 21 Gy, FG: $D90_{GTV}$ 195 ± 60 Gy, $V100_{GTV}$ 94% (71–100), $D2cc_{Rectal}$ 37 ± 21 Gy, $D10_{Urethra}$ 79 ± 33 Gy,	Yes
Banerjee et al. 2015 [15]	Focal	CT	CT	$n = 5$ HDR 7.25 Gy × 6 fx, WG versus HG versus 1/6 gland	WG: D90 109.3% V100 98.7 $D2cc_{Bladder}$ 64.8%, $D2cc_{Rectal}$ 65.3%, $D1cc_{Urethra}$ 103.8%$V75_{Urethra}$ 75% HG: D90 112.7% V100 97.8 $D2cc_{Bladder}$ 56.2%$D2cc_{Rectal}$ 54.2%$D1cc_{Urethra}$ 86.5%$V75_{Urethra}$ 57.1% 1/6 gland: D90 114.7% V100 97.4 $D2cc_{Bladder}$ 24.7%, $D2cc_{Rectal}$ 32.8%, $D1cc_{Urethra}$ 52.1%$V75_{Urethra}$ 14.5%	Yes
Al-Qaisieh et al. 2015 [10]	Focal	MRI/biopsy mapping	MRI reg US	$n = 14$ LDR I^{125} 145 Gy × 1 fx WG versus HG versus FG	WG: D90 181.3 Gy, V100 99.8%, $D2cc_{Rectal}$ 107.5 Gy, $D10_{Urethra}$ 205.9 Gy HG: D90 195.7 Gy, V100 97.8%, $D2cc_{Rectal}$ 77.0 Gy, $D10_{Urethra}$ 191.4 Gy FG: D90 205.9 Gy, V100 99.8%, $D2cc_{Rectal}$ 42.7 Gy, $D10_{Urethra}$ 92.4 Gy	Yes
Mason et al. 2015 [13]	Focused	MRI	MRI reg US	$n = 15$ HDR 15 Gy × 1 fx followed by EBRT 37.5 Gy in 15 fx. WG versus fG	Median values for $PTV_{Focused}$ in WG: D90 18.3 Gy, V150 33.7 Gy, V200 8.9 Gy, $D10_{Urethra}$ 17.1 Gy, $D2cc_{Rectum}$ 8.4 Gy Median values for $PTV_{Focused}$ in fG: D90 24.3 Gy, V150 77.2 Gy, V200 30.2 Gy, $D10_{Urethra}$ 17.2 Gy, $D2cc_{Rectum}$ 8.9 Gy	No

Table 1: Continued.

Author/year	Focal/focused	Tumor imaging	Treatment imaging	Patient number/technique	Dosing data summary	Sal
Moman et al. 2010 [17]	Focal	MRI/biopsy mapping	NR	$n = 3$ HDR 15 Gy × 1 fx WG versus FG post-RT salvage plans	WG: $V100_{GTV}$ 25–53%, $D2cc_{Rectal}$ 5.0–7.2 Gy, $D2cc_{Bladder}$ 6.5–12 Gy FG: $V100_{GTV}$ 93–100%, $D2cc_{Rectal}$ 2.5–6.4 Gy, $D2cc_{Bladder}$ 1.4–4.3 Gy	NA

MRS: magnetic resonance spectroscopy, reg: registered, Sal: salvageable, WG: whole gland, HG: hemigland, FG: focal gland plan, fG: focused gland plan, NR: not reported, and NA: not applicable.

TABLE 2: Summary of clinical manuscripts.

Author/year	Focal/focused	Tumor/treatment imaging	Technique (HDR/LDR)	Dosimetry	Symptoms/outcome	Salv.
DiBiase et al. 2002 [20]	Focused	MRI, Biopsy mapping/MRI	n = 14 LDR I^{125} 145 Gy × 1 fx, LR disease, 130% boost to gross tumor	V100 95% (89–98%) $Dmax_{Urethra}$ 160% (range 131–220%) $Dmax_{Rectal}$ 110% (range 74–150%)	FU duration not recorded, progression not reported GU toxicity grade I 87%, grade II 53% No urinary incontinence, no rectal toxicity	No
Hsu et al. 2013 [22]	Focal	MRI, MRS, biopsy mapping/MRI reg US	n = 15 LDR I^{125} 144 Gy × 1 fx. Post LDR focal salvage, TRUS confirmed disease, 1-2 foci.	$D90_{CTV}$ 187.5 Gy (107.5–247.5) $V100_{CTV}$ 99.0% (91.7–100.0) $V100_{Rectum}$ 5.5% (0.1–18.7)	5 y FU, recurrence (Phoenix criteria): 1 y 0%, 2 y 0%, and 3 y 62.7% Pre-GI grade I, 13.3%, grade II, 6.7%, post-GI grade I, 13.3, grade II, 0% Pre-GU grade I, 33.3%, grade II, 60.0%, grade III, 6.7% Post-GI: grade I, 6.7%, grade II, 60.0%, grade III, 33.3% Pre ED: grade I, 26.7%, grade II, 53.3%, grade III, 0% Post ED: grade I, 13%, grade II, 66.7%, grade III, 13.3%	Yes*
Barret et al. 2013 [23]	Focal	biopsy mapping/TRUS	n = 12 LDR I^{125} compared to other focal techniques in LR disease	NR	FU to one year, PSA change median 6.2 (5–7.9) baseline to 2.5 (0.9–4.4) at 1 year Median $IPSS_{baseline}$ 3 (1–7), median $IPSS_{1\,yr}$ 7 (2–12) Median IIEF-$5_{baseline}$ 21 (10–25), median IIEF-$5_{1\,yr}$ 14 (8–24)	NA
Wallace et al. 2013 [24]	Focal	MRI, biopsy mapping/NR	n = 1 LDR Pd^{103} 124 Gy × 1 fx Single patient s/p EBRT 75 Gy for IR disease, Salvage at 4 years	$D90_{GTV}$ 100%, $V100_{GTV}$ 100% $V100_{rectal}$ 0.00cc $D30_{urethra}$ 54.52%	Median FU 1 month, PSA at one year 0.52 and decreasing Postsalvage: no ED, nocturia 0-1x, 1-2 hr daily voiding AUA 21 from baseline of 5, SHIM score 22 (No ED) 3 months: GU and GI symptoms back to baseline	Yes*
Peters et al. 2014 [16]	Focal	MRI/MRI reg US	n = 20 LDR, LR, IR & HR, I^{125} 144 Gy × 1 fx focal salvage, 35% post LDR, 65% post EBRT, TRUS confirmed unilateral disease 2 y post RT	$D90_{GTV}$ 198 Gy (150–330) $D2cc_{rectum}$ 68 Gy (18–96) $D0.1cc_{rectum}$ 133 Gy (69–207) $D10_{urethral}$ was 132 Gy (100–240)	Median FU 36 months, recurrence (Phoenix criteria): 15% (3 of 6 no initial response) Presalvage ED: grade II, 50%, grade III, 25%, 3 yr ED: grade II, 35%, grade III, 20% Presalvage GI grade I, 45%, grade II, 10%, 3 yr GI grade I, 13.3%, grade II, 15% Presalvage GU grade I, 25%, grade II, 10%, 3 yr GU grade I, 5%, grade II, 15% Only one patient: grade III toxicity (GU) at 3 years FU	No**

Table 2: Continued.

Author/ year	Focal/ focused	Tumor/ treatment imaging	Technique (HDR/LDR)	Dosimetry	Symptoms/outcome	Salv.
Ennis et al. 2015 [21]	Focused	TTI TRUS/TRUS	n = 14 LDR Pd-103, prospective IR patients with Gleason ≤ 6. Total prostate treated with dose painting (GTV goal D100 200% and same OAR constraints as typical plan)	Standard whole gland plan: $V200_{GTV}$ 49% $V150_{Urethra}$ 1% $D1CC_{Rectum}$ 51% Focused plan: $V200_{GTV}$ 97% $V150_{Urethra}$ 11% $D1CC_{Rectum}$ 60%	Biological recurrence: 0% at 31.5 months Acute (less than 6 months), late (greater than 6 months) Acute proctitis grade I, 23%, grade II, 0%, late proctitis grade I, 0%, grade II, 17% Acute urgency/frequency grade I, 54%, grade II, 46% Late urgency/frequency grade I, 58%, grade II, 17% Acute ED: grade I, 31%, grade II, 54%, grade III, 0% Late ED: grade I 33%, grade II, 42%, grade III, 17% No grade III toxicity	No

FU: follow-up, GU: genitourinary, GI: gastrointestinal, Salv.: salvageable, LR: low risk, IR: intermediate risk, HR: high risk, reg: registered, ED: erectile dysfunction, NR: not reported, TTI: tissue-type imaging, IPSS: International Prostate Symptom Score, IIEF-5: 5-item version of the International Index of Erectile Function.

*Would be salvageable given data if not salvage therapy.

**Would not be salvageable given data if not salvage therapy.

stated one major theoretical advantage of focal brachytherapy would be to permit definitive RT salvage in the future; therefore manuscripts were studied to determine salvageability. The authors in two of the publications demonstrated that hemi- and focal treatment plans [14, 15] would be amenable to future salvage. Based on typical OAR constraints three other studies [10, 12, 19] could permit further definitive RT given the significant reduction in OAR dosing achieved from partial therapy.

3.3. Patterns between Selected Clinical Manuscripts. The six manuscripts that included clinical toxicity data of focal/focused brachytherapy were published between 2002 and 2015 with all but one work completed on or after 2013. The number of patients assessed in the manuscripts ranged from 1 to 20 with a mean number of 7 subjects. Two of the six works utilized a focused [20, 21] rather than focal strategy [16, 22–24] (Table 2). The works were evenly divided between salvage treatments [16, 22, 24] and initial treatments [20, 21, 23] with two focused manuscripts being salvage treatments. Planning was based on MRI imaging [16], MRI combined with biopsy data [20, 24], prostate biopsy mapping [23], and MRI combined with both MRS and biopsy data [22]. Treatment imaging utilized MRI registered TRUS [16, 22], MRI [20], and biopsy mapping with TRUS [21]. One manuscript utilized intraoperative planning and treatment guidance with tissue-type imaging (TTI) based TRUS that enables delineation of tumor volumes from US spectra [23]. Wallace et al. did not specify the method of treatment imaging [24]. All of the works employed LDR brachytherapy.

Dosimetric data was compared to consensus prostate brachytherapy constraints [25] to determine if the focal/focused plan was able to increase tumor dose and decrease dose to OARs. All but one clinical work [23] included in this review published dosimetric data. Both focused works were able to achieve OAR doses typical of a standard whole gland treatment, with increased dose to the GTV [20, 21]. Ennis et al. provided examples of what the dosimetry would have been had they employed whole gland rather than focused plans [21]. The focused plans did slightly increase GTV dose than what would have been accomplished in the whole gland plan. Similarly, Peters et al. with focal brachytherapy were able to achieve higher than standard whole gland prostate GTV dosing while remaining within expected OAR tolerances [16]. The two remaining focal manuscripts were able to achieve significantly lower doses to the OARs, while delivering a dose to the target tumor that is comparable to [24] or greater [22] than what would be achieved with whole gland therapy.

Follow-up ranged from 1 to 60 months with a mean of 23 months. Follow-up duration was not published by DiBiase et al., nor was any disease progression information included [20]. There were no recurrences/failures in three manuscripts with median follow-up of 1 month [24], 12 months [23], and 31.5 months [21]. Hsu et al. had a 5-year biological failure rate as determined by Phoenix criteria of 28.6% [22]. Similarly, Peters et al. demonstrated failure via Phoenix criteria of 15% at 36 months, although half of those were patients that did not respond to therapy initially in regard to PSA [16]. When examining the selected publications' toxicity, the overall reported side effects are no more than would be expected for whole gland brachytherapy [26]. Closer examination of focal plans that significantly reduced OARs demonstrated patterns of decreased toxicity. In particular Hsu et al. with an average $V100_{rectum}$ of 5.5% showed only grade I GI toxicity in 13% of the patients [22], while the single subject in the report of Wallace et al. had no long-term side effects at 3 months in the background of significantly reduced rectal and urethra dose [24]. ED was not significantly changed from pre-RT levels in most studies [16, 20, 23, 24] although two had an increase in the proportion of ED being grade III versus grade I/II from the period before to that after treatment [21, 22], with one work achieving otherwise low side effects and low OAR dose [22].

4. Discussion

The dosimetric portion of the studies selected in this systematic review demonstrate that a focal plan is attainable in regard to both GTV dosing and decreasing dose to OARs using either LDR or HDR approaches. Furthermore, there is evidence that such partial gland treatments may permit irradiation of prostate tissue outside the GTV for future definitive, salvage RT [14, 15]. Although the number of clinical studies and the number of treated patients are low, focal and focused plans were able to deliver lower than usual dose to OARs with excellent outcomes from a toxicity standpoint. For example, Ennis et al. were able to achieve a significant reduction to the rectal dose that resulted in less GI toxicity than would have been anticipated by a whole gland treatment [22]. Similar to the dosimetric works, the two focal clinical studies with decreased OAR dose would likely be amenable to future salvage RT or surgery [22, 24]. In our own patient population we have found that select low risk patients are appropriate for focal HDR treatments. Figures 2(a), 2(b), and 2(e) demonstrated an example patient where simulation of focal therapy was able to achieve target dose with minimal exposure to OARs and afford future salvage therapy within OAR and target dose constraints. The ultimate composite between the focal and salvage plan is comparable to standard whole gland therapy (Figures 2(c), 2(d), and 2(e) and Table 3). Based on these results and our own experience, the authors of this work feel that sufficient evidence exists to pursue larger clinical studies of focal therapy for well-selected low risk prostate cancer patients.

In the PSA era there is significant lead-time with the detection of early stage disease [6]. For those patients who have extended life expectancy and low risk disease current options are limited to active surveillance, prostatectomy, or definitive RT [5]. The side effects of both whole gland RT and surgery, including the 50% reported incidence of ED [27], dissuade many patients from therapy who may otherwise be active and healthy. On the other hand there are many patients for whom active surveillance provokes too much anxiety, not to mention the morbidity that potential annual biopsy can induce. Essentially, these patients desire a treatment to halt disease progression with low toxicity. The evidence presented in this manuscript suggests that focal brachytherapy can be

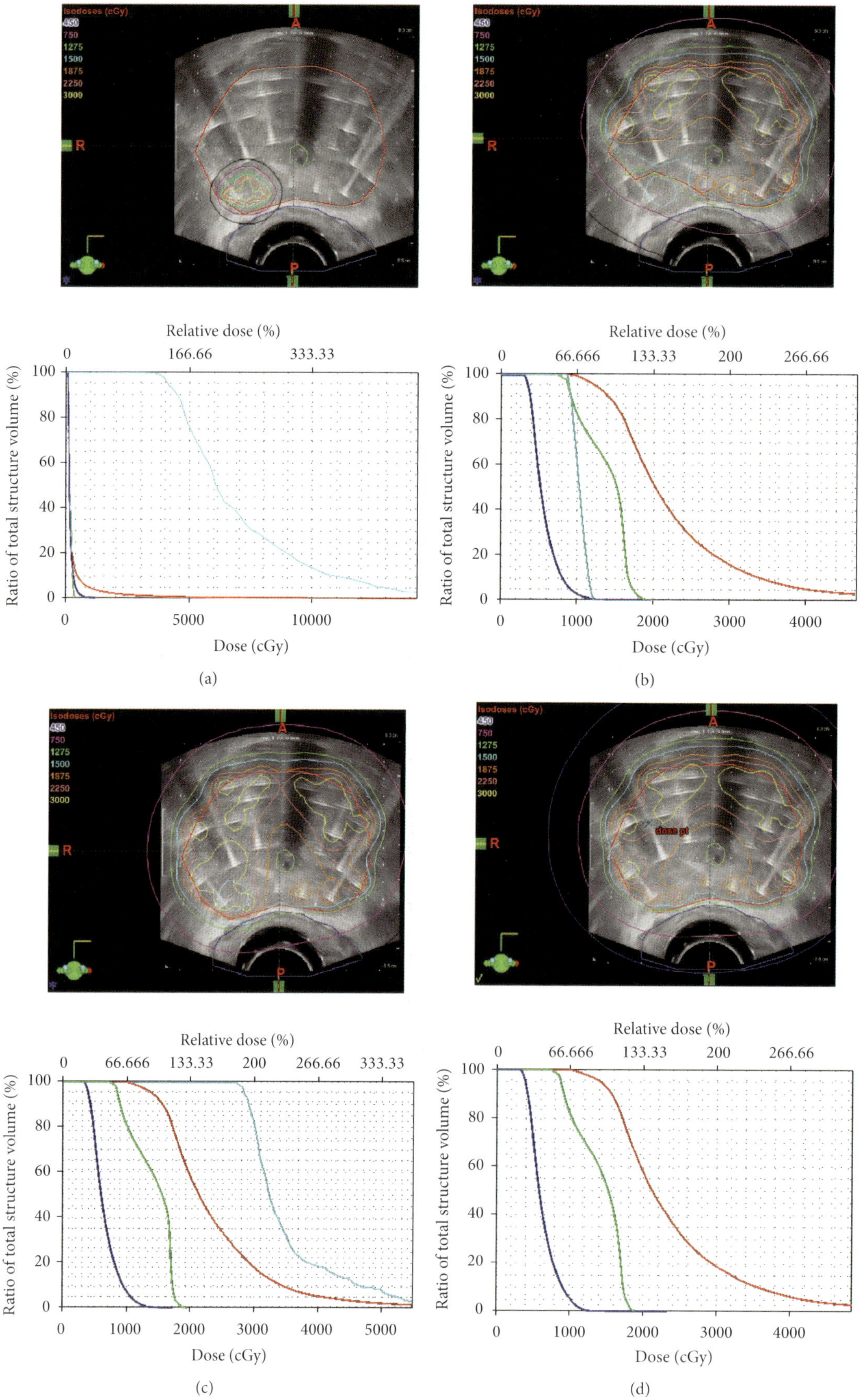

Figure 2: Continued.

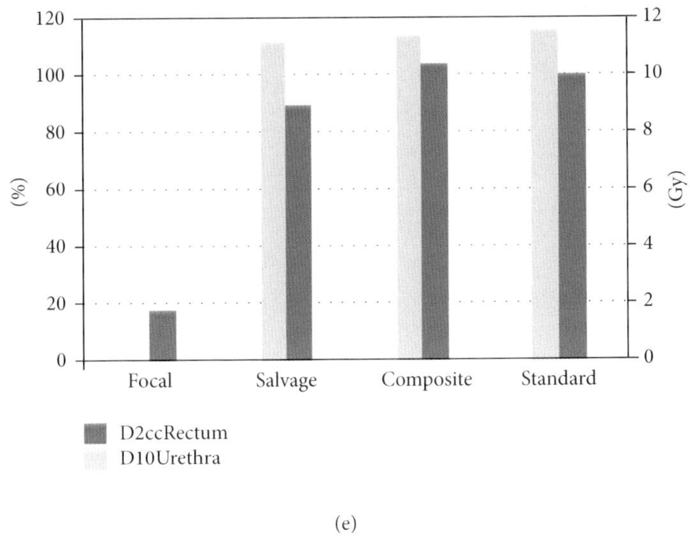

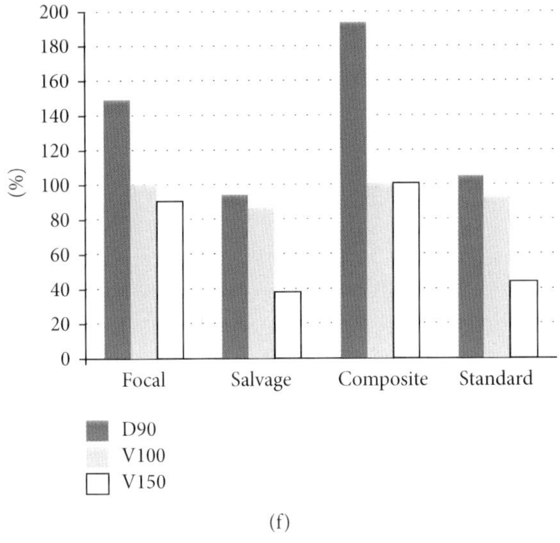

FIGURE 2: Organ/isodose contours, DVH for focal plan (a), salvage plan (b), composite of focal plan and salvage plan (c), and standard whole gland plan (d) of ideal focal HDR patient. Isodose lines are as follows: Black 450 cGy, Magenta 750 cGy, Green 1275 cGy, Cyan 1500 cGy, Orange 1875 cGy, Dark Pink 2250 cGy, and Yellow 3000 cGy. Target (e) and organ at risk doses (f).

TABLE 3: Experimental dose to target and OAR between focal, salvage, and whole gland HDR brachytherapy.

Parameter	Focal	Salvage	Composite	Standard
$D2cc_{Rectum}$ (Gy)	1.76	8.90	10.29	9.98
$D10_{Urethra}$ (%)	0.00	111.66	113.85	115.64
$D90_{PTV}$ (%)	149.30	94.15	193.9	104.54
$V100_{PTV}$ (%)	100.00	86.51	100.00	92.70
$V150_{PTV}$ (%)	89.70	37.89	100.00	43.72

optimized in low risk patients to deliver a fully therapeutic dose to the GTV while avoiding significant side effects. Further this treatment may possibly be salvageable with either surgery or RT with future disease recurrence. While current definitive treatment with surgery or whole gland RT can be technically salvaged, there are issues with both. After whole prostate RT salvage prostatectomy is difficult to perform on what is an extremely fibrotic post-RT prostate and surrounding tissues [28]. Alternatively, salvage RT is more often treating a significantly greater portion of the pelvis with greater side effects than initial whole gland therapy. Focal brachytherapy may be a more salvageable option that could act as a temporizing bridge to definitive therapy. In doing so, focal brachytherapy could be used to extend a period that is free of morbidity before definitive surgery/RT or in the best-case scenario negate any further treatment.

While none of the clinical papers employed HDR brachytherapy, the technique offers theoretical advantages over LDR for focal treatments [7]. First, the treatment volume can be optimized through inverse planning, which allows compensation for suboptimal needle placement and an overall more reliable dose distribution pattern in regard to the PTV [29]. There are fewer radiation concerns in regard to exposure to physician, nurses, and physicists as the source is delivered remotely. Also, there is no need for postimplant dosimetry, which adds to an already efficient planning/treatment delivery system. With the goal to create a salvageable focal plan to spare OAR and maximize dose to the GTV, the flexibility offered by HDR is more optimal. One significant drawback to HDR as monotherapy is that it is traditionally fractionated, which requires multiple needle insertions, or keeping needles placed for prolonged period of times. However, there is some experience with single fraction HDR [30], which likely would suffice for focal therapy given the dosimetric work of Kamrava et al. and Moman et al. [14, 17].

An additional benefit of HDR over LDR is its efficient integration with TRUS guidance, allowing a scan-plan-treat environment [8]. TRUS provides improved visualization of the base and apex of the prostate compared to CT and eliminates the need to move the patient from an imaging room to a brachytherapy suite, saving considerable procedure time. However, one significant drawback is that tumors are not readily visualized and as an imaging modality it takes experience to read. There is (TTI) TRUS which has shown success in delineating tumor from normal prostate [21]; however, the imaging requires some skill with interpretation and as a technique is not in wide use. Alternatively, tumors are readily visualized by MRI. However, the long acquisition time and usually off-site location of MRI scanners preclude them from streamlined HDR simulation, planning, and delivery except at a few specialized centers [20]. As shown by many of the manuscripts selected in this review prior pelvic MRI can be registered to the treatment TRUS, which when combined provides efficient intraprocedural tumor delineation. In regard to focal therapy, Mason et al. confirmed that MRI with T2-weighted, diffusion-weighted, and dynamic-contrast-enhanced sequences can accurately detect tumors, negating biopsy mapping [11]. To combine all of the above technologies together, treatment planning systems such as

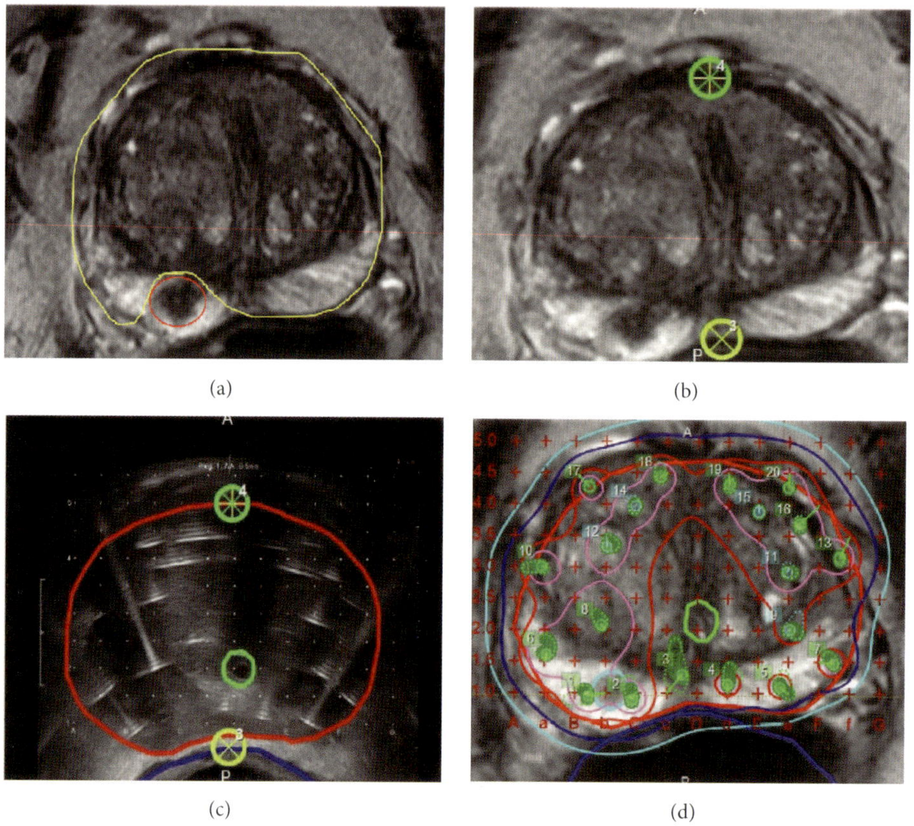

FIGURE 3: (a) Preprocedural MRI demonstrating GTV (yellow) and nondiseased prostate (red). Preprocedural MRI using two anchor points (green and yellow circles) (b) are able to be registered to intraprocedural TRUS with 2.5 mm grid spacing (c). (d) The resulting merge of the TRUS grid and preprocedural MRI with GTV (thick light blue), urethra (thick solid light green), rectum (thick blue line), and isodose lines (thin lines) for typical whole gland plan using 18 HDR catheters.

Vitesse Version 3.0 (Varian, Inc. Palo Alto, CA) that supports HDR intraprocedural TRUS guided needle placement, planning, and delivery already exist which as a software can be readily registered with prior MRI data. This registration has been readily performed experimentally at our own institution as shown in Figure 3. Given the increased utilization of pelvic MRI in prostate cancer workup, MRI registered TRUS is an efficient and reliable focal brachytherapy platform that can be adapted to most brachytherapy centers.

There are areas that, based on this systematic review, require further research to validate focal HDR prostate brachytherapy as a reliable technique. Foremost, the current clinical trials are few in number, have short follow-up duration, and are small in sample size. Therefore, it is a plausible that the clinical results presented in this systematic review may not be accurate representations of the toxicity and efficacy from focal plans. Further, the disease stage varied amongst the papers including those with more advanced disease than low risk prostate cancer that would be more applicable to focal treatments. To the knowledge of the authors, there are also no works that directly compare whole gland to focal treatments in regard to patient toxicity and treatment efficacy. These shortcomings would be clarified with a trial of whole gland and focal brachytherapy that is large enough to permit a comparison of toxicity and efficacy, that is, progression free survival, with significant power. In regard to HDR as monotherapy, single fraction therapy would be more attractive to patients than multiple fractions with either prolonged needle placement or repeat needle application. However, there has been very limited publication experience with single fraction HDR monotherapy, thus requiring more research before application as a part of focal brachytherapy strategy.

5. Conclusion

In this systematic review we demonstrated dosimetrically that focal brachytherapy could be appropriately applied to prostate tumors while decreasing dose to OARs. Clinical studies were also presented that provided evidence that such treatments decreased toxicity over current whole gland therapy. The decreased toxicity and decreased dose to OARs permit potential salvage RT or salvage prostatectomy if there is future recurrence. Given the indolent nature of prostate cancer when caught at an early stage, focal therapy may serve as a temporary and possible permanent measure for low risk prostate cancer that delays/avoids the significant toxicity such as ED that current definitive therapy has. To this end,

HDR brachytherapy allows the dosimetric flexibility required for focal plans. Further, pelvic MRIs, which are increasingly obtained in prostate cancer workup, can be registered to intraprocedural TRUS for an efficient and widely applicable focal brachytherapy platform.

Competing Interests

The authors declare that they have no competing interests.

References

[1] S. Sriprasad, M. R. Feneley, and P. M. Thompson, "History of prostate cancer treatment," *Surgical Oncology*, vol. 18, no. 3, pp. 185–191, 2009.

[2] J. N. Aronowitz, "Whitmore, Henschke, and Hilaris: the reorientation of prostate brachytherapy (1970–1987)," *Brachytherapy*, vol. 11, no. 2, pp. 157–162, 2012.

[3] H. H. Holm, "Interventional ultrasound in Europe," *Ultrasound in Medicine & Biology*, vol. 24, no. 6, pp. 779–791, 1998.

[4] H. Ragde, G. L. Grado, B. Nadir, and A.-A. Elgamal, "Modern prostate brachytherapy," *CA: A Cancer Journal for Clinicians*, vol. 50, no. 6, pp. 380–393, 2000.

[5] National Comprehensive Cancer Network, *Prostate Cancer (Version 1.2015)*, 2015.

[6] J. Hugosson, S. Carlsson, G. Aus et al., "Mortality results from the Göteborg randomised population-based prostate-cancer screening trial," *The Lancet Oncology*, vol. 11, no. 8, pp. 725–732, 2010.

[7] B. Libby, "Implementation of image-guided prostate HDR brachytherapy using MR-ultrasound fusion," in *Proceedings of the 57th Annual Meeting of the AAPM*, Anaheim, Calif, USA, July 2015, *Medical Physics*, vol. 42, no. 6, p. 3572, 2015.

[8] B. Libby, "Real time ultrasound guidance for optimizing high dose rate prostate brachytherapy," in *Proceedings of the 55th Annual Meeting of the AAPM*, Medical Physics 40:6, Invited oral presentation, Indianapolis, Ind, USA, August 2013.

[9] D. Moher, A. Liberati, J. Tetzlaff, and D. G. Altman, "Preferred reporting items for systematic reviews and meta-analyses: the PRISMA statement," *Journal of Clinical Epidemiology*, vol. 62, no. 10, pp. 1006–1012, 2009.

[10] B. Al-Qaisieh, J. Mason, P. Bownes et al., "Dosimetry modeling for focal low-dose-rate prostate brachytherapy," *International Journal of Radiation Oncology, Biology, Physics*, vol. 92, no. 4, pp. 787–793, 2015.

[11] J. Mason, B. Al-Qaisieh, P. Bownes et al., "Multi-parametric MRI-guided focal tumor boost using HDR prostate brachytherapy: a feasibility study," *Brachytherapy*, vol. 13, no. 2, pp. 137–145, 2014.

[12] J. Mason, B. Al-Qaisieh, P. Bownes, D. Thwaites, and A. Henry, "Dosimetry modeling for focal high-dose-rate prostate brachytherapy," *Brachytherapy*, vol. 13, no. 6, pp. 611–617, 2014.

[13] J. Mason, P. Bownes, B. Carey, and A. Henry, "Comparison of focal boost high dose rate prostate brachytherapy optimisation methods," *Radiotherapy and Oncology*, vol. 117, no. 3, pp. 521–524, 2015.

[14] M. Kamrava, M. P. Chung, O. Kayode et al., "Focal high-dose-rate brachytherapy: a dosimetric comparison of hemigland vs. conventional whole-gland treatment," *Brachytherapy*, vol. 12, no. 5, pp. 434–441, 2013.

[15] R. Banerjee, S.-J. Park, E. Anderson, D. J. Demanes, J. Wang, and M. Kamrava, "From whole gland to hemigland to ultra-focal high-dose-rate prostate brachytherapy: a dosimetric analysis," *Brachytherapy*, vol. 14, no. 3, pp. 366–372, 2015.

[16] M. Peters, M. Maenhout, J. R. N. van der Voort Van Zyp et al., "Focal salvage iodine-125 brachytherapy for prostate cancer recurrences after primary radiotherapy: a retrospective study regarding toxicity, biochemical outcome and quality of life," *Radiotherapy and Oncology*, vol. 112, no. 1, pp. 77–82, 2014.

[17] M. R. Moman, C. A. T. van den Berg, A. E. Boeken Kruger et al., "Focal salvage guided by T2-weighted and dynamic contrast-enhanced magnetic resonance imaging for prostate cancer recurrences," *International Journal of Radiation Oncology Biology Physics*, vol. 76, no. 3, pp. 741–746, 2010.

[18] D. A. Todor, I. J. Barani, P.-S. Lin, and M. S. Anscher, "Moving toward focal therapy in prostate cancer: dual-isotope permanent seed implants as a possible solution," *International Journal of Radiation Oncology Biology Physics*, vol. 81, no. 1, pp. 297–304, 2011.

[19] D. L. Polders, M. van Herk, K. Nichol et al., "Establishing implantation uncertainties for focal brachytherapy with I-125 seeds for the treatment of localized prostate cancer," *Acta Oncologica*, vol. 54, no. 6, pp. 839–846, 2015.

[20] S. J. DiBiase, K. Hosseinzadeh, R. P. Gullapalli et al., "Magnetic resonance spectroscopic imaging-guided brachytherapy for localized prostate cancer," *International Journal of Radiation Oncology Biology Physics*, vol. 52, no. 2, pp. 429–438, 2002.

[21] R. D. Ennis, S. A. Quinn, F. Trichter et al., "Phase I/II prospective trial of cancer-specific imaging using ultrasound spectrum analysis tissue-type imaging to guide dose-painting prostate brachytherapy," *Brachytherapy*, vol. 14, no. 6, pp. 801–808, 2015.

[22] C. C. Hsu, H. Hsu, B. Pickett et al., "Feasibility of MR imaging/MR spectroscopy-planned focal partial salvage permanent prostate implant (PPI) for localized recurrence after initial PPI for prostate cancer," *International Journal of Radiation Oncology, Biology, Physics*, vol. 85, no. 2, pp. 370–377, 2013.

[23] E. Barret, Y. Ahallal, R. Sanchez-Salas et al., "Morbidity of focal therapy in the treatment of localized prostate cancer," *European Urology*, vol. 63, no. 4, pp. 618–622, 2013.

[24] T. Wallace, I. Avital, A. Stojadinovic, B. Brucher, E. Coté, and J. Yu, "Multi-parametric mri-directed focal salvage permanent interstitial brachytherapy for locally recurrent adenocarcinoma of the prostate: a novel approach," *Journal of Cancer*, vol. 4, no. 2, pp. 146–151, 2013.

[25] C. Salembier, P. Lavagnini, P. Nickers et al., "Tumour and target volumes in permanent prostate brachytherapy: a supplement to the ESTRO/EAU/EORTC recommendations on prostate brachytherapy," *Radiotherapy and Oncology*, vol. 83, no. 1, pp. 3–10, 2007.

[26] A. Henderson, R. W. Laing, and S. E. M. Langley, "Quality of life following treatment for early prostate cancer: Does Low Dose Rate (LDR) brachytherapy offer a better outcome? a review," *European Urology*, vol. 45, no. 2, pp. 134–141, 2004.

[27] A. L. Potosky, W. W. Davis, R. M. Hoffman et al., "Five-year outcomes after prostatectomy or radiotherapy for prostate cancer: the prostate cancer outcomes study," *Journal of the National Cancer Institute*, vol. 96, no. 18, pp. 1358–1367, 2004.

[28] E. Rogers, M. Ohori, V. S. Kassabian, T. M. Wheeler, and P. T. Scardino, "Salvage radical prostatectomy: outcome measured by serum prostate specific antigen levels," *The Journal of Urology*, vol. 153, no. 1, pp. 104–110, 1995.

[29] D. J. Brenner and E. J. Hall, "Fractionation and protraction for radiotherapy of prostate carcinoma," *International Journal of Radiation Oncology Biology Physics*, vol. 43, no. 5, pp. 1095–1101, 1999.

[30] P. Hoskin, A. Rojas, P. Ostler et al., "High-dose-rate brachytherapy alone given as two or one fraction to patients for locally advanced prostate cancer: acute toxicity," *Radiotherapy and Oncology*, vol. 110, no. 2, pp. 268–271, 2014.

25

Predicting Low-Risk Prostate Cancer from Transperineal Saturation Biopsies

Pim J. van Leeuwen,[1,2] Amila Siriwardana,[1,2,3] Monique Roobol,[4] Francis Ting,[1,2] Daan Nieboer,[5] James Thompson,[1] Warick Delprado,[6] Anne-Marie Haynes,[2] Phillip Brenner,[1,2] and Phillip Stricker[1,2]

[1] *St Vincent's Prostate Cancer Centre, St Vincent's Clinic, Sydney, NSW 2010, Australia*
[2] *Australian Prostate Cancer Research Centre New South Wales, The Garvan Institute of Medical Research, The Kinghorn Cancer Centre, Sydney, NSW 2010, Australia*
[3] *University of New South Wales, Sydney, NSW 2052, Australia*
[4] *Department of Urology, Erasmus University Medical Center, 3015 CE Rotterdam, Netherlands*
[5] *Department of Public Health, Erasmus University Medical Center, 3015 CE Rotterdam, Netherlands*
[6] *University of Notre Dame, Sydney, NSW 2010, Australia*

Correspondence should be addressed to Pim J. van Leeuwen; p.vanleeuwen@erasmusmc.nl

Academic Editor: Cristina Magi-Galluzzi

Introduction. To assess the performance of five previously described clinicopathological definitions of low-risk prostate cancer (PC). *Materials and Methods.* Men who underwent radical prostatectomy (RP) for clinical stage ≤T2, PSA <10 ng/mL, Gleason score <8 PC, diagnosed by transperineal template-guided saturation biopsy were included. The performance of five previously described criteria (i.e., criteria 1–5, criterion 1 stringent (Gleason score 6 + ≤5 mm total max core length PC + ≤3 mm max per core length PC) up to criterion 5 less stringent (Gleason score 6-7 with ≤5% Gleason grade 4) was analysed to assess ability of each to predict insignificant disease in RP specimens (defined as Gleason score ≤6 and total tumour volume <2.5 mL, or Gleason score 7 with ≤5% grade 4 and total tumour volume <0.7 mL). *Results.* 994 men who underwent RP were included. Criterion 4 (Gleason score 6) performed best with area under the curve of receiver operating characteristics 0.792. At decision curve analysis, criterion 4 was deemed clinically the best performing transperineal saturation biopsy-based definition for low-risk PC. *Conclusions.* Gleason score 6 disease demonstrated a superior trade-off between sensitivity and specificity for clarifying low-risk PC that can guide treatment and be used as reference test in diagnostic studies.

1. Introduction

Early detection of prostate cancer (PC) has reduced PC mortality, but at the cost of a substantial increase in overdetection of insignificant disease [1, 2]. As a result, there are concerns about overdiagnosis and overtreatment of PC, and this has led to alternative diagnostic strategies and more conservative approaches, especially in the treatment of low-risk disease. Furthermore, as PC is most frequently a relatively slow-growing tumour, complications of unnecessary curative management in low-risk PC may be obviated by active surveillance (AS) [3]. Over the last decade, this has resulted in a growing acceptance of active surveillance for men diagnosed with low-risk PC [3].

Additionally, the emergence of multiparametric MRI (mpMRI) now allows imaging-based identification of PC, which improves diagnostic accuracy for higher-risk tumours, and might simultaneously reduce the diagnosis of low-risk PCs (overdiagnosis) [4, 5]. Considering the unreliability of PSA testing and 12-core template biopsy in PC diagnosis and risk stratification, the ability to visualise the tumour and then assess tumour grade and volume is of significant clinical benefit. However, to analyse the accuracy of mpMRI, a prospectively validated definition of clinically low-risk PC on saturation template mapping biopsy is required. mpMRI detects both high-grade and larger tumours accurately, which means it may perform particularly well for detection of clinically significant disease [4]. For diagnostic evaluation of mpMRI the ideal reference test would be definitive pathology of whole-mount sections of radical prostatectomy specimens. However, since such a reference test is not applicable in clinical practice, a reference test based on transperineal saturation biopsies would be useful [4].

There are multiple perspectives on low-risk PC (e.g., clinical, epidemiological, and pathological), and several definitions and terminologies are available [6]. The definition of "insignificant" or so-called "low-risk" PC, as well as the selection of men for AS, has been traditionally guided by clinicopathological features found to be predictive of indolent PC based on whole gland histopathology of radical prostatectomy (RP) specimens and defined as an organ-confined, well differentiated tumour (Gleason score ≤3 + 3 or ≤3 + 4) with a total tumour volume not exceeding 0.5–2.5 mL [7, 8]. Obviously, the use of the definition of pathologically insignificant PC requires an examination of the entire prostate. The translation, in clinical terms, of this histopathological definition of insignificant PC has proven to be challenging, owing to inherent inaccuracies of biopsy diagnoses. As a result, these definitions have been criticized for high rates of Gleason upgrading and unfavourable disease at RP [9–11]. Furthermore, it is unclear how to apply eligibility criteria based on 6–12 cores compared to men undergoing saturation biopsy [12–15].

The objective of this study was to assess the utility of five transperineal saturation biopsy-based clinicopathological risk criteria to predict insignificant PC in RP specimens. Thus the most accurate definition of low-risk PC based on transperineal saturation biopsies may be used as the endpoint (reference test) for future diagnostic imaging and biomarker studies. It may also be used to select candidate for AS after a PC diagnosis based on transperineal saturation biopsies.

2. Materials and Methods

2.1. Characterization of the Study Population. Since 2000, data from patients who underwent radical prostatectomy at our centre was collected prospectively in an institutional database. Institutional review board approval was granted and informed consent was obtained in all patients. For the present study, all men aged over 40 years, with PSA ≤10 ng/mL, diagnosed with a clinical T1c or T2, with Gleason <8 PC by transperineal template-guided mapping biopsy, between May 2001 and March 2015, and treated with a radical prostatectomy within 6 months of diagnosis, were included. All patients were reviewed and treated by two urologists at St Vincent's Clinic, Sydney, Australia.

2.2. Study Protocol. All men underwent biopsy for abnormal PSA or DRE. Transperineal template-guided mapping biopsy was performed with a median of 30 cores using 5 mm sampling of the peripheral zone and limited sampling of the transition zone with relative periurethral zone sparing adjusted for volume from 18 template locations. Histopathology from biopsies was processed and reported according to ISUP (International Society of Urological Pathology) protocols by one uropathologist. For all biopsies, the length of cancer was in millimetres (mm) and a primary and secondary Gleason grade were assigned to each cancer-containing core.

Table 1: Five transperineal saturation biopsy-based criteria for low-risk prostate cancer.

Criteria	Definition
Criterion 1	Gleason score 6 + ≤5 mm total max core length PC + ≤3 mm max per core length PC
Criterion 2	Gleason score 6 + <20% of cores positive + <5 mm max core length PC
Criterion 3	Gleason score 6-7 with ≤5% Gleason grade 4 + <20% of cores positive + <7 mm max core length PC
Criterion 4	Gleason score 6
Criterion 5	Gleason score 6-7 with ≤ 5% Gleason grade 4

Subsequently all men underwent nerve sparing radical prostatectomy (open or robotic). Histopathology from radical prostatectomy specimens was processed following previously described protocols [16]. All specimens were fixed, inked, and cut at 3 mm intervals perpendicular to the rectal surface. The apical slice was cut parasagittally at 3 mm intervals. Pathological tumour stage, Gleason score, and surgical margin status were assessed. Tumour areas were marked for each slide and measured using 3D volume estimation.

2.3. Criteria Tested. A literature search was performed to identify published definitions for "insignificant", "indolent", or "low-risk" PC based on transperineal saturation biopsies. In total five clinicopathological definitions of low-risk PC were included and analysed, Table 1 [5, 8, 17]. In the present study, significant PC on radical prostatectomy specimen was defined, using the updated criteria, as PC with Gleason score 3 + 3 = 6 and a total tumour volume of ≥2.5 mL and as any PC of Gleason score 7–10 with greater than 5% Gleason grade 4 or higher and a total tumour volume of ≥0.7 mL [7].

2.4. Development Prediction Model. For descriptive statistical analysis, firstly the rates of significant PC with specific pathologically unfavourable PC characteristics, defined as the presence of either extracapsular extension, seminal vesicle invasion, lymph node invasion, or Gleason score 7–10 that fulfilled the proposed five criteria for low-risk disease, were assessed. Secondly, binary logistic regression was performed to explore the relationship between serum PSA, clinical stage, prostate volume, percentage of positive biopsy cores, and insignificant PC (yes/no) among all patients and individually for the patients that fulfilled the five criteria for low-risk disease. Sensitivity, specificity, negative predictive value (NPV), and positive predictive value (PPV) were assessed for all five criteria to predict insignificant PC in radical prostatectomy specimens.

The discrimination of the various criteria was tested using area under the curve of receiver operating characteristic

Table 2: Patients characteristics.

Variable	All	Criterion 1	Criterion 2	Criterion 3	Criterion 4	Criterion 5
Number of patients	994	52	78	127	219	319
Median (IQR)						
Age	62	60 (57–63)	60 (56–64)	60 (55–64)	59 (55–63)	60 (55–64)
PSA ng/mL	5.5	5.5 (4.0–7.2)	5.5 (4.2–6.8)	5.5 (4.1–7.0)	5.1 (3.8–6.3)	5.1 (3.8–6.3)
Prostate volume	49.0	53.0 (45–69)	53.0 (44–70)	52.0 (44–62)	49.0 (41–57)	48.0 (40–56)
Number of cores	27	28	28	28	28	28
% positive cores	25.0	9.5	11.1	12.5	18.8	21.4
Clinical stage, N (%)						
T1c	537 (54.0)	43 (82.7)	62 (79.5)	93 (73.2)	151 (68.9)	208 (65.2)
T2a	312 (31.4)	5 (9.6)	11 (14.1)	22 (17.3)	47 (21.5)	73 (22.9)
T2b	72 (7.3)	1 (1.9)	2 (3.8)	3 (2.4)	11 (5.0)	15 (4.7)
T2c	73 (7.3)	3 (5.8)	3 (2.6)	9 (7.1)	10 (4.6)	23 (7.2)
Biopsy Gleason score, N (%)						
3 + 3	221 (22.2)	52(100)	78 (100)	99 (78.0)	219 (100)	218 (68.3)
3 + 4	581 (58.5)			28 (22.0)		101 (31.7)
4 + 3	192 (19.3)					

Table 3: Unfavourable pathological characteristics per biopsy criteria.

Variable	Criterion 1	Criterion 2	Criterion 3	Criterion 4	Criterion 5
Number of patients	52	78	127	219	319
Gleason score					
4 + 3 (%)	1 (1.9)	2 (2.6)	1 (0.8)	3 (1.4)	5 (1.6)
≥8 (%)	0 (0.0)	0 (0.0)	2 (1.6)	1 (0.3)	3 (0.9)
ECE (%)	4 (7.7)	6 (7.7)	11 (8.7)	28 (12.8)	55 (17.2)
SVI (%)	0 (0.0)	0 (0.0)	0 (0.0)	0 (0.0)	1 (0.3)
LNI (%)	0 (0.0)	0 (0.0)	0 (0.0)	0 (0.0)	0 (0.0)
Any unfavourable pathological characteristics	5 (9.6)	7 (8.9)	13 (10.2)	29 (13.2)	57 (17.9)

(AUC-ROC) analysis. Discrimination describes the model's ability to differentiate between those with and those without the outcome of interest, in this case the presence of insignificant PC. P values were calculated to indicate whether the AUC was significantly different to the null hypothesis (AUC of 0.5).

Decision curve analysis (DCA) was used to plot the net clinical benefit, measured by weighing the benefits (true positive results) against the harms (false positives), at different probability thresholds, thus yielding the decision curve [18]. Decision curve analysis generated a graph of the net benefit as a function of a threshold probability (p_t) at which an individual considers the potential benefit and harm of surgery to be equivalent. The threshold probability of insignificant cancer is an assumption where the patient would opt for AS. The decision curve is then compared with the two extremes of assuming all or no patients being treated with RP. The net benefit was measured as the rate at which incorporating the decision guide of interest (identifying low-risk PC) would lead to a beneficial decision to diagnose and treat PC without causing any additional harmful decisions to overtreat PC.

For all analyses, two-sided P values <0.05 were considered to be statistically significant. Statistical analyses were performed using SPSS version 21 and the R statistics package.

3. Results

Patient characteristics are presented in Table 2. Between May 2001 and March 2015, in total 3521 men underwent RP. 994 (28.2%) men fulfilled the inclusion criteria (PSA ≤ 10 ng/mL, diagnosed with clinical T1c or T2, Gleason <8 PC based on transperineal template-guided mapping biopsy) and were included for analysis. Of these men, 48 (4.8%) had a previous negative prostate biopsy. In 339 (34.1%) men a bilateral extended pelvic lymph node dissection was performed simultaneously to the RP. Of the 994 men who underwent RP, 143 (14.4%) fulfilled the criteria for insignificant PC at RP. Based on biopsy results, 52 (5.2%) men fulfilled criterion 1, 78 (7.8%) men fulfilled criterion 2, 188 (18.9%) men fulfilled criterion 3, 219 (22.0%) fulfilled men criterion 4, and 319 (32.1%) fulfilled criterion 5.

Table 3 shows the percentages of unfavourable pathological characteristics among the patients that fulfilled the five

Table 4: The ability of the five criteria to predict insignificant PC in RP specimen.

	Specificity	Sensitivity	PPV	NPV
Criterion 1	98	23	63	88
Criterion 2	97	34	63	90
Criterion 3	91	52	46	93
Criterion 4	86	72	47	95
Criterion 5	76	82	37	96

Table 5: Outcomes of area under the receiver operating characteristic analysis of the five biopsy criteria.

	AUC	95% CI	*P* value
Criterion 1	0.604	0.549–0.660	<0.01
Criterion 2	0.654	0.599–0.712	<0.01
Criterion 3	0.641	0.641–0.749	<0.01
Criterion 4	0.792	0.747–0.837	<0.01
Criterion 5	0.790	0.750–0.831	<0.01

low-risk criteria. The number of men with a Gleason ≥4 + 3 at RP specimen and/or extracapsular disease was highest upon applying the least stringent criteria (criterion 5, 17.9%).

3.1. Risk Stratification. Multivariable logistic regression of preoperative clinicopathological parameters predicting insignificant PC at RP was performed. Significant variables predicting insignificant disease among all men included were lower PSA (OR 0.77, 95% CI 0.70–0.86), younger age (OR 0.92, 95% CI 0.92–0.98), larger prostate volume (OR 1.02, 95% CI 1.01–1.04), smaller percentage positive biopsies (OR 0.96, 95% CI 0.95–0.98), and a normal rectal examination (OR 0.56, 95% CI 0.37–0.85). The −2 log likelihood of the model was 689.35, specificity was 98.8%, sensitivity was 8.4%, and overall success rate was 85.8%. Regression coefficients (*B*) were −0.579 for normal rectal examination, −0.255 per ng/mL serum PSA, −0.080 per year of age, −0.039 per % positive biopsies, and 0.024 per cm^3 prostate volume.

3.2. Performance of the 5 Transperineal Saturation Biopsy-Based Criteria. The ability of the five criteria to predict insignificant PC in RP specimen was examined, showing a sensitivity that ranged between 23% (criterion 1) and 82% (criterion 5) and a specificity that varied between 76% (criterion 5) and 98% (criterion 1). The sensitivity, specificity, PPV, NPV, and LR for all five criteria are presented in Table 4. Receiver operator characteristics to assess the performance of the five biopsy-based criteria, to predict insignificant PC in RP, are shown in Table 5. The AUC for each model ranged between 0.604 (criterion 1), 0.654 (criterion 2), 0.741 (criterion 3), 0.790 (criterion 5), and 0.792 (criterion 4), suggesting moderate positive discrimination at best.

A DCA was performed to assess the clinical utility of using each of the five criteria for the definition of low-risk PC to guide the decision of who should not be treated (in order to decrease overtreatment) and/or be selected for AS. Two additional criteria (treatment with RP to all and treatment to none) were added for comparison. The DCA showed that, for threshold probabilities of 0% to 15%, representing a preference to maximize reduction in overtreatment, the net benefit is greatest using criterion 5. In this range of threshold probabilities, patients appear to be more concerned about overtreatment than about missing significant PC. For the midrange, as well as clinically most relevant probabilities of 30% to 50%, criterion 4 was superior to the other criteria. For the higher thresholds (50–75%), at which patients may be more concerned about missing a significant cancer than about unnecessary overtreatment, the more rigorous criteria 1 and 2 should be used. Using a threshold of >75% is best to diagnose and/or treat all patients.

4. Discussion

"Overdiagnosis" and "overtreatment" are defined as the diagnosis and/or treatment of PC that would never cause symptoms or death during the patient's lifetime and may therefore be considered unnecessary [19]. Obviously, both definitions are influenced by disease-related factors and by the natural life expectancy of a patient. "Indolent" PC is defined as a cancer that never becomes locally invasive or metastatic leading to symptoms or death, irrespective of the patient's comorbidities or expected lifespan [6, 8]. This is in contrast to the term "insignificant," which is epidemiologically defined and based on lifetime risk estimations of the occurrence of symptomatic or clinical PC in a population. Consequently, a tumour classified as nonindolent in a patient who dies of an unrelated cause and has not experienced morbidity from PC will also be classified as overdiagnosed. Overdiagnosis has been estimated between 22 and 67% using different screening regimens [2]. In this context, defining low-risk or insignificant PC in a considerable percentage of PCs is an important diagnostic step. In our study cohort, using five different biopsy-based criteria, 6% to 32% of men were classified as having low-risk PC.

In outlining a definition for low-risk PC to reduce overdiagnosis and minimize morbidity associated with overtreatment of PC, the ability to "accurately" select men is paramount. In the present study, we analysed five criteria to predict men with insignificant PC at RP specimen, a surrogate for low-risk PC and/or suitability for AS. Not surprisingly, the specificity was better among the more stringent criteria for low-risk PC (criteria 1 and 2). In contrast the AUCs were found to be significantly higher among the less stringent criteria (criteria 4 and 5). For our specific research question, specificity might take precedence over sensitivity and therefore a DCA was performed to determine clinical utility (Figure 1). Based on clinical acceptance, the criteria with the highest sensitivity by a specificity of 90% would be assumed as the optimal definition for clinical use [2, 3]. As a result, criteria 3 and 4 may be used for further patient selection and validation purposes.

Furthermore, it should be noted that the benefits of early detection and active treatment are limited, and ultimately what is required is improved selection of patients with significant PC who will benefit from immediate active treatment [1, 2]. In this study, it was observed that the application

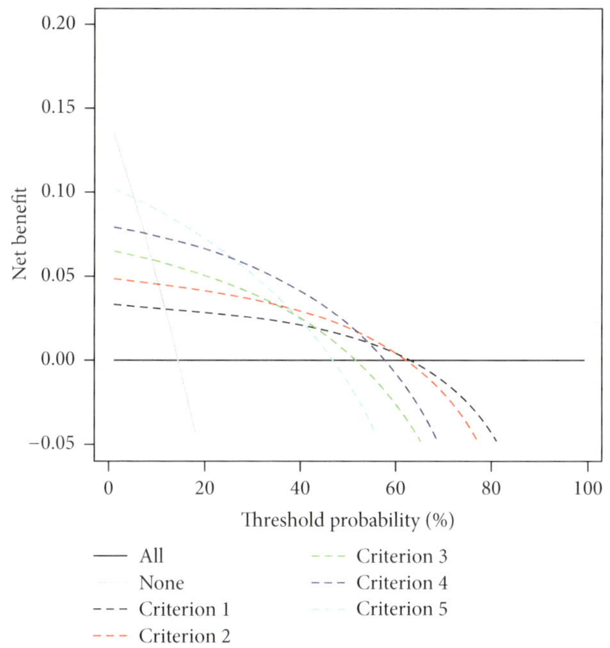

FIGURE 1: Decision curve analysis, demonstrating the net benefit, as measured by rate of nontreating men for low-risk prostate cancer, using the five decision-making strategies as listed in the legend. Threshold probability is the threshold probability of low-risk PC at which an individual considers the benefit of treatment for PC equivalent to the harm of overtreatment for low-risk disease, and thus it reflects how the individual weights the benefits and harms associated with this decision. The highest curve at any given threshold probability is the optimal decision-making strategy to maximize net benefit.

of more liberal criteria would enable 3.6-fold more men to participate in AS program, resulting in a 10% increased risk of underestimating a significant PC (criterion 3 versus criterion 1). In other words, among the present study population, we would decrease the "overdiagnosis" by 13.7% if we only diagnosed insignificant PC using criterion 3 (18.9%) versus criterion 1 (5.2%). In our opinion, these trade-offs could be beneficial, in terms of both quality of life and financial costs related to the early detection of PC [20]. Finally, given the slow evolution of PC, a deferment in definitive treatment would not be likely to substantially alter disease course or limit the patient's chance of complete cure [21].

Finally, the results also showed that, even with the most stringent selection criteria, it is impossible to perfectly differentiate between clinically insignificant and possible life-threatening PC, even after a diagnosis based on transperineal saturation biopsies. Suardi et al. reported rates of 24 to 27.8% of unfavourable PC characteristics in a cohort based on 2 of the most "stringent" criteria looking at 12-core TRUS guided biopsies [9]. Other series reported rates of 8.4–30.5% of unfavourable outcomes in a 12-core TRUS population fulfilling the Epstein criteria [11, 22, 23]. Ultimately, to accurately identify insignificant cancer we will need to look beyond histopathology in isolation, integrating biopsy data with the high-resolution 3D mapping and functional information derived from mpMRI and possibly that from biomarkers (PCA3, pro-2 PSA, and TMPRSS2:erg), mitochondrial RNA mapping (e.g., PC Mitomics Test), epigenetic DNA mapping (e.g., MDx Link), and other emerging predictors of the biologic behaviour of PC in an individualised way [24–28].

Results from the present study may be used for further development of mpMRI protocols. For evaluation of mpMRI performance, ideally inclusion of definitive pathology is required from whole-mount sections of RP specimens as the reference standard [4]. However, since such study designs are not applicable in clinical practice due to the selection biases created by the absence of RP specimens in patients who have no cancer on biopsy low-risk cancer managed with AS or high-risk cancer managed with radiotherapy, an alternative approach is to use transperineal saturation template prostate mapping biopsy instead [4]. Transperineal saturation template mapping biopsy outperforms TRUS guided prostate biopsies, showing an average upgrading in 33% of patients and a change from unilateral to bilateral disease in more than 50% of patients [29]. The present study aids the interpretation of the outcomes of this alternative and demonstrates that saturation biopsy is not a perfect reference standard. Biopsy criterion 3 and criterion 4 showed a specificity and NPV of 86–88% and 93–95%, respectively, for accurately predicting insignificant PC in RP, and therefore may represent clinically relevant definitions for selection of active surveillance patients.

The present study is subject to limitations. Firstly, this was a retrospective analysis of prospectively collected data from only two surgeons in a single centre. Secondly, there is a major selection bias towards higher-risk patients, given that the cohort consists entirely of patients who underwent RP, a decision which may have been driven by unmeasured clinical factors such as a rapidly rising PSA or significant lesions on mpMRI. This could negatively bias the accuracy estimates for each definition. It is a highly selected study population with no control arm. Furthermore, given the long period over which this study data was collected, changes in Gleason reporting for PC may also represent a confounder regarding biopsy and RP specimen pathology. Also, diagnostic performance in terms of sensitivity and specificity are subject to inclusion criteria. We included only low-risk men diagnosed with clinical stage ≤T2, PSA <10 ng/mL, and Gleason score <8 PC in order to estimate the performances of the diagnostic criteria in low-risk patients. Diagnostic performance may differ in higher-risk patients, who are less likely to harbour insignificant disease and are not usually candidates for AS. Furthermore, transperineal saturation biopsies are not generally accepted as a reference test [4], and it is still unclear if transperineal saturation biopsies might detect more insignificant cancers compared to a standard biopsy. Finally, prospective studies that use these biopsy definitions to select patients for AS and then evaluate long-term oncological outcomes will provide a higher level of evidence. However, until such studies are published, retrospective studies such as this can be used to guide patient counselling and treatment decisions.

In conclusion, balancing overtreatment of insignificant PC with undertreatment of significant PC is an ongoing challenge. This study analysed the performance characteristics of various criteria at predicting insignificant PC on transperineal template-guided saturation mapping biopsies in a relatively low-risk PC population who underwent RP. No single definition was superior; however, patients with Gleason 6 disease demonstrated the best trade-off between sensitivity and specificity for clarifying low-risk PC. Depending on patients and physicians preferences, these criteria can be used for treatment decisions and patient counselling and as a reference test in diagnostic studies.

Competing Interests

All authors declare no conflict of interests.

Acknowledgments

This research is funded by the Australian Department of Health and Ageing for its funding of the Australian Prostate Cancer Research Centre NSW, as well as the St Vincent's Prostate Cancer Centre.

References

[1] F. H. Schröder, J. Hugosson, M. J. Roobol et al., "Screening and prostate cancer mortality: results of the European Randomised Study of Screening for Prostate Cancer (ERSPC) at 13 years of follow-up," *The Lancet*, vol. 384, no. 9959, pp. 2027–2035, 2014.

[2] S. Loeb, M. A. Bjurlin, J. Nicholson et al., "Overdiagnosis and overtreatment of prostate cancer," *European Urology*, vol. 65, no. 6, pp. 1046–1055, 2014.

[3] C. H. Bangma, R. Valdagni, P. R. Carroll, H. van Poppel, L. Klotz, and J. Hugosson, "Active surveillance for low-risk prostate cancer: developments to date," *European Urology*, vol. 67, no. 4, pp. 646–648, 2015.

[4] J. J. Fütterer, A. Briganti, P. De Visschere et al., "Can clinically significant prostate cancer be detected with multiparametric magnetic resonance imaging? A systematic review of the literature," *European Urology*, vol. 68, no. 6, pp. 1045–1053, 2015.

[5] J. E. Thompson, D. Moses, R. Shnier et al., "Multiparametric magnetic resonance imaging guided diagnostic biopsy detects significant prostate cancer and could reduce unnecessary biopsies and over detection: a prospective study," *The Journal of Urology*, vol. 192, no. 1, pp. 67–74, 2014.

[6] T. H. van der Kwast and M. J. Roobol, "Defining the threshold for significant versus insignificant prostate cancer," *Nature Reviews Urology*, vol. 10, no. 8, pp. 473–482, 2013.

[7] T. Wolters, M. J. Roobol, P. J. van Leeuwen et al., "A critical analysis of the tumor volume threshold for clinically insignificant prostate cancer using a data set of a randomized screening trial," *The Journal of Urology*, vol. 185, no. 1, pp. 121–125, 2011.

[8] J. I. Epstein, P. C. Walsh, M. Carmichael, and C. B. Brendler, "Pathologic and clinical findings to predict tumor extent of nonpalpable (stage T1c) prostate cancer," *The Journal of the American Medical Association*, vol. 271, no. 5, pp. 368–374, 1994.

[9] N. Suardi, A. Gallina, U. Capitanio et al., "Age-adjusted validation of the most stringent criteria for active surveillance in low-risk prostate cancer patients," *Cancer*, vol. 118, no. 4, pp. 973–980, 2012.

[10] P. Sooriakumaran, A. Srivastava, P. Christos, S. Grover, M. Shevchuk, and A. Tewari, "Predictive models for worsening prognosis in potential candidates for active surveillance of presumed low-risk prostate cancer," *International Urology and Nephrology*, vol. 44, no. 2, pp. 459–470, 2012.

[11] S. E. Lee, D. S. Kim, W. K. Lee et al., "Application of the Epstein criteria for prediction of clinically insignificant prostate cancer in Korean men," *BJU International*, vol. 105, no. 11, pp. 1526–1530, 2010.

[12] M. A. Bjurlin, H. B. Carter, P. Schellhammer et al., "Optimization of initial prostate biopsy in clinical practice: sampling, labeling and specimen processing," *The Journal of Urology*, vol. 189, no. 6, pp. 2039–2046, 2013.

[13] J. I. Epstein, Z. Feng, B. J. Trock, and P. M. Pierorazio, "Upgrading and downgrading of prostate cancer from biopsy to radical prostatectomy: incidence and predictive factors using the modified gleason grading system and factoring in tertiary grades," *European Urology*, vol. 61, no. 5, pp. 1019–1024, 2012.

[14] O. Ukimura, J. A. Coleman, A. de la Taille et al., "Contemporary role of systematic prostate biopsies: indications, techniques, and implications for patient care," *European Urology*, vol. 63, no. 2, pp. 214–230, 2013.

[15] G. Onik, M. Miessau, and D. G. Bostwick, "Three-dimensional prostate mapping biopsy has a potentially significant impact on prostate cancer management," *Journal of Clinical Oncology*, vol. 27, no. 26, pp. 4321–4326, 2009.

[16] D. I. Quinn, S. M. Henshall, A.-M. Haynes et al., "Prognostic significance of pathologic features in localized prostate cancer treated with radical prostatectomy: implications for staging systems and predictive models," *Journal of Clinical Oncology*, vol. 19, no. 16, pp. 3692–3705, 2001.

[17] H. U. Ahmed, Y. Hu, T. Carter et al., "Characterizing clinically significant prostate cancer using template prostate mapping biopsy," *The Journal of Urology*, vol. 186, no. 2, pp. 458–464, 2011.

[18] A. J. Vickers and E. B. Elkin, "Decision curve analysis: a novel method for evaluating prediction models," *Medical Decision Making*, vol. 26, no. 6, pp. 565–574, 2006.

[19] L. J. Esserman, I. M. Thompson Jr., and B. Reid, "Overdiagnosis and overtreatment in cancer: an opportunity for improvement," *The Journal of the American Medical Association*, vol. 310, no. 8, pp. 797–798, 2013.

[20] E. A. M. Heijnsdijk, A. der Kinderen, E. M. Wever, G. Draisma, M. J. Roobol, and H. J. de Koning, "Overdetection, overtreatment and costs in prostate-specific antigen screening for prostate cancer," *British Journal of Cancer*, vol. 101, no. 11, pp. 1833–1838, 2009.

[21] G. Draisma, R. Boer, S. J. Otto et al., "Lead times and overdetection due to prostate-specific antigen screening: estimates from the European randomized study of screening for prostate cancer," *Journal of the National Cancer Institute*, vol. 95, no. 12, pp. 868–878, 2003.

[22] C. Jeldres, N. Suardi, J. Walz et al., "Validation of the contemporary epstein criteria for insignificant prostate cancer in European men," *European Urology*, vol. 54, no. 6, pp. 1306–1313, 2008.

[23] P. J. Bastian, L. A. Mangold, J. I. Epstein, and A. W. Partin, "Characteristics of insignificant clinical T1c prostate tumors: a contemporary analysis," *Cancer*, vol. 101, no. 9, pp. 2001–2005, 2004.

[24] K. Braun, D. D. Sjoberg, A. J. Vickers, H. Lilja, and A. S. Bjartell, "A four-kallikrein panel predicts high-grade cancer

on biopsy: independent validation in a community cohort," *European Urology*, vol. 69, no. 3, pp. 505–511, 2016.

[25] J. K. Rane, M. Scaravilli, A. Ylipää et al., "MicroRNA expression profile of primary prostate cancer stem cells as a source of biomarkers and therapeutic targets," *European Urology*, vol. 67, no. 1, pp. 7–10, 2015.

[26] A. C. Vidal and S. J. Freedland, "Genetic variants in predicting aggressive prostate cancer: 'ready for prime time?'," *European Urology*, vol. 65, no. 6, pp. 1076–1077, 2014.

[27] S. Loeb, M. G. Sanda, D. L. Broyles et al., "The prostate health index selectively identifies clinically significant prostate cancer," *The Journal of Urology*, vol. 193, no. 4, pp. 1163–1169, 2015.

[28] J. K. Parsons, "Novel biomarkers and advanced imaging modalities in the early detection of prostate cancer," *The Journal of Urology*, vol. 193, no. 4, pp. 1084–1085, 2015.

[29] A. V. Taira, G. S. Merrick, R. W. Galbreath et al., "Performance of transperineal template-guided mapping biopsy in detecting prostate cancer in the initial and repeat biopsy setting," *Prostate Cancer and Prostatic Diseases*, vol. 13, no. 1, pp. 71–77, 2010.

26

Emerging Molecularly Targeted Therapies in Castration Refractory Prostate Cancer

Jesal C. Patel,[1] Benjamin L. Maughan,[2] Archana M. Agarwal,[3] Julia A. Batten,[1] Tian Y. Zhang,[2] and Neeraj Agarwal[1]

[1] *Division of Medical Oncology, University of UT Huntsman Cancer Institute, Salt Lake City, Utah 84112, USA*
[2] *Department of Internal Medicine, University of UT, Salt Lake City, Utah 84112, USA*
[3] *Department of Pathology and ARUP Laboratories, University of UT, Salt Lake City, Utah 84108, USA*

Correspondence should be addressed to Neeraj Agarwal; neeraj.agarwal@hci.utah.edu

Academic Editor: William L. Dahut

Androgen deprivation therapy (ADT) with medical or surgical castration is the mainstay of therapy in men with metastatic prostate cancer. However, despite initial responses, almost all men eventually develop castration refractory metastatic prostate cancer (CRPC) and die of their disease. Over the last decade, it has been recognized that despite the failure of ADT, most prostate cancers maintain some dependence on androgen and/or androgen receptor (AR) signaling for proliferation. Furthermore, androgen independent molecular pathways have been identified as drivers of continued progression of CRPC. Subsequently, drugs have been developed targeting these pathways, many of which have received regulatory approval. Agents such as abiraterone, enzalutamide, orteronel (TAK-700), and ARN-509 target androgen signaling. Sipuleucel-T, ipilimumab, and tasquinimod augment immune-mediated tumor killing. Agents targeting classic tumorogenesis pathways including vascular endothelial growth factor, hepatocyte growth factor, insulin like growth factor-1, tumor suppressor, and those which regulate apoptosis and cell cycles are currently being developed. This paper aims to focus on emerging molecular pathways underlying progression of CRPC, and the drugs targeting these pathways, which have recently been approved or have reached advanced stages of development in either phase II or phase III clinical trials.

1. Introduction

Prostate cancer is the most common noncutaneous malignancy and one of the common causes of cancer related deaths among men in the United States [1]. The majority of men are diagnosed with early stage disease. However, approximately a third will eventually develop metastatic disease. The cornerstone of treatment for advanced disease is medical castration by androgen deprivation therapy with a gonadotropin releasing hormone agonist (GnRH) or less commonly, surgical castration with orchiectomy. Despite initial responses, almost all patients will develop disease progression, a stage known as metastatic castration refractory prostate cancer (mCRPC). One of the reasons why prostate cancer continues to progress is the persistence of androgen receptor signaling, despite castrate level of androgens [2]. Additionally, there are androgen independent pathways responsible for prostate cancer progression. This paper summarizes the recent advancements in the development of therapies that target these molecular pathways in CRPC, with an emphasis on agents that are being evaluated in phase II or III clinical trials and those recently approved for the treatment of CRPC (Figure 1, Tables 1 and 2).

2. Targeting Androgen Signaling Pathway

Several mechanisms have been identified to explain persistent androgen signaling in CRPC [2, 3], including increased AR gene expression, mutation of the AR gene, or upregulation of enzymes involved in androgen synthesis [3–6]. Cytochrome P450 17 alpha-hydroxylase and C17,20-lyase (CYP17) are the critical enzymes for synthesis of androgens in the adrenal glands and prostate tumors [6].

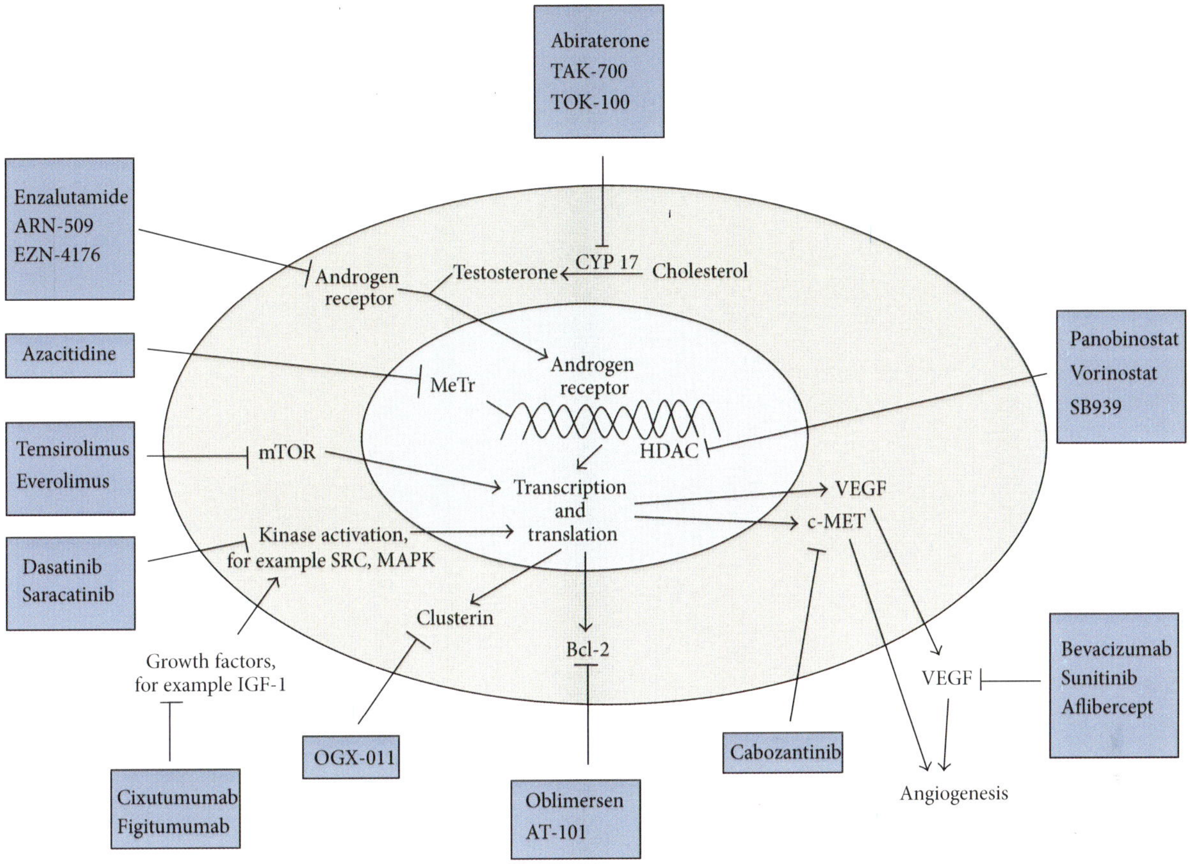

FIGURE 1: Androgen dependent and independent molecular pathways underlying progression of castration refractory prostate cancer and drugs targeting those pathways. CYP17: Cytochrome P450 17 alpha-hydroxylase and C17,20-lyase; mCRPC: metastatic castration refractory prostate cancer; AR: androgen receptor; OS: overall survival; PFS: progression free survival; c-MET: hepatocyte growth factor receptor; VEGF: vascular endothelial growth factor; MeTr: DNA methyl transferase; HDAC: histone deacetylases; Src: Src kinase; MAPK: MAP kinase; IGF-1: insulin like growth factor-1.

Abiraterone acetate, a pregnenolone analog, is an orally administered small molecule that irreversibly inhibits CYP17. Abiraterone was shown to be clinically beneficial and improved overall survival compared to placebo in a landmark phase III trial in patients who had been previously treated with docetaxel (14.8 months versus 10.9 months, $P < 0.0001$) [7]. Abiraterone was well tolerated with mild adverse effects associated with secondary mineralocorticoid excess. In 2011, the FDA approved the use of abiraterone for treatment of CRPC in patients who were previously treated with docetaxel. More recently, another phase III study showed improved radiographic PFS with abiraterone over placebo in men with CRPC who had never received chemotherapy, leading to the regulatory approval of abiraterone in prechemotherapy setting as well [8].

Orteronel (TAK-700), like abiraterone, is a novel inhibitor of the CYP17 pathway. However, TAK-700 more specifically inhibits CYP17, 20 lyase versus CYP17 hydroxylase, and does not generally lead to the syndrome of secondary mineralocorticoid excess. The updated data obtained from phase II portion of a phase I/II study of TAK-700 in chemonaive patients with metastatic CRPC were reported in 2012 Genitourinary Cancers Symposium [9]. Ninety-six chemonaive patients with metastatic CRPC were treated in four TAK-700 dose cohorts. The PSA reduction rates were favorable across all cohorts. Of the 51 patients who had RECIST-evaluable disease, 10 had a partial response, 22 had stable disease, and 15 had disease progression. In a phase II study of patients with nonmetastatic CRPC with biochemical recurrence, 38 patients were treated with TAK-700 at a dose of 300 mg twice daily, without prednisone [10]. Treatment at this dose was feasible with manageable toxicities. After three months of treatment, 16% achieved PSA ≤ 0.2 ng/Ml, 76% achieved $\geq 50\%$ decrease, and 32% achieved a PSA reduction of $\geq 90\%$. Median time to PSA progression was 14.8 months. Currently, there are separate phase 3 trials evaluating TAK-700 in men with progressive CRPC, who are either chemotherapy naïve or posttreatment with docetaxel (Table 1).

Enzalutamide (MDV 3100) is a novel AR antagonist that binds to AR with an eight-times higher affinity than bicalutamide and reduces the efficiency of nuclear translocation of the androgen receptor, DNA binding to androgen response elements, and recruitment of coactivators by the androgen receptor [11]. In contrast to bicalutamide, MDV3100 has no known agonist activity when AR is overexpressed. In a phase

Table 1: Selected ongoing and recently concluded phase III trials in castration refractory prostate cancer.

Target	Drug	Trial	Phase	Primary endpoint	Clinical trial identifier number (accessed on January 22, 2013)	Outcome
Androgen dependent pathways						
CYP17	Orteronel (TAK-700)	Randomized, double-blind, orteronel plus prednisone versus placebo plus prednisone in mCRPC with prior docetaxel therapy	III	OS	NCT01193257	Ongoing
CYP17	Orteronel (TAK-700)	Randomized, double-blind, orteronel plus prednisone versus placebo plus prednisone in progressive, chemotherapy naive mCRPC	III	OS	NCT01193244	Ongoing
CYP17	Abiraterone	Randomized, double-blind, prednisone and abiraterone or placebo and prednisone in mCRPC after failed docetaxel	III	OS	NCT00638690	Improved OS with abiraterone
CYP17	Abiraterone	Randomized, double-blind, prednisone and abiraterone or placebo and prednisone in chemotherapy naive mCRPC	III	PFS	NCT00887198	Improved radiographic PFS with abiraterone
AR	Enzalutamide (MDV 3100)	Randomized, double-blind, MDV3100 versus placebo in chemotherapy naive progressive mCRPC	III	OS, PFS	NCT01212991	Ongoing
AR	Enzalutamide (MDV 3100)	Randomized, double-blind, MDV3100 versus placebo in mCRPC with prior docetaxel	III	OS	NCT00974311	Improved OS with enzalutamide
Androgen independent pathways						
Src kinase	Dasatinib	Randomized, double-blinded, docetaxel, prednisone, and dasatinib versus docetaxel, prednisone, and placebo in mCRPC	III	OS	NCT00744497	No difference in OS
c-MET	Cabozantinib	Randomized, placebo controlled of mitoxantrone and prednisone versus cabozantinib in mCRPC	III	Pain response	NCT01522443	Ongoing
c-MET	Cabozantinib	Randomized, placebo controlled prednisone versus cabozantinib in mCRPC with prior docetaxel and abiraterone or MDV3100	III	OS	NCT01605227	Ongoing

Table 1: Continued.

Target	Drug	Trial	Phase	Primary endpoint	Clinical trial identifier number (accessed on January 22, 2013)	Outcome
Clusterin	Custirsen (OGX-011)	Randomized, open label with cabazitaxel and prednisone with or without custirsen in second line chemotherapy in mCRPC	III	OS	NCT01578655	Ongoing
	Custirsen (OGX-011)	Randomized, docetaxel and prednisone with and without custirsen in chemotherapy naïve mCRPC	III	OS	NCT01188187	Ongoing
	Custirsen (OGX-011)	Randomized, docetaxel retreatment or cabazitaxel and prednisone with and without custirsen in mCRPC	III	Pain response	NCT01083615	Ongoing
VEGF	Bevacizumab (VEGF antibody)	Randomized, double-blinded, docetaxel and prednisone with and without bevacizumab in mCRPC	III	OS	NCT00110214	No difference in OS
	Aflibercept (VEGF trap)	Randomized, double-blind, aflibercept versus placebo in mCRPC with ongoing docetaxel and prednisone	III	OS	NCT00519285	No difference in OS
	Sunitinib (VEGF tyrosine kinase inhibitor)	Randomized, double-blind, sunitinib and prednisone versus prednisone in mCRPC with prior docetaxel	III	OS	NCT00676650	No difference in OS
Immunotherapy	Prostvac-VF	Randomized Prostvac-VF with and without GM-CSF in chemotherapy naive mCRPC	III	OS	NCT01322490	Ongoing
	Ipilimumab	Randomized ipilimumab versus placebo in chemotherapy naive mCRPC	III	OS	NCT01057810	Ongoing
	Ipilimumab	Randomized ipilimumab versus placebo in mCRPC following radiotherapy with prior docetaxel	III	OS	NCT00861614	Ongoing
	Tasquinimod	Randomized tasquinimod versus placebo in chemotherapy naive mCRPC	III	PFS	NCT01234311	Ongoing

CYP17: Cytochrome P450 17 alpha-hydroxylase and C17,20-lyase; mCRPC: metastatic castration refractory prostate cancer; AR: androgen receptor; OS: overall survival; PFS: progression free survival; c-MET: hepatocyte growth factor receptor; VEGF: vascular endothelial growth factor.

TABLE 2: Selected ongoing and recently concluded phase II trials in castration refractory prostate cancer.

Target	Drug	Trial	Phase	Primary endpoint	Clinical trial identifier number
		Androgen dependent pathways			
CYP17	TOK-001 (galeterone)	Single arm, open label, dose escalation, study of TOK-001 in chemotherapy naive mCRPC	I/II	Safety, PSA response (≥50%)	NCT00959959
AR	Enzalutamide (MDV 3100)	Randomized, double-blind, MDV3100 versus bicalutamide in CRPC	II	PFS at 24 months	NCT01664923
	Enzalutamide (MDV 3100)	Randomized, double-blind MDV3100 versus bicalutamide in CRPC	II	PFS at 24 months	NCT01288911
	ARN-509	Open label, single arm, ARN-509 in CRPC	I/II	PSA response	NCT01171898
AR mRNA antagonist	EZN-4176	Open label, single arm study of EZN-4176 in CRPC	I	Maximum tolerated dose, safety	NCT01337518
		Androgen independent pathways			
Src kinase	Dasatinib	Randomized, open label of cediranib and dasatinib versus cediranib and placebo in CRPC resistant to docetaxel	II	PFS	NCT01260688
	Dasatinib	Randomized, open label of abiraterone and prednisone with or without dasatinib in mCRPC	II	PFS	NCT01685125
	Saracatinib	Randomized, double-blind, saracatinib versus placebo in mCRPC with prior docetaxel	II	Time to disease progression, PFS	NCT01267266
	Saracatinib	Single arm, saracatinib in mCRPC	II	PSA response	NCT00513071
mTOR	Everolimus (RAD001)	Single arm, RAD001 in mCRPC	II	Biochemical response rate	NCT00629525
	Everolimus (RAD001)	Single arm, RAD001 with docetaxel and bevacizumab in mCRPC	I/II	Safety	NCT00574769
	Everolimus (RAD001)	Single arm, RAD001 with docetaxel in mCRPC	I/II	Safety, objective response	NCT00459186
	Everolimus (RAD001)	Single arm, carboplatin, everolimus, and prednisone in mCRPC with prior docetaxel	II	Time to progression	NCT01051570
	Temsirolimus	Single arm, cixutumumab with temsirolimus in chemotherapy naive CRPC	I/II	Safety, objective response/PSA response	NCT01026623
	Ridaforolimus	Randomized, placebo controlled, bicalutamide with or without ridaforolimus in mCRPC	II	PSA response, dose limiting toxicities	NCT00777959
IGF-1R	Figitumumab (CP-751871)	Randomized, noncomparative, two arm, open label, docetaxel and prednisone with and without figitumumab in mCRPC	II	PSA response, objective response	NCT00313781
	Cixutumumab (IMC-A12)	Single arm, open label, cixutumumab in chemotherapy naive mCRPC	II	Time to progression, pharmacokinetics	NCT00520481
	Cixutumumab (IMC-A12)	Single arm, cixutumumab with temsirolimus in chemotherapy naive CRPC	I/II	Safety, objective response/PSA response, and time to progression	NCT01026623

Table 2: Continued.

Target	Drug	Trial	Phase	Primary endpoint	Clinical trial identifier number
Bcl-2	Oblimersen	Randomized docetaxel with or without oblimersen in mCRPC	II	PSA response >30%, major toxic event rate <45%[‡]	NCT00085228
	R-(-)-gossypol acetic acid (AT-101)	Randomized, docetaxel and prednisone with or without AT-101 in chemotherapy naive mCRPC	II	OS[*]	NCT00571675
Hsp90	STA-9090	Single arm, open label, STA-9090 in mCRPC with prior docetaxel	II	PFS at 6 months	NCT01270880
Hsp90	AT13387	Two arm, open-label, parallel group, randomized, AT13387 with or without abiraterone in mCRPC progressing on abiraterone	I/II	Safety and tolerability response per PCWG2	NCT01685268
HDAC	Panobinostat (LBH589)	Single arm, panobinostat in mCRPC with prior docetaxel	II	PFS at 24 weeks	NCT00667862
	Panobinostat (LBH589)	Randomized panobinostat at two dose levels combined with bicalutamide for CRPC	I/II	Safety, dosing schedule, proportion free of progression and without symptomatic deterioration at 9 months	NCT00878436
	Vorinostat	Single arm, vorinostat for mCPRC with prior chemotherapy	II	PFS at 6 months[**]	NCT00330161
	SB939	Open label, single arm, SB939 for recurrent or mCRPC	II	PFS PSA response	NCT01075308
DNA methyltransferase	Azacitidine	Single arm, docetaxel retreatment, and prednisone with azacitidine in mCRPC with prior docetaxel	I/II	Safety PSA and objective response	NCT00503984
Immunotherapy	Prostvac-VF	Randomized, open label, flutamide with and without Prostvac-VF in non-mCRPC	II	Time to treatment failure	NCT00450463
	Prostvac-VF	Randomized, open label, docetaxel and prednisone with or without Prostvac-VF in mCRPC	II	OS	NCT01145508
	177Lu radiolabeled monoclonal antibody (Ab) HuJ591 (177Lu-J591)	Randomized ketoconazole and hydrocortisone plus 177Lu-J591 or placebo (111In-J591) in non-mCRPC	II	Proportion free of radiographically evident metastases at 18 months	NCT00859781

CYP17: Cytochrome P450 17 alpha-hydroxylase and C17,20-lyase; mCRPC: metastatic castration refractory prostate cancer; PSA: prostate-specific antigen; AR: androgen receptor; PFS: progression free survival; OS: overall survival; mTOR: mammalian target of rapamycin; IGF-1: insulin like growth factor-1; Hsp: heat shock protein; HDAC: histone deacetylases.

[‡]Primary endpoints not met.

[*]Primary endpoint not met.

[**]Significant toxicities, no one met the primary endpoint.

III trial of men with CRPC with prior docetaxel therapy, enzalutamide when compared to placebo, significantly improved overall survival (18.4 months versus 13.6 months; $P < 0.001$), leading to its regulatory approval in this setting [12]. Another phase III trial of enzalutamide in chemotherapy naïve men with CPRC is currently ongoing (Table 1).

ARN-509 is a novel small molecule AR antagonist, is structurally and mechanistically similar to enzalutamide, and impairs AR nuclear translocation, as well as AR binding to DNA. In phase I/II study of men with metastatic CRPC, ARN-509 was well tolerated and showed pharmacodynamic evidence of AR antagonism with promising clinical activity. Phase II dose was determined to be 240 mg per day. The most common treatment related grade 1-2 side effects were fatigue, nausea, and pain [13] (Table 2). The phase II portion of the study included three distinct population of men with CRPC: nonmetastatic treatment-naïve CRPC, metastatic CRPC (treatment naïve), and metastatic CRPC (with prior treatment with abiraterone acetate). The primary endpoint was PSA response rate at 12 weeks according to the Prostate Cancer Working Group 2 Criteria. Preliminary results were reported at the 2013 genitourinary cancer symposium. Among 47 men with non-metastatic CRPC, the 12-week PSA response was 91%, and the time to PSA progression had not been reached [14]. Among 46 men with metastatic CRPC, 26 were treatment naïve, and 21 had prior treatment with abiraterone acetate. At 12 weeks, the PSA response was 88% in the treatment naïve cohort. Notably, 29% men with prior treatment with abiraterone acetate had PSA response after 12 weeks, thus indicating activity of ARN-509 in the subset of men with CRPC that developed resistance to abiraterone acetate [15].

Other promising rationally designed drugs inhibiting AR signaling include TOK-001 (galeterone), EZN-4176, and EPI-001. TOK-001, formerly known as VN/124-1, inhibits prostate cancer growth by multiple mechanisms. In addition to inhibiting CYP17, it directly antagonizes the AR receptor and also downregulates AR protein expression [16]. A phase I/II trial of TOK-001 has been initiated in chemonaive patients with mCRPC (Table 2). EZN-4176, an AR mRNA antagonist, is a locked nucleic acid (LNA) oligonucleotide that downregulates AR mRNA and is currently ongoing development in a phase I trial of men with CRPC [17]. EPI-001 inhibits the N terminal domain of the AR, which confers transcriptional activity, and has the capability to overcome castration resistance associated with a gain of function mutations of the ligand binding domain, and expression of constitutionally active splice variants of the AR. EPI-001 is currently awaiting clinical trial development in [18].

3. Targeting Androgen Independent Molecular Pathways Implicated in Stromal-Epithelial Crosstalk and in Shaping Tumor Microenvironment

3.1. Targeting Src Kinase Signaling. The Src family of nonreceptor protein tyrosine kinases (SFKs) is upregulated in various human malignancies, including prostate cancer and their expression directly correlates with disease progression and metastasis [19, 20]. In addition, Src signaling plays an important role in normal bone turnover, and is essential for normal osteoclast functioning, as well as osteoblast proliferation, and has been implicated in the promotion of bone metastasis in prostate cancer [20].

Dasatinib (BMS-354825) is a selective small molecule inhibitor of SFKs and other tyrosine kinases, including Bcr-Abl, Kit, and PDGFRβ. A recent phase II study of chemotherapy naïve patients with CRPC has shown promising results. Forty-three percent of patients at week 12 and 19% patients at week 24 had radiographically stable disease. Additionally, at week 12, 51% of patients achieved ≥40% reduction in urinary N-telopeptide, while 60% had reduction in bone alkaline phosphatase. Treatment with dasatinib was generally well tolerated. Based on the positive results from a separate phase I/II study, which combined dasatinib with docetaxel, a randomized phase III study comparing docetaxel with dasatinib to docetaxel with placebo in castration resistant prostate cancer was conducted. The results, however, failed to show an improvement in overall survival [21]. Additionally, dasatinib is being tested in two randomized phase II trials in combination with abiraterone and cediranib (VEGF TKI), respectively (Table 2).

Saracatinib (AZD0530) is an oral non-receptor tyrosine kinase inhibitor targeting Src kinases and has been shown to have activity in orthotopic animal models of CRPC [22]. Two phase II studies of saracatinib in CRPC in chemotherapy naive and postdocetaxel settings, respectively, are underway (Table 1).

3.2. Targeting PI3K/Akt/mTOR Pathway. The phosphatidylinositol 3-kinase (PI3 K)/Akt/mammalian target of rapamycin (mTOR) signaling pathway regulates multiple physiological cell processes, which include metabolism, proliferation, differentiation, survival, migration, and angiogenesis. The lipid and protein phosphatase, PTEN (phosphatase and tensin homology protein), is a key negative regulator of Akt activity. Aberrant expression of PI3K and AKT1 genes or loss of PTEN tumor suppression gene leads to downstream upregulation of mTOR and tumorigenesis. Although, everolimus does not have clear significant single agent activity in CRPC, it holds promise in combination therapy with chemotherapeutics given the fact that it restores sensitivity to chemotherapy as do other drugs within the class [23]. Preliminary results of a phase I/II trial combining docetaxel and temsirolimus have showed acceptable safety and antitumor activity and a phase II expansion cohort is underway [24]. Furthermore, multiple phase II studies of mTOR inhibitors as single agent or in combination with chemotherapeutics or biologic agents are ongoing (Table 2).

3.3. Targeting Vascular Endothelial Growth Factor (VEGF) Pathway. Angiogenesis and neovascularization are necessary for the growth and metastasis of solid tumors. Vascular endothelial growth factor (VEGF) plays a pivotal role in angiogenesis and neovascularization. There is clinical evidence that the simultaneous use of angiogenesis inhibitors and chemotherapeutic drugs may lead to improved outcomes in patients with CRPC [25–27]. Multiple agents have been tested in phase III trials of men with metastatic CRPC.

Bevacizumab is a humanized monoclonal antibody that inhibits angiogenesis by neutralizing circulating vascular endothelial growth factor (VEGF). Sunitinib is a tyrosine kinase inhibitor (TKI) which similarly targets VEGF receptor. Aflibercept (VEGF Trap) is a recombinant humanized fusion protein consisting of the VEGF extracellular domains and the Fc portion of human immunoglobulin IgG1. However, none of these agents have shown overall survival advantage in phase III trials of men with metastatic CRPC (Table 1).

3.4. Targeting Insulin Like Growth Factor (IGF) Pathway. The insulin like growth factor (IGF) pathway, which includes IGF receptor-1 (IGF-1R) and its ligands, IGF-I and IGF-II, not only plays a major role in growth, development, and maintenance of homeostasis in normal cells, but also the proliferation of cancers cells, including prostate cancer cells [28]. Higher levels of circulating IGF-I correlates with increased risk of developing prostate cancer, as well as metastatic disease. Blockade of IGF-IR in combination with chemotherapy leads to chemosensitization in androgen-independent prostate cancer cell lines and improved docetaxel antitumor activity in animal models [28].

Figitumumab and cixutumumab are fully human monoclonal antibodies targeting IGF-1R. In a phase Ib trial, a combination of figitumumab and docetaxel was well tolerated in patients with a variety of solid tumors, with three patients with CRPC demonstrating an objective response [28]. Encouraged by these results, a phase II study of this combination has been initiated in the setting of CRPC (Table 2). In a phase II study, chemotherapy naïve men with metastatic CRPC were treated with cixutumumab at two different dosing schemes in both cohorts. Approximately 30% of patients had disease stabilization for ≥6 months [29]. The most common drug-related adverse events were fatigue and asymptomatic hyperglycemia. Phase II studies of cixutumumab, either as monotherapy or in combination with temsirolimus, are ongoing in men with chemotherapy naïve metastatic CRPC (Table 2).

3.5. Targeting Bcl-2. Overexpression of Bcl-2 is observed in a significant number of men with CRPC. It plays a key role in the onset of castration refractoriness and contributes to the resistance to radiation and docetaxel therapy [30]. Inhibition of Bcl-2 expression leads to increased apoptosis, as well as diminished proliferation and angiogenesis [31].

Oblimersen (Genasense, G3139) is an 18-base synthetic oligonucleotide strand that hybridizes with the first six codons of the Bcl-2 RNA transcript, resulting in degradation by endogenous RNase H and the inhibition of Bcl-2 protein expression [31]. In a multicenter, phase II study men with chemotherapy naïve metastatic CRPC with PSA progression, patients were randomized to receive docetaxel with or without oblimersen [30]. Oblimersen was given on days 1–5 to achieve downregulation of Bcl-2 prior to docetaxel, which was given on day 5. Oblimersen was then continued for two more days after docetaxel to allow for adequate coexposure of the two drugs. However, the primary endpoints of the study (confirmed PSA response rate of >30% and a major toxic event rate <45% in the combination arm) were not met [30].

AT-101 (R—gossypol acetic acid) is a polyphenolic compound derived from the cottonseed plant [32]. Acting as a BH3 mimetic, AT-101 inhibits the function of Bcl-2 family member proteins by preventing their binding with proapoptotic proteins and upregulates proapoptotic factors. In a phase II study, men with progressive metastatic CRPC received docetaxel and prednisone with or without AT-101 [33]. Although, overall survival, the primary endpoint, was not improved, a potential benefit was observed in a subgroup of high-risk patients.

These results suggest that apoptotic failure may result from molecular mechanisms other than Bcl-2 over expression. Men with documented underlying Bcl-2 over expression, as a mechanism of chemoresistance, may be more appropriate candidates for combinatorial regimen employing Bcl-2 targeted therapies.

3.6. Targeting Cytoprotective Chaperone Proteins. Clusterin is a cytoprotective chaperone whose transcription is promoted by the androgen receptor and by heat shock factor-1, a key mediator of carcinogenesis [34]. Over expression of clusterin in prostate cancer has been correlated with progression to CRPC [34, 35].

Custirsen (OGX-011) is an antisense oligonucleotide to the clusterin mRNA translation initiation site that potently inhibits clusterin expression and enhances the efficacy of anticancer therapies in vitro and in vivo. In a phase II study, men with metastatic CRPC were treated with docetaxel and prednisone with or without OGX-011. Although, there was no improvement in PSA response (the primary endpoint), overall survival (secondary endpoint) was improved in the OGX-011 arm (23.8 months versus 16.9 months) [34]. Currently, three phase III trials combing OGX-011 with chemotherapeutic agents are ongoing in metastatic CRPC (Table 1).

HSP-90 is another multifaceted molecular chaperone implicated in the progression of prostate cancer by the induction of several upstream signaling pathways, which promote aberrant androgen receptor activation and stabilize the androgen receptor protein. Phase II trials are currently ongoing in metastatic CRPC using HSP-90 inhibitors (Table 2) [36].

3.7. Targeting Hepatocyte Growth Factor/c-Met Signaling Pathway. Hepatocyte growth factor (HGF) is a potent oncogenic protein, which often acts synergistically with VEGF on endothelial cells, as well as several other cellular signaling pathways, including Ras/MEK pathway and PI3K/AKT pathway [37]. HGF acts through its receptor HGFR, also known as c-Met. The HGF/c-Met pathway is overexpressed in prostate cancer and promotes metastasis. Androgen receptor suppresses c-Met transcription, and c-Met expression is up regulated by castration [38].

Cabozantinib (XL-184) is an inhibitor of c-MET and VEGF receptor tyrosine kinases. In a phase II study of men with metastatic CRPC, treatment with cabozantinib, when compared to placebo, resulted in improved PFS, reduction of soft tissue lesions, resolution of bone scans, and decreased pain [39]. Currently, two phase III trials of cabozantinib are ongoing in men with metastatic CRPC, with prior docetaxel and with prior abiraterone or MDV3100 (Table 1).

3.8. Targeting Epigenetic Pathways. AR, a transcription factor, binds with the androgen response elements (AREs) located throughout the genome and recruits various cofactors, such as histone acetyltransferases (HATs) and histone deacetylases (HDACs). This leads to the formation of multiprotein complexes involved in the AR mediated transcriptional regulation of various genes implicated in prostate cancer growth and proliferation [40]. In prostate cancer, HDAC inhibition leads to decreased proliferation of cell lines and decreased tumor growth in preclinical models [41].

Vorinostat is a small molecule inhibitor of class I and II HDACs and has shown promising antitumor activity in prostate cancer cell lines and animal models of prostate cancer. Unfortunately, a phase II trial in patients with mCRPC showed no PSA or objective response and an unacceptable toxicity profile. Panobinostat, a pan-deacetylase inhibitor, has undergone testing in a phase I trial in combination with docetaxel in CRPC [42]. Furthermore, panobinostat is being tested in a phase I/II study in combination with bicalutamide and in a phase II study, as monotherapy for patients with CRPC (Table 2).

Another epigenetic pathway of interest is DNA methylation. An open chromatin structure induced by hypomethylation facilitates gene transcription, whereas a closed structure inhibits transcription. Azacitidine, an inhibitor of DNA methyltransferase, induces hypomethylation and reverses the silencing of tumor suppressor genes. It has been shown to restore sensitivity to androgen deprivation therapy, as well as chemotherapy in preclinical models of prostate cancer [23]. In a phase II trial of men with chemonaive CRPC progressing on combined androgen blockade, addition of azacitidine significantly prolonged PSA doubling time [43]. Currently, azacitidine is being tested in a phase II trial in combination with docetaxel in CRPC with prior docetaxel therapy (Table 2).

3.9. Targeting Bone Metastasis. The majority of patients with mCRPC develop osteoblastic bone metastasis accompanied by simultaneous bone destruction, due to increased osteoclastic activity. The receptor activator of nuclear factor-kB ligand (RANKL) is critical for the formation, function, and survival of osteoclasts. In preclinical models of prostate cancer, inhibition of osteoclasts leads to improvement of sclerotic changes in the bones [44]. In a phase III trial, zoledronic acid, an inhibitor of osteoclasts, significantly decreased the incidence of skeletal related events (SRE) and increased the median time to the first SRE, over placebo [45].

Denosumab is a monoclonal antibody against RANKL. Compared to zoledronic acid, denosumab improved median time to first SRE in a phase III trial of men with CRPC with bone metastasis (20.7 versus 17.1 months; HR: 0.82; 95% confidence interval, 0.71–0.95; $P = 0.0002$ for noninferiority; $P = 0.008$ for superiority).

Radium-223 chloride (Ra-223), a radiopharmaceutical agent, targets bone metastasis by emitting high energy alpha-particles of extremely short range (<100 μm). In a phase III, placebo controlled trial of men with symptomatic CRPC with bone metastasis, Ra-223 significantly improved overall survival (14.0 versus 11.2 months, two-sided $P = 0.00185$; HR = 0.695; 95% CI, 0.552–0.875) and delayed time to first SRE (13.6 versus 8.4 months, $P = 0.00046$; HR = 0.610; 95% CI, 0.461–0.807) [46].

3.10. Modulating the Immune System. Regulatory approval of sipuleucel-T for mCRPC has validated modulation of the immune system as an effective strategy in prostate cancer. Sipuleucel-T consists of autologous antigen presenting cells enriched for a CD54+ DC fraction that are harvested by leukopheresis and cultured with a fusion protein (PA2024), comprising of prostate acid phosphatase (PAP) and granulocyte-monocyte colony stimulating factor (GM-CSF) [47, 48]. In a phase III trial of men with asymptomatic chemonaïve metastatic CRPC, the median overall survival was significantly improved with sipuleucel-T over placebo (25.8 versus 21.7 months; HR = 0.77; $P = 0.02$), with a relative reduction of 22% in the risk of death in the sipuleucel-T group (HR = 0.78; $P = 0.03$) [48]. Upon disease progression, 64% men in the control arm crossed over to a nonrandomized open-label protocol to receive an investigational autologous immunotherapy made from cryopreserved cells (APC8015F). In an exploratory analysis, after adjusting for the effect of APC8015F and assuming that APC8015F was as effective as sipuleucel-T, the estimated overall benefit with sipuleucel-T was 7.8 months [49].

3.11. Virus-Based Vaccines. The inherent immunogenicity of viruses and the high level of gene expression seen with viral vectors lead to a strong inflammatory response and may lead to an improved immune response against tumor antigens expressed by viruses [50]. Prostvac-VF utilizes a heterologous prime/boost vaccination strategy. It consists of two recombinant viral vectors (vaccinia vector and fowlpox vector), each encoding transgenes for PSA and TRICOM. TRICOM consists of costimulatory molecules, including ICAM (intercellular addition molecules)-1 (CD54), B7.1 (CD80), and leukocyte function-associated antigen-3 (LFA-3)(CD58) [51]. In a randomized phase II trial of men with chemonaïve, minimally symptomatic metastatic CRPC, Prostvac-VF extended overall survival by 8.5 months over placebo (25.1 versus 16.6 months, $P = 0.0061$; HR = 0.56; 95% CI, 0.37–0.85) [52]. Ongoing clinical trials of Prostvac-VF in advanced phases include those in the setting of non-mCRPC, in asymptomatic/minimally symptomatic metastatic CRPC and in symptomatic metastatic CRPC (in combination with docetaxel) (Tables 1 and 2).

3.12. Cytotoxic T Lymphocyte Antigen 4 (CTLA-4) Antibody. Cytotoxic T lymphocyte antigen 4 (CTLA-4) is a key negative regulator of T-cell responses, inhibits recognition of self-antigens by T cells, and can downregulate the antitumor immune response. Ipilimumab and tremelimumab are fully human, monoclonal antibodies against CTLA-4. Objective and PSA responses have been described in phase II studies of ipilimumab in prostate cancer [53, 54]. Recently, two phase III trials of ipilimumab in chemonaive- and postdocetaxel metastatic CRPC settings have completed accrual with results expected in the near future (Table 1).

3.13. Radiolabeled Monoclonal Antibody. Monoclonal antibodies (MoAbs) targeting prostate surface membrane antigen (PSMA) are in advanced phases of development. PSMA is a type II membrane glycoprotein, which is markedly upregulated in prostate cancer [55]. Deimmunized murine MoAb J591 (muJ591) has been chosen as a vehicle to deliver radioisotopes, because of its high affinity for PSMA [56]. Among various radioisotopes used with mu J591, 177 lutetium can be administered in higher doses, with comparatively less radiation to the marrow and because of its gamma emission, it enables imaging to be performed using the treatment doses [55]. A randomized, phase II study is currently evaluating efficacy of 177Lu-J591 (versus placebo, i.e., 111 In-J591) in combination with ketoconazole and hydrocortisone in non-metastatic CRPC (Table 2).

3.14. Tasquinimod. Tasquinimod is a quinoline-3-carboxamide analog that possesses antiangiogenic and immunomodulatory properties [57]. It significantly delayed disease progression, compared to placebo, in a randomized phase II trial of minimally symptomatic men with metastatic CRPC. A phase III, placebo controlled, randomized trial of tasquinimod has recently completed accrual with the primary end-point of progression free survival (Table 1).

4. Conclusions

Herein, we have provided a thorough, but selective list of androgen dependent and independent molecular pathways recognized to drive the progression of CRPC. Additionally, we summarized the novel agents targeting these pathways, which have been recently approved or have reached advanced stages of clinical development. With the discovery of increased intratumoral expression of key enzymes in the steroid synthesis pathway, agents such as abiraterone acetate, orteronel, and TOK-001 were developed to further minimize androgen-driven tumor progression. When AR gene amplification and mutations were shown by in situ studies, enzalutamide and ARN-509 were developed to abrogate the actions of AR in facilitating tumor progression. Regulatory approval of sipuleucel-T for minimally symptomatic mCRPC has revolutionized the way immune therapy is used in management of malignancy in general. Development of other promising immune-modulatory agents such as Prostvac-VF, ipilimumab, and tasquinimod have reached phase III trials. Classic pathways common to many malignancies, such as apoptotic pathways (bcl2), src-kinase, p53, and PTEN, are also dysregulated by mutations, gene duplications/deletions, and chromosomal changes. These discoveries have provided the rationale for testing agents targeting these pathways for treatment of CRPC.

The recent proliferation of therapeutic agents for treatment of metastatic CRPC is indicative of the dramatic changes occurring in the field. Amidst this changing landscape of treatment options for metastatic CRPC, many ongoing trials are likely to result in regulatory approval of newer agents. Advances in evidenced based oncology have led to cost-efficient deep sequencing and individual genome sequencing capability. These and similar tools will give physicians insight into the pathophysiology of the tumors of each individual and help personalize treatment based on the underlying molecular pathway or pathways, driving tumor progression. More rationally designed studies based on predictive biomarkers are needed to guide our way through the changing landscape of treatment and the ever increasing treatment options.

Authors' Contribution

All authors participated in concept and design, collection of data, writing of the paper, and approval of the paper. Jesal C. Patel and Benjamin L. Maughan are equal contributors to the paper.

Acknowledgment

Neeraj Agarwal has received honorarium from Dendreon Inc, Seattle, WA, USA.

References

[1] R. Siegel, D. Naishadham, and A. Jemal, "Cancer statistics," *A Cancer Journal for Clinicians*, vol. 63, no. 1, pp. 11–30, 2013.

[2] Y. Chen, N. J. Clegg, and H. I. Scher, "Anti-androgens and androgen-depleting therapies in prostate cancer: new agents for an established target," *The Lancet Oncology*, vol. 10, no. 10, pp. 981–991, 2009.

[3] A. H. M. Reid, G. Attard, E. Barrie, and J. S. de Bono, "CYP17 inhibition as a hormonal strategy for prostate cancer," *Nature Clinical Practice Urology*, vol. 5, no. 11, pp. 610–620, 2008.

[4] J. Edwards, N. S. Krishna, K. M. Grigor, and J. M. S. Bartlett, "Androgen receptor gene amplification and protein expression in hormone refractory prostate cancer," *British Journal of Cancer*, vol. 89, no. 3, pp. 552–556, 2003.

[5] M. P. Steinkamp, O. A. O'Mahony, M. Brogley et al., "Treatment-dependent androgen receptor mutations in prostate cancer exploit multiple mechanisms to evade therapy," *Cancer Research*, vol. 69, no. 10, pp. 4434–4442, 2009.

[6] N. Agarwal, T. E. Hutson, N. J. Vogelzang, and G. Sonpavde, "Abiraterone acetate: a promising drug for the treatment of castration-resistant prostate cancer," *Future Oncology*, vol. 6, no. 5, pp. 665–679, 2010.

[7] J. S. de Bono, C. J. Logothetis, A. Molina et al., "Abiraterone and increased survival in metastatic prostate cancer.," *The New England Journal of Medicine*, vol. 364, no. 21, pp. 1995–2005, 2011.

[8] C. J. Ryan, M. R. Smith, J. S. de Bono et al., "Abiraterone in metastatic prostate cancer without previous chemotherapy," *The*

New England Journal of Medicine, vol. 368, no. 2, pp. 138–148, 2013.

[9] D. B. Agus, W. M. Stadler, D. H. Shevrin et al., "Efficacy, and pharmacodynamics of the investigational agent orteronel (TAK-700) in metastatic castration-resistant prostate cancer (mCRPC): updated data from a phase I/II study," *Journal of Clinical Oncology*, vol. 30, no. 5, supplement 98, 2012.

[10] M. Hussain, P. Corn, D. Michaelson et al., "Activity and safety of the investigational agent orteronel in men with nonmetastatic castration-resistant prostate cancer and rising prostate-specific antigen: results of a phase 2 study," in *Proceedings of the 27th Annual European Association of Urology*, pp. 24–28, Paris, France, February 2012.

[11] C. Tran, "Development of a second-generation antiandrogen for treatment of advanced prostate cancer," *Science*, vol. 324, no. 5928, pp. 787–790, 2009.

[12] H. I. Scher, K. Fizazi, F. Saad et al., "Increased survival with enzalutamide in prostate cancer after chemotherapy," *The New England Journal of Medicine*, vol. 367, no. 13, pp. 1187–1197, 2012.

[13] D. E. Rathkopf, D. C. Danila, M. J. Morris et al., "Phase I/II safety and pharmacokinetic (PK) study of ARN-509 in patients with metastatic castration-resistant prostate cancer (mCRPC): phase I results of a prostate cancer clinical trials consortium study," *Journal of Clinical Oncology*, vol. 30, 5, 2012.

[14] M. R. Smith, E. S. Antonarakis, C. J. Ryan et al., "ARN-509 in men with high-risk nonmetastatic castration-resistant prostate cancer (CRPC)," *ASCO Meeting Abstracts*, vol. 31, 6, 2013.

[15] D. E. Rathkopf, E. S. Antonarakis, N. D. Shore et al., "ARN-509 in men with metastatic castration-resistant prostate cancer (mCRPC)," *ASCO Meeting Abstracts*, vol. 31, 6, 2013.

[16] T. Vasaitis, A. Belosay, A. Schayowitz et al., "Androgen receptor inactivation contributes to antitumor efficacy of 17α-hydroxylase/17,20-lyase inhibitor 3β-hydroxy-17-(1H-benzimidazole-1-yl)androsta-5,16-diene in prostate cancer," *Molecular Cancer Therapeutics*, vol. 7, no. 8, pp. 2348–2357, 2008.

[17] Y. Zhang, S. Castaneda, M. Dumble et al., "Reduced expression of the androgen receptor by third generation of antisense shows antitumor activity in models of prostate cancer," *Molecular Cancer Therapeutics*, vol. 10, no. 12, pp. 2309–2319, 2011.

[18] R. J. Andersen, N. R. Mawji, J. Wang et al., "Regression of castrate-recurrent prostate cancer by a small-molecule inhibitor of the amino-terminus domain of the androgen receptor," *Cancer Cell*, vol. 17, no. 6, pp. 535–546, 2010.

[19] J. M. Summy and G. E. Gallick, "Src family kinases in tumor progression and metastasis," *Cancer and Metastasis Reviews*, vol. 22, no. 4, pp. 337–358, 2003.

[20] K. Fizazi, "The role of Src in prostate cancer," *Annals of Oncology*, vol. 18, no. 11, pp. 1765–1773, 2007.

[21] J. C. Araujo, G. C. Trudel, F. Saad et al., "Overall survival (OS) and safety of dasatinib/docetaxel versus docetaxel in patients with metastatic castration-resistant prostate cancer (mCRPC): results from the randomized phase III READY trial," *ASCO Meeting Abstracts*, vol. 31, 6, 2013.

[22] M. Karlou, V. Tzelepi, and E. Efstathiou, "Therapeutic targeting of the prostate cancer microenvironment," *Nature Reviews Urology*, vol. 7, no. 9, pp. 494–509, 2010.

[23] E. S. Antonarakis, M. A. Carducci, and M. A. Eisenberger, "Novel targeted therapeutics for metastatic castration-resistant prostate cancer," *Cancer Letters*, vol. 291, no. 1, pp. 1–13, 2010.

[24] I. Duran, C. Montagut, E. Calvo et al., "Overcoming docetaxel resistance in advanced castration-resistant prostate cancer (CRPC): a phase I/II trial of the combination of temsirolimus and docetaxel," *Journal of Clinical Oncology*, vol. 30, 5, 2012.

[25] W. D. Figg, P. Arlen, J. Gulley et al., "A randomized phase II trial of docetaxel (taxotere) plus thalidomide in androgen-independent prostate cancer," *Seminars in Oncology*, vol. 28, no. 4, pp. 62–66, 2001.

[26] W. L. Dahut, J. L. Gulley, P. M. Arlen et al., "Randomized phase II trial of docetaxel plus thalidomide in androgen-independent prostate cancer," *Journal of Clinical Oncology*, vol. 22, no. 13, pp. 2532–2539, 2004.

[27] W. D. Figg, H. Li, T. Sissung et al., "Pre-clinical and clinical evaluation of estramustine, docetaxel and thalidomide combination in androgen-independent prostate cancer," *BJU International*, vol. 99, no. 5, pp. 1047–1055, 2007.

[28] L. R. Molife, P. C. Fong, L. Paccagnella et al., "The insulin-like growth factor-I receptor inhibitor figitumumab (CP-751,871) in combination with docetaxel in patients with advanced solid tumours: results of a phase Ib dose-escalation, open-label study," *British Journal of Cancer*, vol. 103, no. 3, pp. 332–339, 2010.

[29] C. S. Higano, J. J. Alumkal, C. J. Ryan et al., "A phase II study of cixutumumab (IMC-A12), a monoclonal antibody (MAb) against the insulin-like growth factor 1 receptor (IGF-IR), monotherapy in metastatic castration-resistant prostate cancer (mCRPC): feasibility of every 3-week dosing and updated results," *Genitourinary Cancers Symposium*, vol. 189, 2010.

[30] C. N. Sternberg, H. Dumez, H. Van Poppel et al., "Docetaxel plus oblimersen sodium (Bcl-2 antisense oligonucleotide): an EORTC multicenter, randomized phase II study in patients with castration-resistant prostate cancer," *Annals of Oncology*, vol. 20, no. 7, pp. 1264–1269, 2009.

[31] S. Anai, S. Goodison, K. Shiverick, Y. Hirao, B. D. Brown, and C. J. Rosser, "Knock-down of Bcl-2 by antisense oligodeoxynucleotides induces radiosensitization and inhibition of angiogenesis in human PC-3 prostate tumor xenografts," *Molecular Cancer Therapeutics*, vol. 6, no. 1, pp. 101–111, 2007.

[32] G. Liu, W. K. Kelly, G. Wilding, L. Leopold, K. Brill, and B. Somer, "An open-label, multicenter, phase I/II study of single-agent AT-101 in men with castrate-resistant prostate cancer," *Clinical Cancer Research*, vol. 15, no. 9, pp. 3172–3176, 2009.

[33] G. Sonpavde, V. Matveev, J. M. Burke et al., "Randomized phase II trial of docetaxel plus prednisone in combination with placebo or AT-101, an oral small molecule Bcl-2 family antagonist, as first-line therapy for metastatic castration-resistant prostate cancer," *Annals of Oncology*, vol. 23, no. 7, pp. 1803–1808, 2012.

[34] K. N. Chi, S. J. Hotte, E. Y. Yu et al., "Randomized phase II study of docetaxel and prednisone with or without OGX-011 in patients with metastatic castration-resistant prostate cancer," *Journal of Clinical Oncology*, vol. 28, no. 27, pp. 4247–4254, 2010.

[35] A. Zoubeidi, K. Chi, and M. Gleave, "Targeting the cytoprotective chaperone, clusterin, for treatment of advanced cancer," *Clinical Cancer Research*, vol. 16, no. 4, pp. 1088–1093, 2010.

[36] F. Stavridi, E. M. Karapanagiotou, and K. N. Syrigos, "Targeted therapeutic approaches for hormone-refractory prostate cancer," *Cancer Treatment Reviews*, vol. 36, no. 2, pp. 122–130, 2010.

[37] W. K. You and D. M. M, "The hepatocyte growth factor/c-met signaling pathway as a therapeutic target to inhibit angiogenesis," *Journal of Biochemistry and Molecular Biology*, vol. 41, no. 12, pp. 833–839, 2008.

[38] W. H. Tu, C. Zhu, C. Clark, J. G. Christensen, and Z. Sun, "Efficacy of c-Met inhibitor for advanced prostate cancer," *BMC Cancer*, vol. 10, article 556, 2010.

[39] D. C. Smith, M. R. Smith, C. Sweeney et al., "Cabozantinib in patients with advanced prostate cancer: results of a phase II randomized discontinuation trial," *Journal of clinical oncology*, vol. 31, no. 4, pp. 412–419, 2012.

[40] D. N. Lavery and C. L. Bevan, "Androgen receptor signalling in prostate cancer: the functional consequences of acetylation," *Journal of Biomedicine and Biotechnology*, vol. 2011, Article ID 862125, 7 pages, 2011.

[41] D. Bradley, D. Rathkopf, R. Dunn et al., "Vorinostat in advanced prostate cancer patients progressing on prior chemotherapy (National Cancer Institute Trial 6862): trial results and interleukin-6 analysis: a study by the department of defense prostate cancer clinical Trial consortium and university of chicago phase 2 consortium," *Cancer*, vol. 115, no. 23, pp. 5541–5549, 2009.

[42] D. Rathkopf, B. Y. Wong, R. W. Ross et al., "A phase I study of oral panobinostat alone and in combination with docetaxel in patients with castration-resistant prostate cancer," *Cancer Chemotherapy and Pharmacology*, vol. 66, no. 1, pp. 181–189, 2010.

[43] G. Sonpavde, A. M. Aparicio, F. Zhan et al., "Azacitidine favorably modulates PSA kinetics correlating with plasma DNA LINE-1 hypomethylation in men with chemonaive castration-resistant prostate cancer," *Urologic Oncology*, vol. 29, no. 6, pp. 682–689, 2011.

[44] K. Fizazi, M. Carducci, M. Smith et al., "Denosumab versus zoledronic acid for treatment of bone metastases in men with castration-resistant prostate cancer: a randomised, double-blind study," *The Lancet*, vol. 377, no. 9768, pp. 813–822, 2011.

[45] F. Saad, D. M. Gleason, R. Murray et al., "Long-term efficacy of zoledronic acid for the prevention of skeletal complications in patients with metastatic hormone-refractory prostate cancer," *Journal of the National Cancer Institute*, vol. 96, no. 11, pp. 879–882, 2004.

[46] A. O. Sartor, D. Heinrich, S. I. Helle et al. et al., "Radium-223 chloride impact on skeletal-related events in patients with castration-resistant prostate cancer (CRPC) with bone metastases: a phase III randomized trial (ALSYMPCA)," *Journal of Clinical Oncology*, vol. 30, 5, 2012.

[47] N. Agarwal, N. Vogelzang, and N. J, *Development of Novel Immune Interventions For Genito-Urinary Cancers. Cancer Vaccines*, Adrian Bot, Mihail Obrocea & Francesco Marincola, Informa Healthcare, London, UK, 2011.

[48] P. W. Kantoff, C. S. Higano, N. D. Shore et al., "Sipuleucel-T immunotherapy for castration-resistant prostate cancer," *The New England Journal of Medicine*, vol. 363, no. 5, pp. 411–422, 2010.

[49] L. G. Gomella, C. Nabhan, T. DeVries, J. B. Whitmore, M. W. Frohlich, and D. J. George, "Estimating the overall survival benefit of sipuleucel-T in the IMPACT trial accounting for crossover treatment in control subjects with autologous immunotherapy generated from cryopreserved cells," in *American Urological Association Annual Meeting (AUA '12)*, 2012.

[50] J. Schlom, M. Vergati, C. Intrivici, N. Y. Huen, and K. Y. Tsang, "Strategies for cancer vaccine development," *Journal of Biomedicine and Biotechnology*, vol. 2010, Article ID 596432, 13 pages, 2010.

[51] G. Sonpavde, K. M. Slawin, D. M. Spencer, and J. M. Levitt, "Emerging vaccine therapy approaches for prostate cancer," *Reviews in Urology*, vol. 12, no. 1, pp. 25–34, 2010.

[52] P. W. Kantoff, T. J. Schuetz, B. A. Blumenstein et al., "Overall survival analysis of a phase II randomized controlled trial of a poxviral-based PSA-targeted immunotherapy in metastatic castration-resistant prostate cancer," *Journal of Clinical Oncology*, vol. 28, no. 7, pp. 1099–1105, 2010.

[53] L. F. Langer, T. M. Clay, and M. A. Morse, "Update on anti-CTLA-4 antibodies in clinical trials," *Expert Opinion on Biological Therapy*, vol. 7, no. 8, pp. 1245–1256, 2007.

[54] D. O'Mahony, J. C. Morris, C. Quinn et al., "A pilot study of CTLA-4 blockade after cancer vaccine failure in patients with advanced malignancy," *Clinical Cancer Research*, vol. 13, no. 3, pp. 958–964, 2007.

[55] S. T. Tagawa, H. Beltran, S. Vallabhajosula et al., "Anti-prostate-specific membrane antigen-based radioimmunotherapy for prostate cancer," *Cancer*, vol. 116, no. 4, pp. 1075–1083, 2010.

[56] N. H. Bander, D. M. Nanus, M. I. Milowsky, L. Kostakoglu, S. Vallabahajosula, and S. J. Goldsmith, "Targeted systemic therapy of prostate cancer with a monoclonal antibody to prostate-specific membrane antigen," *Seminars in Oncology*, vol. 30, no. 5, pp. 667–677, 2003.

[57] J. T. Isaacs, "The long and winding road for the development of tasquinimod as an oral second-generation quinoline-3-carboxamide antiangiogenic drug for the treatment of prostate cancer," *Expert Opinion on Investigational Drugs*, vol. 19, no. 10, pp. 1235–1243, 2010.

27

Robotic Prostatectomy Has a Superior Outcome in Larger Prostates and PSA Density Is a Strong Predictor of Biochemical Recurrence

S. Bishara, N. Vasdev, T. Lane, G. Boustead, and J. Adshead

Department of Urology, Hertfordshire and South Bedfordshire Robotic Urological Cancer Centre, Lister Hospital, Coreys Mill Lane, Stevenage, Hertfordshire SG1 4AB, UK

Correspondence should be addressed to S. Bishara; bishsam@googlemail.com

Academic Editor: James L. Gulley

Objectives. The aims of this study were to compare the outcomes of robotic assisted laparoscopic prostatectomy (RALP) between patients who had larger (≥75 g) and smaller (<75 g) prostates and to evaluate the performance of PSA density (PSAD) in determining the oncological outcome of surgery. *Methods and Materials.* 344 patients who underwent RALP at a single institution were included in the study. Preoperative risk factors and postoperative, oncological outcomes, erectile function, and continence status were recorded prospectively. *Results.* During a mean follow-up of 20 months, biochemical recurrence (PSA > 0.2) was observed in 15 patients (4.3%). Prostate size ≥75 g was associated with lower Gleason score on final pathology ($P = 0.004$) and lower pathological stage ($P = 0.02$) but an increased length of hospital stay ($P = 0.05$). PSAD on binary logistic regression independently predicted biochemical recurrence (BCR) when defined as postoperative PSA >0.1 ($P = 0.001$) and PSA >0.2 ($P = 0.039$). In both instances PSA was no longer a significant independent predictor. *Conclusions.* RALP in large prostates (≥75 g, <150 g) is as safe as RALP in smaller prostates and is associated with a lower pathological grade and stage. Higher PSAD is independently associated with BCR and is superior to PSA as a predictor of BCR after RALP.

1. Introduction

A number of studies have evaluated the risk factors for biochemical recurrence after radical prostatectomy [1, 2]. PSA, age, Gleason score, and clinical stage have been demonstrated to be independent predictors of outcome. Preoperatively, however, there is considerable risk of under staging of disease, even with the use of multiparametric MRI and increased sampling of the prostate gland on biopsy. A large prostate gland can be surgically challenging at robotic prostatectomy and unsurprisingly is associated with increased operative time, transfusion rate, and risk of postoperative complications [3] but despite this, when evaluated as a prognostic factor it is associated with a superior oncological outcome in terms of positive margin rate and biochemical recurrence [2, 4]. A logical extension of the utilisation of PSA in the preoperative evaluation of patients being considered for RALP is to combine it with prostate size to calculate a PSA density. PSA density is an established prognostic factor that has been widely evaluated but often unused in the diagnostic pathway, particularly as an accurate assessment of prostate size is dependent on MRI or transrectal U/S and therefore the patient is well on the way along the diagnostic pathway before the PSAD is determined. Thus it is unlikely to alter investigative strategy, though it may be a readily available determinant of therapeutic outcomes. Typically PSAD cutoffs of greater than 0.15 have been used to prognosticate higher risk disease in patients undergoing prostatectomy [5].

The principle aims of this study were to record the differences in outcome between smaller <75 g and larger ≥75 g prostates and to test the hypothesis that PSAD is superior to PSA in determining the outcome of RALP for prostate cancer.

Table 1: Preoperative staging.

Prostate size	<75 g, $n = 296$		>75 g, $n = 48$		P
	Mean/proportion	sd/%	Mean/proportion	sd/%	
PSA	8.21	5.3	9.45	5.3	ns
Age	61.4	5.9	63.2	5.7	0.05
Biopsy stage					
T1	139/261	53.3%	25/48	52%	ns
T2	120/261	46%	21/48	43.8%	ns
T3	2/261	0.7%	2/48	4.2%	ns
Biopsy grade					
G6	120/287	41.8%	24/48	50%	ns
G7	147/287	51.2%	21/48	43.8%	ns
G8–10	20/287	6.9%	3/48	6.3%	ns

2. Methods

2.1. Patients. A prospective database of all patients undergoing radical robotic prostatectomy between 2008 and 2013 at a single centre was created. Preoperative status, staging investigations, intraoperative parameters, postoperative outcomes, complications, follow-up biochemical or pathological recurrence, and erectile and continence function were recorded. The patient follow-up schedule was every 3 months for the first year and every 6 months for the second year and yearly thereafter.

2.2. Categorisation and Statistical Analysis. The prostate size was defined according to the pathological specimen weight. PSAD was defined as prostate size divided by the preoperative PSA level. Upstaging was defined as increase in T numerical denomination between clinical and pathological staging. Postoperative complications were defined according to the Clavien Scale and split into two groups: minor (Clavien 1 and 2) and major (Clavien 3 and 4) complications. Continence was classified according to daily pad usage (no pads, 1 pad, 2 pads, 3 pads, and 4 or more pads). Erectile function was categorised in four groups (normal spontaneous erections, good erections with PDE5, partial erections with PDE5, and no erections with PDE5, requiring caverject injections). For comparison of the difference in outcomes according to prostate size, patients were divided into two groups: <75 g and ≥75 g. The difference between the two groups was compared using an unpaired t-test for continuous variables and the Fisher exact test for proportions.

2.3. Evaluation of PSA Density. A multivariate model to predict margin positivity and biochemical recurrence at the PSA > 0.1 level and PSA > 0.2 level was created using the standard preoperative factors: PSA, biopsy Gleason score (<7, 7, >7), clinical stage (T1, T2, T3), and age in addition to PSAD. Analysis was with binary logistic regression.

A second method using Cox proportional hazards was used to evaluate the effect of adding PSAD to a model that contained PSA, biopsy Gleason score, and clinical stage. The strength of these models and the effect of adding PSAD were evaluated by the Chi squared test. In all cases clinical significance was taken as $P \leq 0.05$. Statistical analysis and graphing were carried out by IBM SPSS version 22. Patients were excluded from a statistical analysis when a prerequisite parameter was missing.

3. Results

344 patients were included in the study. 296 patients had a prostate weight of <75 g and 48 a prostate weight of ≥75 g. Mean follow-up of patients amongst the two groups was similar (1.7 years >75 g, 1.6 years ≥75 g, ns).

Preoperative staging (Table 1): patients with prostates ≥75 g were slightly older (63.2 versus 61.4 years, $P = 0.05$) than those with prostates <75 g. Otherwise, there was no significant difference in the preoperative risk factors: PSA, clinical stage, and biopsy Gleason score.

Pathology and oncological outcomes of RALP (Table 2): larger prostates (≥75 g) were more likely to be staged as T1 pathological stage (8.3% versus 1.4%, $P = 0.02$), less likely to be upstaged on final histology (58.3% versus 75.3%, $P = 0.02$), and more likely to have lower grade disease on final histology (41.7% versus 26.4%, $P = 0.04$). There was, however, no difference between these two groups in terms of type of nerve sparing procedure, lymph node dissection rate, positive surgical margin, and biochemical recurrence rate.

Postoperative outcomes and complications of RALP: in Table 3 larger prostates (≥75 g) were associated with a longer operative time (255 versus 222 min, $P = 0.002$), greater blood loss (349 versus 219 mL, $P = 0.0002$), and blood transfusion requirements (0.01 versus 0.13 units per operation, $P = 0.006$). Larger prostates (≥75 g) were associated with a longer postoperative stay (2.82 versus 2.26 days, $P = 0.04$, and longer postoperative catheter time (10.3 versus 9.2 days, $P = 0.05$).

PSAD: mean PSAD was 0.17 ranging from 0.022 to 0.875 and has a positive skew distribution as shown in Figure 1. PSAD alone was predictive of biochemical recurrence as shown in Figure 2, with area under the receiver operated curve of 0.73. A PSAD of >0.136 corresponds to an 85% sensitivity and 51% specificity for detecting biochemical

Table 2: Pathology and oncological outcomes of RALP.

Prostate size	<75 g, n = 296		>75 g, n = 48		P
	Mean/proportion	sd/%	Mean/proportion	sd/%	
Prostate weight	47.48	12.29	97.23	20.7	<0.0001
Nerve spare					
Bilateral NS	92/293	31.4%	15/47	31.9%	ns
Unilateral NS	91/293	31.1%	11/47	23.4%	ns
WLE	100/293	34.1%	21/47	44.6%	ns
Lymph node dissection	34/296	11.5%	4/48	8.3%	ns
Pathological stage					
T1	4/296	1.4%	4/48	8.3%	0.02
T2	226/296	76.4%	32/48	66.7%	ns
T3	64/296	21.6%	12/48	25%	ns
T4	1/296	0.3%	0/48	0%	ns
Positive margin	81/296	27.3%	12/48	25%	ns
Upstage	196/260	75.3%	28/48	58.3%	0.02
SVI[a]	14/296	4.7%	5/48	10.4%	ns
Pathological grade					
G6	78/296	26.4%	20/48	41.7%	0.04
G7	189/296	63.9%	20/48	41.7%	0.004
G8–10	29/296	9.8%	8/48	16.7%	ns
Biochemical recurrence	14/296	4.7%	1/48	2.1%	ns

[a]SVI: seminal vesicle involvement.

Table 3: Postoperative outcomes and complications of RALP.

Prostate size	<75 g, n = 296		>75 g, n = 48		P
	Mean/proportion	sd/%	Mean/proportion	sd/%	
Postop stay/days	2.262	1.62	2.822	2.229	0.04
Catheter time/days	9.166	3.62	10.29	4.177	0.05
Number of pads/day 6 m[a]	0.482	0.781	0.540	0.802	ns
Number of pads/day 12 m[a]	0.2981	0.630	0.117	0.332	ns
ED score 6 m[β]	2.354	0.9377	2.441	0.823	ns
ED score 12 m[β]	2.129	1.049	2	1.061	ns
Operative time	221.7	66	255.4	85.46	0.002
Recorded blood loss	219.4	189.7	348.5	310.3	0.0002
Blood transfusion requirements	0.011	0.1385	0.13	0.62	0.006
Complications					
Clavien 1-2	20/298	6.7%	7/48	14.5%	0.07
Clavien 3-4	13/298	4.3%	4/48	8.3%	ns

[a]Daily pad usage was scored as 0 for no pads, 1 for one pad, 2 for two pads, 3 for three pads, and 4 for four or more pads.
[β]Erectile dysfunction was scored as 0 for normal spontaneous erections, 1 for good erections with PDE5, 2 for partial erections with PDE5, and 3 for no erections with PDE5, requiring caverject injections.

recurrence. The comparable areas under the ROC for predicting biochemical recurrence were 0.69 for PSA, 0.52 for clinical stage, and 0.62 for transrectal biopsy Gleason sum score.

On multivariate analysis of preoperative staging parameters and PSAD, using binary logistic regression (n = 309), Gleason sum score was found to be the only independent predictor of margin positivity (P = 0.013) (Table 4). BCR at PSA >0.1 was only predictable by PSAD (P = 0.001). Likewise BCR at PSA >0.2 was only predictable by PSAD (P = 0.039), despite the inclusion of PSA in both models.

A further analysis using Cox proportional hazards was carried out, where PSAD was added to a model containing Gleason score, clinical stage, and PSA. The effect of adding PSAD to the model increased the predictive power for BCR at PSA >0.1 (Chi square increase from 12.021, df 4, to 19.084, df 5, P = 0.017) and BCR at PSA >0.2 (Chi square increase from 9.832, df 4, to 13.15, df 5, P = 0.110).

Table 4: Multivariate binary logistic regression of preoperative risk factors and outcome of RALP.

Preoperative risk factors	Mean	Margin +ve		BCR PSA > 0.1		BCR PSA > 0.2	
		Coefficient	P value	Coefficient	P value	Coefficient	P value
Age	61.6	−0.029	ns	0.419	ns	0.047	ns
PSA	8.146	0.051	ns	2.983	ns	−0.108	ns
PSA density	0.17	0.526	ns	11.65	0.001	9.022	0.039
Gleason score (<7, 7, and >7)	143, 175, 25	0.63	0.013	3.314	0.069	−0.146	ns
Clinical stage (T1, T2, and T3)	161, 138, 5	−0.164	ns	1.832	ns	0.322	ns

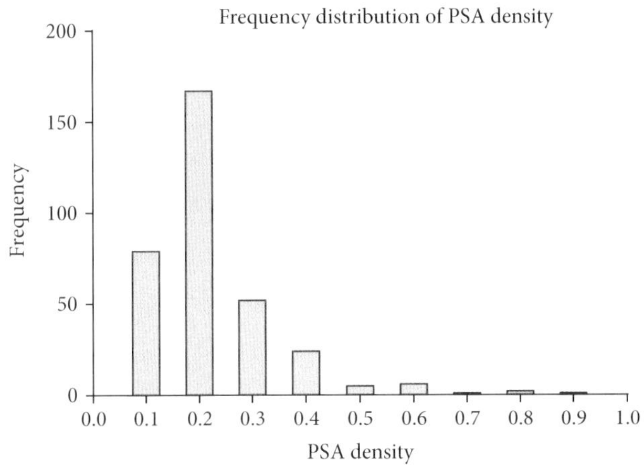

Figure 1

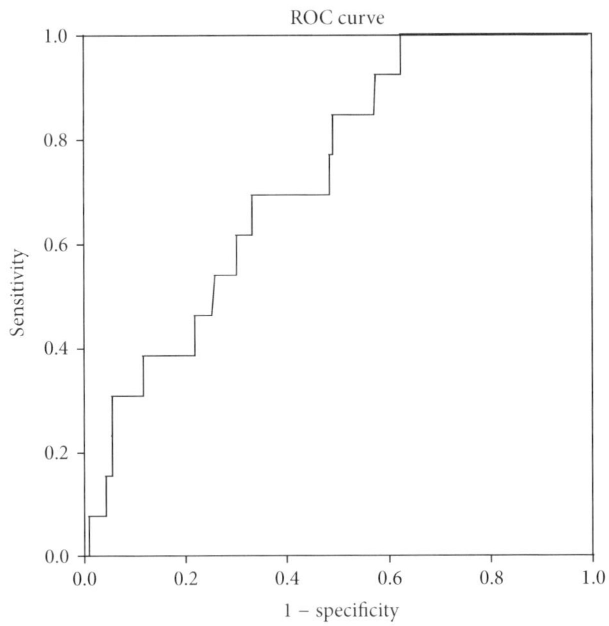

Figure 2: ROC curve for the prediction of biochemical recurrence (PSA > 0.2) by PSA density. $R^2 = 0.73$.

4. Discussion

Whilst larger prostates present a technical challenge at robotic prostatectomy and are associated with a longer operative time [6], greater blood loss, and increased postoperative complications [3, 7], they are associated with a superior oncological outcome in terms of reduced extraprostatic disease, reduced positive margin rate [8–14], and decreased biochemical recurrence rate [3]. In this cohort there was no significant difference between larger prostates (≥75 g) and smaller prostates (<75 g) in terms of the preoperative staging; however, the two groups were markedly different postoperatively. A smaller prostate was associated with a higher Gleason grade and a higher pathological stage at robotic prostatectomy. Smaller prostates were more likely to be upstaged. Whilst this might be counterintuitive, in that a larger prostate is relatively undersampled at TRUS and biopsy, the increased sensitivity of PSA for detecting prostate cancer in smaller glands (as quantified by PSAD) given the lower PSA signal from BPH seems to supervene.

There was a small but statistically significant increase in the length of postoperative stay (0.6 days) and catheter time (1 day) in prostates ≥75 g but no difference between the two groups in terms of postoperative complications, indicating that robotic prostatectomy in large prostates is a safe procedure.

PSAD was first proposed as an enhancement to PSA as a prognostic factor in 1992 by Benson et al. [15] as a means of distinguishing prostate cancer from BPH. Since that time, a number of studies have examined PSAD as a preoperative risk factor in radical prostatectomy [16–20] and more recently robotic prostatectomy [2, 4, 21].

Two previous studies in RALP have demonstrated PSAD as an independent predictor of PSM [4, 16]. In this study, PSAD was not found to be independently predictive of PSM when PSA, biopsy Gleason score, and clinical stage were included in a multivariate model.

This is only the second study which has examined the prognostic power of PSAD in RALP for BCR after the recently published study by Hashimoto et al. [2]. In their study, PSAD was associated with biochemical recurrence but it was not an independent risk factor when PSA was used. In this study PSAD displaces PSA as an independent risk factor for biochemical recurrence. The superiority of PSAD over PSA in the determination of biochemical recurrence in open prostatectomy has previously been examined. Radwan et al. [17] found in their cohort of 1327 radical prostatectomies that a model incorporating PSA density rather than PSA was superior in predicting BCR. Likewise Freedland et al. in 2002 [19] found that PSAD was superior to PSA in determining BCR. However, in a later publication in 2003 [20] this difference was deemed to be clinically insignificant. This is the first paper to demonstrate the superiority of PSAD as a prognostic factor in RALP, in accordance with the findings of Radwan et al. in open prostatectomy [17].

This study has a relatively short median follow-up of 20 months and low recurrence rate of 4.3% at a mean follow-up of 20 months. By comparison a recently published study yielded recurrence rates of 12.8% at median follow-up of 28 months [2]. Despite the low recurrence rate which reduces statistical power, PSAD was able to demonstrate superiority to PSA in detecting BCR at PSA > 0.2. The overall number of patients in this study is less than Radwan and Kundu studies which included 1327 and 1280 patients, respectively, albeit undergoing open prostatectomy, and the number of patients with prostates ≥75 g amounted to only 48.

A further weakness of this study is that the pathological specimen weight was used to calculate PSAD rather than volume on preoperative TRUS or MRI, as these were not always available on account of the initial staging investigations being performed at other hospitals. PSAD has most utility as a preoperative marker; however, TRUS volume and MRI volume demonstrate a strong concordance with prostate specimen weight [22, 23].

In conclusion PSAD is superior to PSA in predicting biochemical recurrence after robotic prostatectomy and should be taken into consideration in the analysis of outcome in any RCT examining treatment alternatives in localised prostate cancer, as it is likely to influence the risk benefit ratio.

References

[1] R. M. Escudero, F. H. Amo, A. P. Borda, and C. H. Fernandez, "Preoperative predictive model for biochemical recurrence in patients with localized prostate cancer treated with radical prostatectomy," *Archivos Espanoles de Urologia*, vol. 66, no. 6, pp. 567–575, 2013.

[2] T. Hashimoto, K. Yoshioka, T. Gondo et al., "Preoperative prognostic factors for biochemical recurrence after robot-assisted radical prostatectomy in Japan," *International Journal of Clinical Oncology*, vol. 19, no. 4, pp. 702–707, 2014.

[3] A. P. Labanaris, V. Zugor, and J. H. Witt, "Robot-assisted radical prostatectomy in patients with a pathologic prostate specimen weight ≥100 grams versus ≤50 grams: surgical, oncologic and short-term functional outcomes," *Urology International*, vol. 90, no. 1, pp. 24–30, 2013.

[4] M. Liss, K. Osann, and D. Ornstein, "Positive surgical margins during robotic radical prostatectomy: a contemporary analysis of risk factors," *BJU International*, vol. 102, no. 5, pp. 603–607, 2008.

[5] A. El Hajj, G. Ploussard, A. de La Taille et al., "Analysis of outcomes after radical prostatectomy in patients eligible for active surveillance (PRIAS)," *BJU International*, vol. 111, no. 1, pp. 53–59, 2013.

[6] D. Z. Yong, M. Tsivian, D. E. Zilberman, M. N. Ferrandino, V. Mouraviev, and D. M. Albala, "Predictors of prolonged operative time during robot-assisted laparoscopic radical prostatectomy," *BJU International*, vol. 107, no. 2, pp. 280–282, 2011.

[7] A. C. Huang, K. J. Kowalczyk, N. D. Hevelone et al., "The impact of prostate size, median lobe, and prior benign prostatic hyperplasia intervention on robot-assisted laparoscopic prostatectomy: technique and outcomes," *European Urology*, vol. 59, no. 4, pp. 595–603, 2011.

[8] P. Sooriakumaran, A. Srivastava, D. Bhagat et al., "Prostate volume and its correlation with histopathological outcomes in prostate cancer," *Urologia Internationalis*, vol. 86, no. 2, pp. 152–155, 2011.

[9] P. E. Marchetti, S. Shikanov, A. A. Razmaria, G. P. Zagaja, and A. L. Shalhav, "Impact of prostate weight on probability of positive surgical margins in patients with low-risk prostate cancer after robotic-assisted laparoscopic radical prostatectomy," *Urology*, vol. 77, no. 3, pp. 677–681, 2011.

[10] S. B. Allaparthi, T. Hoang, N. N. Dhanani, and I. A. Tuerk, "Significance of prostate weight on peri and postoperative outcomes of robot assisted laparoscopic extraperitoneal radical prostatectomy," *Canadian Journal of Urology*, vol. 17, no. 5, pp. 5383–5389, 2010.

[11] L. P. Msezane, O. N. Gofrit, S. Lin, A. L. Shalhav, G. P. Zagaja, and K. C. Zorn, "Prostate weight: an independent predictor for positive surgical margins during robotic-assisted laparoscopic radical prostatectomy," *The Canadian Journal of Urology*, vol. 14, no. 5, pp. 3697–3701, 2007.

[12] P. G. Chu, S. K. Lau, L. M. Weiss et al., "Assessment of low prostate weight as a determinant of a higher positive margin rate after laparoscopic radical prostatectomy: a prospective pathologic study of 1,500 cases," *Surgical Endoscopy and Other Interventional Techniques*, vol. 23, no. 5, pp. 1058–1064, 2009.

[13] K. C. Zorn, M. A. Orvieto, A. A. Mikhail et al., "Effect of prostate weight on operative and postoperative outcomes of robotic-assisted laparoscopic prostatectomy," *Urology*, vol. 69, no. 2, pp. 300–305, 2007.

[14] R. Frota, B. Turna, B. M. R. Santos, Y.-C. Lin, I. S. Gill, and M. Aron, "The effect of prostate weight on the outcomes of laparoscopic radical prostatectomy," *BJU International*, vol. 101, no. 5, pp. 589–593, 2008.

[15] M. C. Benson, C. A. Olsson, D. J. McMahon, and W. H. Cooner, "The use of prostate specific antigen density to enhance the predictive value of intermediate levels of serum prostate specific antigen," *Journal of Urology*, vol. 147, no. 3, pp. 817–821, 1992.

[16] S. Sfoungaristos and P. Perimenis, "PSA density is superior than PSA and Gleason score for adverse pathologic features prediction in patients with clinically localized prostate cancer," *Journal of the Canadian Urological Association*, vol. 6, no. 1, pp. 46–50, 2012.

[17] M. H. Radwan, Y. Yan, J. R. Luly et al., "Prostate-specific antigen density predicts adverse pathology and increased risk of biochemical failure," *Urology*, vol. 69, no. 6, pp. 1121–1127, 2007.

[18] S. D. Kundu, K. A. Roehl, X. Yu, J. A. V. Antenor, B. K. Suarez, and W. J. Catalona, "Prostate specific antigen density correlates with features of prostate cancer aggressiveness," *The Journal of Urology*, vol. 177, no. 2, pp. 505–509, 2007.

[19] S. J. Freedland, J. A. Wieder, G. S. Jack, F. Dorey, J. B. Dekernion, and W. J. Aronson, "Improved risk stratification for biochemical recurrence after radical prostatectomy using a novel risk group system based on prostate specific antigen density and biopsy Gleason score," *The Journal of Urology*, vol. 168, no. 1, pp. 110–115, 2002.

[20] S. J. Freedland, C. J. Kane, J. C. Presti Jr. et al., "Comparison of preoperative prostate specific antigen density and prostate

specific antigen for predicting recurrence after radical prostatectomy: results from the search data base," *Journal of Urology*, vol. 169, no. 3, pp. 969–973, 2003.

[21] J. Uberoi, D. Brison, N. Patel, I. S. Sawczuk, and R. Munver, "Robot-assisted laparoscopic radical prostatectomy in patients with prostate cancer with high-risk features: predictors of favorable pathologic outcome," *Journal of Endourology*, vol. 24, no. 3, pp. 403–407, 2010.

[22] A. Tewari, R. Indudhara, K. Shinohara et al., "Comparison of transrectal ultrasound prostatic volume estimation with magnetic resonance imaging volume estimation and surgical specimen weight in patients with benign prostatic hyperplasia," *Journal of Clinical Ultrasound*, vol. 24, no. 4, pp. 169–174, 1996.

[23] A. Rahmouni, A. Yang, C. M. C. Tempany et al., "Accuracy of in-vivo assessment of prostatic volume by MRI and transrectal ultrasonography," *Journal of Computer Assisted Tomography*, vol. 16, no. 6, pp. 935–940, 1992.

28

Salvage Brachytherapy for Biochemically Recurrent Prostate Cancer following Primary Brachytherapy

John M. Lacy,[1] William A. Wilson,[2] Raevti Bole,[3] Li Chen,[4] Ali S. Meigooni,[5] Randall G. Rowland,[1] and William H. St. Clair[2]

[1] *Department of Urology, University of Kentucky College of Medicine, Lexington, KY 40536, USA*
[2] *Department of Radiation Oncology, University of Kentucky College of Medicine, Lexington, KY 40536, USA*
[3] *University of Kentucky College of Medicine, Lexington, KY 40536, USA*
[4] *Department of Biostatistics, University of Kentucky College of Public Health, Lexington, KY 40536, USA*
[5] *Comprehensive Cancer Centers of Nevada, Las Vegas, NV 89169, USA*

Correspondence should be addressed to William H. St. Clair; stclair@email.uky.edu

Academic Editor: Hendrik Van Poppel

Purpose. In this study, we evaluated our experience with salvage brachytherapy after discovery of biochemical recurrence after a prior brachytherapy procedure. *Methods and Materials.* From 2001 through 2012 twenty-one patients treated by brachytherapy within University of Kentucky or from outside centers developed biochemical failure and had no evidence of metastases. Computed tomography (CT) scans were evaluated; patients who had an underseeded portion of their prostate were considered for reimplantation. *Results.* The majority of the patients in this study (61.9%) were low risk and median presalvage PSA was 3.49 (range 17.41–1.68). Mean follow-up was 61 months. At last follow-up after reseeding, 11/21 (52.4%) were free of biochemical recurrence. There was a trend towards decreased freedom from biochemical recurrence in low risk patients ($p = 0.12$). International Prostate Symptom Scores (IPSS) increased at 3-month follow-up visits but decreased and were equivalent to baseline scores at 18 months. *Conclusions.* Salvage brachytherapy after primary brachytherapy is possible; however, in our experience the side-effect profile after the second brachytherapy procedure was higher than after the first brachytherapy procedure. In this cohort of patients we demonstrate that approximately 50% oncologic control, low risk patients appear to have better outcomes than others.

1. Introduction

The use of interstitial brachytherapy with permanent seed implantation is a well-established means of treating localized prostate cancer [1, 2]. Permanent interstitial brachytherapy for prostate cancer patients involves the insertion of radioactive seeds (containing ^{125}I, ^{103}Pd, or ^{131}Cs), encased in titanium shells, into the prostate gland. Benefits of this treatment modality include a single procedure rather than weeks of daily external beam radiation therapy (EBRT) and equivalent oncologic control for low and intermediate risk disease [1]. Other studies have shown superior quality of life regarding sexual function and urinary bother scores for prostate seed implant compared to prostatectomy [3].

Unfortunately, up to as high as 10% to 15% of men may experience prostate-specific antigen (PSA) failure in five to ten years after interstitial brachytherapy for clinically localized prostate cancer [2, 4]. Some of these men will harbor a component of micrometastatic disease at the time of PSA failure, but a significant number will have a true local-only recurrence and potentially can be cured with a salvage local therapy. Currently, there is no consensus regarding the optimal management of patients who are believed to have a local-only recurrence after prostate radiotherapy. Palliative management options include androgen deprivation therapy or expectant management. A number of salvage therapies with curative intent have also been assessed including cryotherapy, EBRT, high intensity focused ultrasound (HIFU), brachytherapy, and radical prostatectomy [5, 6].

Data on salvage brachytherapy after primary brachytherapy is extremely limited. Much of the data in the current literature comes from patients that were included in cohorts of patients treated with primary radiation therapy with the majority of patients undergoing EBRT. To our knowledge, there are only 2 studies that evaluate salvage brachytherapy for patients who were initially treated with brachytherapy, one in 1990 [7] in the pre-PSA era and one in 2003 [8]. In this single center review of 21 patients, we describe our experience with salvage brachytherapy for prostate cancer patients with biochemical recurrence after primary brachytherapy focusing on oncologic and functional outcomes.

2. Methods and Materials

From July 2001 until February 2012, we reviewed the records of all patients who underwent salvage reimplantation at our center. During this time frame 21 patients underwent a repeat brachytherapy procedure. Of the 21 patients in this analysis, 3 had a biopsy before the repeat brachytherapy procedure and the remainder did not. Of these 21 patients, 14 had their initial brachytherapy procedure performed at the University of Kentucky (UK). One of the patients initially treated at UK was found to have poor coverage at the one-month postimplant CT evaluation and subsequently had a planned reimplantation. The other 13 patients initially treated at UK had adequate postimplant dosimetry; years later they developed a rising PSA. The remaining 7 men in this cohort had their initial brachytherapy procedure at other institutions. One of these 7 patients underwent open brachytherapy procedure in 1984 and many years later developed a rising PSA. Thus, of the patients in this cohort 20 of 21 patients had an acceptable brachytherapy procedure and were later identified as having a biochemical failure defined by either the ASTRO criteria or Phoenix criteria [9]. D'Amico criteria were used to stratify risk category [10]. All patients who met the criteria for biochemical failure had a bone scan and a computed tomography (CT) scan of the abdomen and pelvis to rule out evidence of metastasis. The pelvic CT scan was also evaluated by radiation oncology and urology faculty to assess brachytherapy seed placement within the prostate. If both radiation oncology and urology faculty clinically agreed that a 3-dimensional volume of the prostate was underseeded from the initial brachytherapy procedure and the scans revealed no evidence of metastases, those patients were considered for a brachytherapy salvage procedure. If the prostate appeared to be well seeded with no gaps or evidence of metastasis the patient was excluded from a second brachytherapy procedure. There were no other exclusion criteria, with no restrictions on presalvage PSA or International Prostate Symptom Score (IPSS) survey results.

A preplanning TRUS volume study was performed, and target volumes were outlined by a radiation oncologist with urology collaboration. The target volume to receive radioactive seeds only included the underseeded portion of the prostate with a small margin, of 2 mm. In addition, care was taken to keep the urethral doses low; our goal was to keep the urethral dose to no more than that of the prescribed dose. BrachyVision software was utilized for brachytherapy planning. Sample planning scans are shown in Figure 1(a). All patients were treated using ^{125}I seeds, and the prescribed dose ranged from 108 Gy to 144 Gy (Table 1). When the dosimetric plan was completed, stranded seeds were purchased from a vendor (IsoAid) and the patient returned for implant in approximately 2 weeks.

Epidural anesthesia was administered and patients were placed in the dorsal lithotomy position. A urethral catheter was inserted and instilled with ultrasonic contrast (surgical lubricant with air bubbles) to visualize the urethra. A TRUS probe was placed into the rectum, and the ultrasound images were matched to the preplanned images acquired in the same manner. When the real-time images of the prostate matched the preplan images, the needles carrying the radioactive seeds were inserted and the seeds were placed. Representative postoperative CT images showing seed distribution after reimplantation with and without reimplant isodose distributions are shown in Figure 1(b).

Androgen deprivation therapy (ADT) was concurrently administered at the discretion of the treating physician. Three of 21 (14.3%) patients received one 3-month injection of Lupron along with their salvage brachytherapy. Two of these patients ultimately had biochemical failure after their reseeding.

Patients were followed up in a multidisciplinary urologic oncology clinic by both urology and radiation oncology faculty. PSA values were obtained and patients were questioned regarding potential treatment related toxicity. Lower urinary tract symptoms were evaluated and categorized by their IPSS, which were self-reported by the patients immediately prior to each appointment. Patients were also questioned about gastrointestinal complaints and other concerns and scored according to the RTOG acute and late toxicity criteria.

Summary statistics such as median and range values were calculated for patient characteristics and disease outcomes. Kaplan-Meier curves and Wilcoxon tests were used to evaluate the association between time to biomedical failure and patient categorical characteristics. Paired two-sample t-tests were used to determine the statistical significance of differences in a continuous variable between two different measurement times. Fisher's exact tests were used to determine the statistical significance of differences in binary outcomes between two patient groups. Significance was considered using a two-sided p value <0.05. Statistics were carried out using Microsoft Excel, SAS version 9.2, and R version 3.0.1.

3. Results

Radiation dosing utilized for the salvage therapy in this study is summarized in Table 1. At initial diagnosis of patients in this study, 3 of 21 (14.3%) patients received EBRT with their initial brachytherapy. One of 21 (4.7%) patients underwent open brachytherapy seed placement as his initial brachytherapy. Risk categories were determined based on initial PSA, Gleason score, and initial clinical stage. Thirteen of 21 (61.3%) patients were low risk, and 6 of 21 (28.6%) patients were intermediate risk; 7of 21 (33.3%) patients had initial brachytherapy at other institutions and had incomplete information to adequately calculate their risk category.

Mean presalvage PSA was 3.49 (median 3.6, range 17.41–1.68). PSA dynamics for individual patients during the study

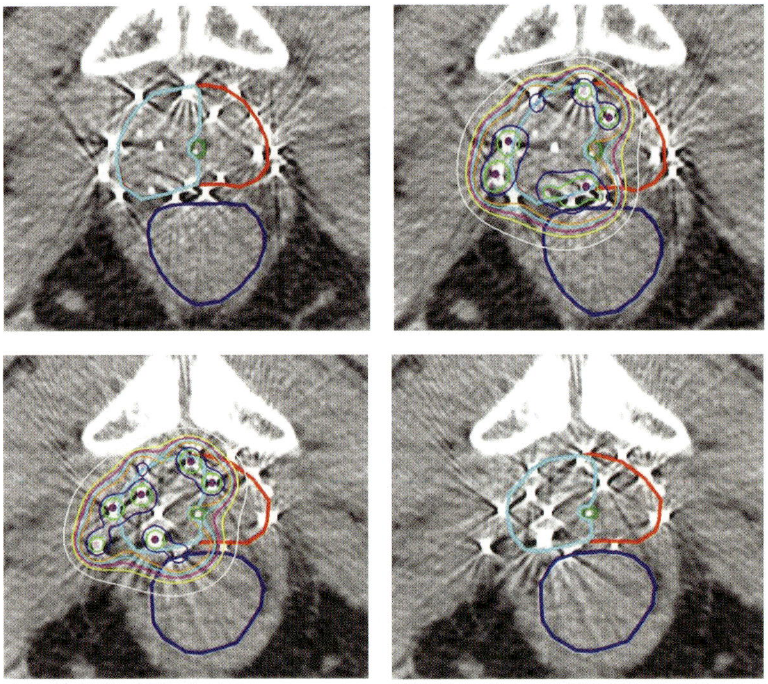

(a)

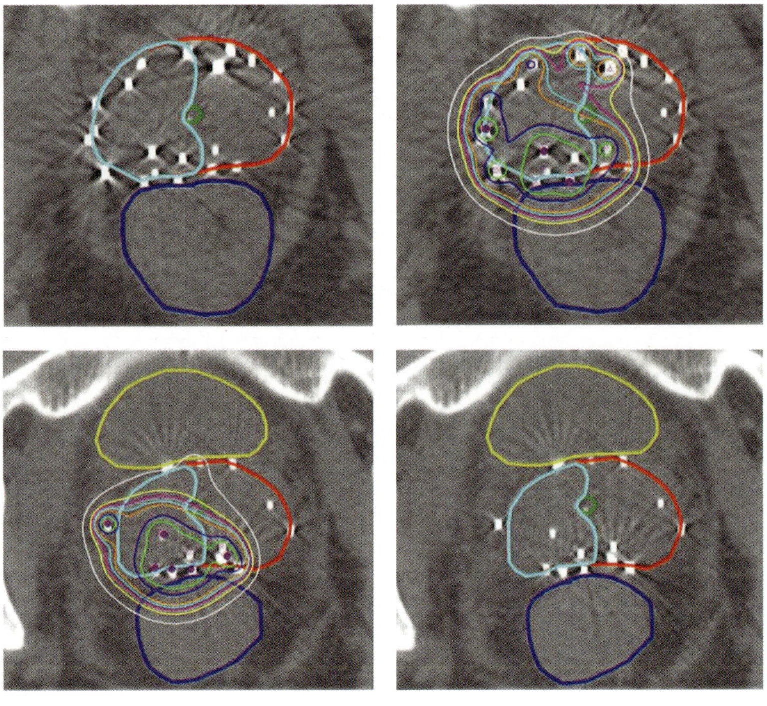

(b)

Figure 1: (a) Sample brachytherapy planning scans using BrachyVision software. (b) CT images showing seed distribution after reimplantation with and without reimplant isodose distributions.

are shown in Table 2. Mean follow-up was 61 months. Median nadir was 0.7 ng/mL (range 2.97–0.01 ng/mL) and median time to nadir was 15 months. All men undergoing a salvage brachytherapy procedure demonstrated an initial decline in their serum PSA. Median time to biochemical failure (according to the Phoenix criteria) of the men failing the second implant was 25 months (range 11–71 months).

3.1. Toxicity. A few patients experienced adverse outcomes following salvage brachytherapy during our study period.

TABLE 1: Radiation dosing.

Patient #	Age at initial treatment (yr)	Prostate cancer risk strata[@]	ADT with BRT #1	ADT with BRT #2	Initial dose	Time b/w Rx (mo)	Salvage dose	Volume treated (cc)
1[‡]	57	Low	No	No	115 Gy	38	144 Gy	21.55
2	61	Low	No	No	144 Gy	32	144 Gy	13.23
3	65	Low	No	Yes	144 Gy	26	144 Gy	7.56
4	63	Intermediate	No	No	144 Gy	34	144 Gy	9.98
5	59	Low	No	No	144 Gy	26	108 Gy	21.58
6[‡]	50	Low	No	Yes	115 Gy	67	108 Gy	26.66
7	48	x	No	No	x	287	108 Gy	21.31
8	60	Low	No	No	144 Gy	123	108 Gy	6.84
9	55	Low	Yes	No	144 Gy	120	108 Gy	7.76
10	57	Low	No	No	144 Gy	19	120 Gy	23.78
11	48	Low	Yes	No	144 Gy	25	125 Gy	16.03
12	66	Low	No	No	144 Gy	46	108 Gy	18.16
13	44	Low	No	No	144 Gy	31	144 Gy	12.05
14	50	Intermediate	No	No	144 Gy	87	144 Gy	15.51
15*	66	Intermediate	Yes	No	108 Gy	42	108 Gy	8.1
16	71	Intermediate	No	No	144 Gy	45	108 Gy	29.36
17*	63	Intermediate	No	Yes	108 Gy	48	108 Gy	9.74
18**	42	x	Yes	No	x	50	120 Gy	12.94
19*	58	Intermediate	Yes	No	108 Gy	105	108 Gy	8.67
20	59	Low	Yes	No	144 Gy	48	144 Gy	27.31
21	72	Low	Yes	No	140 Gy	21	140 Gy	19.93

*Patients who underwent initial external beam radiation therapy.
**Patients who underwent initial open brachytherapy.
‡Patients who had palladium-103 seeds for initial brachytherapy.
x = data point not known.
ADT = androgen deprivation therapy; BRT = brachytherapy.
@ = D'amico risk strata [10].

Two patients experienced Clavien grade I urinary incontinence; one patient experienced each of the following: Clavien grade IIIb bladder neck contracture, rectourethral fistula, and leiomyosarcoma.

Figure 2 depicts urinary tract toxicity obtained from IPSS questionnaires. As expected, IPSS scores increased from a median of 7 to a median of 23 at 3 months following therapy ($p < 0.0001$). Median IPSS dropped to 11 at 9 months ($p = 0.0005$). IPSS continued to decrease at 18 months with a median of 5, which was not significantly different from baseline ($p = 0.294$).

Two of 21 (9.6%) patients developed de novo urinary incontinence, and 1 of 21 (4.8%) developed a rectourethral fistula. One of 21 (4.8%) patients developed bladder outlet obstruction secondary to fibrosis, requiring endoscopic correction (transurethral incision of bladder neck). One patient developed a leiomyosarcoma that ultimately required cystoprostatectomy but had biochemical control of prostate cancer.

Table 3 summarizes changes in sexual function during the study. Eleven of 21 (52.3%) patients had sufficient data to compare pre- and posttherapy sexual function. Six of 11 (54.5%) patients had stable sexual function, and 5 of 11 (45.5%) had decreased sexual function.

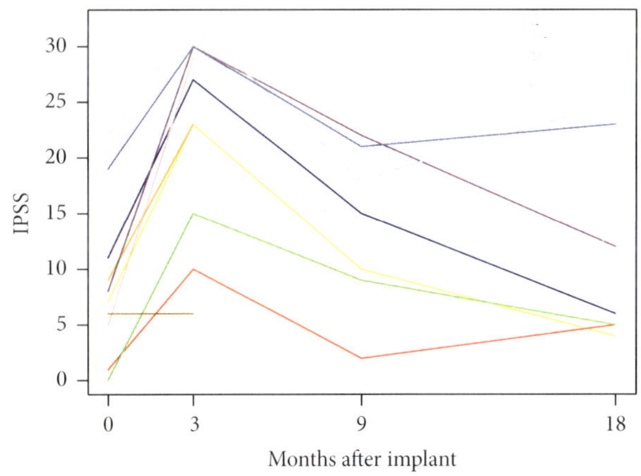

FIGURE 2: IPSS scores throughout follow-up after salvage brachytherapy.

3.2. Time to Failure. The mean decrease in PSA was 4.5 ng/dL (median 3.4, range 0.3–15.0) after salvage brachytherapy. At the time of analysis, 11 of 21 (52.4%) patients had not experienced biochemical recurrence with a mean follow-up of 61 months. Figure 3 shows a Kaplan-Meier curve for time

Table 2: PSA dynamics.

Patient #	Age at initial treatment (yrs)	Time between 1st and 2nd Brachytherapy (mo)	Pre-salvage PSA (ng/mL)	Presalvage PSA (ng/dL)	Follow-up (mo)	Time to nadir (mo)
1	57	38	6.3	3.6	149	21
2	61	32	5.3	3.6	132	31
3	65	26	4.5	4.4	86	73
4	63	34	10	2.5	111	6
5	59	26	4.9	2.7	119	10
6	50	67	8	14.9	83	10
7	48	287	x	8.6	34	22
8	60	123	7.2	17.41	10	9
9	55	120	6.3	1.53	67	7
10	57	19	5.3	3.49	49	48
11	48	25	6.93	2.77	41	41
12	66	4	4.7	1.86	15	4
13	44	31	8.7	2.41	41	29
14	50	87	7.4	7.3	39	33
15	66	42	19.1	1.68	52	9
16	71	45	6.4	3.11	40	5
17	63	48	8.2	13.8	49	3
18	42	50	1	0.98	40	41
19	58	105	x	11.58	52	17
20	59	48	5.7	4.24	25	7
21	72	21	5.8	3.1	21	15
Mean	**57.8**	**62.9**	**6.9**	**5.5**	**61.4**	**20.9**
Median	**59.0**	**45.0**	**6.3**	**3.5**	**49.0**	**15.0**
SD	**8.4**	**60.2**	**3.5**	**4.9**	**37.9**	**18.3**
n	**21**	**21**	**19**	**21**	**21**	**21**

x = data point not known.

to biochemical recurrence based on initial risk category. For the men that failed a second brachytherapy procedure, the median time to failure was 25 months, with a range of 11 to 71 months. There was a trend towards increased time to biochemical failure in the low risk group compared to the intermediate risk group (47 months versus 27 months, $p = 0.12$).

4. Discussion

Prostate cancer patients who experience biochemical failure after initial radiotherapy have a number of options for subsequent treatment: observation, androgen deprivation therapy, salvage radical prostatectomy, salvage cryotherapy, high-intensity focused ultrasound (HIFU), and additional radiotherapy. Salvage therapy is extremely important to control locally recurrent disease and prevent metastases, as lack of further treatment after biochemical recurrence is correlated with the development of clinical disease within 5 years in up to 75% of patients [11].

Biochemical disease-free survival rates of 55–61% at 5-year follow-up have been reported with salvage radical prostatectomy. These were relatively small series with 42, 100, and 138 patients [12–14]. Surgical intervention is even able to achieve a 51% disease-free survival rate at 5-year follow-up in patients with a Gleason score of 8 or higher [15, 16]. However, there are a number of drawbacks to this technique as well. It can be a technically challenging procedure due to residual irradiated tissue damage with increased risk of a number of major complications. Up to 40% of patients are afflicted with urinary incontinence and 25% suffer from bladder neck stricture following this intervention [17]. The risk of rectal injury is 2–9% and urinary fistula is <4% [18].

On the other hand, salvage cryotherapy after initial radiation is a minimally invasive option with improved efficacy, especially following the development of modern techniques to combat issues such as incomplete freezing of tissue. One study reported biochemical disease-free survival, defined as PSA <0.5 ng/mL, at 73% for low risk patients, 45% for intermediate risk patients, and 11% for high risk patients after a median 33.5-months follow-up and actuarial projection of 60 months [19]. Salvage cryotherapy may be a less challenging procedure to perform than salvage radical prostatectomy, giving it minimal variation in outcome across

TABLE 3: Erectile function.

Patient #	Age (yrs)	Baseline ED	18 mo f/u
1	57	1	2
2	61	1	2
3	65	1	3
4	63	1	2
5	59	2	x
6	50	3	x
7	48	1	1
8	60	1	2
9	55	3	x
10	57	x	x
11	48	x	x
12	66	2	2
13	44	2	2
14	50	3	3
15	66	x	2
16	71	2	x
17	63	3	x
18	42	3	3
19	58	2	2
20	59	3	x
21	72	1	x

1 = no difficulty with erection.
2 = erectile function, but not significant enough for penetration.
3 = impotent.
x represents missing data.

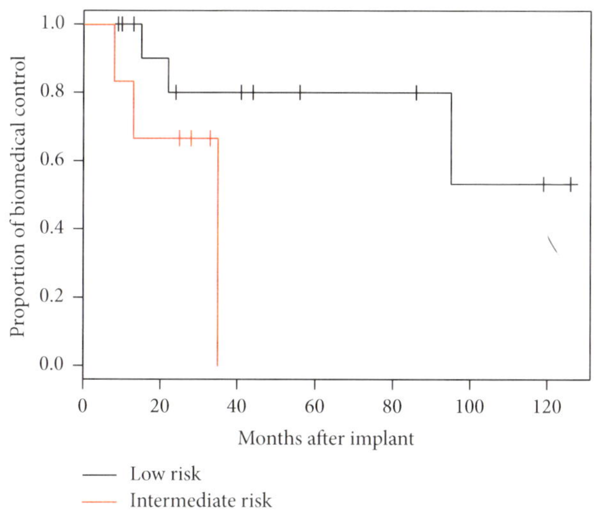

FIGURE 3: Effect of initial risk category on risk of biochemical recurrence.

health providers [20]. In addition, the reported rates of complication are low enough to make it an attractive option for older patients, with urinary incontinence affecting less than 10% of patients [20, 21]. Cryosurgical ablation of the whole prostate gland has also been strongly associated with impotence. Focal cryoablation techniques may limit this adverse effect by relying on targeted image-guided biopsy to guide therapy towards undertreated areas or areas of recurrence, decreasing morbidity [22].

Salvage HIFU has also been studied as a treatment for locally recurrent prostate cancer following external beam radiation therapy (EBRT) only. In a study of 167 European patients, the biochemical disease-free survival was 53%, 42%, and 25% for low, intermediate, and high risk patients, respectively [23]. While the rate of metastatic disease development in this cohort of patients was comparable to that seen in patients treated with other salvage therapies, the complication rate was remarkably low, especially with regard to urinary incontinence and bladder outlet obstruction. Another European study showed that the rate of bladder outlet obstruction decreased from 30% to 15% while the rate of surgical intervention for urinary incontinence decreased from 15% to 5% [24]. Salvage HIFU, however, is not recommended for patients who had initial brachytherapy due to the reflective capacity of the implants, which can redirect excess energy onto surrounding structure such as the rectum and urethra [25].

In recent years, single center brachytherapy studies have shown up to 75% biochemical disease-free survival at 4 years with permanent brachytherapy [17, 26]. In low risk patients who underwent EBRT alone, one recent study showed a biochemical disease control percentage of 85.6% after 5 years [27]. High dose rate (HDR) brachytherapy is now being used as a more customizable form of dosage for patients [28, 29]. However, these doses could cause further toxicity to irradiated damaged tissue and were found in two studies to cause grade 2 urethral strictures in 71% of patients [28, 30]. One prospective study that used MRI-guided seed placement rather than TRUS guidance found that this method was able to keep the incidence of gastrointestinal and genitourinary toxicity requiring surgical treatment at 15% in 4 years [17]. They also found that toxicity was decreased in men who had longer than 4.5-year interval between radiation therapies.

Data on salvage brachytherapy following primary brachytherapy, however, is limited. Studies usually mix patients that were treated with primary brachytherapy with those who initially underwent EBRT. One study from 1990 reported outcomes of salvage brachytherapy seed implantation in 13 patients after initial brachytherapy treatment [31]. Recurrence in this study was detected by digital rectal examination and confirmed with prostate biopsy. A study by Grimm et al. [32] showed that of 31 patients who were reimplanted with seeds for salvage brachytherapy after initial brachytherapy, 87% had biochemical disease control at 31 months using the ASTRO criteria. Interestingly, all but one of these patients underwent 3 months of ADT at the time of salvage brachytherapy. Twenty of 31 (64.5%) of these patients had local recurrence within the prostate, and 11of 31 (35.5%) had disease within the seminal vesicles. Eleven of 31 (35.5%) patients were treated with salvage therapy within 24 months of their primary therapy, and 20 of 31 (64.5%) were treated more than 24 months after their initial therapy. In light of these results, treatment of local recurrence of prostate cancer after initial brachytherapy is an area of evolving interest.

In our series, we show 52.4% freedom from biochemical recurrence with a mean follow-up of 61 months. These data are not as efficacious as those in the Koutrouvelis series, perhaps due to the longer follow-up in our series. It is also possible that 3 months of ADT with salvage brachytherapy led to their superior results, though, in our small subset of patients who received ADT with their salvage therapy, two-thirds of patients had biochemical recurrence during our study. Alternatively, this finding in our study could be due to a selection bias by the treating physician based on the individual patients' risk factors.

When it comes to selecting any salvage therapy modality, accurately characterizing the presence, location, and extent of cancer recurrence in an individual is paramount. Improved cancer targeting and staging techniques significantly improve the risk-benefit ratio for patients with low and intermediate risk disease by allowing physicians to remove malignancy while preserving as much normal tissue and anatomy as possible [33]. In one study, however, the widely used 12-core TRUS biopsy technique was only able to predict unilateral prostate cancer in less than 30% of cases, making it less effective at choosing patients for focal therapy [34]. Instead, using a transperineal template-guided mapping biopsy (TTMB) technique provides better access to the apical and anterior portions of the prostate where up to one-third of significant cancer is located [35, 36]. A recent study used TTMB with multiparametric MRI to assess their combined ability to detect clinically significant cancer, defined as Gleason 6 with tumor length over 3 mm and any Gleason 7 and above [37]. The result of the combined testing was a positive predictive value of 83% and negative predictive value of 91%, which reliably demonstrates the ability to rule out clinically significant prostate cancer [37]. In light of a rising PSA, the negative predictive value of these additional criteria would be helpful in focusing salvage therapy towards patients with clinically significant disease [38].

Alternatively, metabolic imaging offers a less invasive method of detection of both localized and systemic tumor burden. The available literature varies with regard to the optimal PSA value at which to initiate ^{18}F-Choline PET/CT imaging, but there appears to be a strong correlation between increasing PSA values and the positive predictive ability of this tool [39]. In one study of 250 prostate cancer patients with biochemical recurrence, ^{18}F-Choline PET/CT showed 77% sensitivity for cancer detection at a PSA level greater than 0.3 ng/mL and had a particularly high sensitivity in patients treated with ADT as compared to those who did not receive ADT [40].

Our study has several key limitations that warrant discussion. It is a retrospective, nonrandomized study with inherent selection and treatment biases. Patients were treated with salvage therapy based on biochemical recurrence alone, analogous to the delivery of salvage external radiation therapy for a recurrence following a radical prostatectomy. Therefore, the majority of patients did not undergo TTMB or repeat TRUS biopsy prior to salvage therapy, leaving the possibility that their pathology was different from that of their original prostate biopsy and skewing their presalvage risk stratification. Follow-up was not standardized, leading to incomplete data on erectile function, lower urinary tract symptoms, and GI toxicity. Finally, while all patients underwent primary brachytherapy prior to their salvage brachytherapy, the cohort remains somewhat heterogeneous. Three of 21 (14.3%) patients underwent EBRT with their primary brachytherapy. Seven of 21 (33.3%) patients had ADT with primary therapy and 3 of 21 (14.3%) had ADT with their salvage brachytherapy. One of 21 (4.7%) patients had open brachytherapy seed placement as initial treatment.

Salvage brachytherapy is an intriguing treatment option for patients with biochemically recurrent prostate cancer who underwent primary brachytherapy. In our study, this modality appears to provide adequate prostate cancer control in select men with underseeded areas on cross-sectional imaging. There is a trend towards decreased efficacy of salvage brachytherapy in patients who were intermediate risk at initial presentation. Side effects of treatment are higher than expected with a single brachytherapy implantation; out of 21 patients 3 individuals developed grade 3 toxicities. The majority of lower urinary tract symptoms resolve within 9 months of treatment and minimal gastrointestinal side effects. Further studies are warranted to compare this treatment modality to other salvage therapies in patients who underwent primary brachytherapy. Further studies would perhaps be made more meaningful by utilizing more advanced methods to evaluate for location of the recurrence within or beyond the prostate. Technologies have emerged which may be beneficial in better selecting patients for salvage brachytherapy. For example, methods such as transperineal mapping, multiparametric MRI, and/or ^{18}F-Choline PET/CT scans may make partial prostate implants more successful by better localization of the recurrent disease. However, we are unaware of any of these new technologies being used to select patients for salvage prostate brachytherapy. Metabolic imaging using PET/CT likely will increase the detection of metastatic prostate cancer [41] thereby better selecting a population that could benefit from the added brachytherapy procedure.

Abbreviations

CT: Computed tomography scan
PSA: Prostate-specific antigen
TRUS: Transrectal ultrasound
IPSS: International Prostate Symptom Score
EBRT: External beam radiation therapy
HIFU: High-intensity focused ultrasound
ADT: Androgen deprivation therapy
MRI: Magnetic resonance imaging
HDR: High dose rate
GI: Gastrointestinal
GU: Genitourinary
TTMB: Transperineal template-guided mapping biopsy.

Additional Points

In this project, the authors describe the eleven years of experiences at a single institution of salvage therapy in prostate cancer patients with biochemical failure and no evidence of metastatic disease after interstitial brachytherapy. Images from the CT scans were evaluated by radiation oncology and urology faculty. Patients with underseeded areas on the CT images were considered for reimplantation with I-125 interstitial brachytherapy; 21 patients were reimplanted. Our results indicated that the salvage brachytherapy to underseeded areas after primary brachytherapy in patients with biochemical recurrence can be a successful procedure.

Competing Interests

The authors declare that they have no competing interests.

References

[1] N. D. Arvold, M.-H. Chen, J. W. Moul et al., "Risk of death from prostate cancer after radical prostatectomy or brachytherapy in men with low or intermediate risk disease," *Journal of Urology*, vol. 186, no. 1, pp. 91–96, 2011.

[2] A. D. Vassil, E. S. Murphy, C. A. Reddy et al., "Five year biochemical recurrence free survival for intermediate risk prostate cancer after radical prostatectomy, external beam radiation therapy or permanent seed implantation," *Urology*, vol. 76, no. 5, pp. 1251–1257, 2010.

[3] J. B. Malcolm, M. D. Fabrizio, B. B. Barone et al., "Quality of life after open or robotic prostatectomy, cryoablation or brachytherapy for localized prostate cancer," *The Journal of Urology*, vol. 183, no. 5, pp. 1822–1829, 2010.

[4] G. Koukourakis, N. Kelekis, V. Armonis, and V. Kouloulias, "Brachytherapy for prostate cancer: a systematic review," *Advances in Urology*, vol. 2009, Article ID 327945, 11 pages, 2009.

[5] B. Shekarriz, J. Upadhyay, and J. E. Pontes, "Salvage radical prostatectomy," *Urologic Clinics of North America*, vol. 28, no. 3, pp. 545–553, 2001.

[6] P. Russo, "Salvage radical prostatectomy after radiation therapy and brachytherapy," *Journal of Endourology*, vol. 14, no. 4, pp. 385–390, 2000.

[7] K. E. Wallner, D. Nori, M. J. Morse, P. C. Sogani, W. F. Whitmore, and Z. Fuks, "125Iodine reimplantation for locally progressive prostatic carcinoma," *Journal of Urology*, vol. 144, no. 3, pp. 704–706, 1990.

[8] P. Koutrouvelis, F. Hendricks, N. Lailas et al., "Salvage reimplantation in patient with local recurrent prostate carcinoma after brachytherapy with three dimensional computed tomography-guided permanent pararectal implant," *Technology in Cancer Research and Treatment*, vol. 2, no. 4, pp. 339–344, 2003.

[9] M. Roach III, G. Hanks, H. Thames Jr. et al., "Defining biochemical failure following radiotherapy with or without hormonal therapy in men with clinically localized prostate cancer: recommendations of the RTOG-ASTRO Phoenix Consensus Conference," *International Journal of Radiation Oncology, Biology, Physics*, vol. 65, pp. 965–974, 2006.

[10] A. V. D'Amico, R. Whittington, S. Bruce Malkowicz et al., "Biochemical outcome after radical prostatectomy, external beam radiation therapy, or interstitial radiation therapy for clinically localized prostate cancer," *Journal of the American Medical Association*, vol. 280, no. 11, pp. 969–974, 1998.

[11] W. R. Lee, G. E. Hanks, and A. Hanlon, "Increasing prostate-specific antigen profile following definitive radiation therapy for localized prostate cancer: clinical observations," *Journal of Clinical Oncology*, vol. 15, no. 1, pp. 230–238, 1997.

[12] F. J. Bianco Jr., P. T. Scardino, A. J. Stephenson, C. J. DiBlasio, P. A. Fearn, and J. A. Eastham, "Long-term oncologic results of salvage radical prostatectomy for locally recurrent prostate cancer after radiotherapy," *International Journal of Radiation Oncology, Biology, Physics*, vol. 62, no. 2, pp. 448–453, 2005.

[13] J. F. Ward, T. J. Sebo, M. L. Blute, and H. Zincke, "Salvage surgery for radiorecurrent prostate cancer: contemporary outcomes," *Journal of Urology*, vol. 173, no. 4, pp. 1156–1160, 2005.

[14] L. L. Pisters, D. Leibovici, M. Blute et al., "Locally recurrent prostate cancer after initial radiation therapy: a comparison of salvage radical prostatectomy versus cryotherapy," *The Journal of Urology*, vol. 182, no. 2, pp. 517–527, 2009.

[15] A. J. Stephenson and J. A. Eastham, "Role of salvage radical prostatectomy for recurrent prostate cancer after radiation therapy," *Journal of Clinical Oncology*, vol. 23, no. 32, pp. 8198–8203, 2005.

[16] D. C. Chade, S. F. Shariat, A. M. Cronin et al., "Salvage radical prostatectomy for radiation-recurrent prostate cancer: a multi-institutional collaboration," *European Urology*, vol. 60, no. 2, pp. 205–210, 2011.

[17] P. L. Nguyen, M.-H. Chen, A. V. D'Amico et al., "Magnetic resonance image-guided salvage brachytherapy after radiation in select men who initially presented with favorable-risk prostate cancer: a prospective phase 2 study," *Cancer*, vol. 110, no. 7, pp. 1485–1492, 2007.

[18] L. L. Pisters and J. F. Ward, "Salvage therapy after primary non-surgical therapy for prostate cancer," *AUA Update Series*, vol. 33, lesson 2, 2014.

[19] M. Ismail, S. Ahmed, C. Kastner, and J. Davies, "Salvage cryotherapy for recurrent prostate cancer after radiation failure: a prospective case series of the first 100 patients," *BJU International*, vol. 100, no. 4, pp. 760–764, 2007.

[20] L. L. Pisters, J. C. Rewcastle, B. J. Donnelly, F. M. Lugnani, A. E. Katz, and J. S. Jones, "Salvage prostate cryoablation: initial results from the cryo on-line data registry," *Journal of Urology*, vol. 180, no. 2, pp. 559–563, 2008.

[21] A. B. Galosi, F. Lugnani, and G. Muzzonigro, "Salvage cryosurgery for recurrent prostate carcinoma after radiotherapy," *Journal of Endourology*, vol. 21, no. 1, pp. 1–7, 2007.

[22] A. Kanthabalan, M. Arya, S. Punwani et al., "Role of focal salvage ablative therapy in localised radiorecurrent prostate cancer," *World Journal of Urology*, vol. 31, no. 6, pp. 1361–1368, 2013.

[23] F.-J. Murat, L. Poissonnier, M. Rabilloud et al., "Mid-term results demonstrate salvage high-intensity focused ultrasound (HIFU) as an effective and acceptably morbid salvage treatment option for locally radiorecurrent prostate cancer," *European Urology*, vol. 55, no. 3, pp. 640–649, 2009.

[24] S. Crouzet, S. Brown, and V. Berge, "Multicentric oncologic outcomes of salvage HIFU for local failure after external beam radio therapy: 7 years biochemical survival of 929 patients," in *Proceedings of the 27th Annual European Association of Urology Congress*, Paris, France, 2012.

[25] H. U. Ahmed, A. Ishaq, E. Zacharakis et al., "Rectal fistulae after salvage high-intensity focused ultrasound for recurrent prostate cancer after combined brachytherapy and external beam radiotherapy," *BJU International*, vol. 103, no. 3, pp. 321–323, 2009.

[26] R. J. Burri, N. N. Stone, P. Unger, and R. G. Stock, "Long-term outcome and toxicity of salvage brachytherapy for local failure after initial radiotherapy for prostate cancer," *International*

Journal of Radiation Oncology Biology Physics, vol. 77, no. 5, pp. 1338–1344, 2010.

[27] C. Vargas, D. Swartz, A. Vashi et al., "Salvage brachytherapy for recurrent prostate cancer," *Brachytherapy*, vol. 13, no. 1, pp. 53–58, 2014.

[28] B. Lee, K. Shinohara, V. Weinberg et al., "Feasibility of high-dose-rate brachytherapy salvage for local prostate cancer recurrence after radiotherapy: the University of California-San Francisco experience," *International Journal of Radiation Oncology, Biology, Physics*, vol. 67, no. 4, pp. 1106–1112, 2007.

[29] Y. Jo, T. Fujii, R. Hara et al., "Salvage high-dose-rate brachytherapy for local prostate cancer recurrence after radiotherapy-Preliminary results," *BJU International*, vol. 109, no. 6, pp. 835–839, 2012.

[30] M. Tharp, M. Hardacre, R. Bennett, W. T. Jones, D. Stuhldreher, and J. Vaught, "Prostate high-dose-rate brachytherapy as salvage treatment of local failure after previous external or permanent seed irradiation for prostate cancer," *Brachytherapy*, vol. 7, no. 3, pp. 231–236, 2008.

[31] J. C. Blasko, P. D. Grimm, and H. Ragde, "Brachytherapy and organ preservation in the management of carcinoma of the prostate," *Seminars in Radiation Oncology*, vol. 3, no. 4, pp. 240–249, 1993.

[32] P. D. Grimm, J. C. Blasko, and H. Radge, "Ultrasound-guided transperineal implantation of iodine-125 and palladium-103 for the treatment of early stage prostate cancer; technical concepts in planning, operative technique and evaluation," *Atlas of the Urologic Clinics of North America*, vol. 2, pp. 113–125, 1994.

[33] D. W. Smith, D. Stoimenova, K. Eid, and A. Barqawi, "The role of targeted focal therapy in the management of low-risk prostate cancer: update on current challenges," *Prostate Cancer*, vol. 2012, Article ID 587139, 5 pages, 2012.

[34] B. Tareen, G. Godoy, A. Sankin, S. Temkin, H. Lepor, and S. S. Taneja, "Can contemporary transrectal prostate biopsy accurately select candidates for hemi-ablative focal therapy of prostate cancer?" *BJU International*, vol. 104, no. 2, pp. 195–199, 2009.

[35] A. V. Taira, G. S. Merrick, R. W. Galbreath et al., "Performance of transperineal template-guided mapping biopsy in detecting prostate cancer in the initial and repeat biopsy setting," *Prostate Cancer and Prostatic Diseases*, vol. 13, no. 1, pp. 71–77, 2010.

[36] J. E. McNeal, E. A. Redwine, F. S. Freiha, and T. A. Stamey, "Zonal distribution of prostatic adenocarcinoma. Correlation with histologic pattern and direction of spread," *The American Journal of Surgical Pathology*, vol. 12, no. 12, pp. 897–906, 1988.

[37] M. Tran, J. Thompson, M. Böhm et al., "Combination of multiparametric MRI and transperineal template-guided mapping biopsy of the prostate to identify candidates for hemi-ablative focal therapy," *BJU International*, vol. 117, no. 1, pp. 48–54, 2016.

[38] M. Abd-Alazeez, H. U. Ahmed, M. Arya et al., "The accuracy of multiparametric MRI in men with negative biopsy and elevated PSA level—can it rule out clinically significant prostate cancer?" *Urologic Oncology: Seminars and Original Investigations*, vol. 32, no. 1, Article ID e17-22, p. 45, 2014.

[39] S. Chondrogiannis, M. C. Marzola, A. Ferretti et al., "Role of ^{18}F-choline PET/CT in suspicion of relapse following definitive radiotherapy for prostate cancer," *European Journal of Nuclear Medicine and Molecular Imaging*, vol. 40, no. 9, pp. 1356–1364, 2013.

[40] M. Beheshti, S. Haim, R. Zakavi et al., "Impact of 18F-choline PET/CT in prostate cancer patients with biochemical recurrence: influence of androgen deprivation therapy and correlation with PSA kinetics," *Journal of Nuclear Medicine*, vol. 54, no. 6, pp. 833–840, 2013.

[41] B. Tombal and F. Lecouvet, "Modern detection of prostate cancer's bone metastasis: is the bone scan era over?" *Advances in Urology*, vol. 2012, Article ID 893193, 8 pages, 2012.

29

Local Treatment of Metastatic Prostate Cancer: What is the Evidence So Far?

Pedro Leonel Almeida and Bruno Jorge Pereira

Faculdade de Ciências da Saúde, Universidade da Beira Interior (FCS-UBI), Covilhã, Portugal

Correspondence should be addressed to Bruno Jorge Pereira; brunoalexpereira@gmail.com

Academic Editor: Manfred Wirth

Background. Advances in technological, laboratorial, and imaging studies and new treatments available in the last decades significantly improved prostate cancer survival rates. However, this did not occur in metastatic prostate cancer (mPCa) at diagnosis which, in young and fit patients, will become invariably resistant to the established treatments. Progression will lead to an impairment in patients' quality of life and disease-related death. *Methods.* The authors intend to perform a literature review of the advantages of primary treatment of mPCa. Articles were retrieved and filtered for relevance from PubMed, SciELO, and ScienceDirect until March 2017. *Results.* Primary treatment is currently indicated only in cases of nonmetastatic PCa. Nonetheless, there might be some benefits in doing local treatment in mPCa in order to control local disease, prevent new metastasis, and improve the efficacy of chemotherapy and hormonotherapy with similar complications rate when compared to locally confined cancer. Independent factors that have a negative influence are age above 70 years, cT4 stage or high-grade disease, PSA $\geq$ 20 ng/ml, and pelvic lymphadenopathies. The presence of 3 or more of these factors conditions CSS and OS is the same between patients who performed local treatment and those who did not. Metastasis degree and location number can also influence outcome. Meanwhile, patients with visceral metastases have worse results. *Conclusions.* There is growing evidence supporting local treatment in cases of metastatic prostate cancer at diagnosis in the context of a multimodal approach. However, it should be kept in mind that most of the existing studies are retrospective and it would be important to make consistent prospective studies with well-defined patient selection criteria in order to sustain the existing data and understand the main indications to select patients and perform primary treatment in mPCa.

1. Background

Prostate cancer (PCa) is the fourth most common neoplasm worldwide with about 75% of the diagnoses performed in developed countries. Around the world, 307.000 deaths are estimated due to PCa, thus ranking as the fifth cause of death (6.6%). It is the second most common neoplasm in European men above 70 years and the second cause of death due to oncological disease. 10 to 20% may be metastasized at diagnosis [1–3]. This article intends to review the current literature on primary treatment of metastatic prostate cancer, inferring whether there is an advantage in terms of clinical outcome and trying to define criteria for its application.

2. Methods

A vast literature review was carried out using mainly PubMed, SciELO, ScienceDirect, and publications of the International Journal of Urology. During the research, the most relevant articles published were identified, with preference for articles published in the last 10 years, until December 2016.

The research was conducted in the English language, with a free text protocol including preferably the following terms: "metastatic prostate cancer," "primary treatment," "local treatment," "radical prostatectomy," "radiotherapy," "cytoreductive surgery," and "cytoreductive treatment." The references of the articles used were carefully analyzed to find publications with pertinent information, which eventually were included in the present dissertation.

3. Results and Discussion

3.1. Primary Treatment of PCa. Currently, primary treatment in PCa is indicated as first line in cases of nonmetastatic PCa and may be performed as palliative treatment in order to minimize symptoms arising from the underlying pathology, which may occur in cases of metastatic prostate cancer (mPCa) [4].

The primary treatment has been accepted and recommended in other metastatic malignancies with good morbidity and mortality outcomes [5, 6].

Some emerging theories point to the accomplishment of primary therapy, although still without strong scientific evidence.

3.2. Control of Local Disease. Advanced stages of prostate cancer increase patients' morbidity and mortality risk by local progression and/or establishment of metastasis. Local progression may cause invasion of adjacent structures leading to pain, urinary retention due to invasion of the bladder and/or urethra, obstruction of the rectum, establishment of rectourethral or rectovesical fistulas, and infiltration of the pelvic nerve bundles. These factors impair the patients' quality of life and may impact survival. In some cases, it is necessary to perform palliative treatment. The frequency of these complications may be related to whether or not local therapy was performed in a phase of localized disease [7, 8].

It is scientifically plausible that uncontrolled local disease is the source of circulating tumor cells that can establish distant metastases and even recolonize the primary tumor itself with more aggressive and hormone-resistant cell clones [5, 9]. It is also assumed that the primary lesion may produce factors responsible for maintenance of circulating cancer cells' viability [10].

Combination of androgen deprivation therapy (ADT) with a primary treatment (radical prostatectomy or radiotherapy) may be more efficient in terms of local progression control than just isolated ADT. By controlling the local disease through directed local therapy, local symptoms conditioned by the growth and progression of the primary lesion are prevented or delayed [5, 11, 12].

3.3. Metastasis Establishment Prevention/Control. The primary carcinoma, host cells, and metastases are part of a communication circuit connected by molecular pathways, which is responsible for microenvironment changes in certain regions, premetastatic niches, which are responsible for subsequent metastatic pattern. Metastatic establishment seems to occur in pulses [5, 19].

After primary cancer's surgical ablation, circulating tumor cells are unable to establish new metastases. It is biologically plausible that the uncontrolled primary lesion promotes the growth and appearance of new tumoral lesions. However, this capacity is not a unique capacity of the primary lesion, since some metastases may establish and promote the growth of new metastases too. Antwi and Everson also demonstrated that the probability of death from any cause increases with the number of established metastases [4, 9, 20–22].

The abscopal effect, a phenomenon that corresponds to the regression of distant metastases during primary treatment, is another explanation for a potential benefit of local treatment. Radiotherapy promotes antitumor immune reactions directed to the primary lesion and metastases by improving the cross-presentation of antigens by activating cytotoxic CD8+ T cells. Thus, radiotherapy when combined with ADT has an effect on the tumor's genetic expression, potentiating apoptosis [12].

It is logical to think that directed local therapy of primary carcinoma reduces the likelihood of metastasis onset, establishment, and growth through the breakdown of the communication between the different cells involved in the process, not allowing the creation of the necessary environment for implantation of circulating tumor cells in distant sites and preventing signaling that promotes their growth.

3.4. Improved Hormonotherapy and Chemotherapy Efficacy. As stated before, primary treatment with radiotherapy potentiates the effect of hormonal manipulations due to the abscopal effect [12]. The progression of the primary tumor leads to increased genetic and phenotypic heterogeneity, which will lead to appearance of cell colonies with different characteristics: increased proliferative capacity, metastatic potential, and resistance to treatments [7]. Some colonies resistant to castration will be further selected by ADT, which will promote their growth, conditioning the development of resistance to castration, a capacity that many of these tumors show after a few months of conventional therapy [6].

A recent study has shown that primary tumor therapy, whether radical prostatectomy (RP) or radiotherapy (RT), increases the time to the development of castrate-resistant prostate cancer (8 years compared to 4 years in the control group) [23].

Thus, by eliminating the possibility of increased heterogeneity, we may increase the likelihood of long-lasting response to systemic therapies associated with primary treatments, since evidence suggests that the prostate is a focus of resistance to currently recommended regimens, which contributes to accelerating progression [7, 12, 24].

3.5. Results of Primary Therapy Performed in Other Metastatic Cancers. Several studies show that primary tumor therapy is associated with increased survival and better response to systemic treatments in patients diagnosed with metastatic cancer disease, including renal cell carcinoma, colon cancer, breast cancer, ovarian cancer, and glioblastoma. Studies suggest that prostate cancer may have similar behavior [10, 25].

3.6. Radical Prostatectomy and Radiotherapy as Primary Treatment of mPCa. Recent data suggests that performing RP or RT in patients duly selected with mPCa is associated with better oncological outcomes and better overall survival (OS), cancer-specific survival (CSS), and prostate cancer-free survival (PCFS) [4, 25]. Patient survival increases regardless

TABLE 1: Mean survival time and disease-specific mortality by therapeutic modality, adapted from Antwi and Everson (2014) [4].

Therapeutic modality	Average survival time after diagnosis (months)	DSM (%)
RP	29	15,3
BT	31	28,3
NLT	17	45,4

DSM: disease-specific mortality; RP: radical prostatectomy; BT: brachytherapy; NLT: no local treatment.

TABLE 2: Overall survival and cancer-specific survival by therapeutic modality, adapted from Culp et al. (2014) [13].

Therapeutic modality	5-year OS rate (%)	5-year CSS rate (%)
RP	67,4	75,8
BT	52,6	61,3
NLT	22,5	48,7

OS: overall survival; CSS: cancer-specific survival; RP: radical prostatectomy; BT: brachytherapy; NLT: no local treatment.

TABLE 3: Overall survival and disease-specific survival by age and therapeutic modality, adapted from Culp et al. (2014) [13].

Age/therapeutic modality	5-year OS rate (%)	DSS rate (%)		
		1 year	3 years	5 years
<70 years				
NLT	28,9	86,1	57,7	45,8
RP	71,2	96,7	86,9	82,0
BT	57,4	92,2	73,9	65,2
≥70 years				
NLT	18,1	80,1	58,6	49,5
RP	50,3	86,7	70,8	63,5
BT	48,5	86,2	69,9	62,5

OS: overall survival; DSS: disease-specific survival; RP: radical prostatectomy; BT: brachytherapy; NLT: no local treatment.

of M-stage according to American Joint Committee on Cancer (AJCC) [13].

Antwi and Everson conducted a retrospective study using Surveillance, Epidemiology, and End Results Program (SEER) data. Average survival time after diagnosis was 29 months for patients in the RP group, 31 months in brachytherapy (BT) group, and 17 months in no local treatment (NLT) group. It was concluded that patients receiving local therapy had higher survival rates and a lower probability of dying from mPCa (15.3% in the PR group, 28.3% in the BT group, and 45.4% in the NLT group) [4] (Table 1).

Culp et al. through the SEER database compared the results of performing local therapy (RP or BT) versus patients without local treatment. Overall survival at 5 years was 67.4% in the RP group, 52.6% in the BT group, and 22.5% in the NTL group. In the case of specific survival related to PCa, patients in the RP and BT groups showed better results than the NLT group (75.8% and 61.3% compared to 48.7% of the latter group). OS and disease-specific survival (DSS) were higher in patients <70 years, but only OS was significantly higher in patients ≥70 years with local treatment compared to the NLT group. In the prostate-specific antigen (PSA) based groups, OS and DSS were higher in local treatment (LT) group patients with PSA < 20. In the PSA ≥ 20 group, the probability of OS was significantly higher. Considering the extent of metastases, men who underwent RP had decrease in cancer-specific mortality (CSM) not influenced by M-stage and higher OS in groups M1b and M1c. In the case of patients receiving BT, the results were overlapping [13] (Tables 2–5).

Both SEER-based studies excluded external RT from the analysis, since it might be difficult to tell which patients received it with a definitive or palliative intention [13].

Löppenberg et al. in a National Cancer Database (NCDB) based study assessed the impact of local therapy on men with PCa at diagnosis. Overall mortality-free survival (OM-FS) rate was 50% in the total population studied, 63% in LT group, and 48% in NLT group. In the LT group associated with ADT within 6 months of diagnosis, the probability of 3-year survival was 57% and it was 69% in LT group, while in the LT + ADT group it was 48%. When separated by treatment, survival at 3 years was higher in the BT patients (80%) followed by the RP patients (78%) and finally RT patients (60%) [14] (Table 6).

Satkunasivam et al. analyzed data from SEER collected between 2004 and 2009 of men with mPCa, taking into account their treatment modality. OS rate at 3 years was 73% in the RP group, 72% in the intensity-modulated radiotherapy (IMRT), 37% in the conformal radiation therapy (CRT), and 34% in the NTL. DSS at 3 years was 79% in RP group, 82% in IMRT group, 49% in CRT group, and 46% in NLT group [15] (Table 7).

Gratzke et al. followed the same direction of previously published studies using data from the RCM collected between 1998 and 2010. Survival probability at 5 years was superior

Table 4: Overall survival and disease-specific survival by PSA and therapeutic modality, adapted from Culp et al. (2014) [13].

PSA/therapeutic modality	5-year OS rate (%)	DSS rate (%)		
		1 year	3 years	5 years
<20 ng/ml				
NLT	33,7	87,3	66,6	57,9
RP	77,1	96,5	89,9	86,7
BT	71,2	95,3	86,5	82,3
≥20 ng/ml				
NLT	19,8	81,4	55,6	44,8
RP	55,7	88,8	71,3	63,0
BT	37,3	82,9	58,5	48,1

PSA: prostate-specific antigen; OS: overall survival; DSS: disease-specific survival; RP: radical prostatectomy; BT: brachytherapy; NLT: no local treatment.

Table 5: Overall survival and disease-specific survival by stage M according to the AJCC criteria and therapeutic modality, adapted from Culp et al. (2014) [13].

AJCC M-stage/therapeutic modality	5-year OS rate (%)	DSS rate (%)		
		1 year	3 years	5 years
M1a				
NLT	35,1	93,4	73,3	61,4
RP	64,3	98,4	92,9	89,1
BT	54,7	96,3	84,1	76,2
M1b				
NLT	22,9	84,1	59,6	48,4
RP	70,1	94,1	83,4	77,6
BT	55,0	89,2	71,0	61,9
M1c				
NLT	18,6	75,6	50,4	43,0
RP	60,7	91,1	80,0	75,6
BT	53,4	85,4	68,3	62,1

AJCC: American Joint Committee on Cancer; OS: overall survival; DSS: disease-specific survival; RP: radical prostatectomy; BT: brachytherapy; NLT: no local treatment.

Table 6: Overall mortality-free survival and overall survival by therapeutic modality, adapted from Löppenberg et al. (2016) [14].

Therapeutic modality	3-year OM-FS rate (%)	3-year OS rate (%)
TP	50,0	
NLT	48,0	
NLT + ADT		48,0
LT	63,0	69,0
LT + ADT		57,0
RP		78,0
BT		80,0
RT		60,0

OM-FS: overall mortality-free survival; OS: overall survival; TP: total population; NLT: no local treatment; ADT: androgen deprivation therapy; RP: radical prostatectomy; BT: brachytherapy; RT: radiotherapy.

Table 7: Overall survival and disease-specific survival by therapeutic modality, adapted from Satkunasivam et al. (2015) [15].

Therapeutic modality	3-year OS rate (%)	3-year DSS rate (%)
NLT	34	46,0
CRT	37	49,0
IMRT	72,0	82,0
RP	73,0	79,0

OS: overall survival; DSS: disease-specific survival; NLT: no local treatment; CRT: conformal radiation therapy; IMRT: intensity-modulated radiotherapy; RP: radical prostatectomy.

TABLE 8: Overall survival and biochemical failure free survival by therapeutic modality, adapted from Cho et al. (2016) [16].

Therapeutic modality	3-year OS rate (%)	BCFFS (%)
TP	48,2	25,0
RT	69,0	52,0
NLT	43,0	16,0
Palliative RT	50,0	10,0
Without palliative RT	40,0	20,0

OS: overall survival; BCFFS: biochemical failure-free survival; TP: total population; RT: radiotherapy; NLT: no local treatment.

TABLE 9: Overall survival and overall survival rates by therapeutic modality, adapted from Rusthoven et al. (2016) [17].

	OS (months)	3-year OS rate (%)	5-year OS rate (%)	8-year OS rate (%)
RT + ADT	53	62,0	49,0	33,0
ADT	29	43,0	25,0	13,0

OS: overall survival; RT: radiotherapy; ADT: androgen deprivation therapy.

TABLE 10: Overall survival and surgery-free survival rate by therapeutic modality, adapted from Heidenreich et al. [18].

Therapeutic modality	OS rate (%)	CSS rate (%)	Surgery-free survival rate
RP	91,3	95,6	100,0
NLT	78,9	84,2	71,1

OS: overall survival; CSS: cancer-specific survival; RP: radical prostatectomy; NLT: no local treatment.

in the RP group compared to NLT group (55% versus 21%) [26].

Cho et al. carried out a cohort study with the purpose of analyzing the efficacy and safety of RT treatment in mPCa patients. The established indications for RT included metastatic lesions conditioning pain, fracture risk, and neurological complications. Virtually all patients (96%) started ADT at diagnosis. RT group had a 69% OS at 3 years, which was significantly higher than the 43% of the NLT group. Biochemical failure-free survival (BCFFS) value at 3 years was also higher in the RT group when compared to NLT group (52% and 16%, resp.) [16] (Table 8).

Rusthoven et al. looked through the data recorded between 2004 and 2012 in NCDB to evaluate the outcome of RT therapy in patients with mPCa at diagnosis. ADT combined with prostate-directed RT had longer OS (53 months) versus 29 months of isolated ADT therapy. Patients who received ADT + RT had an OS probability of 62% at 3 years, 49% at 5 years, and 33% at 8 years compared to 43%, 25%, and 13%, respectively, for those who received ADT only [17] (Table 9).

Heidenreich et al. developed the first case-control study addressing this subject and although with a small population, the criteria used to select individuals allowed to reach important conclusions. Group 1 included 23 patients with mPCa with low volume bone metastases who underwent cytoreductive radical prostatectomy (CRP), since 6 defined criteria were satisfied: completely resectable PCa assessed by transrectal ultrasonography and rectal examination, three or less bone metastases, absence of retroperitoneal lymphatic metastases, absence of pelvic lymphadenopathy greater than 3 centimeters, absence of visceral metastases, and signed informed consent. This group has been given luteinizing hormone-releasing hormone (LHRH) analogues for at least 6 months in combination with bicalutamide. A second control group (group 2) consisted of 38 men treated with ADT, without any local therapy until there was progression and were submitted to intervention only if local symptoms were present. Comparing the two groups according to OS rate and CSS rate, group 1 had 91,3% OS rate and group 2 78,9%. CSS rate was 95,6% in group 1 and 84,2% in group 2 [18] (Table 10).

3.7. Complications of Local Treatment in mPCa. Primary treatment modalities that may be offered in cases of PCa also entail complications. However, current evidence shows that these are not worse than those usually seen in these procedures for primary localized disease.

Considering the postoperative complications over a 90-day period, according to a 2015 study, 79.2% of patients did not experience any complication. Of the 106 men, only 21 (19.8%) experienced complications, 9 (8.5%) had lymphocele, 7 (6.6%) had anastomotic leakage, and 5 (4.7%) had a surgical scar infection. Six (27.3%) of the patients had 2 complications. M1a and M1b (19.4% versus 21.4% of patients) did not differ significantly. Postsurgical urinary continence at 90 days revealed that 38 (64.4%) of the 59 patients reported were reestablished, and only 11 (18.6%) of the 59 patients had moderate-to-severe incontinence. Based on these data, RP in cases of mPCa is safe and reliable and does not lead to more complications or increased mortality compared to nonmetastatic patients [27].

In Heidenreich et al.'s study, the mean time of hospitalization was 7.8 days with an average of 5.6 days of bladder catheterization. Intraoperatively, the blood loss had an average value of 335 ml, with preoperative and postoperative hemoglobin values of 13.1 mg/dl and 11.8 mg/dl, respectively.

Three patients (13%) who developed lymphocele were found, of which 2 (8.7%) were resolved by percutaneous drainage and 1 (4.3%) by laparoscopic marsupialization. Two patients (8.7%) developed deep vein thrombosis (DVT) and one of them had pulmonary embolism. Analyzing the data on urinary continence, 91.3% presented urinary continence with 1 or fewer diapers per day [18].

Cho et al. evaluated the toxicity of RT follow-up and weekly hematologic evaluation. None of the 38 patients who performed RT directed to the primary lesion had severe effects due to this therapeutic modality. However, 4 men (11%) had grade 3 thrombocytopenia and 3 (8%) had grade 3 leukocytopenia [16].

3.8. Identify Candidates for Local Treatment of mPCa at Diagnosis. First of all, the primary tumor should have characteristics that allow local treatment to be performed. When opting for a surgical modality, the primary neoplastic lesion should be resected with appropriate safety margins. If the lesion is too extensive, neoadjuvant ADT followed by a local therapeutic modality chosen (radical prostatectomy or targeted radiotherapy) may be considered [7].

Independent factors that have a negative influence are age above 70 years, cT4 stage or high-grade disease, PSA $\geq$ 20 ng/ml, and pelvic lymphadenopathies. The presence of 3 or more of these factors conditions CSS and OS is the same between patients who performed local treatment and those who did not [13]. Metastasis degree, location, and number can also influence outcome. Meanwhile, patients with visceral metastases have worse results [16, 28].

4. Conclusion

In recent years, there has been growing interest with the possibility of offering treatments directed to the primary tumor in cases of metastatic prostate carcinoma at diagnosis. It is thus sought to achieve local disease control and consequent control of systemic disease by performing radical prostatectomy or targeted radiation therapy. There are several rational-based explanations and strong evidences that support this new stream of thought.

Several studies have suggested the advantages in patient overall survival and cancer-specific survival when compared to current therapeutic approaches. In virtually all studies, radical prostatectomy has a slight advantage over directed radiotherapy. However, caution should be exercised when analyzing existing data because we based our review on retrospective studies that scrutinized information from databases in which it is not always possible to obtain all relevant information about all patients. The authors themselves generally point out this gap in their studies, which does not allow conclusions to be drawn with high scientific evidence. Selection bias and previous or concomitant treatments are the general limitations of the studies databases.

At this point, one of the biggest questions is to realize which patients may actually benefit from local radical therapies. The studies analyzed in general indicate factors that condition less favorable prognoses that may in the future be the basis for the selection criteria.

On the other hand, recently published data for the treatment of mPCa (CHAARTED, STAMPEDE, and LATITUDE trials) bring some more confounding variables and systemic medication might be more beneficial than local treatments in the metastatic setting.

By now, it is impossible to say with certainty that there is an obvious advantage in performing primary treatment in metastatic prostate carcinoma. However, it is possible to affirm that the evidence begins to point in this direction and that we may be close to a paradigm shift. Prospective multicentric studies are indubitably needed in this field at the same time that new standard therapies (docetaxel or abiraterone plus hormonotherapy) will make recruitment for local treatments more difficult.

References

[1] P. Filippou, J. E. Ferguson, and M. E. Nielsen, "Epidemiology of Prostate and Testicular Cancer," *Seminars in Interventional Radiology*, vol. 33, no. 3, pp. 182–185, 2016.

[2] P. Nunes, F. L. Pimentel, F. Pina, and F. Rolo, "Registo Nacional de Cancro da Próstata, em Portugal - ReNaCaP," *Acta Urológica*, no. 3, pp. 39–45, 2010, http://www.apurologia.pt/acta/3-2010/renacap.pdf.

[3] Programa Nacional para as Doenças Oncológicas, *Doenças Oncológicas em números*, vol. 11, Ministério da Saúde - Direção-Geral Saúde, 2014.

[4] S. Antwi and T. M. Everson, "Prognostic impact of definitive local therapy of the primary tumor in men with metastatic prostate cancer at diagnosis: A population-based, propensity score analysis," *Cancer Epidemiology*, vol. 38, no. 4, pp. 435–441, 2014.

[5] C. E. Bayne, S. B. Williams, M. R. Cooperberg et al., "Treatment of the primary tumor in metastatic prostate cancer: current concepts and future perspectives," *European Urology*, vol. 69, no. 5, pp. 775–787, 2016.

[6] R. Mathieu, S. M. Korn, K. Bensalah, G. Kramer, and S. F. Shariat, "Cytoreductive radical prostatectomy in metastatic prostate cancer: Does it really make sense?" *World Journal of Urology*, pp. 1–11, 2016.

[7] E. Canby-Hagino, G. Swanson, E. Crawford, J. Basler, J. Hernandez, and I. Thompson, "Local and systemic therapy for patients with metastatic prostate cancer: should the primary tumor be treated?" *Current Prostate Reports*, vol. 3, pp. 153–159, 2005.

[8] C. Piper, D. Porres, D. Pfister, and A. Heidenreich, "The role of palliative surgery in castration-resistant prostate cancer," *Current Opinion in Supportive and Palliative Care*, vol. 8, no. 3, pp. 250–257, 2014.

[9] G. Gundem, P. Van Loo, B. Kremeyer, L. B. Alexandrov, J. M. C. Tubio, E. Papaemmanuil et al., "The evolutionary history of lethal metastatic prostate cancer," *Nature*, vol. 520, no. 7547, pp. 353–357, 2015.

[10] G. Swanson, I. Thompson, J. Basler, and E. D. Crawford, "Metastatic prostate cancer-does treatment of the primary tumor matter?" *The Journal of Urology*, vol. 176, no. 4, pp. 1292–1298, 2006.

[11] M. Y. Kim, T. Oskarsson, S. Acharyya et al., "Tumor self-seeding by circulating cancer cells," *Cell*, vol. 139, no. 7, pp. 1315–1326, 2009.

[12] S. Arcangeli, T. Zilli, B. De Bari, and F. Alongi, ""Hit the primary": A paradigm shift in the treatment of metastatic prostate cancer?" *Critical Review in Oncology/Hematology*, vol. 97, pp. 231–237, 2016.

[13] S. H. Culp, P. F. Schellhammer, and M. B. Williams, "Might men diagnosed with metastatic prostate cancer benefit from definitive treatment of the primary tumor? A SEER-based study," *European Urology*, vol. 65, no. 6, pp. 1058–1066, 2014.

[14] B. Löppenberg, D. Dalela, P. Karabon, A. Sood, J. D. Sammon, C. P. Meyer et al., "The impact of local treatment on overall survival in patients with metastatic prostate cancer on diagnosis: a national cancer data base analysis," *European Urology*, pp. 2–7, 2016.

[15] R. Satkunasivam, A. E. Kim, M. Desai, M. M. Nguyen, D. I. Quinn, L. Ballas et al., "Radical prostatectomy or external beam radiation therapy vs no local therapy for survival benefit in metastatic prostate cancer: A SEER-Medicare Analysis," *Journal of Urology*, vol. 194, no. 2, pp. 378–385, 2015.

[16] Y. Cho, J. S. Chang, K. H. Rha et al., "Does radiotherapy for the primary tumor benefit prostate cancer patients with distant metastasis at initial diagnosis?" *PLoS ONE*, vol. 11, no. 1, Article ID 0147191, 2016.

[17] C. G. Rusthoven, B. L. Jones, T. W. Flaig et al., "Improved survival with prostate radiation in addition to androgen deprivation therapy for men with newly diagnosed metastatic prostate cancer," *Journal of Clinical Oncology*, vol. 34, no. 24, pp. 2835–2842, 2016.

[18] A. Heidenreich, D. Pfister, and D. Porres, "Cytoreductive radical prostatectomy in patients with prostate cancer and low volume skeletal metastases: Results of a feasibility and case-control study," *The Journal of Urology*, vol. 193, no. 3, pp. 832–838, 2016.

[19] R. N. Kaplan, S. Rafii, and D. Lyden, "Preparing the "soil": the premetastatic niche," *Cancer Research*, vol. 66, no. 23, pp. 11089–11093, 2006.

[20] F. Reeves and A. J. Costello, "Is there a place for cytoreduction in metastatic prostate cancer?" *BJU International*, vol. 118, no. 1, pp. 14-15, 2015.

[21] D. Weckermann, B. Polzer, T. Ragg, A. Blana, G. Schlimok, H. Arnholdt et al., "Perioperative activation of disseminated tumor cells in bone marrow of patients with prostate cancer," *Journal of Clinical Oncology*, vol. 27, no. 10, pp. 1549–1556, 2009.

[22] L. Resel Folkersma, L. San José Manso, I. Galante Romo, J. Moreno Sierra, and C. Olivier Gómez, "Prognostic significance of circulating tumor cell count in patients with metastatic hormone-sensitive prostate cancer," *Urology*, vol. 80, no. 6, pp. 1328–1332, 2012.

[23] A. C. M. Won, H. Gurney, G. Marx, P. De Souza, and M. I. Patel, "Primary treatment of the prostate improves local palliation in men who ultimately develop castrate-resistant prostate cancer," *BJU International*, vol. 112, no. 4, pp. E250–E255, 2013.

[24] C. J. Logothetis and A. M. Aparicio, "Is it time to re-examine the prostate cancer treatment paradigm by targeting the interaction between the prostate and metastases?" *Journal of Clinical Oncology*, vol. 34, no. 24, pp. 2810-2811, 2016.

[25] F. Aoun, A. Peltier, and R. van Velthoven, "A comprehensive review of contemporary role of local treatment of the primary tumor and/or the metastases in metastatic prostate cancer," *BioMed Research International*, vol. 2014, Article ID 501213, pp. 1–12, 2014.

[26] C. Gratzke, J. Engel, and C. G. Stief, "Role of radical prostatectomy in metastatic prostate cancer: Data from the munich cancer registry," *European Urology*, vol. 66, no. 3, pp. 602-603, 2014.

[27] P. Sooriakumaran, J. Karnes, C. Stief et al., "A Multi-institutional analysis of perioperative outcomes in 106 men who underwent radical prostatectomy for distant metastatic prostate cancer at presentation," *European Urology*, vol. 69, no. 5, pp. 788–794, 2016.

[28] D. Moon, N. J. Sathianathen, N. Lawrentschuk, D. A. Moon, and D. G. Murphy, "Role of cytoreductive prostatectomy in non-organ confined prostate cancer," *Forum Role of Cytoreductive Prostatectomy*, p. 24, 2015.

Advances in Robotic-Assisted Radical Prostatectomy over Time

Emma F. P. Jacobs, Ronald Boris, and Timothy A. Masterson

Department of Urology, Indiana University Medical Center, 535 N. Barnhill Drive, Suite 420, Indianapolis, IN 46202, USA

Correspondence should be addressed to Emma F. P. Jacobs; jacobemi@iupui.edu

Academic Editor: J. W. Moul

Since the introduction of robot-assisted radical prostatectomy (RALP), robotics has become increasingly more commonplace in the armamentarium of the urologic surgeon. Robotic utilization has exploded across surgical disciplines well beyond the fields of urology and prostate surgery. The literature detailing technical steps, comparison of large surgical series, and even robotically focused randomized control trials are available for review. RALP, the first robot-assisted surgical procedure to achieve widespread use, has recently become the primary approach for the surgical management of localized prostate cancer. As a result, surgeons are constantly trying to refine and improve upon current technical aspects of the operation. Recent areas of published modifications include bladder neck anastomosis and reconstruction, bladder drainage, nerve sparing approaches and techniques, and perioperative and postoperative management including penile rehabilitation. In this review, we summarize recent advances in perioperative management and surgical technique for RALP.

1. Introduction

Prostate cancer is the most common visceral malignancy diagnosed in American men. The American Cancer Society estimates 241,740 new diagnoses of prostate cancer [1]. It remains the second most common cause of cancer death in American men [1]. Although controversies remain over ideal diagnostic and treatment strategies for prostate cancer, complete removal of the prostate remains the gold standard in the surgical management of localized disease.

Hugh Hampton Young first described the perineal prostatectomy over 100 years ago in 1905 [2]. Subsequently, the first retropubic radical prostatectomy (RRP) was performed by Millin in 1947 [3]. Anatomic studies in the 1970s and early 1980s led to improved appreciation of periprostatic features (dorsal venous complex, endopelvic fascia, autonomic innervation, and striated sphincter) to decrease morbidity of surgery and improve overall outcomes [4, 5]. More recently, in 1997, Schuessler et al. described the first LRP reporting the feasibility of technique despite its association with long operative times [6]. Since that time, numerous European and US centers continued to improve and refine technical aspects of the laparoscopic approach [7, 8].

Several robotic systems were introduced around the turn of the century. The da Vinci system (Intuitive Surgical Inc, CA, USA) was first introduced in 1999. Following a merger with Computer Motion Inc. (AESOP and ZEUS systems) in 2003, Intuitive Surgical has become the sole producer of robotic surgical devices [9]. After initially embarking into cardiothoracic surgery, the da Vinci robot found popularity within the urological community. From the initial descriptions of RALP in 2000 [10, 11], it has become widely adopted by urologists. By 2008, roughly 80% of RPs in the United States were performed robotically [12]. RALP has continued to evolve rapidly since that time with contributions including procedural step by steps, technical modifications, and outcomes data from various surgeons throughout the literature. In this review, we summarize the recent advances in surgical technique and perioperative management of patients undergoing RALP. An overview of significant contributions can be found in Table 1. Major areas of interest which we will address include urinary continence and the vesicourethral anastomosis, bladder and abdominal drainage, modifications to the procedure to minimize erectile dysfunction, and perioperative considerations such as positioning, incision choice, and thromboembolic prophylaxis.

Table 1: Modifications to RALP.

	Modifications	Year introduced	References
Urinary continence	Sling construction	1997	Jorion [18]
	Bladder neck preservation	2002	Deliveliotis et al. [16], Selli et al. [15], and von Bodman et al. [85]
	Intraoperative cooling	2009	Finley et al. [29]
	Pubovesical complex sparing	2011	Asimakopoulos et al. [28]
UVA	Posterior reconstruction	2008	Rocco et al. [19, 86], Coelho et al. [87]
	Anterior reconstruction	2009	Campenni et al. [20], Patel et al. [21]
	Double layer anastomosis	2009	Menon et al. [22], Sammon et al. [23], and Joshi et al. [25], Sutherland et al. [24], Sammon et al. [23], and Hurtes et al. [88]
	Barbed suture	2011	Sammon et al. [26], and Kaushik et al. [27]
NVB sparing	NVB sparing	1991	Quinlan et al. [36], Catalona et al. [39], Dubbelman et al. [38], Rabbani et al. [37], and Walsh et al. [40]
	Veil of Aphrodite	2002	Menon et al. [41, 45]
	Athermal dissection	2007	Tewari et al. [52], Mandhani et al. [56], and Khan et al. [57], Ahlering et al. [58], Chien et al. [59], and Gill et al. [60]
	Tension-free	2007	Kowalczyk et al. [53], Mattei et al. [55]
Bladder drainage	SP drainage	2009	Krane et al. [31], Sammon et al. [32], and Tewari et al. [33]

2. Methods

A comprehensive review of the published literature was performed using the PubMed search engine. Search terms included robotic prostatectomy, laparoscopic prostatectomy, robotic complications, and robotic technique. English-language search results were reviewed for relevance and then used appropriately. We focused on articles that have been published in the last 5 years, with some review of older sources for a historic perspective.

2.1. Urinary Continence and the Urethrovesical Anastomosis. Urinary continence remains a significant source of morbidity and concern for patients with prostate cancer. Major advances are detailed in Tables 2 and 3. Quality of life questionnaires have demonstrated that urinary control postoperatively may have the greatest impact on a patient's perception of his recovery [13, 14]. As a result, a number of surgical modifications in technique have been used in an attempt to improve early return and overall continence following surgery. Despite numerous published outcomes supporting outstanding recovery of continence following surgery, lack of standardization has led to some controversy. Definitions of continence have ranged from 0 to 1 pad use, 0 pads including a "security pad", 0 pads, and "leak free, pad free" (LFPF). Additionally, patient-recorded outcomes via questionnaire may significantly differ from surgeon perception. Standardization of RALP outcome definitions (such as continence) is imperative before adequate comparisons of these variables can be made.

A variety of surgical techniques have been employed in an attempt to improve early return of continence after RP (both open and minimally invasive), including bladder neck (BN) preservation [15, 16], intussusception of the BN [17], puboprostatic ligament sparing, sling construction [18], incorporation of the striate urethral sphincter to the anastomosis, and tubularization of the bladder neck. Historically, the actual benefits of these modifications have been somewhat controversial. Many of the surgical reconstruction techniques for RALP have been based on the posterior reconstruction described by Rocco and colleagues in 2001 [19]. In posterior reconstruction, the posterior rhabdosphincter is joined to the posterior Denonvilliers' fascia and fixed to the bladder wall 1-2 cm cranial to the new bladder neck to avoid caudal retraction of the urethrosphincteric complex, prior to completing the standard vesicourethral anastomosis. Additional modifications have been described as posterior (PR), anterior (AR), or complete reconstruction and have been employed with subtle variances by numerous open and minimally invasive prostate surgeons.

The anterior fixation stitch or urethropexy can be performed either prior to or after the anastomosis. As documented by Campenni et al., some patients who have had an anterior urethropexy stitch placed appear to increase continence as measured by leak-point pressures [20]. This maneuver has been described to increase overall continence and decrease time to return of continence [21]. Although many published reconstruction modifications have suggested improved time to continence for RALP, the vast majority have been observational studies with low levels of evidence. By contrast, Menon et al. used a randomized controlled trial to demonstrate no improvement in continence combining an AR and PR (double layered anastomosis) with his standard anastomosis [22]. There were 57 patients randomized to the single and 59 to the double layer anastomotic groups. The study was powered to detect a 30% difference in urinary continence measured in pad weight at various time intervals following surgery. No significant difference between groups was noted. A followup study was performed at two years confirming the author's earlier findings showing excellent urinary control for patients with or without the additional reconstruction [23]. Patients without the double layered technique did demonstrate a higher anastomotic leak rate, but this was not clinically significant. Similar negative results were reproduced in smaller series by Sutherland et al. and

TABLE 2: Urinary continence.

Modification	Primary author	Results
Sling construction	Jorion [18]	Fascial sling suspension after anastomosis in RRP resulted in earlier and more complete continence.
Bladder neck preservation	Deliveliotis [16]	Return of continence was earlier after RRP in bladder neck preservation group compared to puboprostatic ligament sparing or both techniques used together. Final continence rates were unchanged.
	Selli [15]	Bladder neck preservation in RRP leads to faster return of continence but does not affect long-term recovery.
	von Bodman [85]	Anatomic variables membranous urethral length, urethral volume, and an anatomically close relation between the levator muscle and membranous urethra on preoperative magnetic resonance imaging are independent predictors of continence recovery after radical prostatectomy.
Intraoperative cooling	Finley [29]	Regional pelvic cooling during RRP was associated with early return of continence. Longer and deeper cooling improved continence.
Pubovesical complex-sparing	Asimakopoulos [28]	128 patients were randomized to LRP or RALP. Erectile function at 12 months was better in the RALP group. Oncologic outcomes and continence were similar between the two groups.

TABLE 3: Urethrovesical anastomosis.

Modification	Primary author	Results
Posterior reconstruction	Rocco [19, 86]	Posterior reconstruction in RRP was associated with improved time to return to continence.
	Coelho [87]	Posterior reconstruction in RALP had faster return of continence and fewer anastomotic leaks.
Anterior reconstruction	Campenni [20]	Anterior anastomotic urethral suspension sutures increase Valsalva LLP and may speed the return of continence.
	Patel [21]	Suspension stitch in RALP leads to improved continence at 3 months.
Double layer anastomosis	Menon [22]	No improvement in continence was seen with reconstruction.
	Sammon [23]	Single or double layer anastomosis did not correlate to urinary outcomes at 2 years.
	Joshi [25]	Posterior reconstruction did not improve continence after RALP.
	Sutherland [24]	Posterior reconstruction did not increase early return of continence after RALP.
	Hurtes [88]	Early return of continence after RALP was improved with anterior suspension combined with posterior reconstruction.
Barbed suture	Sammon [26]	RALP using v-lock suture showed a decrease in anastomotic time without change in outcomes.

Joshi et al. evaluating 94 and 107 patients, respectively [24, 25].

Barbed suture has been theorized to simplify and decrease time for the BN anastomosis. A randomized clinical trial was recently conducted at the Vattikuti Institute in Detroit with 64 patients [26]. Posterior reconstruction was done using a single barbed, 3–0 polyglyconate suture. The urethrovesical anastomosis (UVA) and PR were completed separately using double loaded barbed suture. Knots were not required due to the gripping properties of the suture. The control arm used similar technique with the exception of tying the suture and using an assistant to provide tension on the running anastomosis. The anastomosis was completed more efficiently in the barbed suture arm (4.7 minutes time difference overall). They found no difference in leaks, bladder neck contractures, patient symptoms, or other outcome measures. Kaushik et al. examined the effect of robotic manipulation on unidirectional barbed suture and did find minor structural damage to the barbs and suture on electron microscopy. This was not felt to be clinically significant [27].

Additional published modifications to RALP technique for the improvement of continence include a "pubovesical complex sparing technique" and the use of intraoperative hypothermia. In a small sample of patients, Asimakopoulos et al. described their anatomic dissection plane ventrally between the detrusor apron and the prostate to spare the plexus of Santorini, essentially leaving the dorsal vein complex intact [28]. Using an intraoperative cooling balloon in 109 patients, hypothermia was introduced by Finley et al. to potentially better recover both continence and potency after surgery in a prospective study with a historic control group [29]. The median temperature achieved was 25.5°C. Long-term followup showed that the time to 0 pad status at 3 and 12 months was 81% to 89% and 100% for the initial and extended cooling groups compared with 69% and 89% in the control group, respectively. Return to continence was also faster in the cooling group (39 versus 62 days to zero pads). Although there was some debate as to the ideal temperature goal, duration of cooling, and reproducibility of technique, patients tolerated hypothermia without side effects and early results were encouraging. It is unclear if the authors are continuing to use hypothermia routinely with RALP to date.

Traditionally with RRP, the bladder has been drained via urethral catheter for a finite period of time to maintain urethral patency. Historically, after RRP, catheters were left in place for 2-3 weeks [4]. Despite this precaution, BN contractures were reported in 5–32% of patients [30]. With the running anastomosis and the improved visualization of mucosa to mucosa suturing, postoperative bladder neck contractures have been significantly reduced with RALP to 0–3% [30]. The desire by both patient and surgeon for early catheter removal, or perhaps to obviate the need for urethral stenting altogether, has led to novel methods of bladder drainage. The group at the Vattikuti Urology Institute in Detroit determined that the indwelling urethral catheter was the least tolerated aspect for patients after RALP [31]. This led to the introduction of a 14F suprapubic tube (SP) placed under direct vision following the anastomosis. Patients began cycling their bladder by day 5. The SP was removed when PVRs were less than 30 mL, typically on day 7. Cystography was not used routinely [32]. Continence and stricture rates were similar between this group and historical controls [31]. Another study looked at a custom SP with a small bladder neck anastomotic splint which could be retracted. This pilot study found earlier return of continence and decreased patient discomfort [33]. Longer followup with larger cohorts will be needed to evaluate the possible downstream effects of the total removal of urethral catheterization (continence rates, leak rates, and bladder neck contracture rates) following RALP, but early results are intriguing.

In summary, the overwhelming majority of patients will eventually recover continence after RALP. Despite this notion, time to continence and achievement of a true "pad free, leak free" state may be impacted by numerous factors and frequently subject to poor reporting, patient and physician biases, and limited utilization of accepted quality of life questionnaires. As the vast majority of patients undergoing RP will ultimately succumb to diseases other than prostate cancer, recovery of functional outcomes after surgery may have more impact on the "perceived success" of surgery compared to surgery for any other surgical malignancy. Hence, we continue to strive to find new ways to deliver continence quicker and better despite an acceptable status quo demonstrated in most post-RP health related quality of life studies [34]. Whether or not these described technical modifications to RALP truly improve recovery of continence, they appear safe, are relatively easy to perform, and carry little risk.

2.2. Erectile Dysfunction. Several surgical modifications in the technical approach to RALP have resulted in vast improvements in understanding the neuropathic basis behind the development of erectile dysfunction. Prominent studies are detailed in Table 4. Historical rates of erectile dysfunction after RRP were near universal until the neuroanatomy of the pelvic plexus responsible for physiological erections was described by Walsh and Donker [35]. In the subsequent era of the anatomic RRP, erectile dysfunction rates improved dramatically. Clinical features that predict better outcomes for sexual function recovery include patient age, quality of erections prior to surgery, clinical stage, and the quality and extent of neurovascular bundle preservation [36–38]. While reported rates vary, centers of excellence achieve 12-month potency rates with or without the use of phosphodiesterase-5 inhibitors ranging from 68% up to 91% with bilateral nerve sparing using RRP techniques [36, 37, 39, 40]. While disparate data exists with outcomes for sexual function after RALP, high volume centers have published comparable outcomes ranging from 70% to 80% at one year [41–43].

Several centers, including the group at Henry Ford Hospital in Detroit, Michigan, have offered their experience in surgical technique leading to the evolution of RALP. The VIP approach to RALP was first described in 2002 [44], followed by several refinements leading to the current description [41]. Among these refinements are the development and preservation of the lateral prostatic fascia (i.e., veil of Aphrodite). This involves releasing the lattice or curtain of cavernosal nerve tissue extending along the posterolateral aspects of the prostate bilaterally, up to the fibrous stroma of the dorsal vein complex anteriorly overlying the apex of the prostate [41]. In a more recent modification, a "superveil" technique was developed for select patients with favorable anatomy allowing for further extension anteriorly of the dissection to preserve the pubovesical ligaments and dorsal vein complex [45]. In both circumstances, erectile function recovery rates in the most favorable patient groups were 93% and 94%, respectively.

The rationale for these modifications was based upon cadaveric dissections suggesting that smaller nerves of the pelvic neurovascular plexus exist along the prostatic and Denonvilliers' fascia [46]. Further cadaveric studies have supported the concept of a neural "hammock" extending from the posterior surface of the seminal vesicles down along the posterolateral aspects of the mid-prostate, and diverging anterolaterally near the membranous urethra [47–49]. Based upon these studies, a "trizonal" neural hammock concept including the proximal neurovascular plate posterior to the seminal vesicles, the predominant neurovascular bundle along the posterolateral aspect of the prostate, and the accessory neural pathway was characterized [50]. Using similar concepts, Srivastava and colleagues recently published a review of their current technique for neurovascular bundle (NVB) preservation [51]. Building upon basic tenants of the RRP, their approach includes avoiding unnecessary traction and thermal injury to the neurovascular bundle throughout the trizonal region. Through a medial to lateral approach beginning with the seminal vesicles and extending along the posterolateral aspect of the prostate, the authors used sharp, athermal dissection and small pedicle clipping to facilitate intrafascial dissection. Once released posterolaterally, further dissection allows easy mobilization of the anterolateral lattice of accessory nerves from the base towards the membranous urethra. In their retrospective analysis of 2317 consecutive patients undergoing RALP, 91% of men with the most favorable characteristics undergoing these technical modifications reported the ability to engage in sexual intercourse [52]. For

Table 4: Neurovascular bundle sparing.

Veil of Aphrodite	Menon et al. [41]	VIP with veil nerve sparing has comparable outcomes to traditional RALP.
	Menon et al. [45]	VIP had improved erectile function compared to RALP.
Athermal dissection	Tewari et al. [52]	Neural hammock sparing improves return to baseline erectile function without affecting other outcomes.
	Khan et al. [57]	Heat sink demonstrated in this porcine model suggests that the vascular pedicle should be protective of the NVB.
	Ahlering et al. [58]	Avoiding thermal injury leads to earlier return of sexual function.
	Chien et al. [59]	Antegrade athermal dissection may lead to earlier return of erectile function.
Tension-free	Kowalczyk et al. [53]	Avoidance of countertraction on the NVB leads to earlier return of erectile function.
	Mattei et al. [55]	This lateral approach to the NVB is tension-free and athermal.

men aged 60 years or less, rates of erectile function recovery beyond 12 months were 95% with grade 1 NVB preservation. These rates incrementally deteriorated with progressively wider planes of dissection resulting in greater degrees of NVB resection (i.e., grades 2–4).

The impact of countertraction on NVB injury and secondary neuropraxia has been further emphasized in a recent report by Kowalczyk and colleagues [53]. In their single surgeon experience among 610 patients undergoing RALP, 342 of the procedures were performed while avoiding assistant and/or surgeon countertraction of the NVB during nerve sparing RP. This was accomplished by placing traction on the prostate itself and dissecting it away from the NVB. These patients experienced earlier time sexual function recovery (45% versus 28% at 5 months), but overall potency rates at one year were similar between groups. This is in line with similar results reported with RRP in techniques developed to avoid traction on the NVB [54]. The investigators from Bordeaux, France, reported on their lateral technique to NVB preservation [55]. In their approach, the NVB is released prior to division of the bladder neck fibers and seminal vesicle dissection to facilitate a tension-free release to the NVB preservation. While no comparison cohort is offered, they report a high rate of spontaneous erections (not necessarily sufficient for intercourse) in 46% of patients within one week after catheter removal. Additionally, 65% of patients were considered potent at the 4-month followup visit. No results at the 12-month time period were reported for comparison.

Regarding the effect of thermal energy on the recovery of potency after RALP, limited clinical data exists to draw significant conclusions. While monopolar cautery is generally accepted to be associated with significant thermal injury to nervous tissue when applied, equipoise remains as to the impact of bipolar cautery during NVB preservation. In a study utilizing thermal probes intraoperatively during RALP, Mandhani et al. demonstrate a substantial increase in regional temperature of the NVB when bipolar cautery was used compared to monopolar current [56]. While differences in its impact on sexual function have not been reported, the author raises the question as to whether bipolar current is truly safer. Questions as to the importance of thermal injury were also raised by Khan et al. Using fiber optic thermometry, they found that when bipolar and monopolar currents were applied to the anterior abdominal wall, the inferior epigastrics were able to act as a heat sink. This was extrapolated to suggest that the prostatic pedicle should be protective of the neurovascular bundle during bladder neck dissection [57]. Nevertheless, it is easy to suspect that thermal injury may contribute to loss of potency at some level. Subsequently, several investigators have attempted to determine the feasibility of performing completely athermal RALP. Ahlering et al. reported that utilizing bulldog clamps on the hypogastric vessels to potentially eliminate the need for cautery during prostate dissection was feasible and resulted in a nearly 5-fold rate of improvement in sexual function recovery [58]. Similarly, Chien et al. from Chicago reported similar findings during a completely athermal RALP, stating that their results led to a quicker return and preservation of potency [59]. Most recently, Gill et al. demonstrated using real-time Doppler transrectal ultrasound that bulldog clamping of the lateral vascular pedicle preserved NVB blood flow while minimizing cautery need [60].

Overall, general principles of NVB preservation remain steadfast. Prospective anatomic identification of location and routes of primary and accessory neurovascular bundles combined with the minimization of countertraction, tension, and thermal injury to these bundles will optimize the technical success of the operation in preserving and recovering sexual function in well-selected patients.

3. Perioperative Considerations

As with all major operations, surgeons constantly strive to minimize perioperative complications and their associated morbidity from the time the patient enters the operating room until their recovery is complete. In some circumstances, prevention of complications can begin prior to surgery. Because RALP is an overall well-tolerated procedure for a relatively healthy patient population for a malignancy associated with high survival rates, perioperative morbidity is highly scrutinized. Potentially devastating consequences may occur from subtle nuances associated with the use (or absence) of venous thromboembolism prophylaxis, patient padding and positioning, operative times, and trocar placement and/or incision choice.

The incidence of venous thromboembolism (VTE) associated with robotic or laparoscopic prostatectomy is roughly 0.5% [61]. Additionally, the actual incidence is likely much higher as VTE is typically only reported when it is symptomatic. The Best Practice Statement on deep venous thrombosis recommends intermittent pneumatic compression (IPC) for laparoscopic and robotic procedures, with the possible addition of chemoprophylaxis in high risk groups [62]. A large multi-institutional retrospective review concluded that VTE prophylaxis is not indicated in RALP (without additional risk factors) [61]. Preoperative prophylaxis may lead to significantly increased blood loss [61]; however, the increased morbidity and mortality associated with VTE certainly makes it an issue of concern. The mortality of RRP overall is 0.1%, which is increased to 6% in patients with VTE. Risk factors include malignancy, immobility in the perioperative period, and medical comorbidities. A recent study by Schmitges et al. found that the surgeon's overall annual caseload also had an effect on the rate of DVT and PE [63]. They found a rate of 0.1% with surgeons doing more than 24 RALPs yearly, 0.3% with 10–24 cases, and 0.3% with less than 10 cases. These authors also did not find a difference in the incidence of VTE between open and minimally invasive techniques. As more patients undergo extended lymph node dissection during RALP, it remains unclear what if any impact this will have on the future rates of VTE in this patient population. Without question, future investigation will be needed to better define which patients are best candidates for VTE prophylaxis and at what doses and durations should patients be treated.

During standard RALP, the patient is typically secured with his legs apart in the split-leg position or in dorsal lithotomy, followed by transitioning into a steep Trendelenburg position (25–35 degrees). This allows for positioning of the robot system, as well as providing access for the assistant to manipulate the catheter during the anastomosis [64]. Proper padding, positioning, and assuring that the robot remains a safe distance from the patient are key components to avoid compartment syndromes and other compressive injuries, which can ultimately lead to myonecrosis and renal insult. The hallmark of compartment syndromes on physical exam is pain on passive stretch. The rate of lower extremity neuropathies in split-leg position is roughly 1.3%, with increased intraoperative time being the only factor studied which increased risk [65]. This position increases the risk of injury to the femoral nerve [65]. At 3 hours, significant ischemia-reperfusion injury occurs [66]. Modified lithotomy, heel support, and avoidance of the Trendelenburg position and ankle dorsiflexion, as well as the use of intermittent compression devices (many of these features not feasible with RALP), have all been found to reduce the risk of intraoperative compartment syndromes [67]. Although rare, case reports of gluteal compartment syndromes have been associated with dorsal lithotomy positioning and may occur bilaterally with untoward results [68]. Statistics on the incidence of myonecrosis after RALP are not available in the literature, although it can be presumed to be a rare and largely preventable complication.

The need for placement of an abdominal drain for the potential collection of urinary extravasation prior to closure has become somewhat controversial in RALP. Despite being relatively well tolerated, most drains play little role in the postoperative course of men undergoing RALP. Drains are commonly removed within 24 hours prior to discharge whenever placed and are many times already out in the unusual circumstance when a patient re-presents with symptoms of urinary ascites. Sharma et al.'s 2007 review of 225 open and 100 robotic cases did not find that drainage improved recovery or complication rates in either group [69]. Selective drain placement when the integrity of the anastomosis is in doubt was supported by another review from Lahey Clinic [70]. The overall trend supports moving away from routine abdominal drainage.

The rate of incisional hernias after RALP is poorly defined, largely because it is not followed as a long-term endpoint. Most hernias develop at the periumbilical incision, although more rarely the smaller port sites have developed hernias as well [71]. Port site hernias may have significant morbidity as the smaller size of the defect can lead to entrapment and strangulation of bowel and omentum. The risk of a trocar site hernia is 0.8–1.2% [72]. The rate of hernia occurrence is higher with 12 mm trocars (as opposed to 10 mm or 5 mm) [73] and with cutting trocars (as opposed to blunt or radially expanding) [74]. However, overall hernia incidence has been estimated at 3.3–16.7%, with great variation found between different methods of followup [75]. Factors that can contribute to hernia development include patient comorbidities, technical issues with wound closure, and the choice of incision. Previous review in the surgical literature [76] has suggested that a transverse incision has a statistically significant advantage in terms of hernia occurrence. Beck et al. [75] found that a transverse incision in RALP can reduce the rate of hernias. Fuller et al. determined that closure of the midline incision with nonabsorbable suture using interrupted stitches can decrease hernia occurrence [71]. Early recognition is a key in preventing severe complications secondary to postoperative hernias. Instrument and suture selection, as well as careful wound closure, can avoid these complications.

Inguinal hernias have been reported as a complication of RRP, originally reported as appearing in 12% of postprostatectomy patients as opposed to 5% in the male population [77]. Rabbani et al. concluded that risk factors included advanced age, low BMI, prior inguinal hernia repair, and bladder neck contracture [78]. This has been theorized to be due to the lower midline incision and subsequent weakening of the abdominal wall [79]. Nerve sparing prostatectomies (open, laparoscopic, and robotic) have also been associated with higher rates of inguinal hernias requiring operative repair [80].

Perioperative complications can often be reduced by awareness and attention to details. Careful positioning, reduced operative time, selection of operative equipment and suture, and prophylaxis in some circumstances can avoid preventable complications.

4. Robotic Technologic Advances

Continued advances in both modern medicine and technology constantly drive change of current technique. As we continue to emphasize a shift toward "minimally invasive surgery," industry has developed new concepts employing fewer ports and tinier incisions while trying to maintain similar outcomes. Laparoendoscopic single site surgery (LESS) has yet to become widespread in urology but is gaining ground in the robotics arena. Currently, single-site robotic instruments and techniques have been better described for upper tract and pediatric indications [81] than pelvic and/urologic surgery. White et al. concluded after a retrospective review of 50 robotic LESS procedures that a redesigned or task specific robotic platform would be required before this technique could be adopted for widespread use [82]. LESS RALP was described in 2010 using multiple ports in a single umbilical incision. Of 20 patients undergoing this procedure, 2 required additional ports and 1 was converted to a traditional RALP [83]. Challenges with LESS surgery include adjusting to the necessary curved instruments and the limited range of motion. Florescent-sensitive cameras are a recent innovation which may provide functional intraoperative imaging. Protoporphyrin IX (PpIX) precursors delta-aminolevulinic acid (δALA) and hexyl aminolevulinate (HAL), fluorescein, and indocyanine green (ICG) have been approved by the FDA for clinical use. ALA has been used experimentally to visualize prostate tissue [84]. Newer daVinci equipment is florescence capable. The clinical applications of this have not been fully established.

5. Conclusions

Over the past ten years, both domestically and worldwide, there has been explosive growth in the use of robotic-assisted laparoscopic prostatectomy as an alternative to open radical retropubic prostatectomy. Some advantages of the minimally invasive approach have been well established, while others, particularly those associated with functional outcomes, remain controversial. Multiple factors, including the drive to improve oncologic outcome, patient comfort, and quality of life, have driven refinement in technique as well as perceived "success" of the operation. Our review outlines the evolution of robotic prostatectomy through both improvements in functional outcomes as well as the minimization of patient discomfort and overall morbidity. Whether or not these described technical modifications to RALP truly improve upon these elements remains unknown. Surgeons should be encouraged to evaluate their own results and introduce any one or more of these changes if their results are below standard of care.

Abbreviations

AR: Anterior reconstruction
CR: Complete reconstruction
BN: Bladder neck
ED: Erectile dysfunction
LESS: Laparoendoscopic single site surgery
LFLP: Leak free, pad free
NVB: Neurovascular bundle
MUL: Membranous urethral length
PR: Posterior reconstruction
RALP: Robot-assisted laparoscopic (radical) prostatectomy
LRP: Laparoscopic radical prostatectomy
RP: Radical prostatectomy
RRP: Radical retropubic prostatectomy
SHIM: Sexual Health Inventory for Men
SP: Suprapubic
VIP: Vattikuti Institute Prostatectomy
VTE: Venous thromboembolism
UVA: Urethrovesical anastomosis.

References

[1] American Cancer Society, *Facts and Figures*, American Cancer Society, Atlanta, Ga, USA, 2012.

[2] H. Young, "The early diagnosis and radical cure of carcinoma of the prostate: being a study of 40 cases and presentations of a radical operation which was carried out in 4 cases," *Bulletin of the Johns Hopkins Hospital*, vol. 16, p. 315, 1905.

[3] T. Millin, *Retropubic Urinary Surgery*, Livingstone, London, UK, 1947.

[4] P. Walsh, "Anatomic radical prostatectomy: evolution of the surgical technique," *Journal of Urology*, vol. 160, no. 6, pp. 2418–2424, 1998.

[5] F. J. Bianco Jr., P. T. Scardino, and J. A. Eastham, "Radical prostatectomy: long-term cancer control and recovery of sexual and urinary function ('trifecta')," *Urology*, vol. 66, supplement 5, pp. 83–94, 2005.

[6] W. W. Schuessler, P. G. Schulam, R. V. Clayman, and L. R. Kavoussi, "Laparoscopic radical prostatectomy: initial short-term experience," *Urology*, vol. 50, no. 6, pp. 854–857, 1997.

[7] B. Guillonneau, X. Cathelineau, E. Barret, F. Rozet, and G. Vallancien, "Laparoscopic radical prostatectomy: technical and early oncological assessment of 40 operations," *European Urology*, vol. 36, no. 1, pp. 14–20, 1999.

[8] K. Touijer, K. Kuroiwa, J. W. Saranchuk et al., "Quality improvement in laparoscopic radical prostatectomy for pT2 prostate cancer: impact of video documentation review on positive surgical margin," *Journal of Urology*, vol. 173, no. 3, pp. 765–768, 2005.

[9] D. R. Yates, C. Vaessen, and M. Roupret, "From Leonardo to da Vinci: the history of robot-assisted surgery in urology," *BJU International*, vol. 108, no. 11, pp. 1708–1714, 2011.

[10] C. C. Abbou, A. Hoznek, L. Salomon et al., "Laparoscopic radical prostatectomy with a remote controlled robot," *Journal of Urology*, vol. 165, no. 6, part 1, pp. 1964–1966, 2001.

[11] J. Binder and W. Kramer, "Robotically-assisted laparoscopic radical prostatectomy," *BJU International*, vol. 87, no. 4, pp. 408–410, 2001.

[12] M. P. Freire, W. W. Choi, Y. Lei, F. Carvas, and J. C. Hu, "Overcoming the learning curve for robotic-assisted laparoscopic radical prostatectomy," *Urologic Clinics of North America*, vol. 37, no. 1, pp. 37–47, 2010.

[13] G. Katz and R. Rodriguez, "Changes in continence and health-related quality of life after curative treatment and watchful waiting of prostate cancer," *Urology*, vol. 69, no. 6, pp. 1157–1160, 2007.

[14] M. Jønler, O. S. Nielsen, and H. Wolf, "Urinary symptoms, potency, and quality of life in patients with localized prostate cancer followed up with deferred treatment," *Urology*, vol. 52, no. 6, pp. 1055–1063, 1998.

[15] C. Selli, P. De Antoni, U. Moro, A. Macchiarella, G. Giannarini, and A. Crisci, "Role of bladder neck preservation in urinary

continence following radical retropubic prostatectomy," *Scandinavian Journal of Urology and Nephrology*, vol. 38, no. 1, pp. 32–37, 2004.

[16] C. Deliveliotis, V. Protogerou, E. Alargof, and J. Varkarakis, "Radical prostatectomy: bladder neck preservation and puboprostatic ligament sparing—effects on continence and positive margins," *Urology*, vol. 60, no. 5, pp. 855–858, 2002.

[17] P. C. Walsh and P. Marschke, "Intussusception of the reconstructed bladder neck leads to earlier continence after radical prostatectomy," *Urology*, vol. 59, no. 6, pp. 934–938, 2002.

[18] J. L. Jorion, "Rectus fascial sling suspension of the vesicourethral anastomosis after radical prostatectomy," *Journal of Urology*, vol. 157, no. 3, pp. 926–928, 1997.

[19] F. Rocco, F. Gadda, P. Acquati et al., "Personal research: reconstruction of the urethral striated sphincter," *Archivio Italiano di Urologia, Andrologia*, vol. 73, no. 3, pp. 127–137, 2001.

[20] M. A. Campenni, J. D. Harmon, P. C. Ginsberg, and R. C. Harkaway, "Improved continence after radical retropubic prostatectomy using two pubo-urethral suspension stitches," *Urologia Internationalis*, vol. 68, no. 2, pp. 109–112, 2002.

[21] V. R. Patel, R. F. Coelho, K. J. Palmer, and B. Rocco, "Periurethral suspension stitch during robot-assisted laparoscopic radical prostatectomy: description of the technique and continence outcomes," *European Urology*, vol. 56, no. 3, pp. 472–478, 2009.

[22] M. Menon, F. Muhletaler, M. Campos, and J. O. Peabody, "Assessment of early continence after reconstruction of the periprostatic tissues in patients undergoing computer assisted (Robotic) prostatectomy: results of a 2 group parallel randomized controlled trial," *Journal of Urology*, vol. 180, no. 3, pp. 1018–1023, 2008.

[23] J. D. Sammon, F. Muhletaler, J. O. Peabody, M. Diaz-Insua, R. Satyanaryana, and M. Menon, "Long-term functional urinary outcomes comparing single- vs double-layer urethrovesical anastomosis: two-year follow-up of a two-group parallel randomized controlled trial," *Urology*, vol. 76, no. 5, pp. 1102–1107, 2010.

[24] D. E. Sutherland, B. Linder, A. M. Guzman et al., "Posterior rhabdosphincter reconstruction during robotic assisted radical prostatectomy: results from a phase II randomized clinical trial," *Journal of Urology*, vol. 185, no. 4, pp. 1262–1267, 2011.

[25] N. Joshi, W. de Blok, E. van Muilekom, and H. van der Poel, "Impact of posterior musculofascial reconstruction on early continence after robot-assisted laparoscopic radical prostatectomy: results of a prospective parallel group trial," *European Urology*, vol. 58, no. 1, pp. 84–89, 2010.

[26] J. Sammon, T. Kim, Q. Trinh et al., "Anastomosis during robot-assisted radical prostatectomy: randomized controlled trial comparing barbed and standard monofilament suture," *Urology*, vol. 78, no. 3, pp. 572–579, 2011.

[27] D. Kaushik, K. Clay, S. G. Hossain, E. Park, C. A. Nelson, and C. A. Lagrange, "Effect of robotic manipulation on unidirectional barbed suture integrity: evaluation of tensile strength and sliding force," *Journal of Endourology*, vol. 26, no. 6, pp. 711–715, 2012.

[28] A. D. Asimakopoulos, C. Pereira Fraga, F. Annino, P. Pasqualetti, A. A. Calado, and C. Mugnier, "Randomized comparison between laparoscopic and robot-assisted nerve-sparing radical prostatectomy," *Journal of Sexual Medicine*, vol. 8, no. 5, pp. 1503–1512, 2011.

[29] D. S. Finley, K. Osann, A. Chang, R. Santos, D. Skarecky, and T. E. Ahlering, "Hypothermic robotic radical prostatectomy: impact on continence," *Journal of Endourology*, vol. 23, no. 9, pp. 1443–1450, 2009.

[30] L. P. Msezane, W. Reynolds, O. N. Gofrit, A. L. Shalhav, G. P. Zagaja, and K. C. Zorn, "Bladder neck contracture after robot-assisted laparoscopic radical prostatectomy: evaluation of the incidence, risk factors, and impact on urinary function," *Journal of Endourology*, vol. 22, no. 2, pp. 377–383, 2008.

[31] L. S. Krane, M. Bhandari, J. O. Peabody, and M. Menon, "Impact of percutaneous suprapubic tube drainage on patient discomfort after radical prostatectomy," *European Urology*, vol. 56, no. 2, pp. 325–331, 2009.

[32] J. D. Sammon, Q. Trinh, S. Sukumar et al., "Long-term follow-up of patients undergoing percutaneous suprapubic tube drainage after robot-assisted radical prostatectomy (RARP)," *BJU International*, vol. 110, no. 4, pp. 580–585, 2012.

[33] A. Tewari, S. Rao, and A. Mandhani, "Catheter-less robotic radical prostatectomy using a custom-made synchronous anastomotic splint and vesical urinary diversion device: report of the initial series and perioperative outcomes," *BJU International*, vol. 102, no. 8, pp. 1000–1004, 2008.

[34] P. Walsh, "Radical prostatectomy for localized prostate cancer provides durable cancer control with excellent quality of life: a structured debate," *Journal of Urology*, vol. 163, no. 6, pp. 1802–1807, 2000.

[35] P. Walsh and P. Donker, "Impotence following radical prostatectomy: insight into etiology and prevention. 1982," *Journal of Urology*, vol. 167, no. 2, pp. 1005–1010, 2002.

[36] D. M. Quinlan, J. Epstein, B. S. Carter, and P. C. Walsh, "Sexual function following radical prostatectomy: influence of preservation of neurovascular bundles," *Journal of Urology*, vol. 145, no. 5, pp. 998–1002, 1991.

[37] F. Rabbani, A. Stapleton, M. W. Kattan, T. M. Wheeler, and P. T. Scardino, "Factors predicting recovery of erections after radical prostatectomy," *Journal of Urology*, vol. 164, no. 6, pp. 1929–1934, 2000.

[38] Y. D. Dubbelman, G. R. Dohle, and F. H. Schröder, "Sexual function before and after radical retropubic prostatectomy: a systematic review of prognostic indicators for a successful outcome," *European Urology*, vol. 50, no. 4, pp. 711–720, 2006.

[39] W. J. Catalona, G. Carvalhal, D. E. Mager, and D. S. Smith, "Potency, continence and complication rates in 1,870 consecutive radical retropubic prostatectomies," *Journal of Urology*, vol. 162, no. 2, pp. 433–438, 1999.

[40] P. C. Walsh, P. Marschke, D. Ricker, and A. L. Burnett, "Use of intraoperative video documentation to improve sexual function after radical retropubic prostatectomy," *Urology*, vol. 55, no. 1, pp. 62–67, 2000.

[41] M. Menon, A. Shrivastava, S. Kaul et al., "Vattikuti institute prostatectomy: contemporary technique and analysis of results," *European Urology*, vol. 51, no. 3, pp. 648–658, 2007.

[42] V. R. Patel, R. Thaly, and K. Shah, "Robotic radical prostatectomy: outcomes of 500 cases," *BJU International*, vol. 99, no. 5, pp. 1109–1112, 2007.

[43] K. C. Zorn, O. Gofrit, M. A. Orvieto, A. A. Mikhail, G. P. Zagaja, and A. L. Shalhav, "Robotic-assisted laparoscopic prostatectomy: functional and pathologic outcomes with interfascial nerve preservation," *European Urology*, vol. 51, no. 3, pp. 755–763, 2007.

[44] M. Menon, A. Tewari, J. Peabody et al., "Vattikuti Institute prostatectomy: technique," *Journal of Urology*, vol. 169, no. 6, pp. 2289–2292, 2003.

[45] M. Menon, A. Shrivastava, M. Bhandari, R. Satyanarayana, S. Siva, and P. K. Agarwal, "Vattikuti institute prostatectomy: technical modifications in 2009," *European Urology*, vol. 56, no. 1, pp. 89–96, 2009.

[46] A. Tewari, J. O. Peabody, M. Fischer et al., "An operative and anatomic study to help in nerve sparing during laparoscopic and robotic radical prostatectomy," *European Urology*, vol. 43, no. 5, pp. 444–454, 2003.

[47] A. J. Costello, M. Brooks, and O. J. Cole, "Anatomical studies of the neurovascular bundle and cavernosal nerves," *BJU International*, vol. 94, no. 7, pp. 1071–1076, 2004.

[48] K. Kiyoshima, A. Yokomizo, T. Yoshida et al., "Anatomical features of periprostatic tissue and its surroundings: a histological analysis of 79 radical retropubic prostatectomy specimens," *Japanese Journal of Clinical Oncology*, vol. 34, no. 8, pp. 463–468, 2004.

[49] C. Eichelberg, A. Erbersdobler, U. Michl et al., "Nerve distribution along the prostatic capsule," *European Urology*, vol. 51, no. 1, pp. 105–111, 2007.

[50] A. Tewari, A. Takenaka, E. Mtui et al., "The proximal neurovascular plate and the tri-zonal neural architecture around the prostate gland: importance in the athermal robotic technique of nerve-sparing prostatectomy," *BJU International*, vol. 98, no. 2, pp. 314–323, 2006.

[51] A. Srivastava, S. Grover, P. Sooriakumaran, G. Tan, A. Takenaka, and A. K. Tewari, "Neuroanatomic basis for traction-free preservation of the neural hammock during athermal robotic radical prostatectomy," *Current Opinion in Urology*, vol. 21, no. 1, pp. 49–59, 2011.

[52] A. K. Tewari, A. Srivastava, M. W. Huang et al., "Anatomical grades of nerve sparing: a risk-stratified approach to neural-hammock sparing during robot-assisted radical prostatectomy (RARP)," *BJU International*, vol. 108, no. 6, part 2, pp. 984–992, 2011.

[53] K. J. Kowalczyk, A. C. Huang, N. D. Hevelone et al., "Stepwise approach for nerve sparing without countertraction during robot-assisted radical prostatectomy: technique and outcomes," *European Urology*, vol. 60, no. 3, pp. 536–547, 2011.

[54] T. A. Masterson, A. M. Serio, J. P. Mulhall, A. J. Vickers, and J. A. Eastham, "Modified technique for neurovascular bundle preservation during radical prostatectomy: association between technique and recovery of erectile function," *BJU International*, vol. 101, no. 10, pp. 1217–1222, 2008.

[55] A. Mattei, R. Naspro, F. Annino, D. Burke, R. Guida Jr., and R. Gaston, "Tension and energy-free robotic-assisted laparoscopic radical prostatectomy with interfascial dissection of the neurovascular bundles," *European Urology*, vol. 52, no. 3, pp. 687–695, 2007.

[56] A. Mandhani, P. J. Dorsey Jr., R. Ramanathan et al., "Real time monitoring of temperature changes in neurovascular bundles during robotic radical prostatectomy: thermal map for nerve-sparing radical prostatectomy," *Journal of Endourology*, vol. 22, no. 10, pp. 2313–2317, 2008.

[57] F. Khan, E. Rodriguez, D. S. Finley, D. W. Skarecky, and T. E. Ahlering, "Spread of thermal energy and heat sinks: implications for nerve-sparing robotic prostatectomy," *Journal of Endourology*, vol. 21, no. 10, pp. 1195–1198, 2007.

[58] T. E. Ahlering, E. Rodriguez, and D. W. Skarecky, "Overcoming obstacles: nerve-sparing issues in radical prostatectomy," *Journal of Endourology*, vol. 22, no. 4, pp. 745–749, 2008.

[59] G. W. Chien, A. A. Mikhail, M. A. Orvieto et al., "Modified clipless antegrade nerve preservation in robotic-assisted laparoscopic radical prostatectomy with validated sexual function evaluation," *Urology*, vol. 66, no. 2, pp. 419–423, 2005.

[60] I. S. Gill, O. Ukimura, M. Rubinstein et al., "Lateral pedicle control during laparoscopic radical prostatectomy: refined technique," *Urology*, vol. 65, no. 1, pp. 23–27, 2005.

[61] F. P. Secin, T. Jiborn, A. S. Bjartell et al., "Multi-institutional study of symptomatic deep venous thrombosis and pulmonary embolism in prostate cancer patients undergoing laparoscopic or robot-assisted laparoscopic radical prostatectomy," *European Urology*, vol. 53, no. 1, pp. 134–145, 2008.

[62] J. B. Forrest, J. Q. Clemens, P. Finamore et al., "AUA best practice statement for the prevention of deep vein thrombosis in patients undergoing urologic surgery. Urologic laparoscopic and/or robotically assisted urologic laparoscopic procedures," *Journal of Urology*, vol. 181, no. 3, pp. 1170–1177, 2009.

[63] J. Schmitges, Q. Trinh, M. Sun et al., "Venous thromboembolism after radical prostatectomy: the effect of surgical caseload," *BJU International*, vol. 110, no. 6, pp. 828–833, 2012.

[64] A. Cestari, N. M. Buffi, E. Scapaticci et al., "Simplifying patient positioning and port placement during robotic-assisted laparoscopic prostatectomy," *European Urology*, vol. 57, no. 3, pp. 530–533, 2010.

[65] G. Koc, N. Tazeh, F. N. Joudi, H. N. Winfield, C. R. Tracy, and J. A. Brown, "Lower extremity neuropathies after robot-assisted laparoscopic prostatectomy on a split-leg table," *Journal of Endourology*, vol. 26, no. 8, pp. 1026–1029, 2012.

[66] M. Belkin, R. D. Brown, J. G. Wright, W. W. LaMorte, and R. W. Hobson II, "A new quantitative spectrophotometric assay of ischemia-reperfusion injury in skeletal muscle," *American Journal of Surgery*, vol. 156, no. 2, pp. 83–86, 1988.

[67] I. M. Anusionwu and E. J. Wright, "Compartment syndrome after positioning in lithotomy: what a urologist needs to know," *BJU International*, vol. 108, no. 4, pp. 477–478, 2011.

[68] R. Keene, J. M. Froelich, J. C. Milbrandt, and O. B. Idusuyi, "Bilateral gluteal compartment syndrome following robotic-assisted prostatectomy," *Orthopedics*, vol. 33, no. 11, p. 852, 2010.

[69] S. Sharma, H. L. Kim, and J. L. Mohler, "Routine pelvic drainage not required after open or robotic radical prostatectomy," *Urology*, vol. 69, no. 2, pp. 330–333, 2007.

[70] D. Canes, M. S. Cohen, and I. A. Tuerk, "Laparoscopic radical prostatectomy: omitting a pelvic drain," *International Braz J Urol*, vol. 34, no. 2, pp. 151–158, 2008.

[71] A. Fuller, A. Fernandez, and S. E. Pautler, "Incisional hernia after robot-assisted radical prostatectomy-predisposing factors in a prospective cohort of 250 cases," *Journal of Endourology*, vol. 25, no. 6, pp. 1021–1024, 2011.

[72] B. J. Leibl, C. Schmedt, J. Schwarz, K. Kraft, and R. Bittner, "Laparoscopic surgery complications associated with trocar tip design: review of literature and own results," *Journal of Laparoendoscopic and Advanced Surgical Techniques A*, vol. 9, no. 2, pp. 135–140, 1999.

[73] N. Kadar, H. Reich, C. Y. Liu, G. F. Manko, and R. Gimpelson, "Incisional hernias after major laparoscopic gynecologic procedures," *American Journal of Obstetrics and Gynecology*, vol. 168, no. 5, pp. 1493–1495, 1993.

[74] S. Bhoyrul, J. Payne, B. Steffes, L. Swanstrom, and L. W. Way, "A randomized prospective study of radially expanding trocars in laparoscopic surgery," *Journal of Gastrointestinal Surgery*, vol. 4, no. 4, pp. 392–397, 2000.

[75] S. Beck, D. Skarecky, K. Osann, R. Juarez, and T. E. Ahlering, "Transverse versus vertical camera port incision in robotic radical prostatectomy: effect on incisional hernias and cosmesis," *Urology*, vol. 78, no. 3, pp. 586–590, 2011.

[76] S. R. Brown and P. B. Goodfellow, "Transverse verses midline incisions for abdominal surgery," *Cochrane Database of Systematic Reviews*, vol. 19, no. 4, Article ID CD005199, 2005.

[77] T. C. Regan, R. M. Mordkin, N. L. Constantinople, I. J. Spence, and S. W. Dejter Jr., "Incidence of inguinal hernias following radical retropubic prostatectomy," *Urology*, vol. 47, no. 4, pp. 536–537, 1996.

[78] F. Rabbani, L. Yunis, K. Touijer, and M. S. Brady, "Predictors of inguinal hernia after radical prostatectomy," *Urology*, vol. 77, no. 2, pp. 391–395, 2011.

[79] J. Stranne, J. Hugosson, and P. Lodding, "Inguinal hernia is a common complication in lower midline incision surgery," *Hernia*, vol. 11, no. 3, pp. 247–252, 2007.

[80] J. H. Ku, C. W. Jeong, Y. H. Park, M. C. Cho, C. Kwak, and H. H. Kim, "Nerve-sparing procedure in radical prostatectomy: a risk factor for hernia repair following open retropubic, pure laparoscopic and robot-assisted laparoscopic procedures," *Scandinavian Journal of Urology and Nephrology*, vol. 45, no. 3, pp. 164–170, 2011.

[81] G. Haber, M. White, R. Autorino et al., "Novel robotic da vinci instruments for laparoendoscopic single-site surgery," *Urology*, vol. 76, no. 6, pp. 1279–1282, 2010.

[82] M. A. White, R. Autorino, G. Spana, S. Hillyer, R. J. Stein, and J. H. Kaouk, "Robotic laparoendoscopic single site urological surgery: analysis of 50 consecutive cases," *Journal of Urology*, vol. 187, no. 5, pp. 1696–1701, 2012.

[83] M. A. White, G. Haber, R. Autorino et al., "Robotic laparoendoscopic single-site radical prostatectomy: technique and early outcomes," *European Urology*, vol. 58, no. 4, pp. 544–550, 2010.

[84] N. S. van den Berg, F. W. B. van Leeuwen, and H. G. van der Poel, "Fluorescence guidance in urologic surgery," *Current Opinion in Urology*, vol. 22, no. 2, pp. 109–120, 2012.

[85] C. von Bodman, K. Matsushita, C. Savage et al., "Recovery of urinary function after radical prostatectomy: predictors of urinary function on preoperative prostate magnetic resonance imaging," *Journal of Urology*, vol. 187, no. 3, pp. 945–950, 2012.

[86] F. Rocco, L. Carmignani, P. Acquati et al., "Restoration of posterior aspect of rhabdosphincter shortens continence time after radical retropubic prostatectomy," *Journal of Urology*, vol. 175, no. 6, pp. 2201–2206, 2006.

[87] R. F. Coelho, S. Chauhan, M. A. Orvieto et al., "Influence of modified posterior reconstruction of the rhabdosphincter on early recovery of continence and anastomotic leakage rates after robot-assisted radical prostatectomy," *European Urology*, vol. 59, no. 1, pp. 72–80, 2011.

[88] X. Hurtes, M. Rouprêt, C. Vaessen et al., "Anterior suspension combined with posterior reconstruction during robot-assisted laparoscopic prostatectomy improves early return of urinary continence: a prospective randomized multicentre trial," *BJU International*, vol. 110, no. 6, pp. 875–883, 2012.

Permissions

All chapters in this book were first published in PC, by Hindawi Publishing Corporation; hereby published with permission under the Creative Commons Attribution License or equivalent. Every chapter published in this book has been scrutinized by our experts. Their significance has been extensively debated. The topics covered herein carry significant findings which will fuel the growth of the discipline. They may even be implemented as practical applications or may be referred to as a beginning point for another development.

The contributors of this book come from diverse backgrounds, making this book a truly international effort. This book will bring forth new frontiers with its revolutionizing research information and detailed analysis of the nascent developments around the world.

We would like to thank all the contributing authors for lending their expertise to make the book truly unique. They have played a crucial role in the development of this book. Without their invaluable contributions this book wouldn't have been possible. They have made vital efforts to compile up to date information on the varied aspects of this subject to make this book a valuable addition to the collection of many professionals and students.

This book was conceptualized with the vision of imparting up-to-date information and advanced data in this field. To ensure the same, a matchless editorial board was set up. Every individual on the board went through rigorous rounds of assessment to prove their worth. After which they invested a large part of their time researching and compiling the most relevant data for our readers.

The editorial board has been involved in producing this book since its inception. They have spent rigorous hours researching and exploring the diverse topics which have resulted in the successful publishing of this book. They have passed on their knowledge of decades through this book. To expedite this challenging task, the publisher supported the team at every step. A small team of assistant editors was also appointed to further simplify the editing procedure and attain best results for the readers.

Apart from the editorial board, the designing team has also invested a significant amount of their time in understanding the subject and creating the most relevant covers. They scrutinized every image to scout for the most suitable representation of the subject and create an appropriate cover for the book.

The publishing team has been an ardent support to the editorial, designing and production team. Their endless efforts to recruit the best for this project, has resulted in the accomplishment of this book. They are a veteran in the field of academics and their pool of knowledge is as vast as their experience in printing. Their expertise and guidance has proved useful at every step. Their uncompromising quality standards have made this book an exceptional effort. Their encouragement from time to time has been an inspiration for everyone.

The publisher and the editorial board hope that this book will prove to be a valuable piece of knowledge for researchers, students, practitioners and scholars across the globe.

List of Contributors

Joy L. Kovar and Lael L. Cheung
Translational Research, LI-COR Biosciences, 4647 Superior Street, Lincoln, NE 68504, USA

Melanie A. Simpson
Department of Biochemistry, University of Nebraska, Lincoln, NE 68588-0664, USA

D. Michael Olive
SVS Consulting, Lincoln, NE 68516, USA

Diego J. Laderach, Lucas Gentilini, Felipe M. Jaworski and Daniel Compagno
Laboratorio de GlicÓmica Funcional, IQUIBICEN-CONICET, Departamento de QÚımica BiolÓgica, Facultad de Ciencias Exactas y Naturales, Universidad de Buenos Aires, C1428, Buenos Aires, Argentina

Victoria Hale and Jong Y. Park
Department of Cancer Epidemiology, Moffitt Cancer Center, 12902 Magnolia Drive, Tampa, FL 33612, USA

Maren Weischer
Department of Clinical Biochemistry, Herlev Hospital, 2730 Herlev, Denmark

Shyam K. Tanguturi
Harvard Radiation Oncology Program, Harvard Medical School, Boston, MA 02115, USA
Brigham andWomen's Hospital, 75 Francis Street, ASB1 L2, Boston, MA 02115, USA

Ming-Hui Chen
Department of Statistics, University of Connecticut, Storrs, CT 06269, USA

Jerome P. Richie
Lank Center for Genitourinary Oncology, Dana Farber Cancer Institute, Boston, MA 02115, USA

Marian Loffredo and Anthony V. D'Amico
Lank Center for Genitourinary Oncology, Dana Farber Cancer Institute, Boston, MA 02115, USA
Department of Radiation Oncology, Dana Farber Cancer Institute and Brigham and Women's Hospital, Boston, MA 02115, USA

Pedro Fernandez and Andre van der Merwe
Division of Urology and Tygerberg Hospital, Stellenbosch University, Cape Town 8000, South Africa

Muneeb Salie
SA MRC Centre for TB Research and DST/NRF Centre of Excellence for Biomedical Tuberculosis Research, Division of Molecular Biology and Human Genetics, Stellenbosch University, Cape Town 8000, South Africa

Danielle du Toit
Unistel Medical Laboratories, Cape Town 8000, South Africa

J. Caon
BC Cancer Agency Radiation Therapy Program, BC Cancer Agency, Vancouver Centre, 600West 10th Avenue, Vancouver, BC, Canada V5Z 4E6

M. Paquette
University of British Columbia, 2329West Mall, Vancouver, BC, Canada V6T 1Z4

T. Pickles
BC Cancer Agency Radiation Therapy Program, BC Cancer Agency, Vancouver Centre, 600West 10th Avenue, Vancouver, BC, Canada V5Z 4E6
University of British Columbia, 2329West Mall, Vancouver, BC, Canada V6T 1Z4

J. Hamm
Cancer Surveillance and Outcomes, Population Oncology, BC Cancer Agency, 600West 10th Avenue, Vancouver, BC, Canada V5Z 4E6

Matthew E. Johnson and Mark K. Buyyounouski
Department of Radiation Oncology, Fox Chase Cancer Center, Philadelphia, PA 19111, USA

Emma Roberts and Davina A. F. Cossigny
Spinal Biology Research Laboratory, University of Melbourne, Department of Surgery, Austin Health

Gerald M. Y. Quan
Spinal Biology Research Laboratory, University of Melbourne, Department of Surgery, Austin Health
Department of Spinal Surgery, Austin Health, Heidelberg, VIC 3084, Australia

Dima Y. Jadaan
University College Dublin, Belfield, Dublin, Ireland

Mutaz M. Jadaan and John P. McCabe
Department of Orthopaedic Surgery, Galway University Hospitals, Galway, Ireland

Ömer Acar
Department of Urology, VKF American Hospital, 34365 Istanbul, Turkey

TarJk Esen
Department of Urology, VKF American Hospital, 34365 Istanbul, Turkey
School ofMedicine, KocUniversity, 34450 Istanbul, Turkey

L. Michael Carastro and Kaia K. Hampton
Department of Chemistry, Biochemistry and Physics, University of Tampa, Tampa, FL 33606, USA

Hui-Yi Lin
Department of Biostatistics, Moffitt Cancer Center, Tampa, FL 33612, USA

Hyun Y. Park, Selina Radlein and Jong Y. Park
Department of Cancer Epidemiology, Moffitt Cancer Center, 12902 Magnolia Drive, Tampa, FL 33612, USA

Donghwa Kim
Department of Molecular Oncology, Moffitt Cancer Center, Tampa, FL 33612, USA

Ardeshir Hakam
Department of Anatomic Pathology, Moffitt Cancer Center, Tampa, FL 33612, USA

Babu Zachariah
Genitourinary Program, James Haley VA Hospital, Tampa, FL 33612, USA

Julio Pow-Sang
Genitourinary Program, Moffitt Cancer Center, Tampa, FL 33612, USA

Anselm J. M. Hennis
Chronic Disease Research Centre, The University of the West Indies, Jemmott's Lane, St. Michael, BB11115, Barbados
Department of Preventive Medicine, Stony Brook University, Stony Brook, NY 11794-8036, USA
Ministry of Health, Frank Walcott Building, Culloden Road, St. Michael, BB14001, Barbados
Faculty of Medical Sciences, Cave Hill Campus, The University of the West Indies, St. Michael, BB11000, Barbados

Suh-Yuh Wu, Barbara Nemesure and M. Cristina Leske
Department of Preventive Medicine, Stony Brook University, Stony Brook, NY 11794-8036, USA

Ernest K. Amankwah
Department of Cancer Epidemiology, Moffitt Cancer Center, Tampa, FL 33612, USA

Ganna Chornokur, CatherineM. Phelan Nagi B. Kumar and Jong Y. Park
Department of Cancer Epidemiology, Moffitt Cancer Center, Tampa, FL 33612, USA
The Center for EqualHealth, Tampa, FL 33612, USA

Stacy N. Davis
Department of Health Outcomes and Behavior, Moffitt Cancer Center, Tampa, FL 33612, USA

Julio Pow-Sang
Department of Genitourinary Oncology, Moffitt Cancer Center, Tampa, FL 33612, USA

Ksenija Limani
Department of Urology, Jules Bordet Institute, 1 Rue Héger-Bordet, 1000 Brussels, Belgium

Fouad Aoun, Alexandre Peltier and Roland van Velthoven
Department of Urology, Jules Bordet Institute, 1 Rue Héger-Bordet, 1000 Brussels, Belgium
Université Libre de Bruxelles, 50 Franklin Roosevelt Avenue, 1050 Brussels, Belgium

Serge Holz
Department of Urology, Jules Bordet Institute, 1 Rue Héger-Bordet, 1000 Brussels, Belgium

Marianne Paesmans
Department of Data Management, Jules Bordet Institute, 1 Rue Héger-Bordet, 1000 Brussels, Belgium

Sean Woolen, Cameron Holzmeyer and Emily Nesbitt
Research Institute of Deaconess Clinic, 421 Chestnut Street, Evansville, IN 47713, USA

Paul F. Siami
Department of Urology, Deaconess Clinic, 421 Chestnut Street, Evansville, IN 47713, USA

Lior Z. Braunstein
Harvard Radiation Oncology Program, Brigham andWomen's Hospital, ASB-I Radiation Oncology L2, 75 Francis Street, Boston, MA 02115, USA

Ming-Hui Chen
Department of Statistics, University of Connecticut, 215 Glenbrook Road, U-4120, Storrs, CT 06269-4120, USA

Marian Loffredo and Anthony V. D'Amico
Lank Center for Genitourinary Oncology, Dana-Farber Cancer Institute, Mailstop Dana 1230, 450 Brookline Avenue, Boston, MA 02215, USA
Department of Radiation Oncology, Dana-Farber/ Brigham and Women's Hospital, ASB-I Radiation Oncology L2, 75 Francis Street, Boston, MA 02115, USA

Philip W. Kantoff
Lank Center for Genitourinary Oncology, Dana-Farber Cancer Institute, Mailstop Dana 1230, 450 Brookline Avenue, Boston, MA 02215, USA

TerrenceM. Vance, Sang Gil Lee, Sung I. Koo and Ock K. Chun
Department of Nutritional Sciences, University of Connecticut, Storrs, CT 06269, USA

Gissou Azabdaftari and Elena A. Pop
Roswell Park Cancer Institute, Buffalo, NY 14263, USA

James L. Mohler
Roswell Park Cancer Institute, Buffalo, NY 14263, USA
School of Public Health, University of North Carolina at Chapel Hill, Chapel Hill, NC 27599, USA

L. Joseph Su
Epidemiology and Genomics Research Program, Division of Cancer Control and Population Sciences, National Cancer Institute, Bethesda, MD 20892, USA

Elizabeth T. H. Fontham
School of PublicHealth, Louisiana State University Health Sciences Center, NewOrleans, LA 70112, USA

Jeannette T. Bensen
School of Public Health, University of North Carolina at Chapel Hill, Chapel Hill, NC 27599, USA

Susan E. Steck
Department of Epidemiology and Biostatistics, Cancer Prevention and Control Program, University of South Carolina, Columbia, SC 29208, USA

Lenore Arab
David Geffen School of Medicine, University of California, Los Angeles, CA 90095, USA

Ming-Hui Chen
Department of Statistics, University of Connecticut, Storrs, CT 06269, USA

Shahana Sarwar
Department of Biochemistry, Owaisi Group of Hospitals, DCMS, Hyderabad, Telangana, India

Mohammed Abdul Majid Adil
Department of Urology, Owaisi Group of Hospitals, DCMS, Hyderabad, Telangana, India

Parveen Nyamath and Mohammed Ishaq
Salar-e-Millat Research Centre, PEH, DCMS, Hyderabad, Telangana, India

Henrique B. da Silva, Eduardo P. Amaral and Nathalia C. de Victo
Departamento de Imunologia, Instituto de Ciências Biomédicas, Universidade de São Paulo, Avenida Prof. Lineu Prestes 1730, 05508-900 São Paulo, SP, Brazil

Eduardo L. Nolasco
Departamento de Análises Clínicas e Toxicológicas, Faculdade de Ciências Farmacêuticas, Universidade de Sáo Paulo, Avenida Prof. Lineu Prestes 580, 05508-000 São Paulo, SP, Brazil

Rodrigo Atique and Valesca Anschau
Departamento de Genética e Biologia Evolutiva, Instituto de Biociências, Universidade de São Paulo, Rua do Matão 277, 05508-900 São Paulo, SP, Brazil

Carina C. Jank
Departamento de Imunologia, Instituto de Ciências Biomédicas, Universidade de São Paulo, Avenida Prof. Lineu Prestes 1730, 05508-900 São Paulo, SP, Brazil
Instituto Israelita de Ensino e Pesquisa Albert Einstein, Avenida Albert Einstein 627/701, 05652-000 São Paulo, SP, Brazil

Luiz F. Zerbini
International Center for Genetic Engineering and Biotechnology (ICGEB), Cancer Genomics Group and Division of Medical Biochemistry, University of Cape Town, Cape Town 7925, South Africa

Ricardo G. Correa
Sanford-Burnham Medical Research Institute, 10901 North Torrey Pines Road, La Jolla, CA 92037, USA

Francis Ting, Pim J. Van Leeuwen and Phillip D. Stricker
St. Vincent's Prostate Cancer Centre, darlinghurst, NSW2010, Australia
Garvan Institute of Medical Research, The Kinghorn Cancer Centre, Darlinghurst, NSW2010, Australia

James Thompson
St. Vincent's Prostate Cancer Centre, Darling Hurst, NSW2010, Australia
Garvan Institute of Medical Research, The Kinghorn Cancer Centre, Darlinghurst, NSW2010, Australia
School of Medicine, University of New South Wales, Kensington, NSW2052, Australia

Ron Shnier
Southern Radiology, Rand wick, NSW 2031, Australia

Daniel Moses
School of Medicine, University of New South Wales, Kensington, NSW2052, Australia
Spectrum Radiology, Rand wick, NSW 2031, Australia

Warick Delprado
Douglas Hanly Moir Pathology, Macquarie Park, NSW2113, Australia

Mankgopo M. Kgatle
Division of Hepatology and Liver Research, Department of Medicine, Faculty of Health Sciences, University of Cape Town and Groote Schuur Hospital, Observatory, Western Cape 7925, South Africa

Asgar A. Kalla
Division of Rheumatology, Department of Medicine, Faculty of Health Sciences, University of Cape Town and Groote Schuur Hospital, Observatory, Western Cape 7925, South Africa

Muhammed M. Islam
Department of Integrative Biomedical Sciences, Institute of Infectious Disease and Molecular Medicine, Faculty of Health Sciences, University of Cape Town, Observatory, Western Cape 7925, South Africa

Mike Sathekge
Department of Nuclear Medicine, University of Pretoria and Steve Biko Academic Hospital, Private Bag X169, Pretoria, Gauteng 0001, South Africa

Razia Moorad
Department of Surgery, Faculty of Health Science, University of Cape Town and Groote Schuur Hospital, Observatory, Western Cape 7925, South Africa

Andrew Leone, Katherine Rotker and Stephen F. Schiff
Division of Urology, Rhode Island Hospital and TheWarren Alpert Medical School of Brown University, Providence, RI 02905, USA

Christi Butler
The Warren Alpert Medical School of Brown University, Providence, RI 02905, USA

Anthony Mega
Department of Hematology/Oncology, The Miriam Hospital, Providence, RI 02905, USA

Jianhong Li and Ali Amin
Pathology and Laboratory Medicine, Rhode Island Hospital, Providence, RI 02905, USA

Gyan Pareek, Dragan Golijanin and Joseph F. Renzulli II
Section of Minimally Invasive Urology, TheWarren Alpert Medical School of Brown University, Providence, RI 02905, USA

Dianne van Strijp, Christiane de Witz, Pieter C. Vos, Eveline den Biezen-Timmermans, Anne van Brussel and Janneke Wrobel
Philips Research Europe, High Tech Campus 34, 5656AE Eindhoven, Netherlands

Ralf Hoffmann
Philips Research Europe, High Tech Campus 34, 5656AE Eindhoven, Netherlands
Institute of Cardiovascular and Medical Science, University of Glasgow, G12 8TA Glasgow, Scotland, UK

George S. Baillie
Institute of Cardiovascular and Medical Science, University of Glasgow, G12 8TA Glasgow, Scotland, UK

Pierre Tennstedt
Martini-Klinik Prostate Cancer Center, University Medical Center Hamburg-Eppendorf, 20246 Hamburg, Germany

Thorsten Schlomm
Klinik für Urologie, Charité–Universit¨atsmedizin Berlin, 10117 Berlin, Germany

Birthe Heitkötter and Sebastian Huss
Gerhard-Domagk-Institute of Pathology, University Hospital M¨unster, 48149 Münster, Germany

Martin Bögemann and Axel Semjonow
Prostate Center, University Hospital M¨unster, 48149 Münster, Germany

Miles D. Houslay
Institute of Pharmaceutical Science, King's College London, WC2R 2LS London, UK
Mironid Ltd, Bio City Scotland, ML1 5UHNewhouse, Scotland, UK

Chris Bangma
Department of Urology, 3000CA Erasmus Medical Center, Rotterdam, Netherlands

M. Sean Peach, Daniel M. Trifiletti and Bruce Libby
Department of Radiation Oncology, University of Virginia School of Medicine, Charlottesville, VA 22908, USA

James Thompson
St Vincent's Prostate Cancer Centre, St Vincent's Clinic, Sydney, NSW 2010, Australia

Anne-Marie Haynes
Australian Prostate Cancer Research Centre New South Wales, The Garvan Institute of Medical Research, The Kinghorn Cancer Centre, Sydney, NSW 2010, Australia

Pim J. van Leeuwen, Francis Ting, Phillip Brenner and Phillip Stricker
St Vincent's Prostate Cancer Centre, St Vincent's Clinic, Sydney, NSW 2010, Australia
Australian Prostate Cancer Research Centre New South Wales, The Garvan Institute of Medical Research, The Kinghorn Cancer Centre, Sydney, NSW 2010, Australia

Amila Siriwardana
St Vincent's Prostate Cancer Centre, St Vincent's Clinic, Sydney, NSW 2010, Australia
Australian Prostate Cancer Research Centre New South Wales, The Garvan Institute of Medical Research, The Kinghorn Cancer Centre, Sydney, NSW 2010, Australia
University of New South Wales, Sydney, NSW2052, Australia

Monique Roobol
Department of Urology, Erasmus University Medical Center, 3015 CE Rotterdam, Netherlands

Daan Nieboer
Department of Public Health, Erasmus University Medical Center, 3015 CE Rotterdam, Netherlands

Warick Delprado
University of Notre Dame, Sydney, NSW 2010, Australia

Jesal C. Patel, Julia A. Batten and Neeraj Agarwal
Division of Medical Oncology, University of UT Huntsman Cancer Institute, Salt Lake City, Utah 84112, USA

Benjamin L. Maughan and Tian Y. Zhang
Department of Internal Medicine, University of UT, Salt Lake City, Utah 84112, USA

Archana M. Agarwal
Department of Pathology and ARUP Laboratories, University of UT, Salt Lake City, Utah 84108, USA

S. Bishara, N. Vasdev, T. Lane, G. Boustead and J. Adshead
Department of Urology, Hertfordshire and South Bedfordshire Robotic Urological Cancer Centre, Lister Hospital, Coreys Mill Lane, Stevenage, Hertfordshire SG1 4AB, UK

John M. Lacy and Randall G. Rowland
Department of Urology, University of Kentucky College of Medicine, Lexington, KY 40536, USA

William A. Wilson and William H. St. Clair
Department of Radiation Oncology, University of Kentucky College of Medicine, Lexington, KY 40536, USA

Raevti Bole
University of Kentucky College of Medicine, Lexington, KY 40536, USA

Li Chen
Department of Biostatistics, University of Kentucky College of Public Health, Lexington, KY 40536, USA

Ali S. Meigooni
Comprehensive Cancer Centers of Nevada, Las Vegas, NV 89169, USA

Emma F. P. Jacobs, Ronald Boris and Timothy A. Masterson
Department of Urology, Indiana University Medical Center, 535 N. Barnhill Drive, Suite 420, Indianapolis, IN 46202, USA

Index